"十三五"国家重点出版物出版规划项目

总 主 编　刘树伟

副总主编　赵　斌　柳　澄　李振平　徐以发

Color Atlas of Digital Human Cross Sectional Anatomy
Thorax

数字人连续横断层解剖学彩色图谱
胸部分册

主编　孟海伟　张忠和　左一智

山东科学技术出版社

图书在版编目（CIP）数据

数字人连续横断层解剖学彩色图谱. 胸部分册 / 孟海伟, 张忠和, 左一智主编. -- 济南：山东科学技术出版社, 2020.12
ISBN 978-7-5723-0676-1

Ⅰ.①数… Ⅱ.①孟… ②张… ③左… Ⅲ.①胸—计算机X线扫描体层摄影—断面解剖学—图谱 Ⅳ.①R814.42-64

中国版本图书馆CIP数据核字(2020)第166506号

数字人连续横断层解剖学彩色图谱·胸部分册
SHUZIREN LIANXU HENGDUANCENG JIEPOUXUE CAISE TUPU·XIONGBU FENCE

责任编辑：魏　然　徐日强
装帧设计：侯　宇　李晨溪

主管单位：山东出版传媒股份有限公司
出 版 者：山东科学技术出版社
　　　　　地址：济南市市中区英雄山路189号
　　　　　邮编：250002　电话：（0531）82098088
　　　　　网址：www.lkj.com.cn
　　　　　电子邮件：sdkj@sdcbcm.com
发 行 者：山东科学技术出版社
　　　　　地址：济南市市中区英雄山路189号
　　　　　邮编：250002　电话：（0531）82098071
印 刷 者：济南新先锋彩印有限公司
　　　　　地址：济南市工业北路188-6号
　　　　　邮编：250101　电话：（0531）88615699

规格：8开（285mm×420mm）
印张：28.25　　字数：283千　　印数：1~2000
版次：2020年12月第1版　2020年12月第1次印刷
定价：340.00元

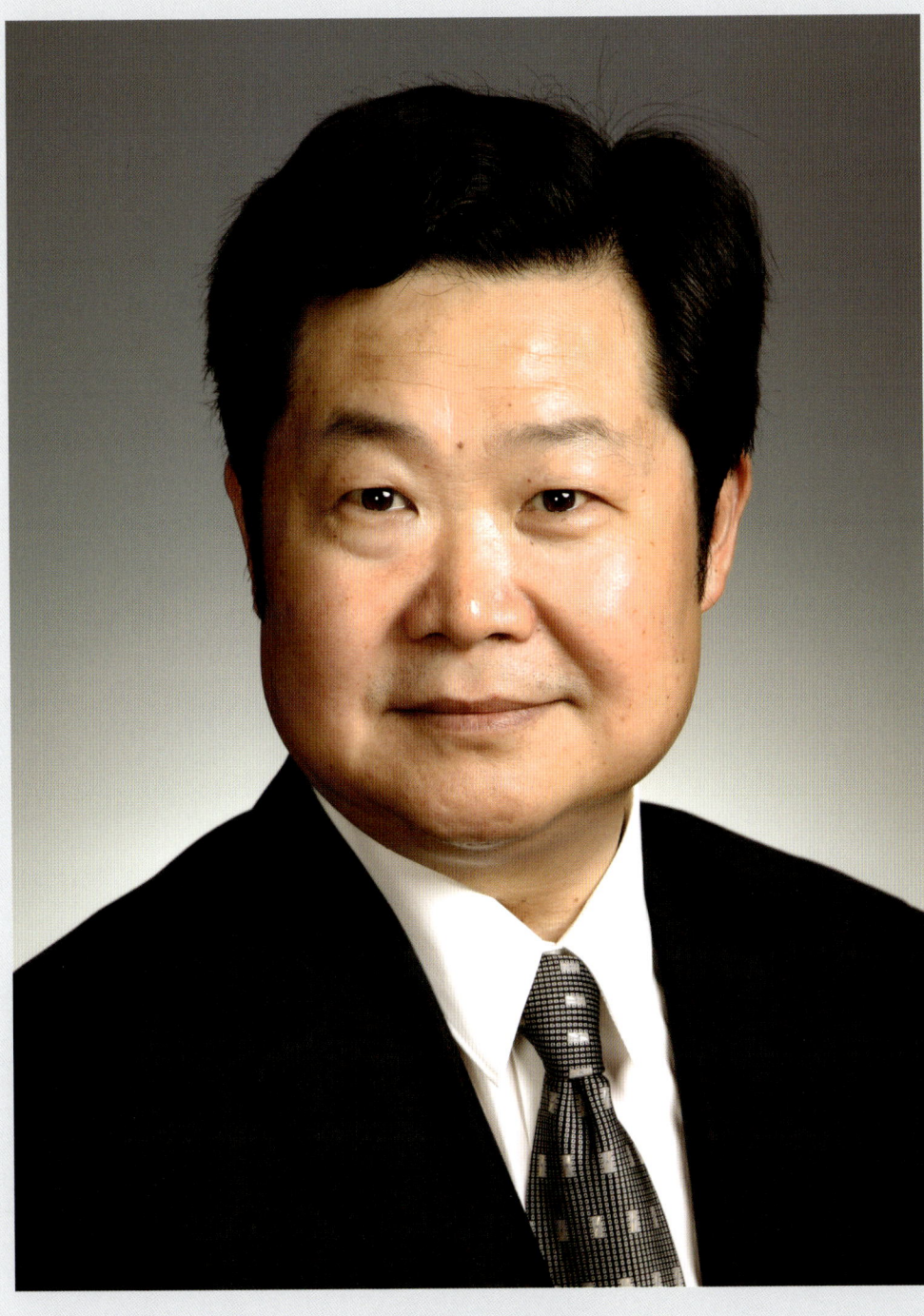

总主编　刘树伟

刘树伟，医学博士，山东大学基础医学院解剖学与神经生物学系教授、博士生导师，山东大学断层影像解剖学研究中心主任，山东大学数字人研究院院长，山东大学脑与类脑科学研究院副院长。曾任山东大学研究生院常务副院长、医学院副院长、人体解剖与组织胚胎学系主任等职，兼任亚洲临床解剖学会副主席、中国解剖学会副理事长和断层影像解剖学分会主任委员、中华医学会数字医学分会常务委员等职。获"卫生部有突出贡献的中青年专家"和"山东省教学名师"称号，享受国务院政府特殊津贴。潜心断层影像解剖学、数字人体和计算神经科学研究，承担国家及省部级课题20余项，在 Radiology、NeuroImage 和 Cerebral Cortex 等杂志发表论文320余篇（其中SCI收录70余篇），主编《人体断层解剖学》《临床中枢神经解剖学》和《功能神经影像学》等著作40余部，获省部级科技进步奖4项（其中一等奖1项）。长期从事人体解剖学教学，主持的"顺应现代影像学发展，创建断层解剖学课程"教学改革项目于1997年获山东省教学成果奖一等奖和国家级教学成果奖二等奖，主持完成的"我国数字解剖学教学体系创建与推广"教学研究项目于2018年获山东省教学成果奖特等奖和国家级教学成果奖二等奖。

主要学术著作、论文如下：

1. 刘树伟. 断层解剖学. 北京：人民卫生出版社, 1998.
2. 刘树伟. 人体断层解剖学图谱. 济南：山东科学技术出版社, 2003.
3. 刘树伟. 人体断层解剖学. 北京：高等教育出版社, 2006.
4. 刘树伟，柳澄，胡三元. 腹部外科临床解剖学图谱. 济南：山东科学技术出版社, 2006.
5. 刘树伟，王怀经. 应用解剖学（全六册）. 北京：高等教育出版社, 2007.
6. 刘树伟，尹岭，唐一源. 功能神经影像学. 济南：山东科学技术出版社, 2011.
7. 刘树伟，李瑞锡. 局部解剖学. 8版. 北京：人民卫生出版社, 2013.
8. 刘树伟，杨晓飞，邓雪飞. 临床解剖学·腹盆部分册. 2版. 北京：人民卫生出版社, 2014.
9. 刘树伟. 断层解剖学. 3版. 北京：高等教育出版社, 2017.
10. 刘树伟，林祥涛. 影像解剖学系列图谱（全六册）. 济南：山东科学技术出版社, 2020.
11. Tang Y, Hojatkashani C, Dinov ID, Sun B, Fan L, Lin X, Qi H, Hua X, Liu S*, Toga AW*. The construction of a Chinese MRI brain atlas: a morphometric comparison study between Chinese and Caucasian cohorts. NeuroImage, 2010, 51(1): 33-41.
12. Liu F, Zhang Z, Lin X, Teng G, Meng H, Yu T, Fang F, Zang F, Li Z, Liu S*. Development of the human fetal cerebellum in the second trimester: a post mortem magnetic resonance imaging evaluation. J Anat, 2011, 219: 582–588.
13. Zuo Y, Liu C, Liu S*. Pulmonary intersegmental planes: imaging appearance and possible reasons leading to their visualization. Radiology, 2013, 267(1): 267-275.
14. Yin X, Han Y, Ge H, Xu W, Huang R, Zhang D, Xu J, Fan L, Pang Z, Liu S*. Inferior frontal white matter asymmetry correlates with executive control of attention. Hum Brain Mapp, 2013, 34(4): 796-813.
15. Zhan J, Dinov ID, Li J, Zhang Z, Hobel S, Shi Y, Lin X, Zamanyan A, Lei F, Teng G, Fang F, Tang Y, Zang F, Toga AW*, Liu S*. Spatial-temporal atlas of fetal brain development during the early second trimester. NeuroImage, 2013, 82:115-126.
16. Ge X, Shi Y, Li J, Zhang Z, Lin X, Zhan J, Ge H, Xu J, Yu Q, Leng Y, Teng G, Feng L, Meng H, Tang Y, Zang F, Toga AW*, Liu S*. Development of the human fetal hippocampal formation during early second trimester. NeuroImage, 2015, 119: 33-43.
17. Xu J, Yin X, Ge H, Han Y, Pang Z, Liu B*, Liu S*, Friston K. Heritability of the effective connectivity in the resting-state default mode network. Cerebral Cortex, 2017, 27(12): 5626-5634.
18. Tang Y, Zhao L, Lou Y, Shi Y, Fang R, Lin X, Liu S*, Toga AW. Brain structure differences between Chinese and Caucasian cohorts: A comprehensive morphometry study. Hum Brain Mapp, 2018, 39(5): 2147-2155.
19. Li Z, Xu F, Zhang Z, Lin X, Teng G, Zang F, Liu S*. Morphologic evolution and coordinated development of the fetal lateral ventricles in the second and third trimesters. Am J Neuroradiol, 2019, 40(4): 718-725.
20. Xu F, Ge X, Shi Y, Zhang Z, Tang Y, Lin X, Teng G, Zang F, Gao N, Liu H, Toga AW*, Liu S*. Morphometric development of the human fetal cerebellum during the early second trimester. NeuroImage, 2020, 207: 116372.

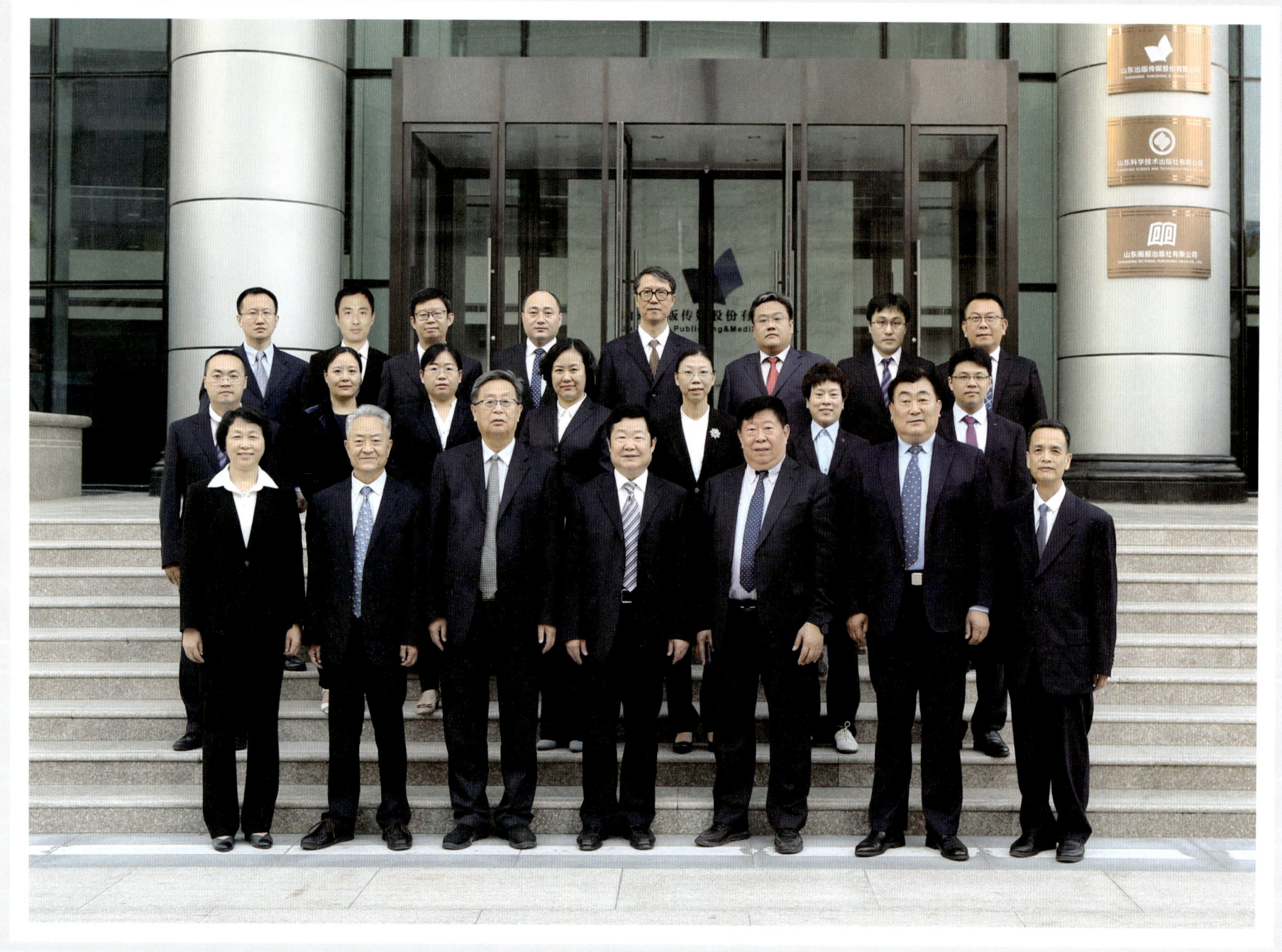

编委会全体人员合影

前排（从左至右）：王 青　李振平　柳 澄　刘树伟　赵 斌　徐以发　林祥涛
中排（从左至右）：孙 博　孟海伟　冯 蕾　张 杨　吴凤霞　王韶玉　任福欣
后排（从左至右）：侯中煜　左一智　于德新　汤煜春　于台飞　张忠和　于乔文　王增涛

《数字人连续横断层解剖学彩色图谱》编委会

总 主 编 刘树伟

副总主编 赵　斌　柳　澄　李振平　徐以发

编　　委（以姓氏笔画为序）

于台飞（山东省医学影像学研究所）	汤煜春（山东大学齐鲁医学院）
于乔文（山东省立医院）	吴凤霞（山东大学齐鲁医学院）
于德新（山东大学齐鲁医院）	张　杨（山东大学齐鲁医院）
王　青（山东大学齐鲁医院）	张忠和（山东省立医院）
王韶玉（山东大学齐鲁医院）	李振平（山东大学齐鲁医学院）
王增涛（山东大学齐鲁医学院，山东省立医院）	孟海伟（山东大学齐鲁医学院）
刘树伟（山东大学齐鲁医学院）	林祥涛（山东大学齐鲁医学院，山东省立医院）
冯　蕾（山东大学齐鲁医学院）	赵　斌（山东省医学影像学研究所）
左一智（南京医科大学）	柳　澄（山东省医学影像学研究所）
孙　博（山东省医学影像学研究所）	侯中煜（山东省立医院）
任福欣（山东省医学影像学研究所）	徐以发（山东省数字人工程技术研究中心）

胸部分册

主　　编　孟海伟　张忠和　左一智

编　　者　（以姓氏笔画为序）

左一智（南京医科大学）　　　　　　　　　孟海伟（山东大学齐鲁医学院）

李　雷（南京医科大学）　　　　　　　　　陈云超（山东省立医院）

刘海蓝（山东大学齐鲁医学院）　　　　　　梅艺璇（山东大学齐鲁医学院）

张忠和（山东省立医院）　　　　　　　　　Emmanuel Suluba（山东大学齐鲁医学院）

冷　媛（山东大学第二医院）

标本图像处理

魏　昱（山东省数字人工程技术研究中心）

李照群（山东省数字人工程技术研究中心）

任晓雪（山东省数字人工程技术研究中心）

总前言

"图谱是表达断层解剖的最好形式。"这是我的导师四川大学王永贵教授34年前的谆谆教诲,当时只是一名硕士研究生的我并未完全理解。随着岁月的磨炼,我逐渐认识到这真是一句至理名言。时间进入21世纪,尤其是近10年间,人体断层解剖学发展迅速。在断层数据的获取方面,数控冷冻铣削技术使标本断层层厚达到了亚毫米水平,以CT和MRI为代表的医学影像设备的扫描速度更快、层厚更薄、分辨力更高;在断层图像的处理方面,多平面重组、三维重建、多模态影像融合、虚拟现实、增强现实和生物学计量等技术的发展更加深入、应用更趋广泛;在研究内容方面,对人体局部断层解剖信息的要求更加精细,形态与功能的结合更加密切,临床应用的针对性更强。在这种学术背景下,无论是人体解剖学工作者,还是临床医师,均呼唤着层厚在毫米级的薄层连续人体断层解剖学彩色图谱的出版。"好雨知时节,当春乃发生。"这部《数字人连续横断层解剖学彩色图谱》应运而生,既是人体解剖学领域最重要的前沿进展之一,又迎合了临床医师尤其是医学影像学医师的祈盼,还实现了本人的终生夙愿。

《数字人连续横断层解剖学彩色图谱》共包括头颈部、胸部、腹部、盆部与会阴、上肢和下肢6个分册,图像共4 519幅(含断层标本彩色图像917幅、螺旋CT图像1 753幅、3T MR图像1 841幅、其他图像8幅),文字约170万字。从图像采集到全书定稿,主要由山东大学数字人研究院完成。我们的目标是把本套图谱打造成断层解剖学的传世经典、解剖学工作者案头必备的工具书、临床工作者爱不释手的阅片指南。努力追求做到以下四个突出。第一,突出薄层断层解剖。以往的厚片断层解剖切片多在厘米级,许多解剖结构难以显示。本图谱标本断层层厚为0.1 mm,每隔20层选用1层,因此可充分展示一些细小的解剖结构。在标注和文字描述中,重点突出那些以往厚片无法展示的解剖细节,使断层解剖学为之一新。第二,突出解剖与影像的融合。标本断层和影像断层是断层解剖学两大支柱内容,在以往的研究中往往强调相互对照,而融合不够。本图谱不但强调二者之间的相互匹配,而且更强调二者的融合,旨在给出关键结构影像学表现的精准解剖学阐释。第三,突出断层解剖学规律的总结。以往的许多图谱,只注重断层结构的标注,而忽略了解剖结构在连续断层中的变化规律。本图谱每一断层均有300~500字的总结性短文,以讨论关键结构的断层形态变化规律、类型、大小、位置、毗邻、分区、发育、变异、影像学特征、生理功能、诊断和治疗意义等,以期将具体知识总结升华为断层解剖学理论。第四,突出基础理论与临床应用的结合。伟大导师恩格斯说过:"没有解剖学就没有医学。"因此,解剖学知识只有应用于临床才能显示出其巨大实用意义和社会价值。书中关键结构的选择以临床需要为标准,在写作中强调精选内容,重点讨论关键结构在疾病诊断、介入治疗和外科手术中的应用价值。

"雄关漫道真如铁,而今迈步从头越。"在全书即将付梓之际,心中百感交集,思绪万千。我要衷心感谢国家自然科学基金委员会和山东省科技厅,是其立项的科研项目使本图谱使用的原始数据得以成功获取;我要衷心感谢我的同事们和研究生们,是大家齐心协力、忘我无私的工作,才使本书得以完成;我要衷心感谢中国工程院钟世镇院士、张运院士、顾晓松院士及西安交通大学刘军教授,是他们的推荐意见和序,照亮了我前进的道路;我要衷心感谢我的解剖学、影像学和外科学同仁,他们富有建设性的意见和建议使得本书内容在解剖学与临床的结合上更加紧密;我要衷心感谢山东科学技术出版社,是其领导和编辑们的视野、耐心和意志使得本图谱历尽千辛万苦而得以出版并入选"十三五"国家重点出版物出版规划项目。书是在使用中日臻完善的。最后,我衷心希望和感谢广大读者,不断提出您的意见和需求,以使本书更具理论价值和临床适用性。

2020年是中国解剖学会成立100周年。特将本部图谱献给中国解剖学会,以隆重纪念其百年华诞。

总主编 刘树伟

2020年10月15日

前 言

《数字人连续横断层解剖学彩色图谱·胸部分册》是系列图谱之一，主要介绍了胸部连续横断层标本及 CT、MRI 解剖结构及其变化规律。本图谱标本图像来源于数字人女性标本 1 号，该标本铣切层厚 0.1 mm，每隔 20 层选取 1 层，分辨率高达 16 000 像素 ×26 000 像素，且动、静脉分别用红色和蓝色染料灌注，血管走行，动、静脉的分、属支显示清晰，方便连续追踪观察。本图谱的图像自第 1 胸椎上缘平面开始，至第 10-11 胸椎椎间盘层面肺下缘消失为止，共获取横断面图像 101 幅。胸部影像学检查以 CT 应用最为广泛，MR 亦具备一定优势。本图谱同时匹配与标本断面解剖结构相接近的连续胸部 CT 纵隔窗强化图像和肺窗图像各 101 幅，以及包括胸部纵隔淋巴结、心血管或特征性病变在内的 MR T1WI 和 T2WI 图像 202 幅，共有图像 505 幅，文字约 28 万字。

CT 和 MR 图像采集自山东省立医院医学影像科，分别来自不同的个体。双源 CT 扫描仪为 SIEMENS Force，3.0T MR 扫描仪为 SIEMENS Prisma。CT 和 MR 图像尽量做到与断层标本结构契合，但由于 CT、MR 图像是在活体状态下获取，肺部气体比较饱满，因此，下胸段影像学肺部图像与标本存在一定差异。

本图谱具有三个特点。第一，标注细致，结构全面，且中英文对照。图谱写作以标本图像为主体，对上纵隔结构、胸部血管、心腔结构、肺内管道和肺段及脊柱区结构进行了详细的追踪观察及描述。尤其对一些其他标本不容易观察到的细小结构，我们做了详细标注及连续追踪并进行了规律性总结，如心包膈血管、迷走神经、胸导管、胸交感干等。每一断层概述性描述该断层中结构的整体配布规律，并结合文献讨论关键结构的断层形态变化规律，如关键结构的位置、毗邻、大小、分区、影像学特征、生理功能、临床诊断和诊疗意义等。对应的 CT 及 MR 图像的中英文标注，以同一断层标本图像标注为标准，同时兼顾标本与活体状态器官的位置差异及个体差异。第二，密切联系临床，加强断层结构的临床应用。除常规的胸部 CT 纵隔窗、肺窗及 MR T1WI 或 T2WI 图像外，书中还配有常见的胸部疾病的影像图与正常图像相对照，如肿瘤、炎症、动脉夹层、冠脉狭窄、胸膜炎、心包或胸膜腔积液等。为更好地理解冠状动脉血管的横断层变化，选配有部分冠状动脉 CTA 的断面或重建图像及 DSA 图像等，以加深理解。对纵隔淋巴结的分区，采用新的国际肺癌研究协会（International Association for the Study of Lung Cancer, IASLC）分区方法，并配有相应区域的增大淋巴结 CT 图像加以对比并详细介绍。第三，总结整体规律，从断层中学习整体观。本图谱通过追踪分析连续断层的结构特点，系统介绍了上纵隔结构、心脏、纵隔淋巴结、肺门和肺段等结构，构建断层解剖学的理论体系。为方便读者查阅，体现图谱的可拓展性，正文后附有权威的、近期的参考文献。

尽管我们努力工作、反复校对，但是由于结构繁多、细小及作者水平所限，难免会有错误和不足之处，望读者尤其专家们多多指正，以便改进和不断完善。

孟海伟　张忠和　左一智
2020 年 11 月 15 日

目 录

胸部连续横断层解剖

胸部连续横断层 1（FH.13490） 2
胸部连续横断层 2（FH.13470） 4
胸部连续横断层 3（FH.13450） 6
胸部连续横断层 4（FH.13430） 8
胸部连续横断层 5（FH.13410） 10
胸部连续横断层 6（FH.13390） 12
胸部连续横断层 7（FH.13370） 14
胸部连续横断层 8（FH.13350） 16
胸部连续横断层 9（FH.13330） 18
胸部连续横断层 10（FH.13310） 20
胸部连续横断层 11（FH.13290） 22
胸部连续横断层 12（FH.13270） 24
胸部连续横断层 13（FH.13250） 26
胸部连续横断层 14（FH.13230） 28
胸部连续横断层 15（FH.13210） 30
胸部连续横断层 16（FH.13190） 32
胸部连续横断层 17（FH.13170） 34
胸部连续横断层 18（FH.13150） 36
胸部连续横断层 19（FH.13130） 38
胸部连续横断层 20（FH.13110） 40
胸部连续横断层 21（FH.13090） 42
胸部连续横断层 22（FH.13070） 44
胸部连续横断层 23（FH.13050） 46
胸部连续横断层 24（FH.13030） 48
胸部连续横断层 25（FH.13010） 50
胸部连续横断层 26（FH.12990） 52
胸部连续横断层 27（FH.12970） 54
胸部连续横断层 28（FH.12950） 56
胸部连续横断层 29（FH.12930） 58
胸部连续横断层 30（FH.12910） 60
胸部连续横断层 31（FH.12890） 62
胸部连续横断层 32（FH.12870） 64
胸部连续横断层 33（FH.12850） 66
胸部连续横断层 34（FH.12830） 68
胸部连续横断层 35（FH.12810） 70
胸部连续横断层 36（FH.12790） 72
胸部连续横断层 37（FH.12770） 74
胸部连续横断层 38（FH.12750） 76
胸部连续横断层 39（FH.12730） 78
胸部连续横断层 40（FH.12710） 80
胸部连续横断层 41（FH.12690） 82
胸部连续横断层 42（FH.12670） 84
胸部连续横断层 43（FH.12650） 86
胸部连续横断层 44（FH.12630） 88

胸部连续横断层 45（FH.12610）..................90
胸部连续横断层 46（FH.12590）..................92
胸部连续横断层 47（FH.12570）..................94
胸部连续横断层 48（FH.12550）..................96
胸部连续横断层 49（FH.12530）..................98
胸部连续横断层 50（FH.12510）..................100
胸部连续横断层 51（FH.12490）..................102
胸部连续横断层 52（FH.12470）..................104
胸部连续横断层 53（FH.12450）..................106
胸部连续横断层 54（FH.12430）..................108
胸部连续横断层 55（FH.12410）..................110
胸部连续横断层 56（FH.12390）..................112
胸部连续横断层 57（FH.12370）..................114
胸部连续横断层 58（FH.12350）..................116
胸部连续横断层 59（FH.12330）..................118
胸部连续横断层 60（FH.12310）..................120
胸部连续横断层 61（FH.12290）..................122
胸部连续横断层 62（FH.12270）..................124
胸部连续横断层 63（FH.12250）..................126
胸部连续横断层 64（FH.12230）..................128
胸部连续横断层 65（FH.12210）..................130
胸部连续横断层 66（FH.12190）..................132
胸部连续横断层 67（FH.12170）..................134
胸部连续横断层 68（FH.12150）..................136
胸部连续横断层 69（FH.12130）..................138
胸部连续横断层 70（FH.12110）..................140
胸部连续横断层 71（FH.12090）..................142
胸部连续横断层 72（FH.12070）..................144
胸部连续横断层 73（FH.12050）..................146
胸部连续横断层 74（FH.12030）..................148

胸部连续横断层 75（FH.12010）..................150
胸部连续横断层 76（FH.11990）..................152
胸部连续横断层 77（FH.11970）..................154
胸部连续横断层 78（FH.11950）..................156
胸部连续横断层 79（FH.11930）..................158
胸部连续横断层 80（FH.11910）..................160
胸部连续横断层 81（FH.11890）..................162
胸部连续横断层 82（FH.11870）..................164
胸部连续横断层 83（FH.11850）..................166
胸部连续横断层 84（FH.11830）..................168
胸部连续横断层 85（FH.11810）..................170
胸部连续横断层 86（FH.11790）..................172
胸部连续横断层 87（FH.11770）..................174
胸部连续横断层 88（FH.11750）..................176
胸部连续横断层 89（FH.11730）..................178
胸部连续横断层 90（FH.11710）..................180
胸部连续横断层 91（FH.11690）..................182
胸部连续横断层 92（FH.11670）..................184
胸部连续横断层 93（FH.11650）..................186
胸部连续横断层 94（FH.11630）..................188
胸部连续横断层 95（FH.11610）..................190
胸部连续横断层 96（FH.11590）..................192
胸部连续横断层 97（FH.11570）..................194
胸部连续横断层 98（FH.11550）..................196
胸部连续横断层 99（FH.11530）..................198
胸部连续横断层 100（FH.11510）..................200
胸部连续横断层 101（FH.11490）..................202

参考文献..................204
索　引..................207

胸部分册
胸部连续横断层解剖

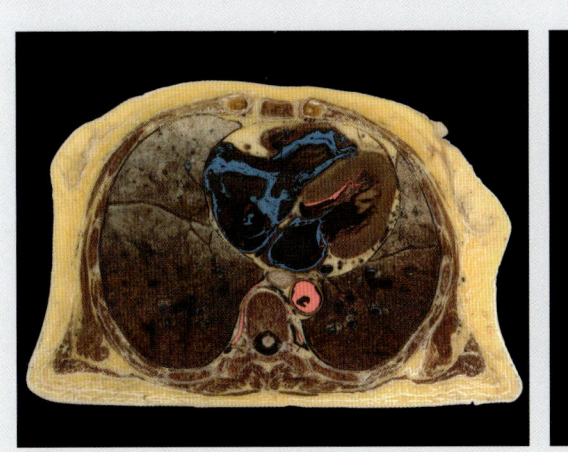
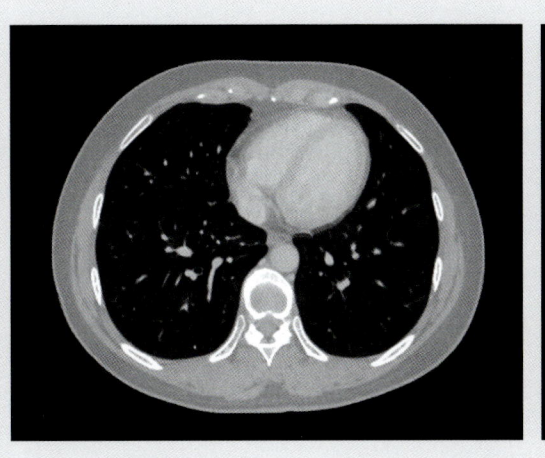
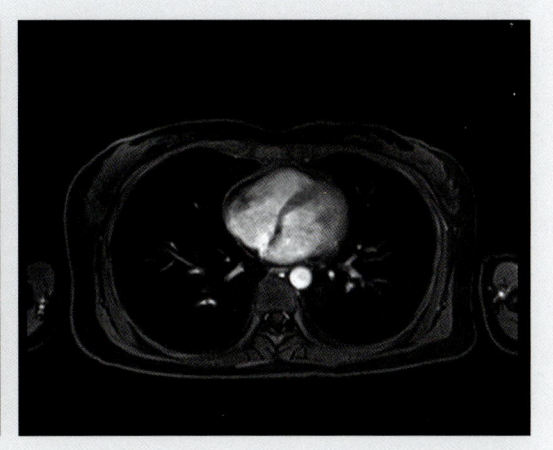

胸部连续横断层 1（FH.13490）

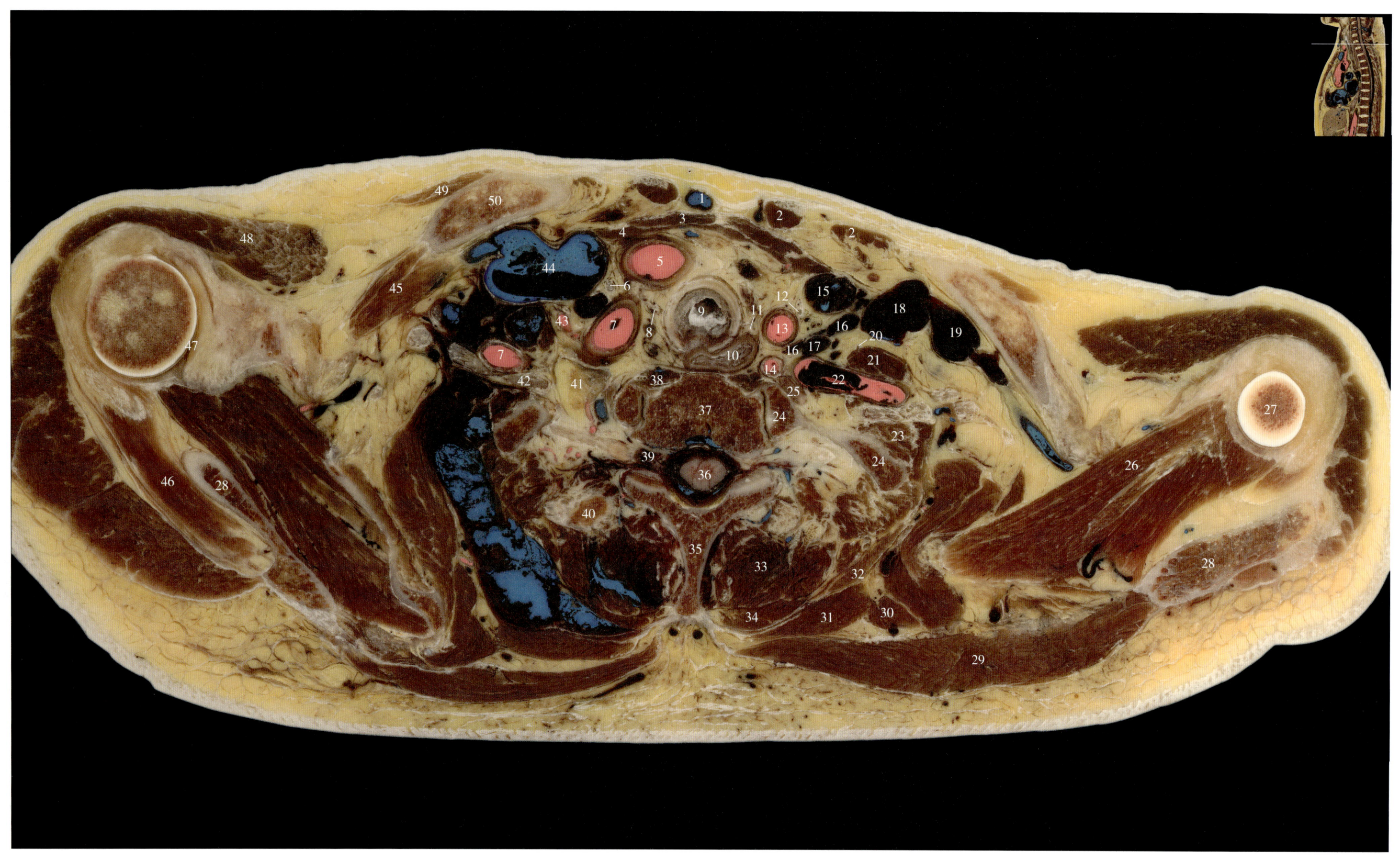

A. 断层标本图像

1. 颈前静脉 anterior jugular vein
2. 胸锁乳突肌 sternocleidomastoid
3. 胸骨舌骨肌 sternohyoid
4. 胸骨甲状肌 sternothyroid
5. 右颈总动脉 right common carotid artery
6. 右迷走神经 right vagus nerve
7. 右锁骨下动脉 right subclavian artery
8. 右喉返神经 right recurrent laryngeal nerve
9. 气管 trachea
10. 食管 esophagus
11. 左喉返神经 left recurrent laryngeal nerve
12. 左迷走神经 left vagus nerve
13. 左颈总动脉 left common carotid artery
14. 左椎动脉 left vertebral artery
15. 左颈内静脉 left internal jugular vein
16. 胸导管 thoracic duct
17. 左椎静脉 left vertebral vein
18. 左锁骨下静脉 left subclavian vein
19. 颈外静脉 external jugular vein
20. 膈神经 phrenic nerve
21. 前斜角肌 scalenus anterior
22. 左锁骨下动脉 left subclavian artery
23. 中斜角肌 scalenus medius
24. 第1肋骨 1st costal bone
25. 星状神经节 stellate ganglion
26. 冈上肌 supraspinatus
27. 肱骨头 head of humerus
28. 肩胛冈 spine of scapula
29. 斜方肌 trapezius
30. 肩胛提肌 levator scapulae
31. 菱形肌 rhomboideus
32. 上后锯肌 serratus posterior superior
33. 竖脊肌 erector spinae
34. 颈夹肌 splenius cervicis
35. 棘突 spinous process
36. 脊髓 spinal cord
37. 第1胸椎椎体 body of 1st thoracic vertebra
38. 颈长肌 longus colli
39. 椎间孔 intervertebral foramen
40. 横突 transverse process
41. 胸膜顶 cupula of pleura
42. 臂丛 brachial plexus
43. 右胸廓内动脉 right internal thoracic artery
44. 右头臂静脉 right brachiocephalic vein
45. 锁骨下肌 subclavius
46. 冈下肌 infraspinatus
47. 肩关节腔 cavity of shoulder joint
48. 三角肌 deltoid
49. 胸大肌 pectoralis major
50. 锁骨 clavicle

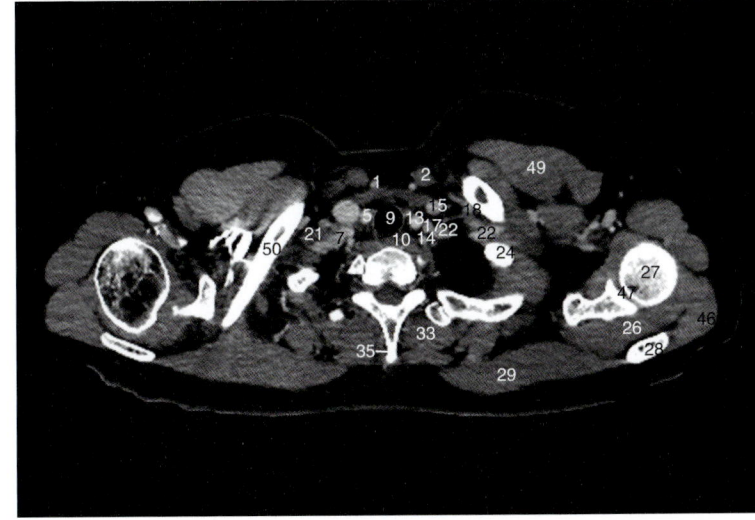

B. CT 纵隔窗增强图像

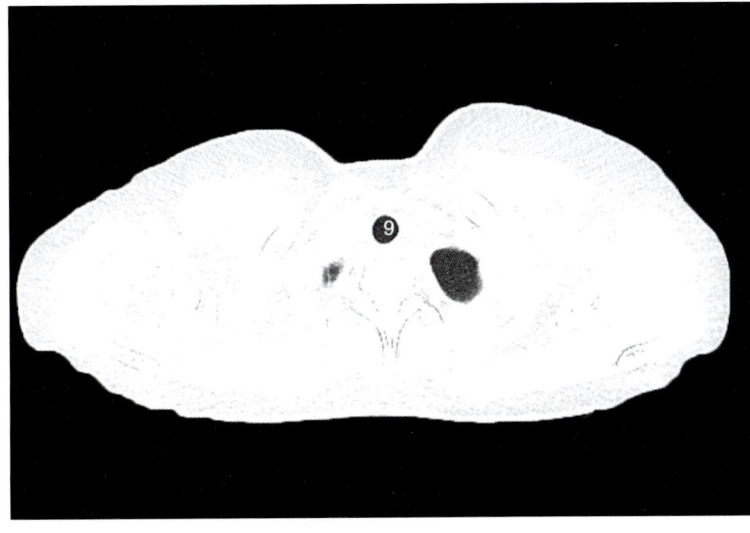

C. CT 肺窗图像

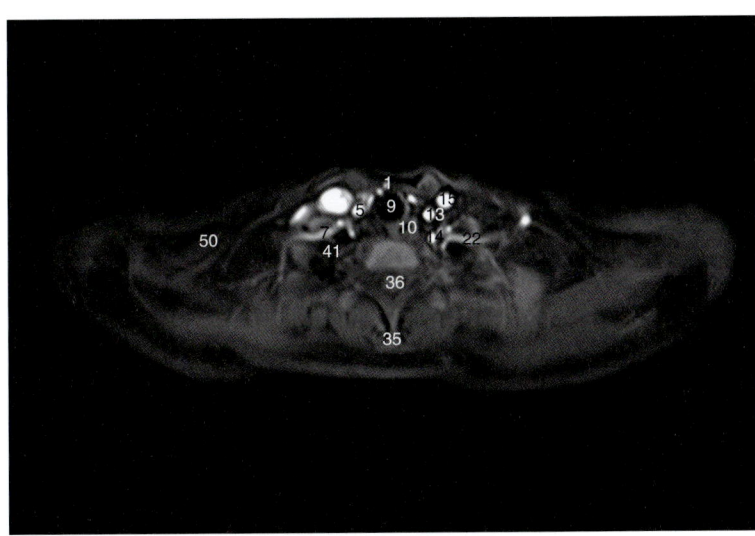

D. MR T1WI 增强图像

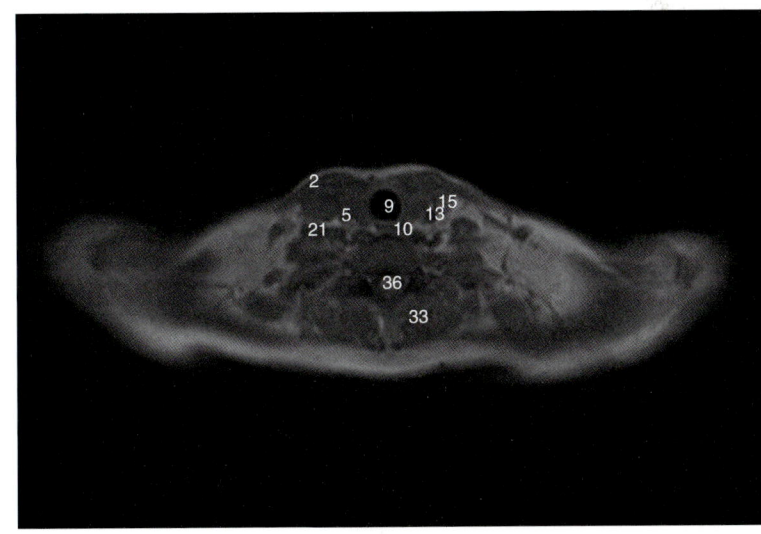

E. MR T1WI 平扫图像

关键结构：颈动脉鞘，斜角肌间隙，第 1 肋。

此断面经第 1 胸椎椎体上份。

第 1 胸椎椎体两侧与第 1 肋头形成肋头关节。气管位于上纵隔中心位置，食管位于气管左后方。胸锁乳突肌内侧可见颈前静脉。胸锁乳突肌深面可见颈动脉鞘、颈总动脉、颈内静脉和迷走神经。颈动脉鞘上起自颅底，下续纵隔，与颈筋膜各层存在密切的联系。颈筋膜中层和椎前筋膜浅层是构成颈动脉鞘的主体。椎动、静脉位于颈动脉鞘的后方。颈内静脉外侧依次为锁骨下静脉与颈外静脉，后 2/3 为第 1 胸椎椎体及项部肌和前、中斜角肌。斜角肌间隙位于颈根部，由前、中斜角肌和第 1 肋围成，内有臂丛及锁骨下动脉等重要结构[1]。临床上，因锁骨下动脉紧贴前斜角肌后面外行，故前斜角肌病变导致上肢血运障碍并不罕见。因锁骨下静脉在前斜角肌止点前面横跨第 1 肋，故无论锁骨、第 1 肋或前斜角肌的病变都有可能首先影响该静脉，导致患病上肢肿胀和淤血。第 1 肋骨扁、宽而短，无肋角和肋沟，分为上、下面和内、外缘；上面内缘处有前斜角肌结节，为前斜角肌附着处，其前、后方分别有锁骨下静脉和锁骨下动脉走行。

胸部连续横断层 2（FH.13470）

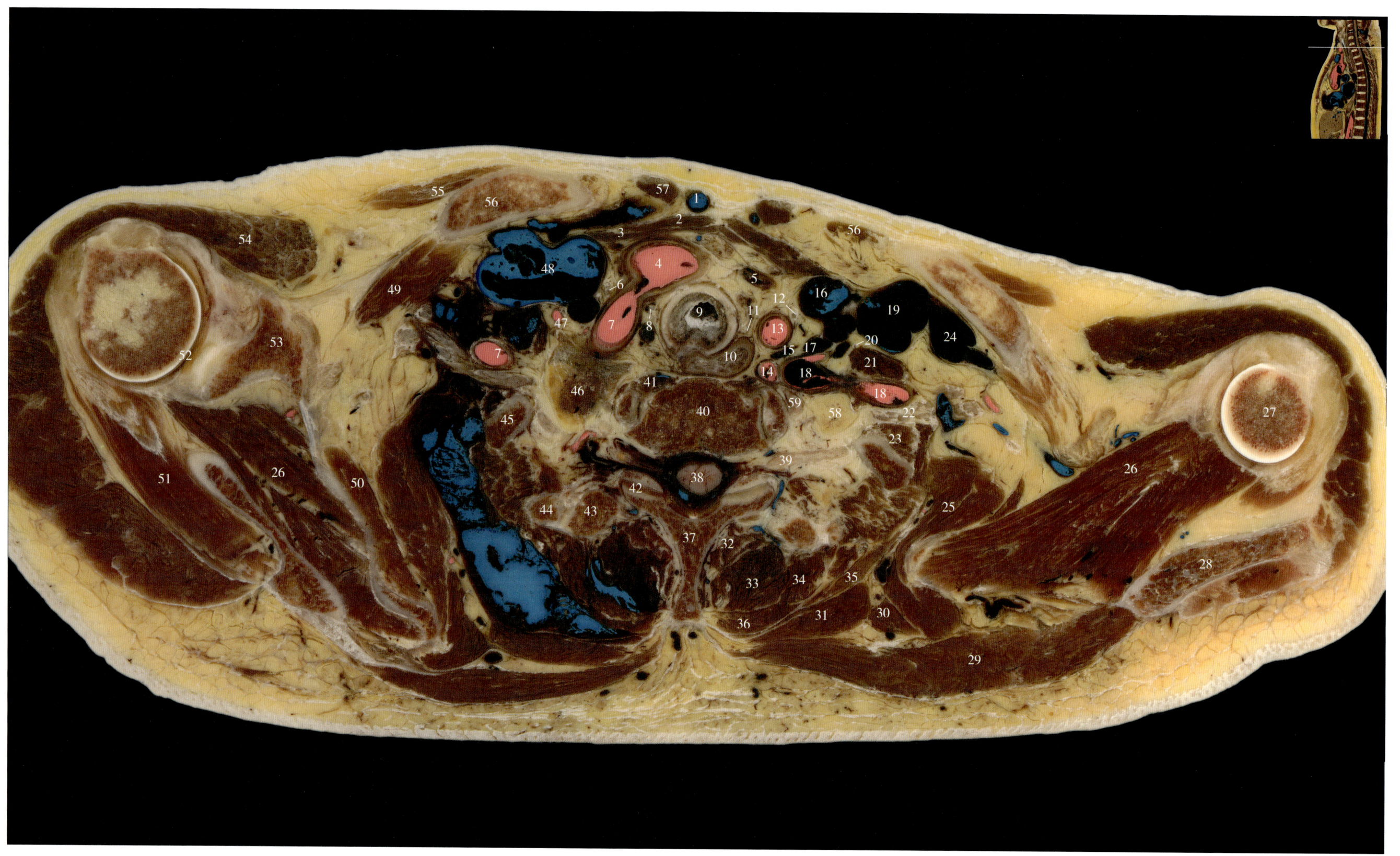

A. 断层标本图像

1. 颈前静脉 anterior jugular vein
2. 胸骨舌骨肌 sternohyoid
3. 胸骨甲状肌 sternothyroid
4. 右颈总动脉 right common carotid artery
5. 甲状腺下静脉 inferior thyroid vein
6. 右迷走神经 right vagus nerve
7. 右锁骨下动脉 right subclavian artery
8. 右喉返神经 right recurrent laryngeal nerve
9. 气管 trachea
10. 食管 esophagus
11. 左喉返神经 left recurrent laryngeal nerve
12. 左迷走神经 left vagus nerve
13. 左颈总动脉 left common carotid artery
14. 左椎动脉 left vertebral artery
15. 胸导管 thoracic duct
16. 左颈内静脉 left internal jugular vein
17. 左椎静脉 left vertebral vein
18. 左锁骨下动脉 left subclavian artery
19. 左锁骨下静脉 left subclavian vein
20. 膈神经 phrenic nerve
21. 前斜角肌 scalenus anterior
22. 臂丛 brachial plexus
23. 中斜角肌 scalenus medius
24. 颈外静脉 external jugular vein
25. 前锯肌 serratus anterior
26. 冈上肌 supraspinatus
27. 肱骨头 head of humerus
28. 肩胛冈 spine of scapula
29. 斜方肌 trapezius
30. 肩胛提肌 levator scapulae
31. 菱形肌 rhomboideus
32. 横突棘肌 transversospinales
33. 棘肌 spinales
34. 最长肌 longissimus
35. 上后锯肌 serratus posterior superior
36. 颈夹肌 splenius cervicis
37. 棘突 spinous process
38. 脊髓 spinal cord
39. 第8颈神经 8th spinal nerve
40. 第1胸椎椎体 body of 1st thoracic vertebra
41. 颈长肌 longus colli
42. 关节突关节 zygapophysial joint
43. 横突 transverse process
44. 第2肋骨 2nd costal bone
45. 第1肋骨 1st costal bone
46. 右肺尖 apex of right lung
47. 胸廓内动脉 internal thoracic artery
48. 右头臂静脉 right brachiocephalic vein
49. 锁骨下肌 subclavius
50. 肩胛下肌 subscapularis
51. 冈下肌 infraspinatus
52. 肩关节腔 cavity of shoulder joint
53. 肩胛骨 scapula
54. 三角肌 deltoid
55. 胸大肌 pectoralis major
56. 锁骨 clavicle
57. 胸锁乳突肌 sternocleidomastoid
58. 胸膜顶 cupula of pleura
59. 星状神经节 stellate ganglion

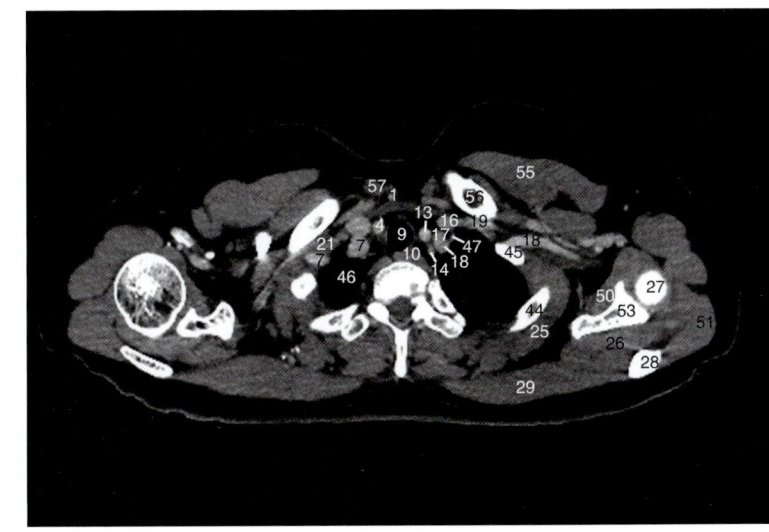

B. CT 纵隔窗增强图像

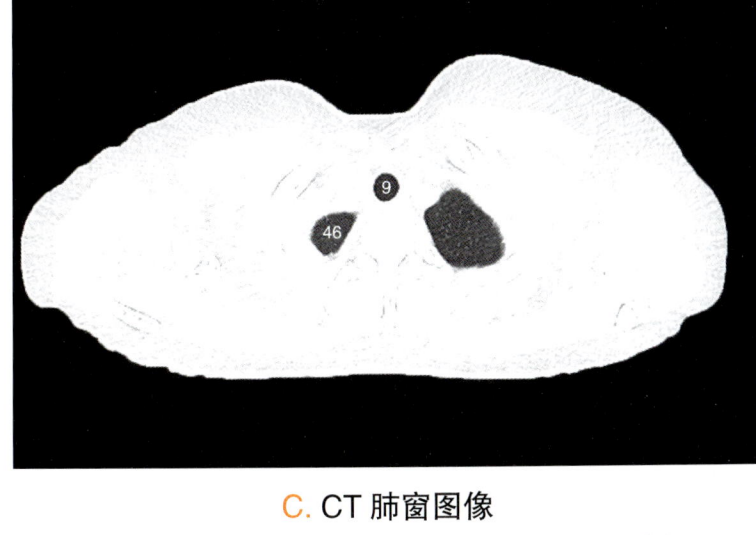

C. CT 肺窗图像

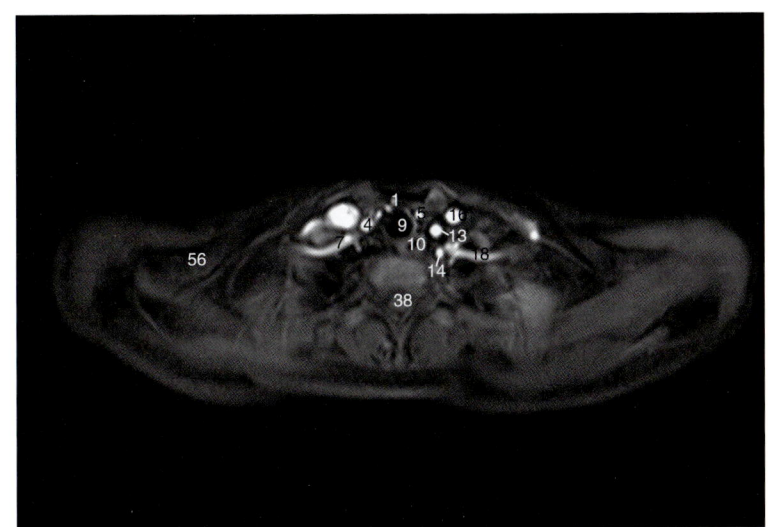

D. MR T1WI 增强图像

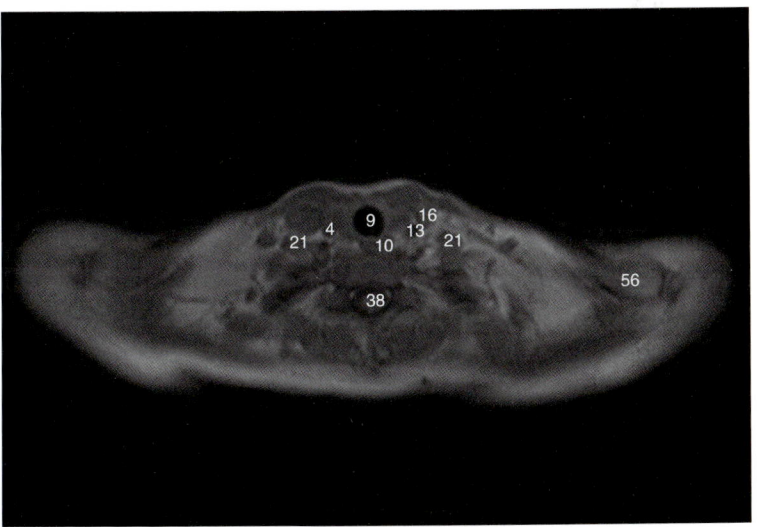

E. MR T1WI 平扫图像

关键结构：星状神经节，第8颈神经，胸膜顶。

此断面经第1胸椎椎体上部。

前部为颈根部结构，两侧见胸膜顶和肺尖，脊柱两侧有膨大的星状神经节。星状神经节是颈部交感神经节之一，又称颈胸神经节，其中心位置位于第1肋骨颈水平，毗邻肺尖、斜角肌、锁骨下动脉、颈总动脉和椎动脉等。星状神经节一般由颈下神经节与第1胸交感神经节融合而形成，这种融合出现的概率是75%~80%[2]。由C8~T1节段脊髓灰质中间外侧核发出的交感神经节前纤维，在星状神经节换元发出节后纤维，支配头面、颈项、上肢及胸内的心脏、血管等多个器官组织。星状神经节大小平均约为2.5 cm，25%的个体出现明显左右不对称。明确星状神经节的位置对于理解胸廓入口处的复杂结构及顺利实施星状神经节阻滞术具有重要意义。第8颈神经在C7-T1椎间孔穿出，第2胸椎体后上侧方可见。胸膜顶，又称颈胸膜，为覆盖在肺尖上方的壁胸膜，位于第1肋所围成的骨环内，被胸膜上膜、斜角肌和斜角肌筋膜所限制；其前方为臂丛和锁骨下动脉，后方与第1肋相邻，内侧有胸椎椎体和星状神经节，外侧可见第2肋间隙、臂丛。胸膜顶的最高点在腹侧相当于第1肋软骨上方3~4 cm处，背侧约与第1肋骨颈下缘的平面一致。一般右侧胸膜顶稍高于左侧。胸膜顶的体表投影为胸锁关节与锁骨内、中1/3交点间一个凸向上的弧形线，最凸点在锁骨上方2.5（1~4）cm处。

胸部连续横断层 3（FH.13450）

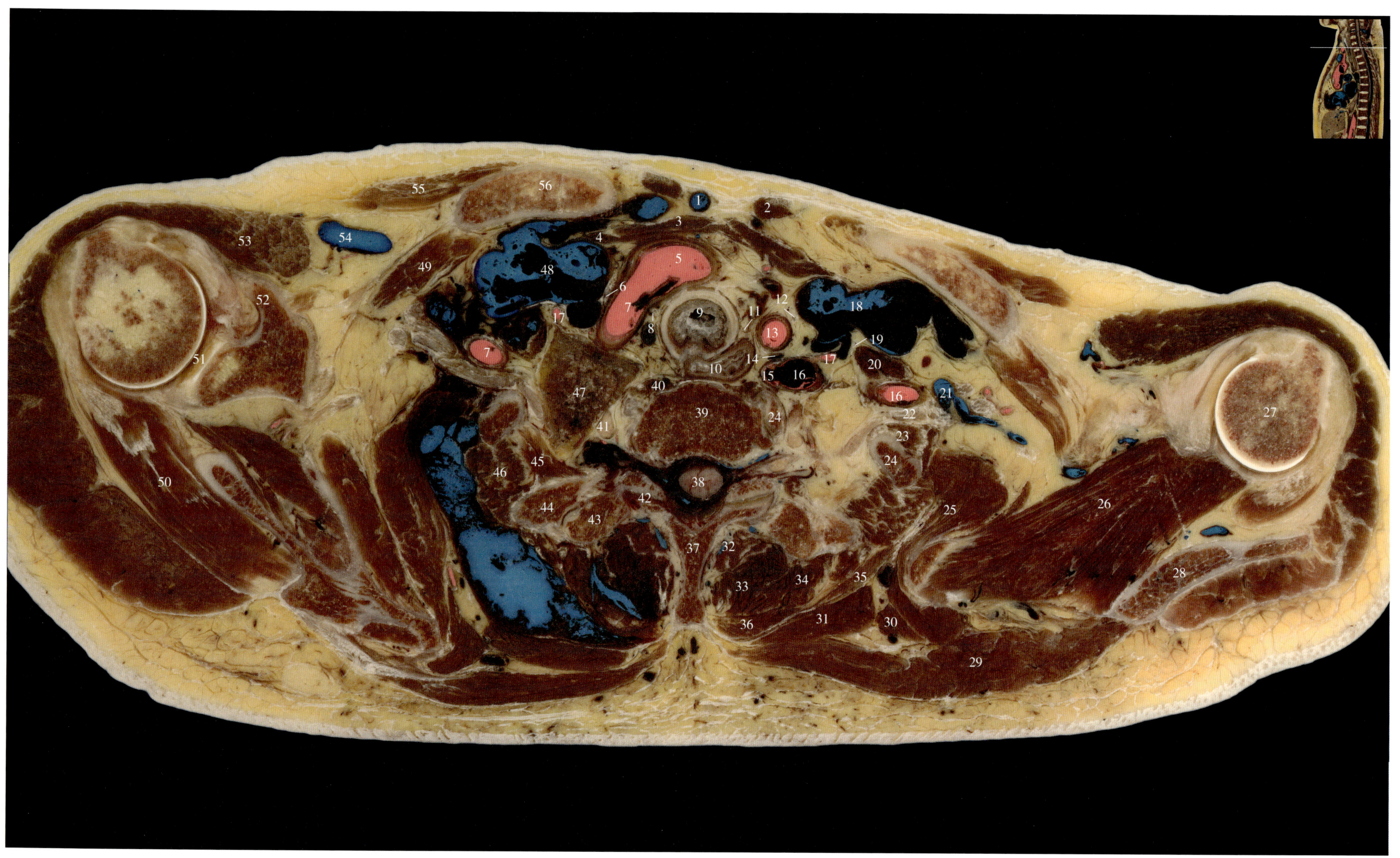

A. 断层标本图像

1. 颈前静脉 anterior jugular vein
2. 胸锁乳突肌 sternocleidomastoid
3. 胸骨舌骨肌 sternohyoid
4. 胸骨甲状肌 sternothyroid
5. 头臂干 brachiocephalic trunk
6. 右迷走神经 right vagus nerve
7. 右锁骨下动脉 right subclavian artery
8. 右喉返神经 right recurrent laryngeal nerve
9. 气管 trachea
10. 食管 esophagus
11. 左喉返神经 left recurrent laryngeal nerve
12. 左迷走神经 left vagus nerve
13. 左颈总动脉 left common carotid artery
14. 胸导管 thoracic duct
15. 左椎动脉 left vertebral artery
16. 左锁骨下动脉 left subclavian artery
17. 胸廓内动脉 internal thoracic artery
18. 左头臂静脉 left brachiocephalic vein
19. 膈神经 phrenic nerve
20. 前斜角肌 scalenus anterior
21. 肩胛上静脉 suprascapular vein
22. 臂丛 brachial plexus
23. 中斜角肌 scalenus medius
24. 第 1 肋骨 1st costal bone
25. 前锯肌 serratus anterior
26. 冈上肌 supraspinatus
27. 肱骨头 head of humerus
28. 肩胛冈 spine of scapula
29. 斜方肌 trapezius
30. 肩胛提肌 levator scapulae
31. 菱形肌 rhomboideus
32. 横突棘肌 transversospinales
33. 棘肌 spinales
34. 最长肌 longissimus
35. 上后锯肌 serratus posterior superior
36. 颈夹肌 splenius cervicis
37. 棘突 spinous process
38. 脊髓 spinal cord
39. 第 1 胸椎椎体 body of 1st thoracic vertebra
40. 颈长肌 longus colli
41. 胸交感神经节 thoracic sympathetic ganglion
42. 关节突关节 zygapophysial joint
43. 横突 transverse process
44. 第 2 肋骨 2nd costal bone
45. 肋间最内肌 intercostales intimi
46. 肋间内、外肌 intercostales interni and externi
47. 右肺尖 apex of right lung
48. 右头臂静脉 right brachiocephalic vein
49. 锁骨下肌 subclavius
50. 冈下肌 infraspinatus
51. 肩关节腔 cavity of shoulder joint
52. 喙突 coracoid process
53. 三角肌 deltoid
54. 头静脉 cephalic vein
55. 胸大肌 pectoralis major
56. 锁骨 clavicle

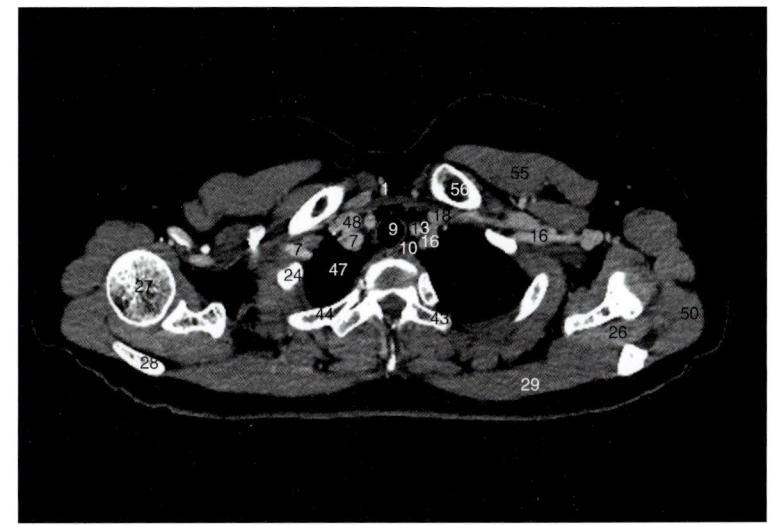

B. CT 纵隔窗增强图像

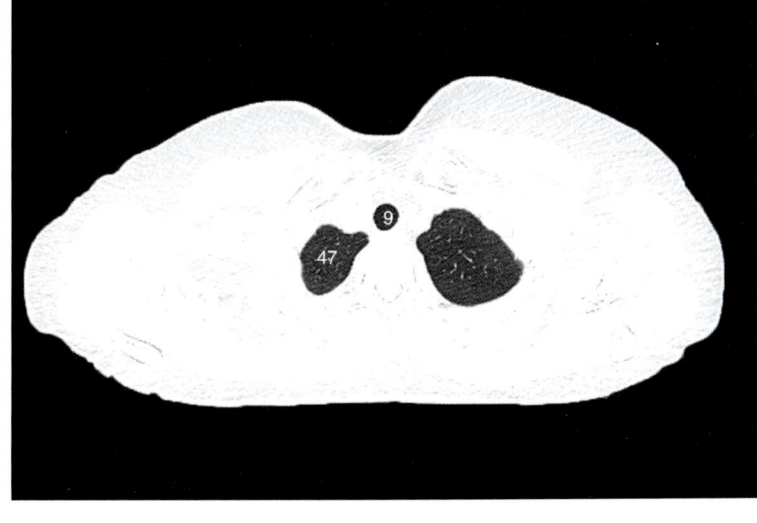

C. CT 肺窗图像

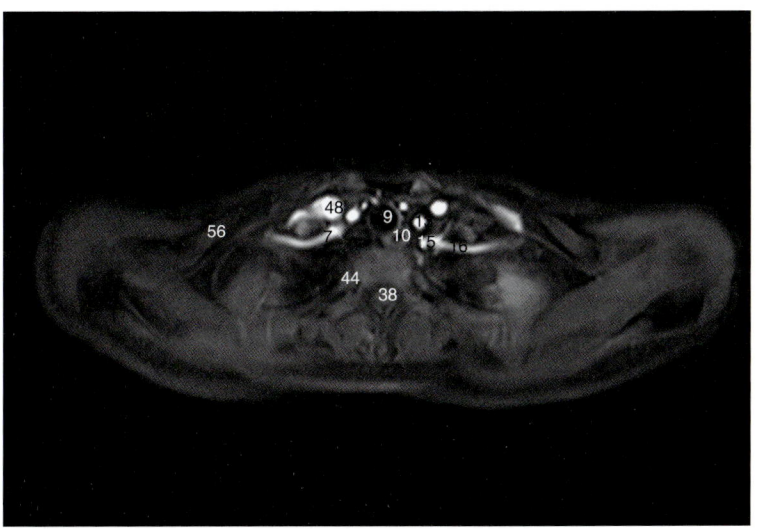

D. MR T1WI 增强图像

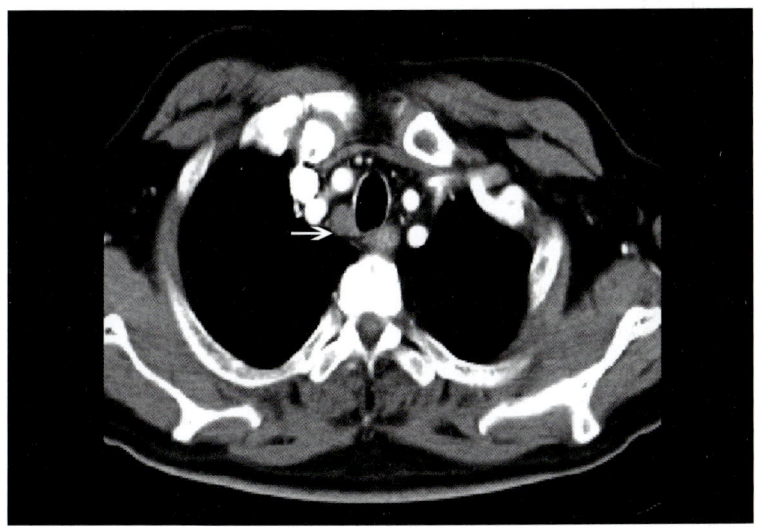

E. 1 区淋巴结转移 CT 图像

关键结构：锁骨下肌，胸廓内动脉，锁骨上淋巴结。

此断面经第 1 胸椎椎体中份。

锁骨由外侧向内侧移动。锁骨下肌附着点起于第 1 肋与肋软骨的交界处，一般止于喙锁韧带锁骨止部的内侧，大致位于锁骨下缘中外 1/3 处，部分位于喙突的前内侧缘锁骨下缘中外 1/3 处，与胸大肌、胸小肌、锁胸筋膜共同形成腋窝前壁。锁骨下肌伴行锁骨走行，位于锁骨与锁骨下静脉之间，部分位置紧贴锁骨及锁骨下静脉。其主要作用于胸锁关节和肩锁关节，功能为从下方固定锁骨，上抬第 1 肋和协助肩胛骨向前下拉肩部。胸廓内动脉在胸膜顶前方，正对椎动脉起始处，发自锁骨下动脉的下壁，在锁骨下静脉后方和胸膜顶前方降入胸腔，最后可分为 3 个分支：①穿膈肌胸肋角进入腹前壁的腹直肌鞘内移行为腹壁上动脉，并与腹壁下动脉吻合；②胸廓内动脉的上部可发出分支心包膈动脉，伴膈神经分布于膈、胸膜和心包；③至第 6 肋软骨深面分出肌膈动脉，沿肋弓后面行向外下方，沿途发支分布于下位 5 个肋间隙与膈。根据国际肺癌研究学会（International Association for the Study of Lung Cancer, IASLC）提出的肺癌淋巴结分区，此区域可见 1 区淋巴结，称为锁骨上淋巴结（如 1 区淋巴结转移 CT 图像中箭头所示）。1 区淋巴结意味着淋巴结的较远处转移，属于 N3 期淋巴结，提示预后不良[3]。

胸部连续横断层 4 （FH.13430）

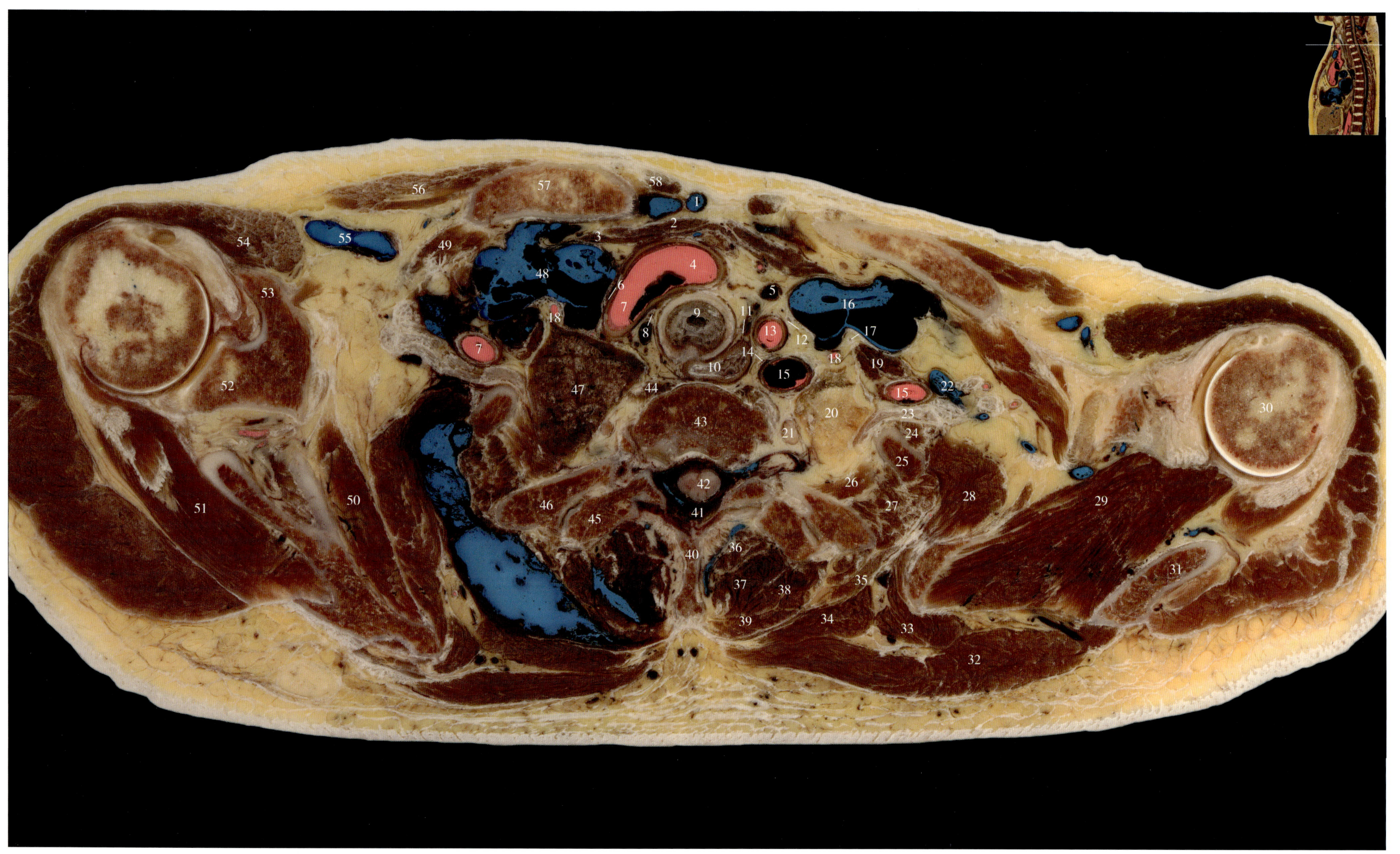

A. 断层标本图像

1. 颈前静脉 anterior jugular vein
2. 胸骨舌骨肌 sternohyoid
3. 胸骨甲状肌 sternothyroid
4. 头臂干 brachiocephalic trunk
5. 甲状腺下静脉 inferior thyroid vein
6. 右迷走神经 right vagus nerve
7. 右锁骨下动脉 right subclavian artery
8. 右喉返神经 right recurrent laryngeal nerve
9. 气管 trachea
10. 食管 esophagus
11. 左喉返神经 left recurrent laryngeal nerve
12. 左迷走神经 left vagus nerve
13. 左颈总动脉 left common carotid artery
14. 胸导管 thoracic duct
15. 左锁骨下动脉 left subclavian artery
16. 左头臂静脉 left brachiocephalic vein
17. 膈神经 phrenic nerve
18. 胸廓内动脉 internal thoracic artery
19. 前斜角肌 scalenus anterior
20. 左胸膜顶 left cupula of pleura
21. 胸交感神经节 thoracic sympathetic ganglion
22. 肩胛上静脉 suprascapular vein
23. 臂丛 brachial plexus
24. 中斜角肌 scalenus medius
25. 第1肋骨 1st costal bone
26. 肋间最内肌 intercostales intimi
27. 肋间内、外肌 intercostales interni and externi
28. 前锯肌 serratus anterior
29. 冈上肌 supraspinatus
30. 肱骨头 head of humerus
31. 肩胛冈 spine of scapula
32. 斜方肌 trapezius
33. 肩胛提肌 levator scapulae
34. 菱形肌 rhomboideus
35. 上后锯肌 serratus posterior superior
36. 横突棘肌 transversospinales
37. 棘肌 spinales
38. 最长肌 longissimus
39. 颈夹肌 splenius cervicis
40. 棘突 spinous process
41. 硬膜外隙 epidural space
42. 脊髓 spinal cord
43. 第1胸椎体 body of 1st thoracic vertebra
44. 颈长肌 longus colli
45. 横突 transverse process
46. 第2肋骨 2nd costal bone
47. 右肺尖 apex of right lung
48. 右头臂静脉 right brachiocephalic vein
49. 锁骨下肌 subclavius
50. 肩胛下肌 subscapularis
51. 冈下肌 infraspinatus
52. 肩胛骨 scapula
53. 喙突 coracoid process
54. 三角肌 deltoid
55. 头静脉 cephalic vein
56. 胸大肌 pectoralis major
57. 锁骨 clavicle
58. 胸锁乳突肌 sternocleidomastoid

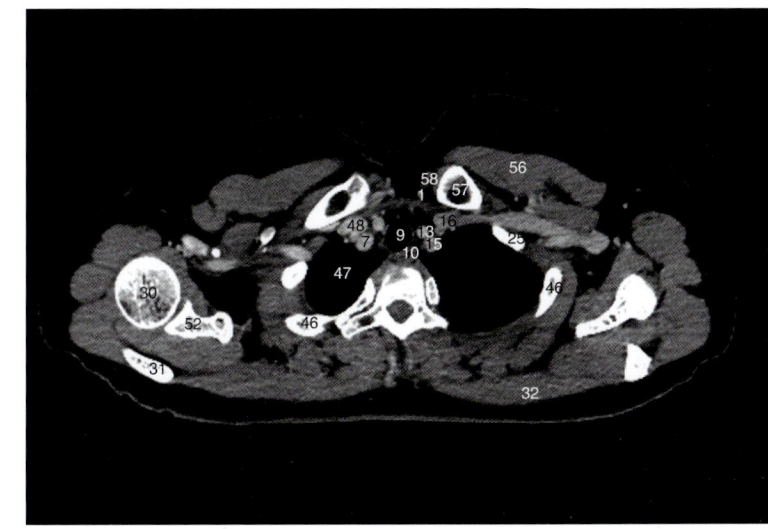

B. CT 纵隔窗增强图像

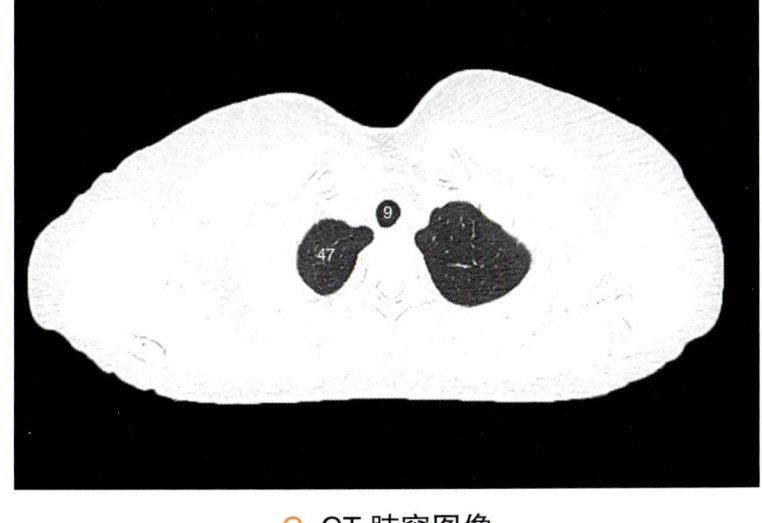

C. CT 肺窗图像

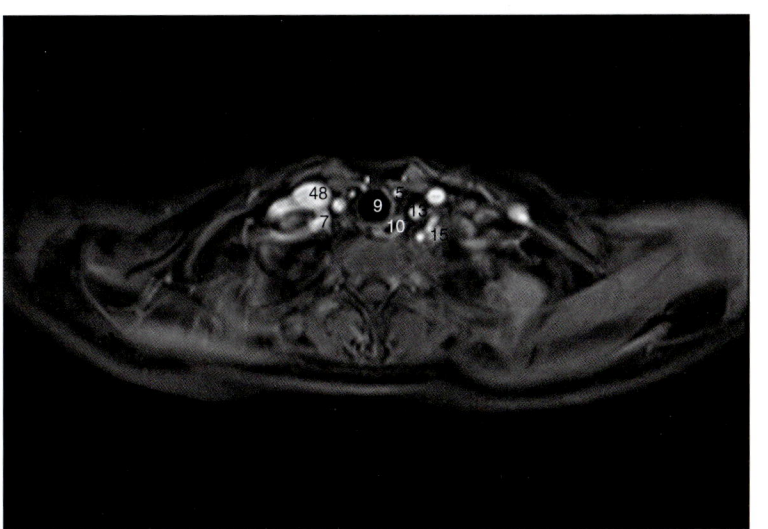

D. MR T1WI 增强图像

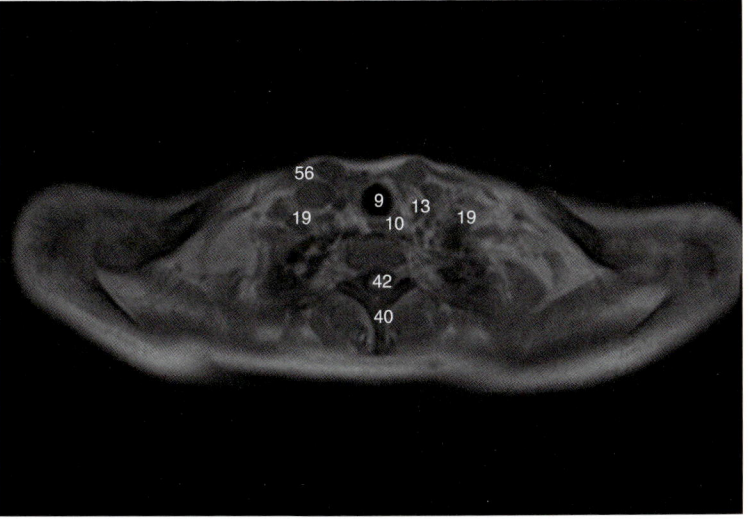

E. MR T1WI 平扫图像

关键结构：头臂干，锁骨下动脉，静脉角。

此断面经第1肋胸椎椎体下份。

右颈总动脉与右锁骨下动脉汇合形成头臂干。头臂干（又称无名动脉）发自主动脉弓，而后发出右颈总动脉和右锁骨下动脉。左锁骨下动脉直接起自主动脉弓。锁骨下动脉自胸锁关节后方行向外，斜越胸膜顶的前面，弓形向外穿过斜角肌间隙，行于锁骨后下方，至第1肋外侧缘，进入腋窝移行为腋动脉。锁骨下动脉主要分支有椎动脉、胸廓内动脉、甲状颈干、肋颈干、颈横动脉等，分布于头颈、胸腹壁等区域。于锁骨上窝中点处向下压此动脉于第1肋上，可达到止血的目的。两侧锁骨后可见左右头臂静脉，在头臂静脉的内侧可见左、右迷走神经，后侧可见胸廓内动、静脉与膈神经。同侧的颈内静脉和锁骨下静脉在胸锁关节的后方汇合而成头臂静脉（又称无名静脉），汇合处的夹角称静脉角。左、右静脉角分别有胸导管和右淋巴导管注入。锁骨下静脉内有多个静脉瓣，有颈外静脉、颈横静脉和椎静脉汇入。锁骨下静脉常呈开放状态，其原因一是管壁与周围筋膜紧密附着，二是与上述静脉从不同方向汇入有关。气管位于食管右前方，紧贴二者左右两侧有喉返神经。在纵隔的右侧面可见右头臂静脉、气管、食管的右侧壁和椎体的右缘。右肺紧贴气管的右侧壁。在纵隔的左侧面，可见左头臂静脉、左锁骨下动脉和椎体的左缘。

胸部连续横断层 5（FH.13410）

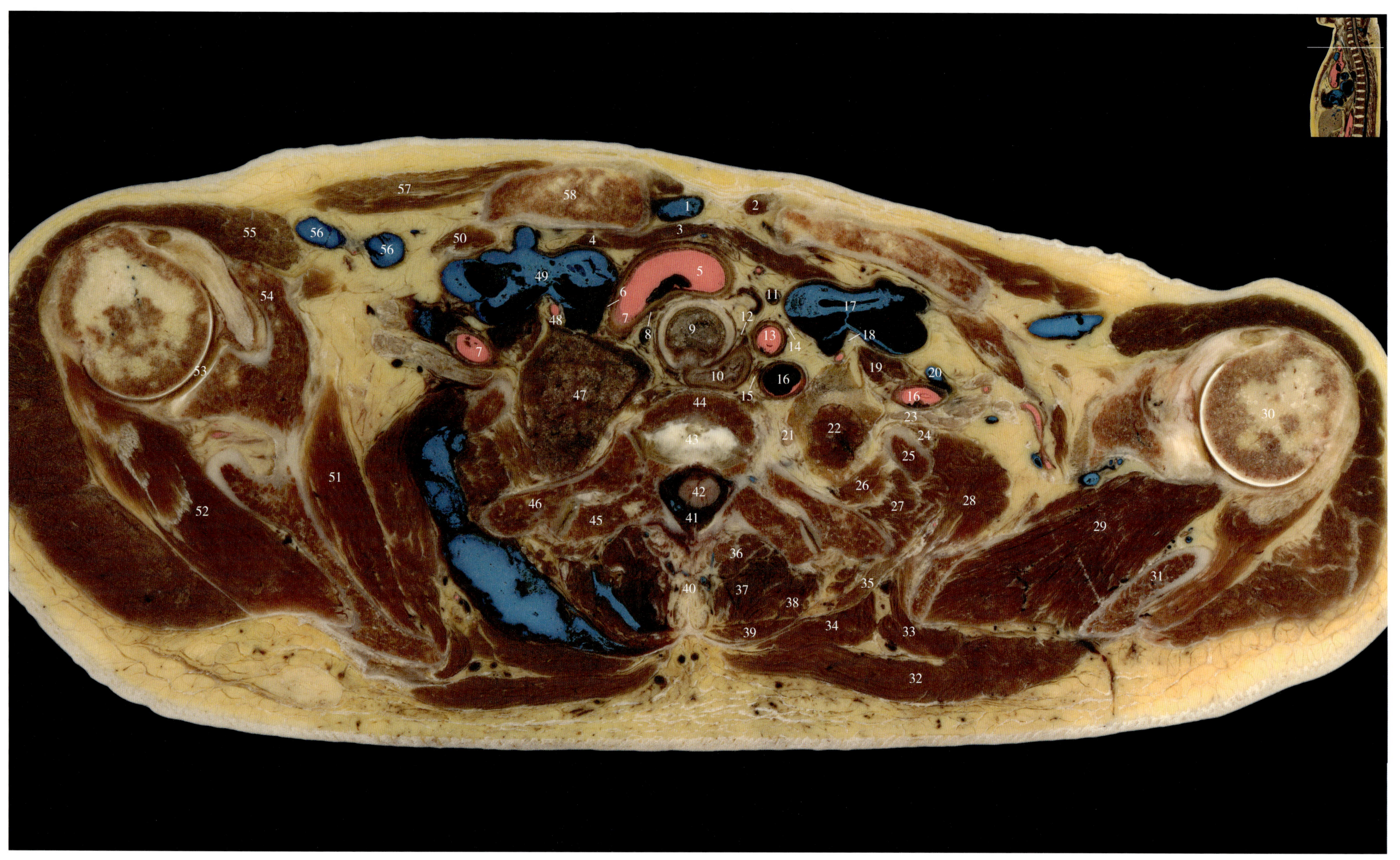

A. 断层标本图像

1. 颈前静脉 anterior jugular vein
2. 胸锁乳突肌 sternocleidomastoid
3. 胸骨舌骨肌 sternohyoid
4. 胸骨甲状肌 sternothyroid
5. 头臂干 brachiocephalic trunk
6. 右迷走神经 right vagus nerve
7. 右锁骨下动脉 right subclavian artery
8. 右喉返神经 right recurrent laryngeal nerve
9. 气管 trachea
10. 食管 esophagus
11. 甲状腺下静脉 inferior thyroid vein
12. 左喉返神经 left recurrent laryngeal nerve
13. 左颈总动脉 left common carotid artery
14. 左迷走神经 left vagus nerve
15. 胸导管 thoracic duct
16. 左锁骨下动脉 left subclavian artery
17. 左头臂静脉 left brachiocephalic vein
18. 膈神经 phrenic nerve
19. 前斜角肌 scalenus anterior
20. 肩胛上静脉 suprascapular vein
21. 胸交感神经节 thoracic sympathetic ganglion
22. 左肺尖 apex of left lung
23. 臂丛 brachial plexus
24. 中斜角肌 scalenus medius
25. 第 1 肋骨 1st costal bone
26. 肋间最内肌 intercostales intimi
27. 肋间内、外肌 intercostales interni and externi
28. 前锯肌 serratus anterior
29. 冈上肌 supraspinatus
30. 肱骨头 head of humerus
31. 肩胛冈 spine of scapula
32. 斜方肌 trapezius
33. 肩胛提肌 levator scapulae
34. 菱形肌 rhomboideus
35. 上后锯肌 serratus posterior superior
36. 横突棘肌 transversospinales
37. 棘肌 spinales
38. 最长肌 longissimus
39. 颈夹肌 splenius cervicis
40. 棘间韧带 interspinous ligament
41. 硬膜外隙 epidural space
42. 脊髓 spinal cord
43. T1-2 椎间盘 T1-2 intervertebral disc
44. 第 1 胸椎椎体 body of first thoracic vertebra
45. 横突 transverse process
46. 第 2 肋骨 2nd costal bone
47. 右肺尖 apex of right lung
48. 胸廓内动脉 internal thoracic artery
49. 右头臂静脉 right brachiocephalic vein
50. 锁骨下肌 subclavius
51. 肩胛下肌 subscapularis
52. 冈下肌 infraspinatus
53. 肩关节腔 cavity of shoulder joint
54. 喙突 coracoid process
55. 三角肌 deltoid
56. 头静脉 cephalic vein
57. 胸大肌 pectoralis major
58. 锁骨 clavicle

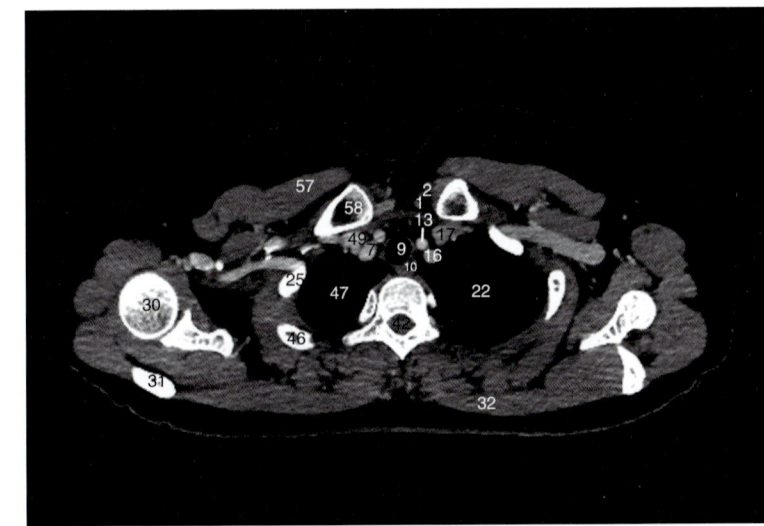

B. CT 纵隔窗增强图像

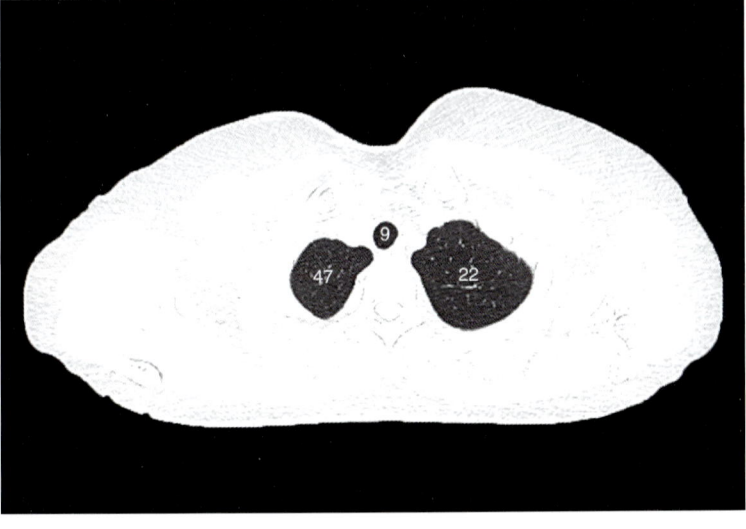

C. CT 肺窗图像

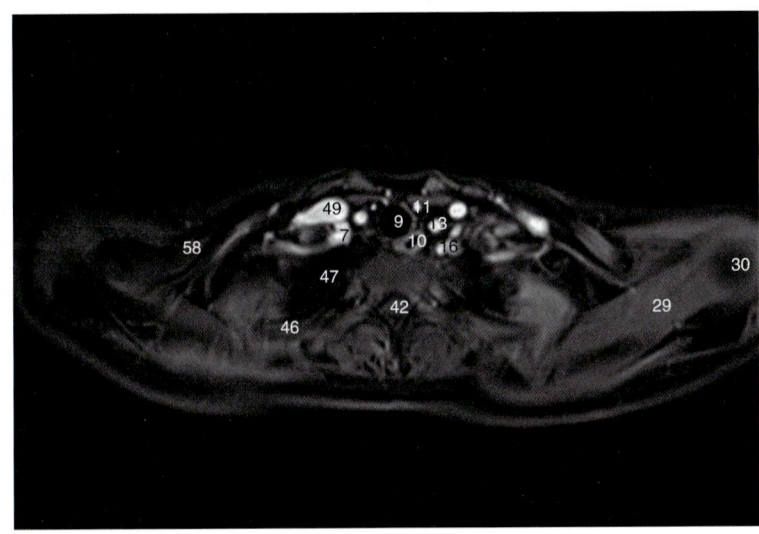

D. MR T1WI 增强图像

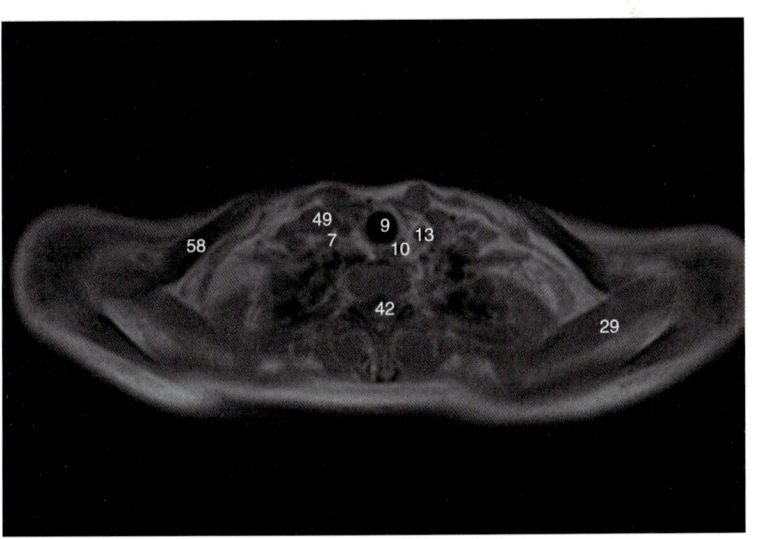

E. MR T1WI 平扫图像

关键结构：胸导管，肺尖，头静脉。

此断面经 T1-2 椎间盘上部。

食管左侧、左颈内动脉后侧与左锁骨下动脉内侧之间可见胸导管。胸导管是全身最长的淋巴导管，又称左淋巴导管，全长 30~40 cm，直径约为 3 mm，管腔内瓣膜较少，收纳两下肢、盆部、腹部、左胸部、左上肢、左头颈部的淋巴液。胸导管上段和下段与纵隔胸膜相贴，故胸导管损伤伴有纵隔胸膜破损时可引起左侧或右侧乳糜胸。头静脉是上肢的浅静脉之一，起自手背静脉网的桡侧，沿前臂桡侧上行至肘窝，通过正中静脉与贵要静脉吻合，再沿肱二头肌的外侧上行，在三角肌与胸大肌之间穿深筋膜注入锁骨下静脉或腋静脉。头静脉是临床进行静脉穿刺常用的静脉之一，比如进行抽血、输血、输液时常用。椎体两侧可见胸交感神经节，两侧肺尖体积亦增大。肺上沟癌是发生于肺尖部的周围型肺癌，易侵犯邻近的组织和器官，引起一系列特殊的临床表现，即 Pancoast 综合征[4]，表现为患侧颈、胸、背部及上肢疼痛，运动障碍和感觉过敏或丧失。此外，还因侵犯神经而引起相应的症状，如声音嘶哑、膈肌阵挛等。大多数病例胸部 X 线检查可发现肺尖部肿块影，但有 20%~40% 的病例仅表现为肺尖帽征，约有 6% 的病例胸部 X 线检查示无明显异常，CT 检查可清晰地显示肿块的特征及其与周围组织的关系。

胸部连续横断层9（FH.13330）

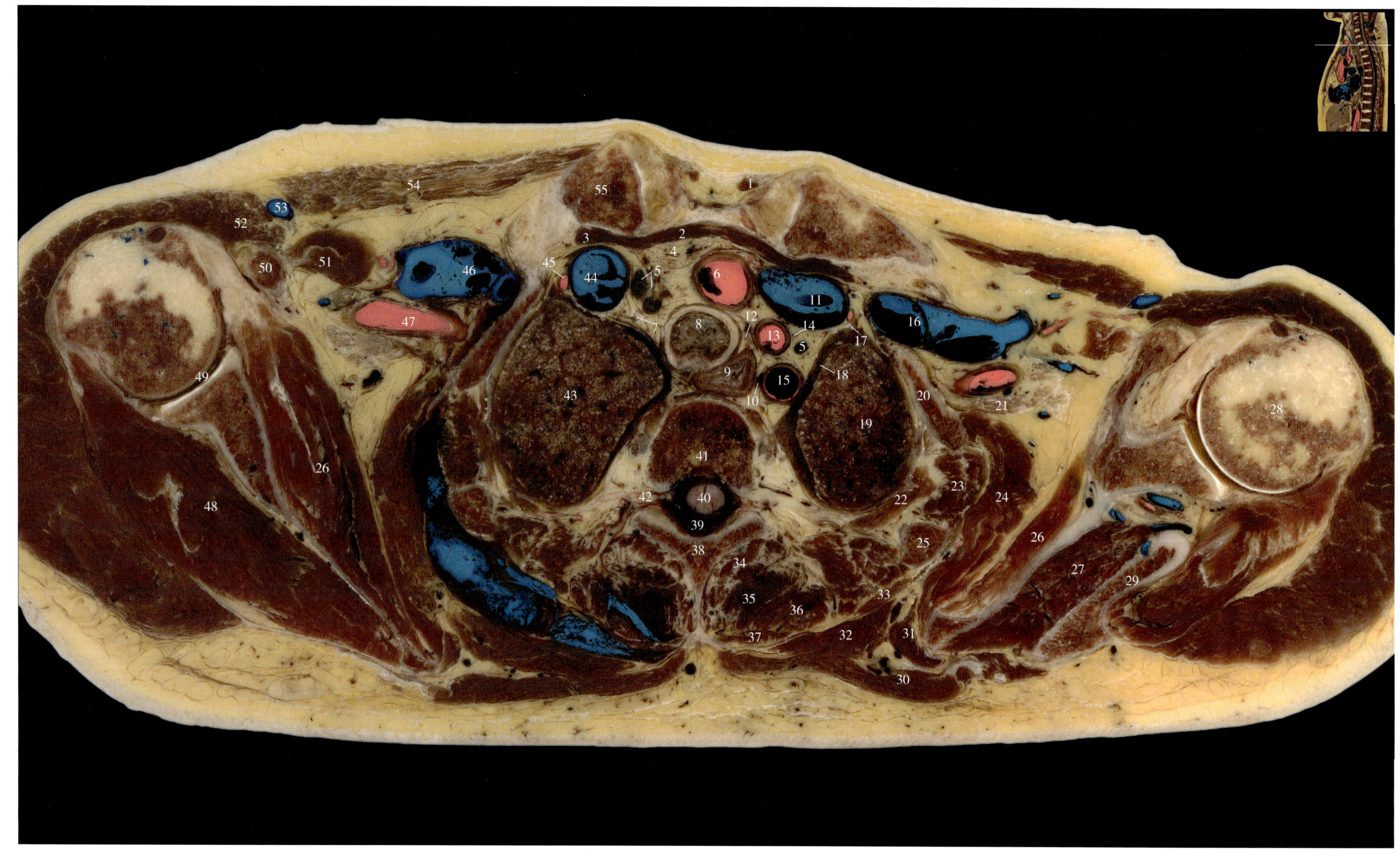

A. 断层标本图像

1. 胸锁乳突肌 sternocleidomastoid
2. 胸骨舌骨肌 sternohyoid
3. 胸骨甲状肌 sternothyroid
4. 胸腺 thymus
5. 上气管旁淋巴结（2区）upper paratracheal lymph nodes
6. 头臂干 brachiocephalic trunk
7. 右迷走神经 right vagus nerve
8. 气管 trachea
9. 食管 esophagus
10. 胸导管 thoracic duct
11. 左头臂静脉 left brachiocephalic vein
12. 左喉返神经 left recurrent laryngeal nerve
13. 左颈总动脉 left common carotid artery
14. 左迷走神经 left vagus nerve
15. 左锁骨下动脉 left subclavian artery
16. 左锁骨下静脉 left subclavian vein
17. 膈神经 phrenic nerve
18. 胸膜腔 pleural cavity
19. 左肺尖 apex of left lung
20. 第1肋骨 1st costal bone
21. 臂丛 brachial plexus
22. 肋间最内肌 intercostales intimi
23. 肋间内、外肌 intercostales interni and externi
24. 前锯肌 serratus anterior
25. 第2肋骨 2nd costal bone
26. 肩胛下肌 subscapularis
27. 冈上肌 supraspinatus
28. 肱骨头 head of humerus
29. 肩胛冈 spine of scapula
30. 斜方肌 trapezius
31. 肩胛提肌 levator scapulae
32. 菱形肌 rhomboideus
33. 上后锯肌 serratus posterior superior
34. 横突棘肌 transversospinales
35. 棘肌 spinales
36. 最长肌 longissimus
37. 颈夹肌 splenius cervicis
38. 椎弓板 lamina of vertebral arch
39. 硬膜外隙 epidural space
40. 脊髓 spinal cord
41. 第2胸椎椎体 body of 2nd thoracic vertebra
42. 椎间孔 intervertebral foramen
43. 右肺上叶 superior lobe of right lung
44. 右头臂静脉 right brachiocephalic vein
45. 胸廓内动脉 internal thoracic artery
46. 腋静脉 axillary vein
47. 腋动脉 axillary artery
48. 冈下肌 infraspinatus
49. 肩关节腔 cavity of shoulder joint
50. 喙突 coracoid process
51. 胸小肌 pectoralis minor
52. 三角肌 deltoid
53. 头静脉 cephalic vein
54. 胸大肌 pectoralis major
55. 锁骨 clavicle

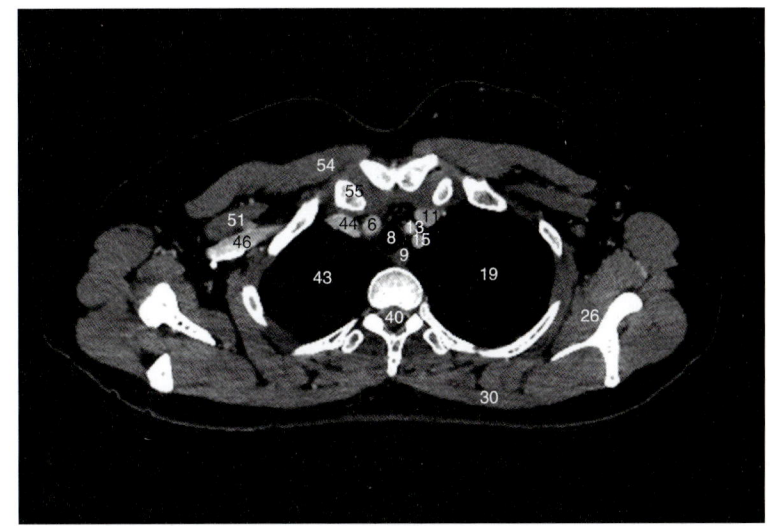

B. CT 纵隔窗增强图像

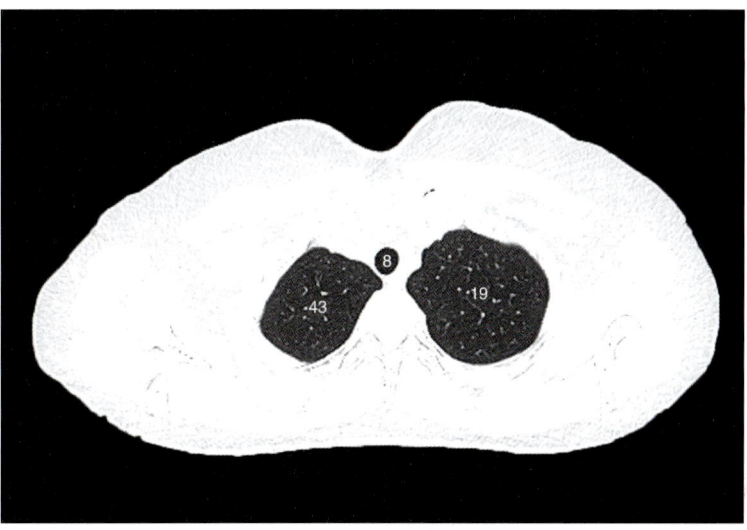

C. CT 肺窗图像

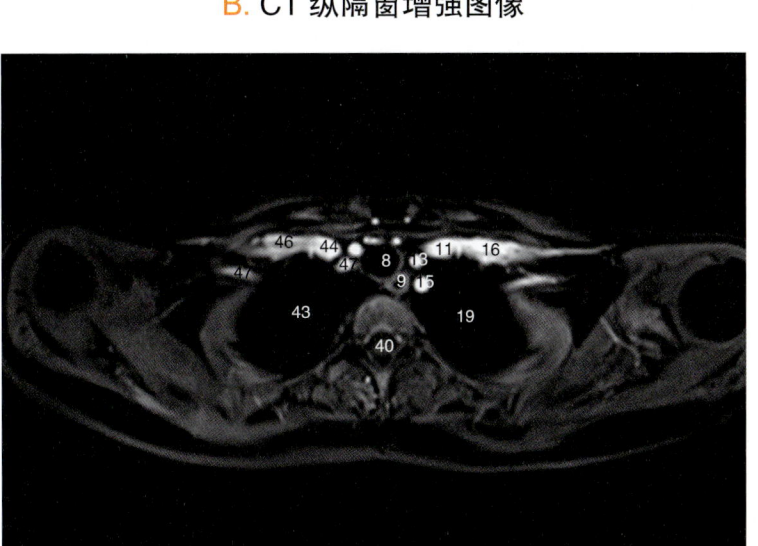

D. MR T1WI 增强图像

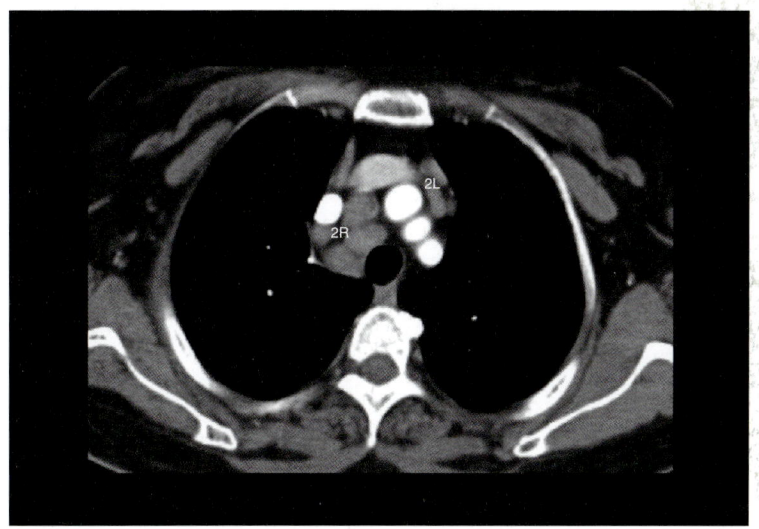

E. 2L、2R 区淋巴结转移 CT 图像

关键结构：上气管旁淋巴结（2区），血管前间隙，胸导管，气管，食管。

此断面经第2胸椎椎体上份。

前方出现胸锁关节。胸骨后上纵隔内即血管前间隙区可见胸腺。纵隔淋巴结在 CT 上表现为纵隔一定部位内出现的伴强化的软组织密度影，多呈圆形或椭圆形。在 CT 上正确认识纵隔淋巴结对于肺癌术前的分期诊断有重要的意义。根据 IASLC 提出的肺癌淋巴结分区，上气管旁淋巴结（2区）为锁骨上至主动脉弓上方的淋巴结，以气管左缘为界，可分为左、右群（2L、2R）[10]。2L 区淋巴结位于左头臂静脉与主动脉弓顶之间；2R 区淋巴结位于胸骨上切迹与上腔静脉起始部之间。如图 E 所示，可见增大的 2R、2L 区淋巴结。血管前间隙位于胸骨柄的后方、大血管的前方，两侧为纵隔胸膜，内含舌骨下肌群、成人有残存胸腺（小儿含胸腺）、脂肪、淋巴结、低位的甲状腺。食管与左锁骨下动脉之间可见胸导管。胸导管是全身最长的淋巴导管，收纳左半身上半身及腹部、两下肢的淋巴液。胸导管一般在第1和第2腰椎前方形成起始部，此处称"乳糜池"。胸导管向上穿膈的主动脉裂孔进入胸腔，注入左静脉角。如发生阻塞、破裂，可导致乳糜胸、乳糜腹。

胸部连续横断层 10（FH.13310）

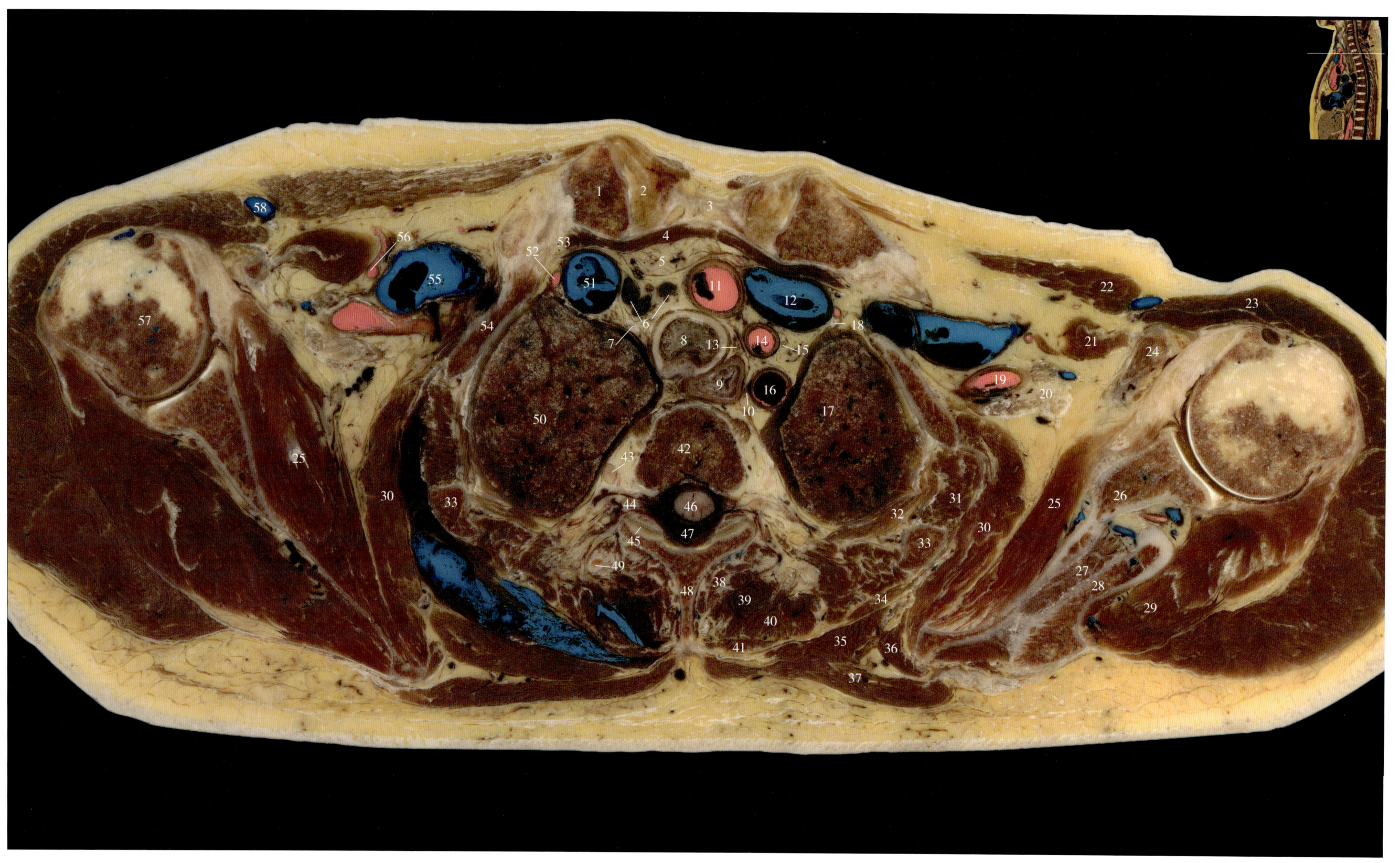

A. 断层标本图像

1. 锁骨胸骨端 sternal end of clavicle
2. 关节盘 articular disc
3. 胸骨柄 manubrium sterni
4. 胸骨舌骨肌 sternohyoid
5. 胸腺 thymus
6. 右上气管旁淋巴结（2R）right upper paratracheal lymph nodes
7. 右迷走神经 right vagus nerve
8. 气管 trachea
9. 食管 esophagus
10. 胸导管 thoracic duct
11. 头臂干 brachiocephalic trunk
12. 左头臂静脉 left brachiocephalic vein
13. 左喉返神经 left recurrent laryngeal nerve
14. 左颈总动脉 left common carotid artery
15. 左迷走神经 left vagus nerve
16. 左锁骨下动脉 left subclavian artery
17. 左肺尖 apex of left lung
18. 膈神经 phrenic nerve
19. 腋动脉 axillary artery
20. 臂丛 brachial plexus
21. 胸小肌 pectoralis minor
22. 胸大肌 pectoralis major
23. 三角肌 deltoid
24. 喙突 coracoid process
25. 肩胛下肌 subscapularis
26. 肩胛骨 scapula
27. 冈上肌 supraspinatus
28. 肩胛冈 spine of scapula
29. 冈下肌 infraspinatus
30. 前锯肌 serratus anterior
31. 肋间内、外肌 intercostales interni and externi
32. 肋间最内肌 intercostales intimi
33. 第 2 肋骨 2nd costal bone
34. 上后锯肌 serratus posterior superior
35. 菱形肌 rhomboideus
36. 肩胛提肌 levator scapulae
37. 斜方肌 trapezius
38. 横突棘肌 transversospinales
39. 棘肌 spinales
40. 最长肌 longissimus
41. 颈夹肌 splenius cervicis
42. 第 2 胸椎椎体 body of 2nd thoracic vertebra
43. 胸交感神经节 thoracic sympathetic ganglion
44. 第 2 胸神经 2nd thoracic nerve
45. 关节突关节 zygapophysial joint
46. 脊髓 spinal cord
47. 硬膜外隙 epidural space
48. 棘突 spinous process
49. 第 3 肋骨 3rd costal bone
50. 右肺尖 apex of right lung
51. 右头臂静脉 right brachiocephalic vein
52. 胸廓内动脉 internal thoracic artery
53. 胸骨甲状肌 sternothyroid
54. 第 1 肋骨 1st costal bone
55. 腋静脉 axillary vein
56. 胸肩峰动脉 thoracoacromial artery
57. 肱骨 humerus
58. 头静脉 cephalic vein

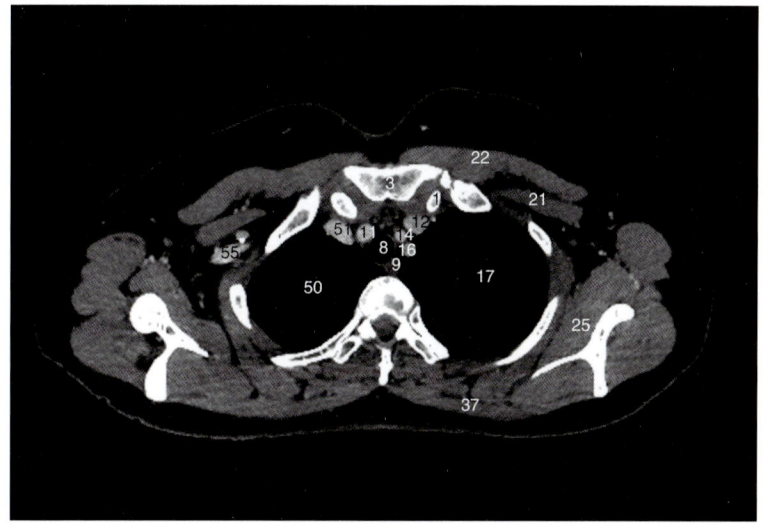

B. CT 纵隔窗增强图像

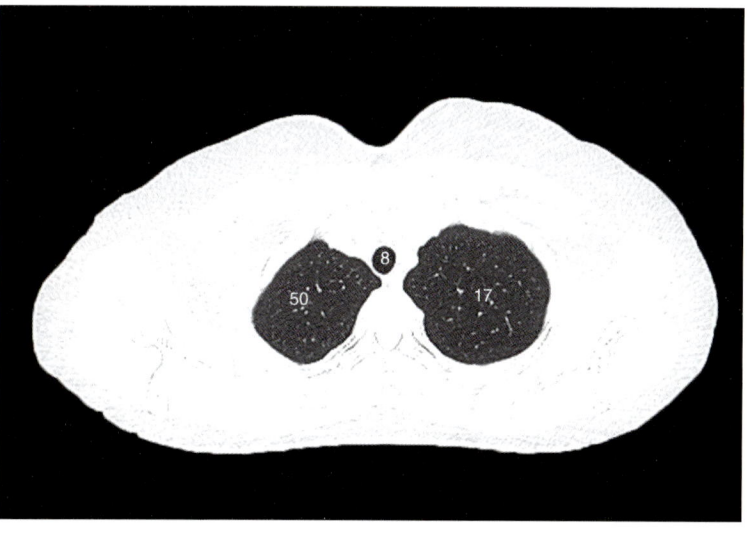

C. CT 肺窗图像

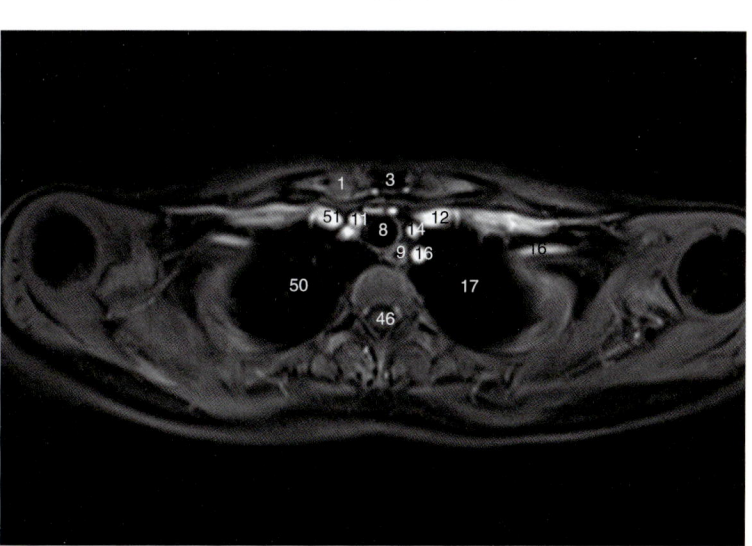

D. MR T1WI 增强图像

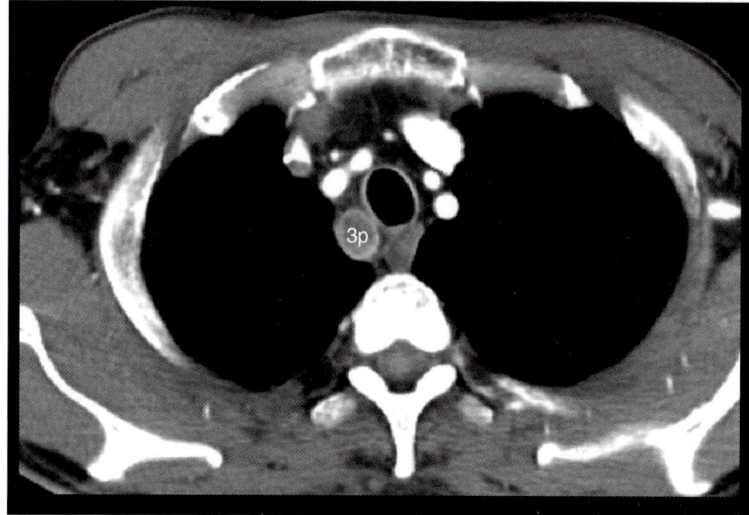

E. 3p 区淋巴结转移 CT 图像

关键结构：胸腺，血管前淋巴结，气管后淋巴结。

此断面前方经胸锁关节，后方经第 2 胸椎椎体中份。

气管前方为头臂干，左邻左颈总动脉，其后外侧为左锁骨下动脉，腋动脉由锁骨下动脉延伸而来，锁骨下动脉在越过第 1 肋骨外侧缘后即变为腋动脉，腋静脉与其伴行。胸腺位于胸腔前纵隔上部，胸骨柄后方，呈扁长条状，分左右叶。胸腺的形态各年龄组变异较大，但 9 岁以下大多数呈方形、梯形，10 岁以后大多数呈箭头形，部分呈新月形、烧杯形。另外，还发现 40 岁及以下胸腺的长轴夹角多成锐角，40 岁以上多成钝角。胸腺在 19 岁以前主要呈软组织密度；19 岁以后，胸腺逐渐退化，由脂肪置换，且随年龄增加，脂肪置换的比例也增高，虽仍可保持其原有形态，但分叶变得不明显，仅在脂肪背景上见到散在的残余胸腺组织，呈片絮状或弧状、点状、条状密度增高影（相对于脂肪背景），若显示为软组织密度影，应考虑为异常。早产儿胸腺体积变小；胸腺体积减小也是自发性早产的一个预测因素；胸腺体积可能是胎儿宫内炎症反应的一个反应标志[11]。胸腺区淋巴结为 3a 区淋巴结，3 区包括血管前淋巴结（3a）和气管后淋巴结（3p）。3a 区淋巴结右侧上界为胸膜顶，下界为隆突水平，前界为胸骨后，后界为上腔静脉前缘，左侧组后界为左颈总动脉。3p 区淋巴结上界为胸膜顶，下界为隆突水平，如图 E 所示。

胸部连续横断层 12（FH.13270）

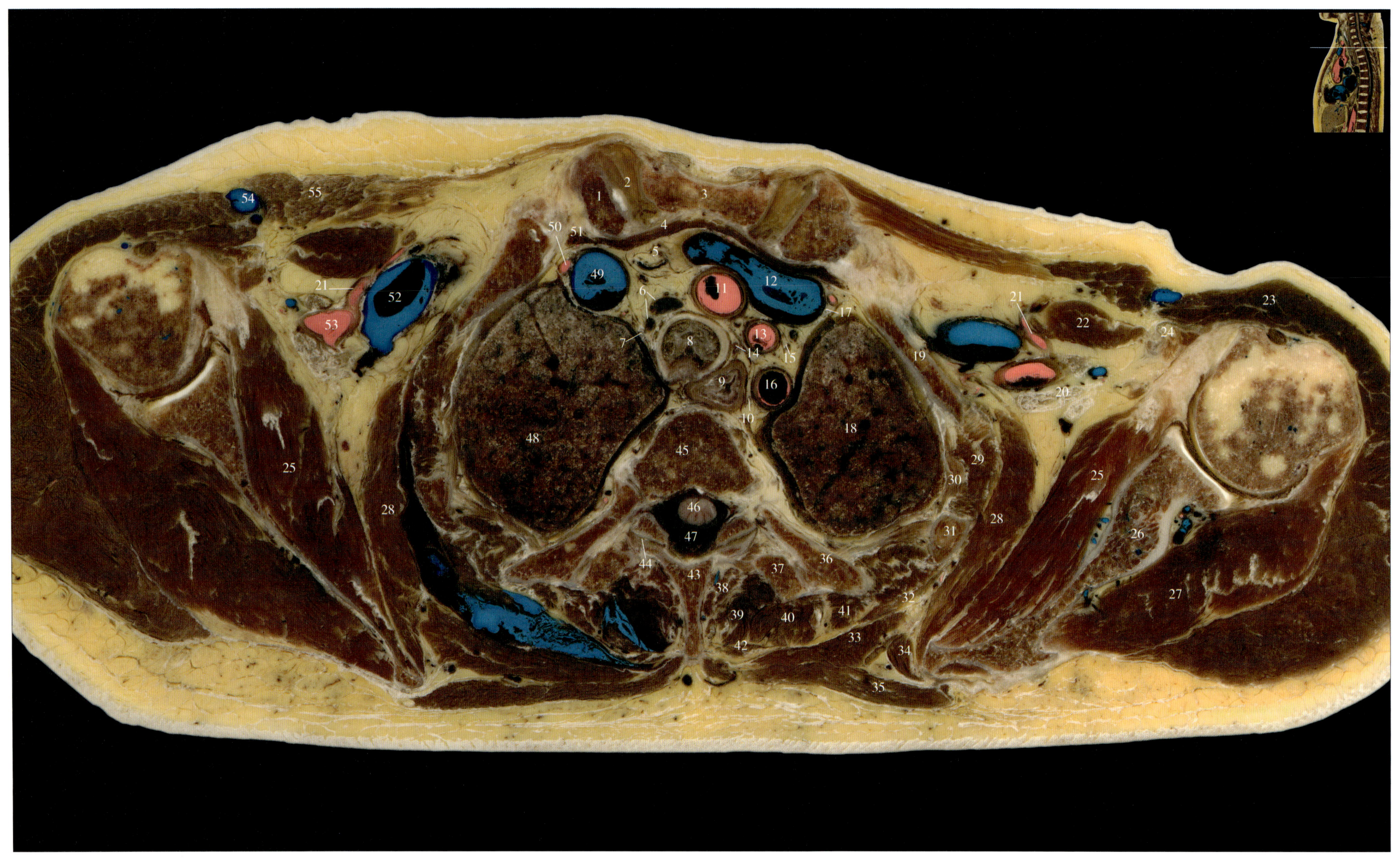

A. 断层标本图像

1. 锁骨胸骨端 sternal end of clavicle
2. 关节盘 articular disc
3. 胸骨柄 manubrium sterni
4. 胸骨舌骨肌 sternohyoid
5. 胸腺 thymus
6. 右上气管旁淋巴结（2R）right upper paratracheal lymph nodes
7. 右迷走神经 right vagus nerve
8. 气管 trachea
9. 食管 esophagus
10. 胸导管 thoracic duct
11. 头臂干 brachiocephalic trunk
12. 左头臂静脉 left brachiocephalic vein
13. 左颈总动脉 left common carotid artery
14. 左喉返神经 left recurrent laryngeal nerve
15. 左迷走神经 left vagus nerve
16. 左锁骨下动脉 left subclavian artery
17. 膈神经 phrenic nerve
18. 左肺上叶 superior lobe of left lung
19. 第1肋骨 1st costal bone
20. 臂丛 brachial plexus
21. 胸肩峰动脉 thoracoacromial artery
22. 胸小肌 pectoralis minor
23. 三角肌 deltoid
24. 喙突 coracoid process
25. 肩胛下肌 subscapularis
26. 肩胛骨 scapula
27. 冈下肌 infraspinatus
28. 前锯肌 serratus anterior
29. 肋间内、外肌 intercostales interni and externi
30. 肋间最内肌 intercostales intimi
31. 第2肋骨 2nd costal bone
32. 上后锯肌 serratus posterior superior
33. 菱形肌 rhomboideus
34. 肩胛提肌 levator scapulae
35. 斜方肌 trapezius
36. 第3肋骨 3rd costal bone
37. 横突 transverse process
38. 横突棘肌 transversospinales
39. 棘肌 spinales
40. 最长肌 longissimus
41. 髂肋肌 iliocostalis
42. 颈夹肌 splenius cervicis
43. 棘突 spinous process
44. 关节突关节 zygapophysial joint
45. 第2胸椎椎体 body of 2nd thoracic vertebra
46. 脊髓 spinal cord
47. 硬膜外隙 epidural space
48. 右肺上叶 superior lobe of right lung
49. 右头臂静脉 right brachiocephalic vein
50. 胸廓内动脉 internal thoracic artery
51. 胸骨甲状肌 sternothyroid
52. 腋静脉 axillary vein
53. 腋动脉 axillary artery
54. 头静脉 cephalic vein
55. 胸大肌 pectoralis major

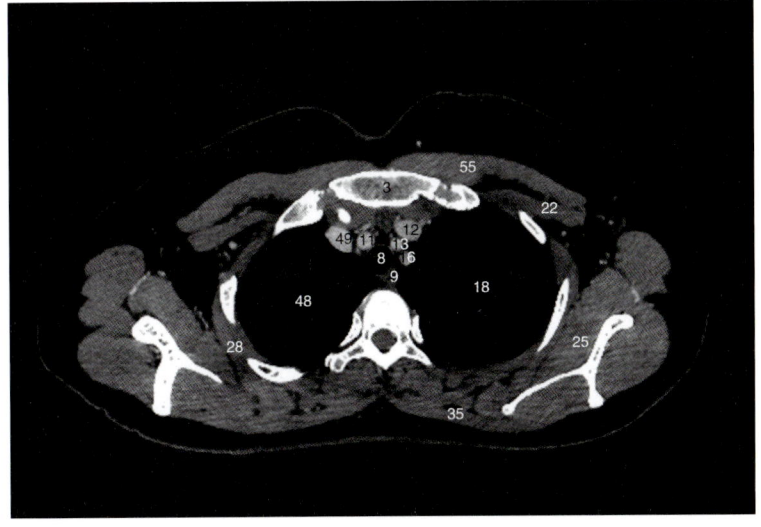

B. CT 纵隔窗增强图像

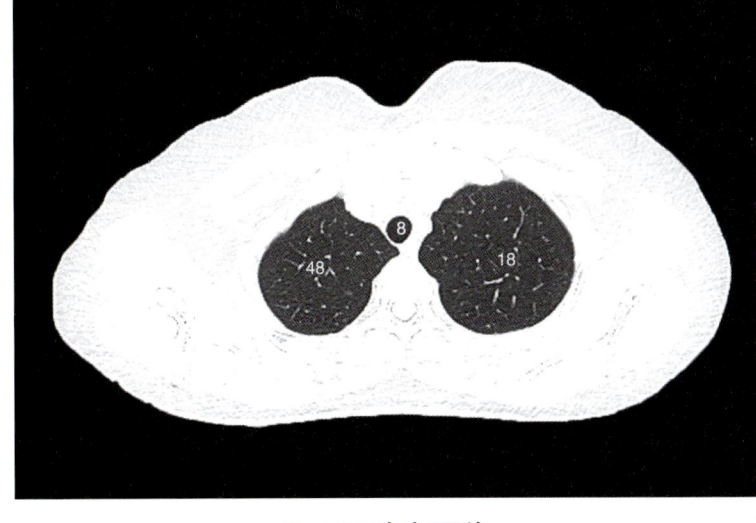

C. CT 肺窗图像

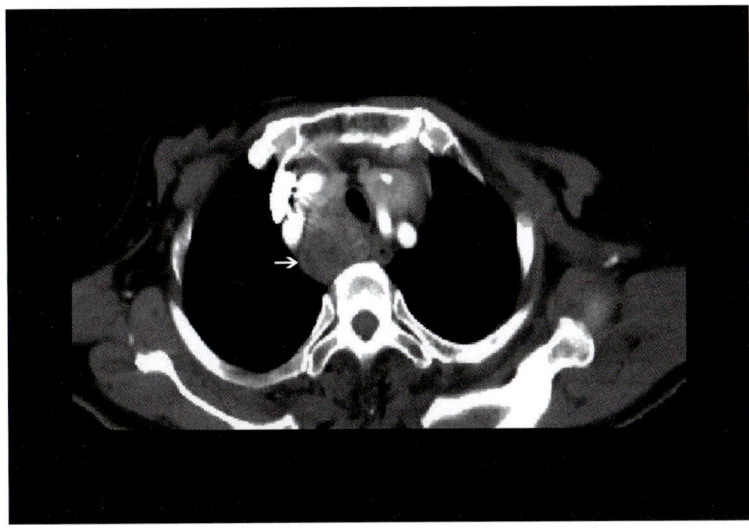

D. 胸骨后甲状腺肿 CT 图像

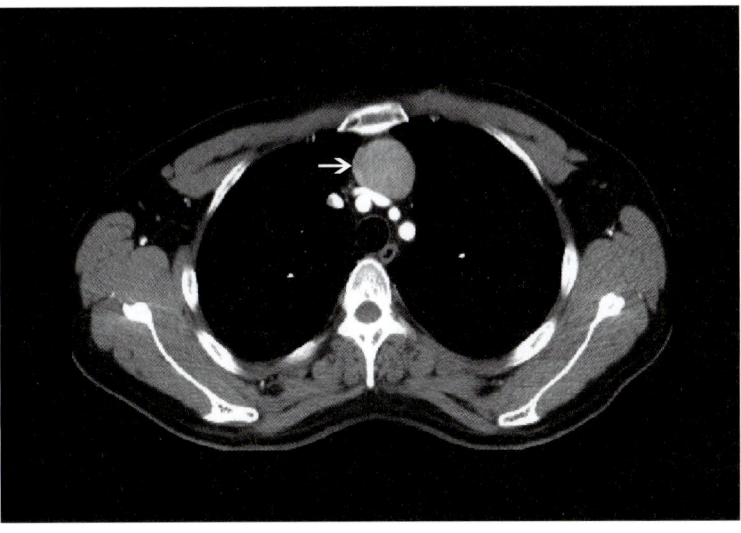

E. 胸腺瘤 CT 图像

关键结构：纵隔胸膜，右上气管旁淋巴结。

此断面经第2胸椎椎体下份。

胸导管位于食管、左锁骨下动脉和左肺之间，紧贴纵隔胸膜，左侧胸膜的病变常累及胸导管。气管的右侧壁与右纵隔胸膜紧贴，而左侧则隔以大动脉。上纵隔内血管的横轴断面较多，易与淋巴结相混淆，增强扫描有助于淋巴结的诊断。2区淋巴结属于N2期淋巴结，常为食管癌、肺癌转移与判断愈后的标志[12]。右上气管旁淋巴结（2R）发育一般较左侧好，平均数目为2~4个，正常平均短横径为3.5~3.7 mm。上纵隔常见变异是胸骨后甲状腺肿，占纵隔肿瘤的5.3%。胸骨后甲状腺肿位于颈前两深筋膜间，两侧受颈前肌限制，因甲状腺自身重力的作用，逐渐下坠，进入胸廓入口，受到胸腔内负压的吸引，使正常或肿大的甲状腺部分或完全坠入胸骨后间隙内，故又可称为坠入性胸腔内甲状腺肿。临床主要表现为肿块压迫周围器官引起的相关症状。如压迫气管引起呼吸困难、喘鸣；压迫上腔静脉引起上胸部及颈部表浅静脉怒张、上肢水肿等上腔静脉综合征；压迫食管引起吞咽困难，症状的轻重与肿块的大小、部位有关。左头臂静脉是区别胸骨后甲状腺肿的要点，其前方是胸腺，后面是异常的甲状腺。

胸部连续横断层 13（FH.13250）

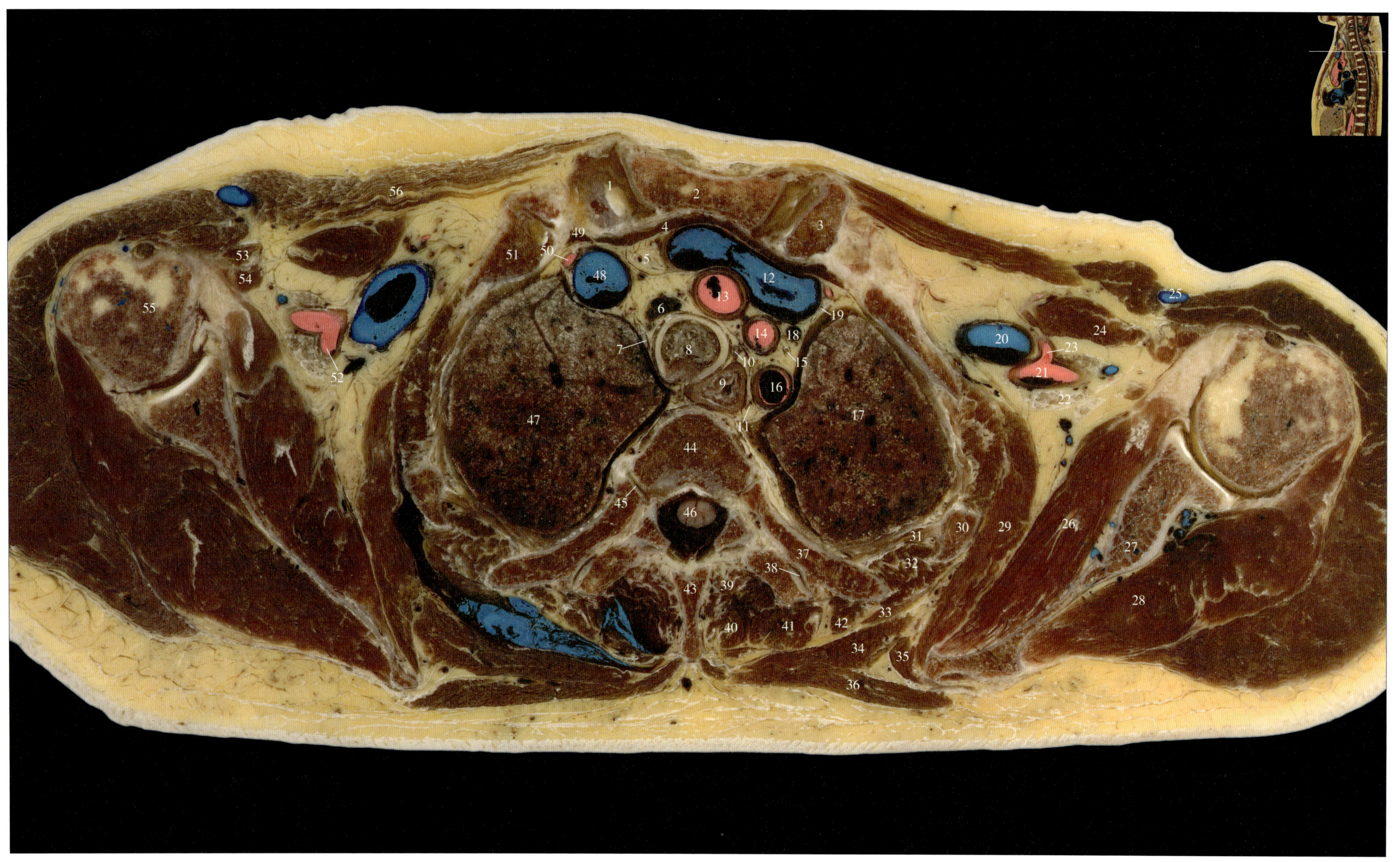

A. 断层标本图像

1. 胸锁关节 sternoclavicular joint
2. 胸骨柄 manubrium sterni
3. 锁骨胸骨端 sternal end of clavicle
4. 胸骨舌骨肌 sternohyoid
5. 胸腺 thymus
6. 右上气管旁淋巴结（2R）right upper paratracheal lymph nodes
7. 右迷走神经 right vagus nerve
8. 气管 trachea
9. 食管 esophagus
10. 左喉返神经 left recurrent laryngeal nerve
11. 胸导管 thoracic duct
12. 左头臂静脉 left brachiocephalic vein
13. 头臂干 brachiocephalic trunk
14. 左颈总动脉 left common carotid artery
15. 左迷走神经 left vagus nerve
16. 左锁骨下动脉 left subclavian artery
17. 左肺上叶 superior lobe of left lung
18. 左上气管旁淋巴结（2L）left upper paratracheal lymph nodes
19. 膈神经 phrenic nerve
20. 腋静脉 axillary vein
21. 腋动脉 axillary artery
22. 臂丛 brachial plexus
23. 胸肩峰动脉 thoracoacromial artery
24. 胸小肌 pectoralis minor
25. 头静脉 cephalic vein
26. 肩胛下肌 subscapularis
27. 肩胛骨 scapula
28. 冈下肌 infraspinatus
29. 前锯肌 serratus anterior
30. 第 2 肋骨 2nd costal bone
31. 肋间最内肌 intercostales intimi
32. 肋间内、外肌 intercostales interni and externi
33. 上后锯肌 serratus posterior superior
34. 菱形肌 rhomboideus
35. 肩胛提肌 levator scapulae
36. 斜方肌 trapezius
37. 第 3 肋骨 3rd costal bone
38. 肋横突关节 costotransverse joint
39. 横突棘肌 transversospinales
40. 棘肌 spinales
41. 最长肌 longissimus
42. 髂肋肌 iliocostalis
43. 棘突 spinous process
44. 第 2 胸椎椎体 body of 2nd thoracic vertebra
45. 肋头关节 joint of costal head
46. 脊髓 spinal cord
47. 右肺上叶 superior lobe of right lung
48. 右头臂静脉 right brachiocephalic vein
49. 胸骨甲状肌 sternothyroid
50. 胸廓内动脉 internal thoracic artery
51. 第 1 肋骨 1st costal bone
52. 肩胛下动脉 subscapular artery
53. 肱二头肌短头 short head of biceps brachii
54. 喙肱肌 coracobrachialis
55. 肱骨 humerus
56. 胸大肌 pectoralis major

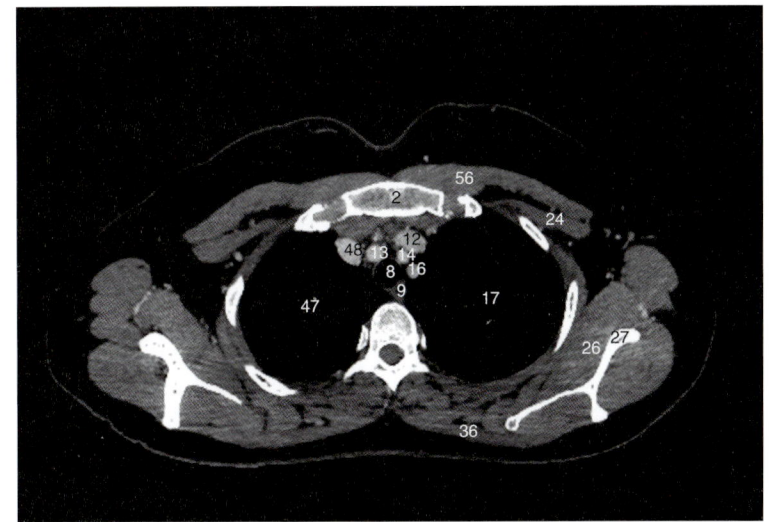

B. CT 纵隔窗增强图像

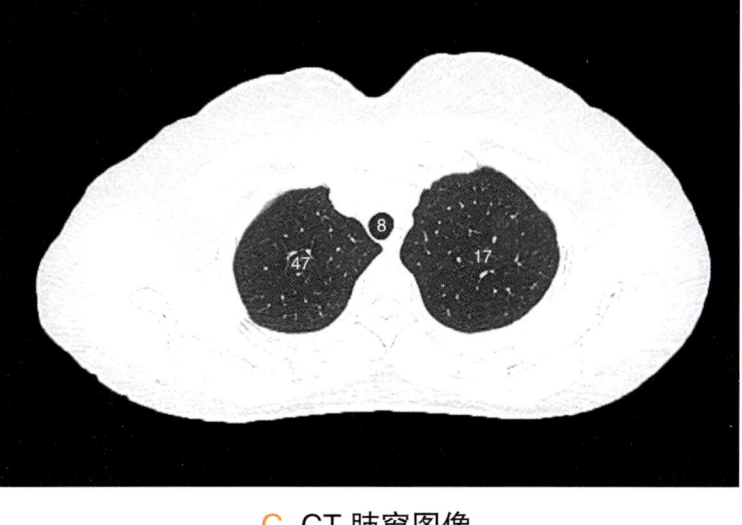

C. CT 肺窗图像

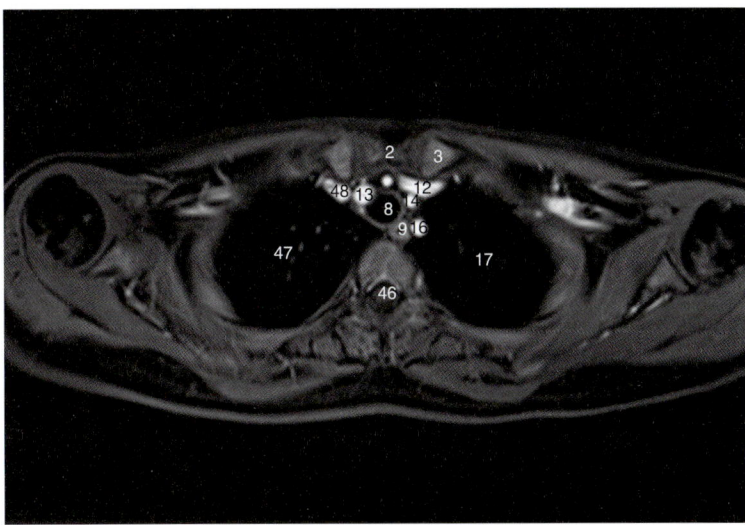

D. MR T1WI 增强图像

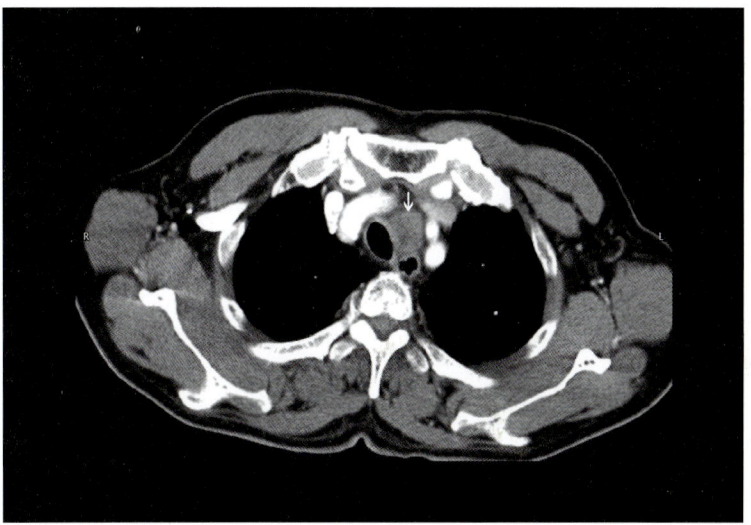

E. 2L 区淋巴结转移 CT 图像

关键结构：臂丛，上气管旁淋巴结。

本面经第 2 胸椎椎体下份。

臂丛是由第 5~8 颈神经前支和第 1 胸神经前支的大部分纤维组成的，经斜角肌间隙走出，行于锁骨下动脉后上方，经锁骨后方进入腋窝。臂丛的分支分布于胸上肢肌，上肢带肌、背浅层肌（斜方肌除外）以及臂、前臂、手的肌、关节、骨和皮肤。组成臂丛的神经根先合成上、中、下三个干，每个干在锁骨上方或后方又分为前、后两股，由上、中干的前股合成外侧束，下干前股自成内侧束，三干后股汇合成后束。三束分别从内、外、后三面包围腋动脉。臂丛在锁骨中点后方比较集中，位置浅表，容易摸到，常作为臂丛阻滞麻醉的部位。根据 IASLC 提出的肺癌淋巴结分区，此断面 2 区左右两组淋巴结均可显示。E 图白色箭头所示为 2L 区增大淋巴结。由于转移性淋巴结在形态、密度等方面与非转移性淋巴结难以区分，只能用大小来界定是否可能为转移性淋巴结。大部分文献倾向于短径 ≥ 10 mm，有些文献倾向于 8 mm 为转移性的淋巴结[13]。现阶段，单靠测量数值的界定尚不能确切反映是否为转移性淋巴结。淋巴结的大小常以短轴直径为标准。动态观察是比较确切地诊断转移性淋巴结的方法。

胸部连续横断层 14（FH.13230）

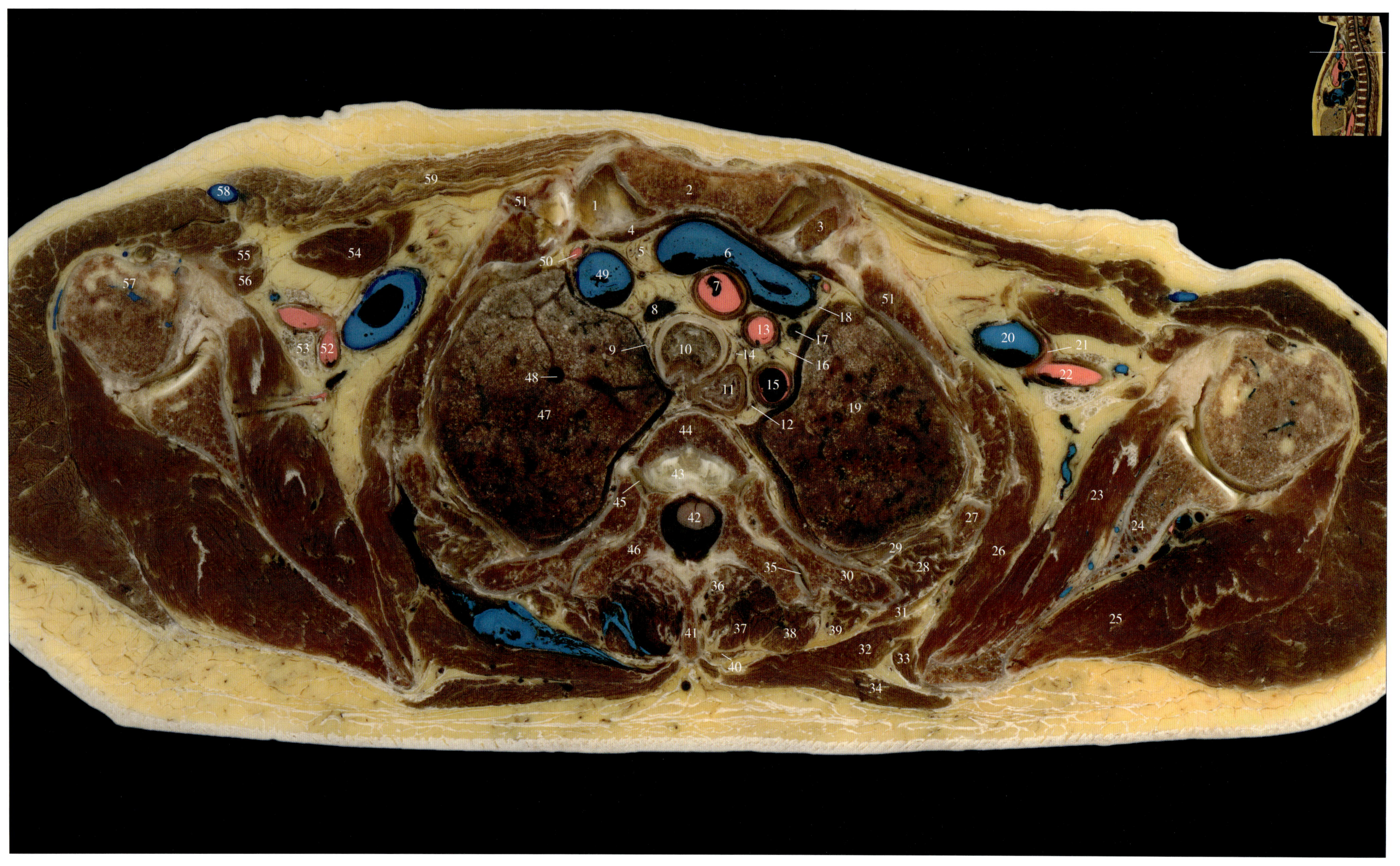

A. 断层标本图像

1. 胸锁关节腔 cavity of sternoclavicular joint
2. 胸骨柄 manubrium sterni
3. 锁骨胸骨端 sternal end of clavicle
4. 胸骨舌骨肌 sternohyoid
5. 胸腺 thymus
6. 左头臂静脉 left brachiocephalic vein
7. 头臂干 brachiocephalic trunk
8. 右上气管旁淋巴结（2R）right upper paratracheal lymph nodes
9. 右迷走神经 right vagus nerve
10. 气管 trachea
11. 食管 esophagus
12. 胸导管 thoracic duct
13. 左颈总动脉 left common carotid artery
14. 左喉返神经 left recurrent laryngeal nerve
15. 左锁骨下动脉 left subclavian artery
16. 左迷走神经 left vagus nerve
17. 左上气管旁淋巴结（2L）left upper paratracheal lymph nodes
18. 膈神经 phrenic nerve
19. 左肺上叶 superior lobe of left lung
20. 腋静脉 axillary vein
21. 胸肩峰动脉 thoracoacromial artery
22. 腋动脉 axillary artery
23. 肩胛下肌 subscapularis
24. 肩胛骨 scapula
25. 冈下肌 infraspinatus
26. 前锯肌 serratus anterior
27. 第2肋骨 2nd costal bone
28. 肋间内、外肌 intercostales interni and externi
29. 肋间最内肌 intercostales intimi
30. 第3肋骨 3rd costal bone
31. 上后锯肌 serratus posterior superior
32. 菱形肌 rhomboideus
33. 肩胛提肌 levator scapulae
34. 斜方肌 trapezius
35. 肋横突关节 costotransverse joint
36. 横突棘肌 transversospinales
37. 棘肌 spinales
38. 最长肌 longissimus
39. 髂肋肌 iliocostalis
40. 颈夹肌 splenius cervicis
41. 棘突 spinous process
42. 脊髓 spinal cord
43. T2-3 椎间盘 T2-3 intervertebral disc
44. 第2胸椎椎体 body of 2nd thoracic vertebra
45. 肋头关节 joint of costal head
46. 横突 transverse process
47. 右肺上叶 superior lobe of right lung
48. 尖段静脉尖支（V1）apical branch of apical segmental vein
49. 右头臂静脉 right brachiocephalic vein
50. 胸廓内动脉 internal thoracic artery
51. 第1肋骨 1st costal bone
52. 肩胛下动脉 subscapular artery
53. 臂丛 brachial plexus
54. 胸小肌 pectoralis minor
55. 肱二头肌短头 short head of biceps brachii
56. 喙肱肌 coracobrachialis
57. 肱骨 humerus
58. 头静脉 cephalic vein
59. 胸大肌 pectoralis major

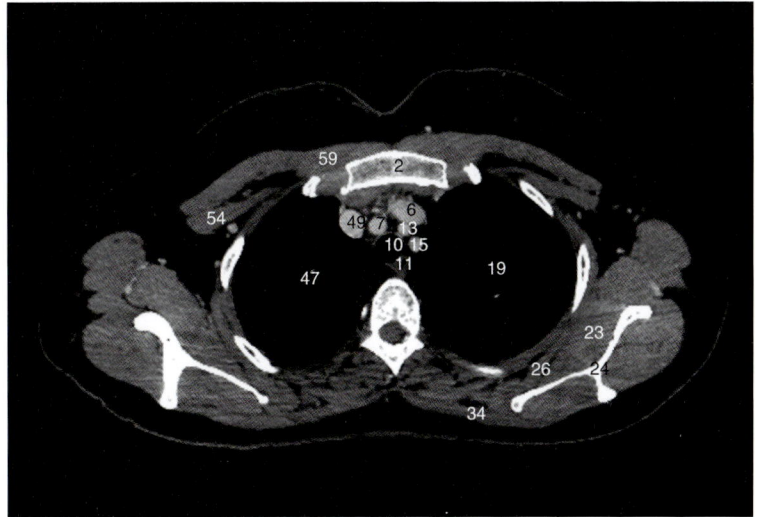

B. CT 纵隔窗增强图像

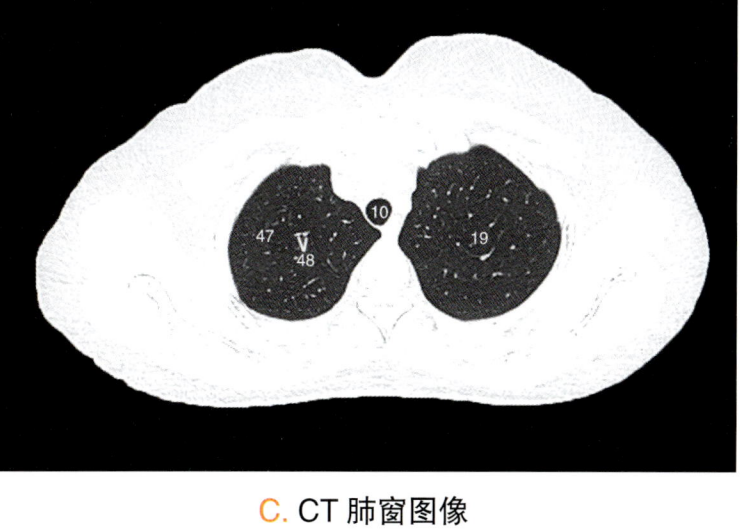

C. CT 肺窗图像

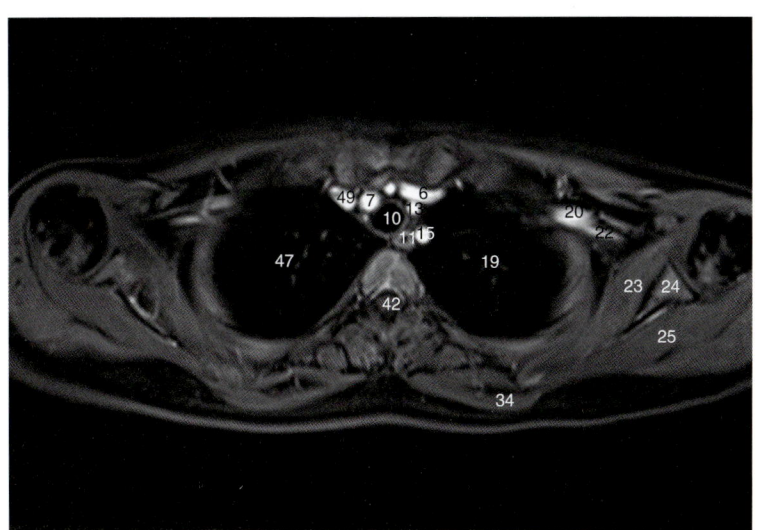

D. MR T1WI 增强图像

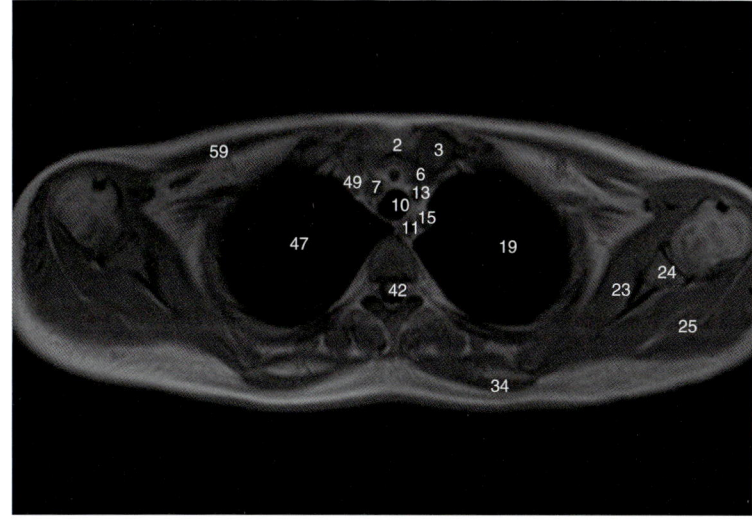

E. MR T1WI 平扫图像

关键结构：胸锁关节，肩胛下动脉，头臂静脉。

此断面经 T2-3 椎间盘上份。

前方由锁骨的胸骨端、胸骨的锁切迹和第1肋软骨的上面共同构成胸锁关节，此关节是上肢骨与躯干骨连结的唯一关节。胸锁关节是人体最稳定的关节之一，脱位并不常见，仅占肩关节脱位总数的 3%[14]。肩胛下动脉是腋动脉最大的分支，以粗大的短干在肩胛下肌下缘附近起自腋动脉第三段，行向内下，沿窝后壁肩胛下肌外侧缘下行，先发出小支至肩胛下肌，继而分为旋肩胛动脉和胸背动脉，供应肩胛下肌、大圆肌、前锯肌和背阔肌。

旋肩胛动脉弯向后，经三边孔绕过肩胛骨外侧缘进入冈下窝，分布于冈下肌、肩胛下肌和大、小圆肌等，并与肩胛上动脉吻合；胸背动脉沿肩胛骨外侧缘下降，主要分支分布于背阔肌。胸骨后左头臂静脉逐步右移，向右头臂静脉靠近。气管前方为头臂干，其由前向后外侧排列依次为左颈总动脉、左锁骨下动脉。气管在不同的平面与不同的结构相毗邻，但后面恒定地与食管相毗邻。正常气管的形态变化较大，多数呈马蹄形或"C"形，慢性阻塞性肺疾病气管常呈军刀鞘样，其横断面上的特点是前后径大于左右径1倍以上。

胸部连续横断层 15（FH.13210）

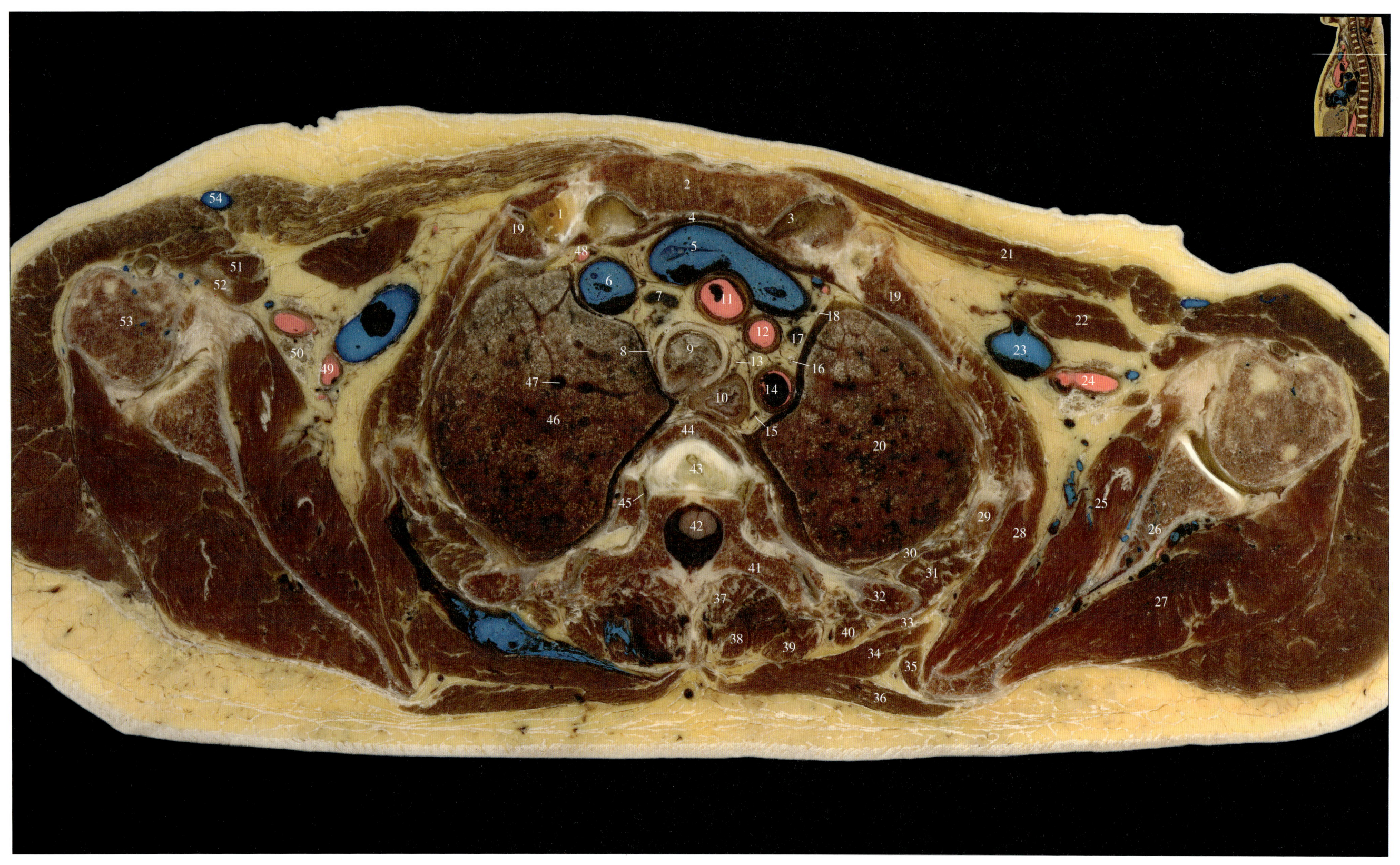

A. 断层标本图像

1. 第1肋软骨 1st costal cartilage
2. 胸骨柄 manubrium sterni
3. 胸锁关节 sternoclavicular joint
4. 胸骨舌骨肌 sternohyoid
5. 左头臂静脉 left brachiocephalic vein
6. 右头臂静脉 right brachiocephalic vein
7. 右上气管旁淋巴结（2R）right upper paratracheal lymph nodes
8. 右迷走神经 right vagus nerve
9. 气管 trachea
10. 食管 esophagus
11. 头臂干 brachiocephalic trunk
12. 左颈总动脉 left common carotid artery
13. 左喉返神经 left recurrent laryngeal nerve
14. 左锁骨下动脉 left subclavian artery
15. 胸导管 thoracic duct
16. 左迷走神经 left vagus nerve
17. 左上气管旁淋巴结（2L）left upper paratracheal lymph nodes
18. 膈神经 phrenic nerve
19. 第1肋骨 1st costal bone
20. 左肺上叶 superior lobe of left lung
21. 胸大肌 pectoralis major
22. 胸小肌 pectoralis minor
23. 腋静脉 axillary vein
24. 腋动脉 axillary artery
25. 肩胛下肌 subscapularis
26. 肩胛骨 scapula
27. 冈下肌 infraspinatus
28. 前锯肌 serratus anterior
29. 第2肋骨 2nd costal bone
30. 肋间最内肌 intercostales intimi
31. 肋间内、外肌 intercostales interni and externi
32. 第3肋骨 3rd costal bone
33. 上后锯肌 serratus posterior superior
34. 菱形肌 rhomboideus
35. 肩胛提肌 levator scapulae
36. 斜方肌 trapezius
37. 横突棘肌 transversospinales
38. 棘肌 spinales
39. 最长肌 longissimus
40. 髂肋肌 iliocostalis
41. 横突 transverse process
42. 脊髓 spinal cord

43. T2-3椎间盘 T2-3 intervertebral disc
44. 第2胸椎椎体 body of 2nd thoracic vertebra
45. 肋头关节 joint of costal head
46. 右肺上叶 superior lobe of right lung
47. 尖段静脉尖支（V1）apical branch of apical segmental vein
48. 胸廓内动脉 internal thoracic artery
49. 肩胛下动脉 subscapular artery
50. 臂丛 brachial plexus
51. 肱二头肌短头 short head of biceps brachii
52. 喙肱肌 coracobrachialis
53. 肱骨 humerus
54. 头静脉 cephalic vein

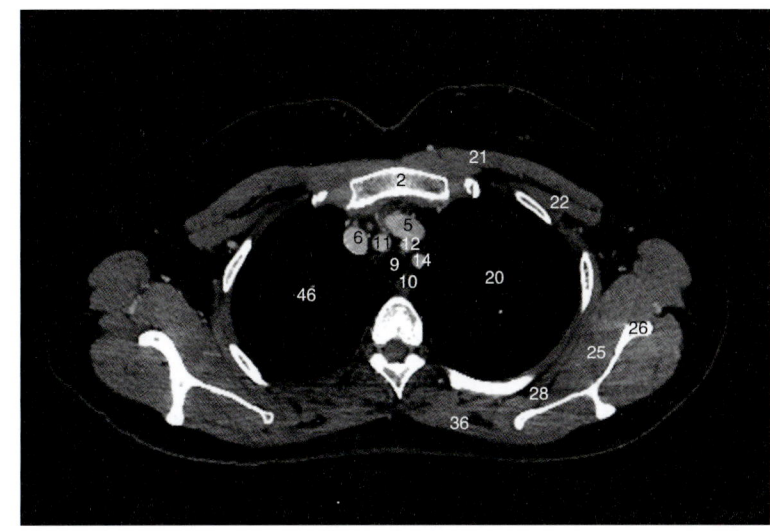

B. CT 纵隔窗增强图像

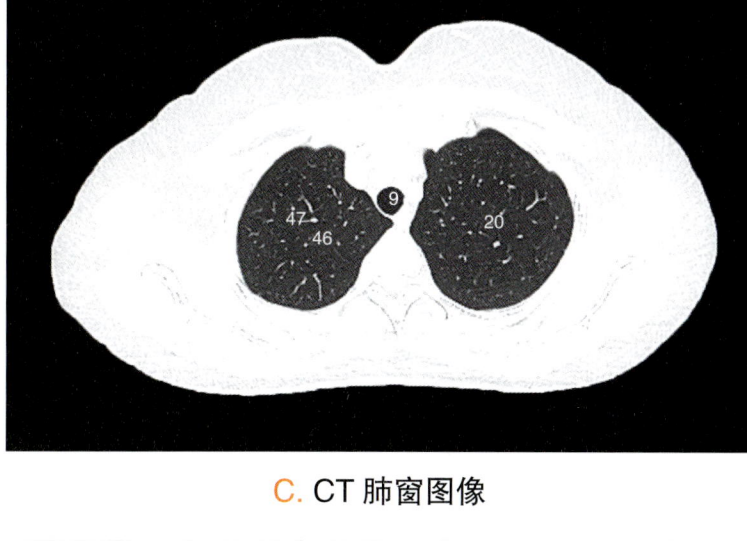

C. CT 肺窗图像

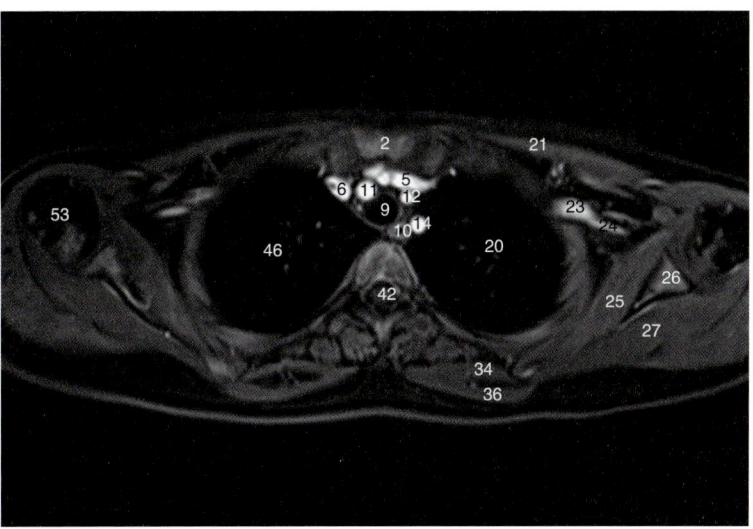

D. MR T1WI 增强图像

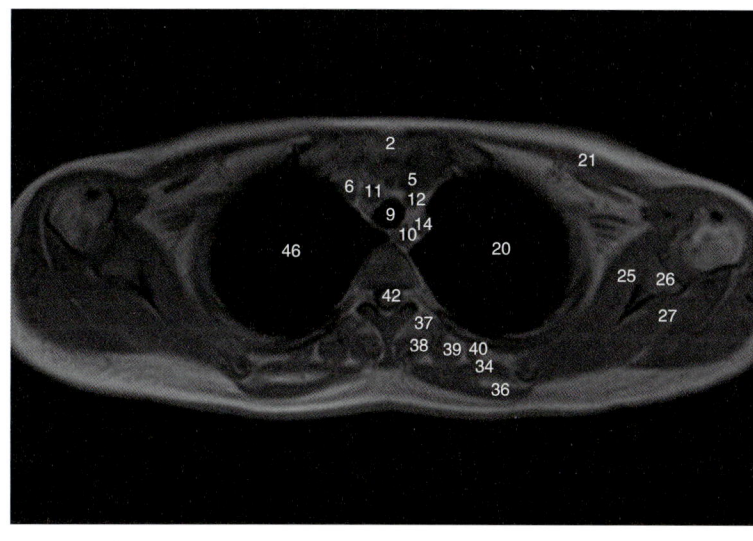

E. MR T1WI 平扫图像

关键结构：胸骨柄，第1胸肋结合，右迷走神经，胸导管。

此断面经T2-3椎间盘中份。

前方经第1肋软骨和胸骨柄，二者之间的连结称为第1胸肋结合，是特殊的不动关节。而第2至第7肋软骨与相应的肋切迹构成的胸肋关节属于微动关节。胸骨柄位于胸骨的上部，外形略呈六角形。胸骨柄和体相连接处，形成一个稍向前突的钝角，称胸骨角。其上缘中部为颈静脉切迹，在成人约平T2-3椎间盘，上缘两侧的卵圆形关节面，称为锁切迹，与锁骨的胸骨端相关节；下缘与胸骨体相连。胸骨柄也常被用于胸骨穿刺的部位。上纵隔内，头臂干位于气管的前方，左颈总动脉位于气管的左侧，前邻左头臂静脉，该静脉逐步右移靠近右头臂静脉，上纵隔结构逐渐失去典型的倒置三角形外观。左锁骨下动脉位于气管的左侧，紧贴左纵隔胸膜。右迷走神经离开右头臂静脉的深面逐渐至气管的右侧，左迷走神经和左喉返神经位置不变。胸导管位于食管、左锁骨下动脉和左肺之间，紧贴纵隔胸膜，左侧胸膜的病变常累及胸导管。胸导管在此或相近断面损伤常可引起左侧乳糜胸。

胸部连续横断层 16（FH.13190）

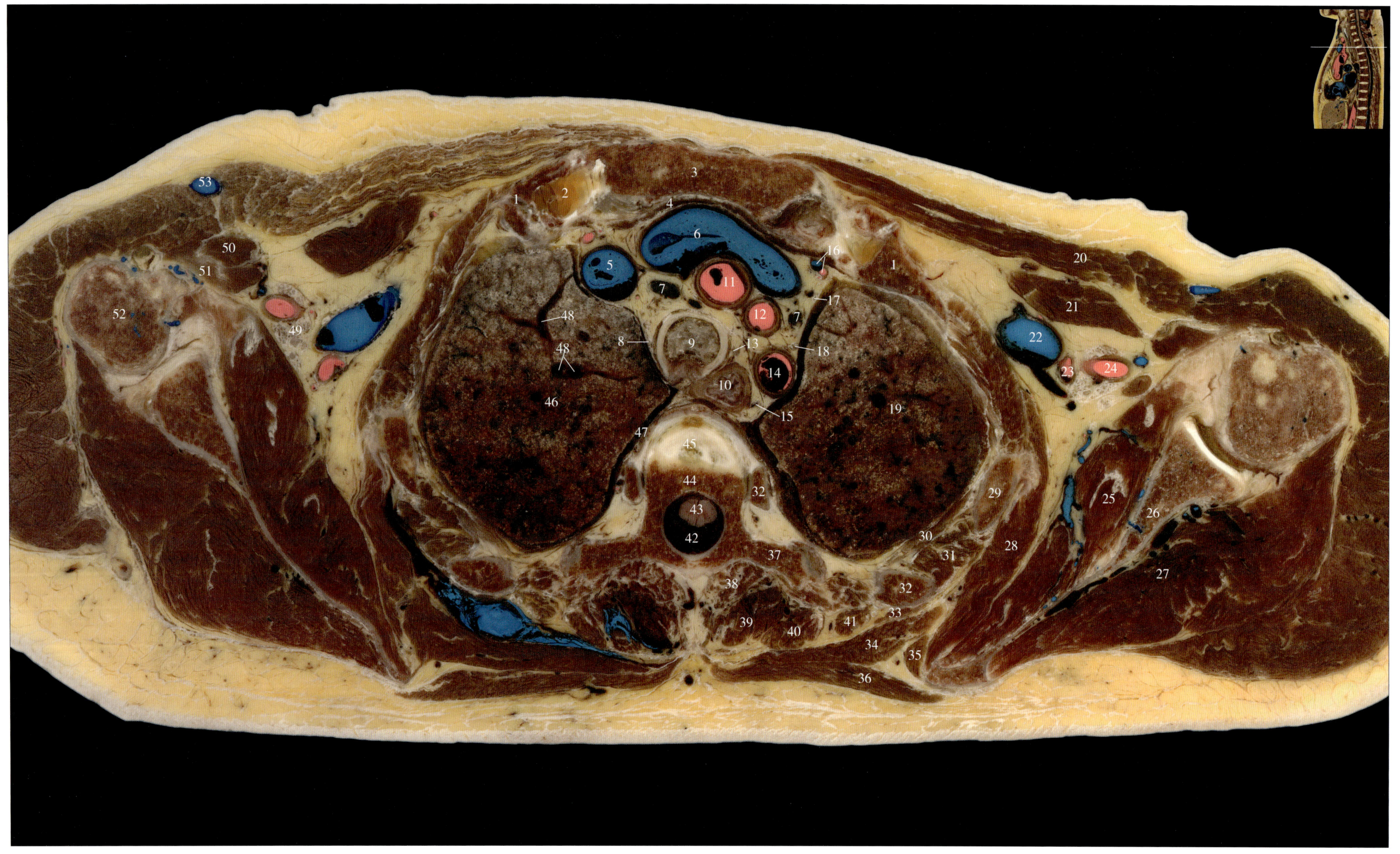

A. 断层标本图像

1. 第1肋骨 1st costal bone
2. 第1肋软骨 1st costal cartilage
3. 胸骨柄 manubrium sterni
4. 胸骨舌骨肌 sternohyoid
5. 右头臂静脉 right brachiocephalic vein
6. 左头臂静脉 left brachiocephalic vein
7. 上气管旁淋巴结（2区）upper paratracheal lymph nodes
8. 右迷走神经 right vagus nerve
9. 气管 trachea
10. 食管 esophagus
11. 头臂干 brachiocephalic trunk
12. 左颈总动脉 left common carotid artery
13. 左喉返神经 left recurrent laryngeal nerve
14. 左锁骨下动脉 left subclavian artery
15. 胸导管 thoracic duct
16. 胸廓内动、静脉 internal thoracic artery and vein
17. 膈神经 phrenic nerve
18. 左迷走神经 left vagus nerve
19. 左肺上叶 superior lobe of left lung
20. 胸大肌 pectoralis major
21. 胸小肌 pectoralis minor
22. 腋静脉 axillary vein
23. 肩胛下动脉 subscapular artery
24. 腋动脉 axillary artery
25. 肩胛下肌 subscapularis
26. 肩胛骨 scapula
27. 冈下肌 infraspinatus
28. 前锯肌 serratus anterior
29. 第2肋骨 2nd costal bone
30. 肋间最内肌 intercostales intimi
31. 肋间内、外肌 intercostales interni and externi
32. 第3肋骨 3rd costal bone
33. 上后锯肌 serratus posterior superior
34. 菱形肌 rhomboideus
35. 肩胛提肌 levator scapulae
36. 斜方肌 trapezius
37. 横突 transverse process
38. 横突棘肌 transversospinales
39. 棘肌 spinales
40. 最长肌 longissimus
41. 髂肋肌 iliocostalis
42. 硬膜外隙 epidural space
43. 脊髓 spinal cord

44. 第3胸椎椎体 body of 3rd thoracic vertebra
45. T3-4椎间盘 T3-4 intervertebral disc
46. 右肺上叶 superior lobe of right lung
47. 胸膜腔 pleural cavity
48. 尖段静脉尖支（V1）apical branch of apical segmental vein
49. 臂丛 brachial plexus
50. 肱二头肌短头 short head of biceps brachii
51. 喙肱肌 coracobrachialis
52. 肱骨 humerus
53. 头静脉 cephalic vein

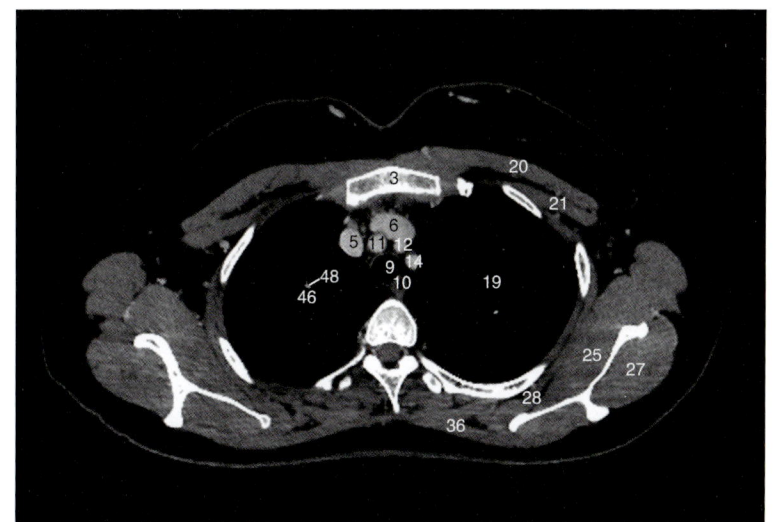

B. CT 纵隔窗增强图像

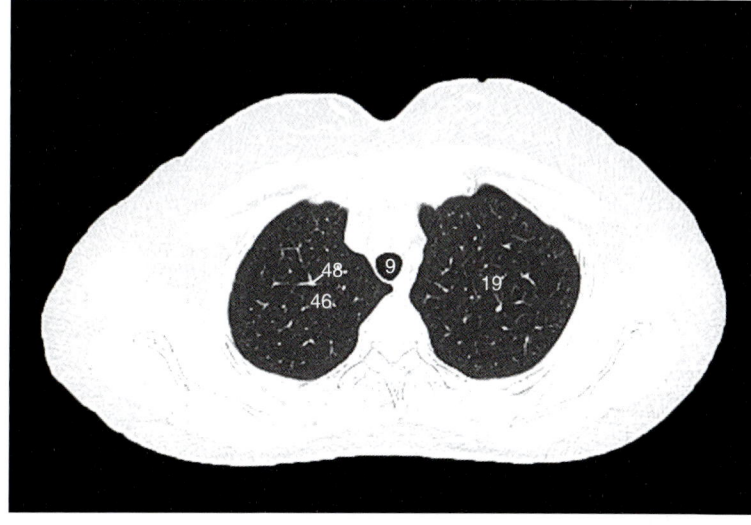

C. CT 肺窗图像

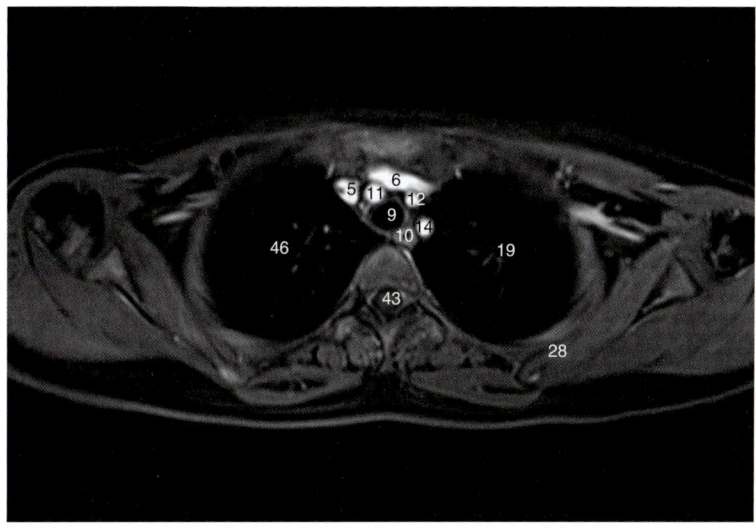

D. MR T1WI 增强图像

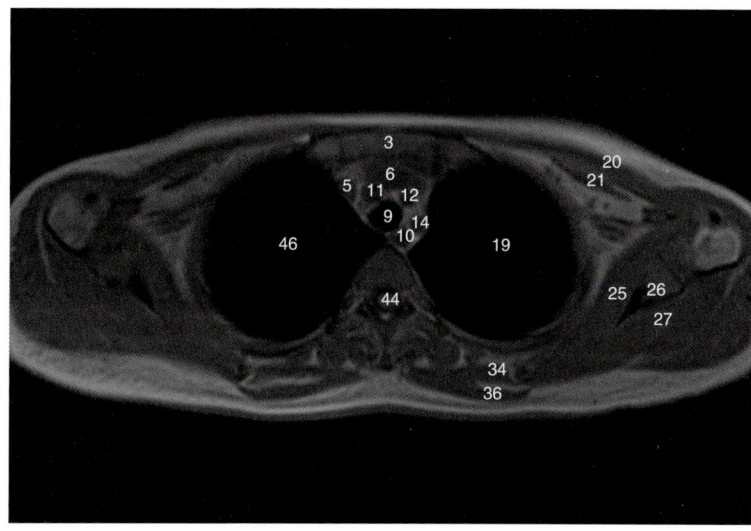

E. MR T1WI 平扫图像

关键结构：前锯肌。

断面后方经过第3胸椎椎体上份。

前锯肌为胸上肢肌之一，贴附在胸廓侧壁表面，以肌齿起自第1~9肋骨，止于肩胛骨的脊柱缘。各个肌束呈多指状排列，根据肌束走行及所附着的肋骨位置，可以把前锯肌分为上、中、下三个部分。上部起自第1~2肋和肋间，由1~2个肌齿构成；中部起自第3~5肋，由2~3个肌齿构成；上部和中部肌束近于横行走向后内方，止于肩胛骨内侧缘；下部起自第6~9肋或第10肋，由4~5个肌齿构成，止于肩胛下角。从上至下肌束逐渐变大变长，下部肌束相对较厚。支配前锯肌的神经来自胸长神经，胸长神经从前锯肌的上端入肌，入肌后沿肌前面中间向肌下部走行，肌内神经整体呈树枝样分布。胸长神经在前锯肌上部和中部分别发出4~6和7~9支分支，在下部发出分支较少，仅2~3支。当支配前锯肌的胸长神经损伤时，出现肩胛骨脊柱缘和下角向后外翘起，形成"翼状肩胛"。前锯肌平面阻滞是一种新的区域阻滞技术，能阻滞肋间神经外侧皮支，提供良好的前外侧胸壁镇痛效果。前锯肌平面阻滞已用于开胸术后镇痛和肋骨骨折的疼痛治疗[15]。

胸部连续横断层 17（FH.13170）

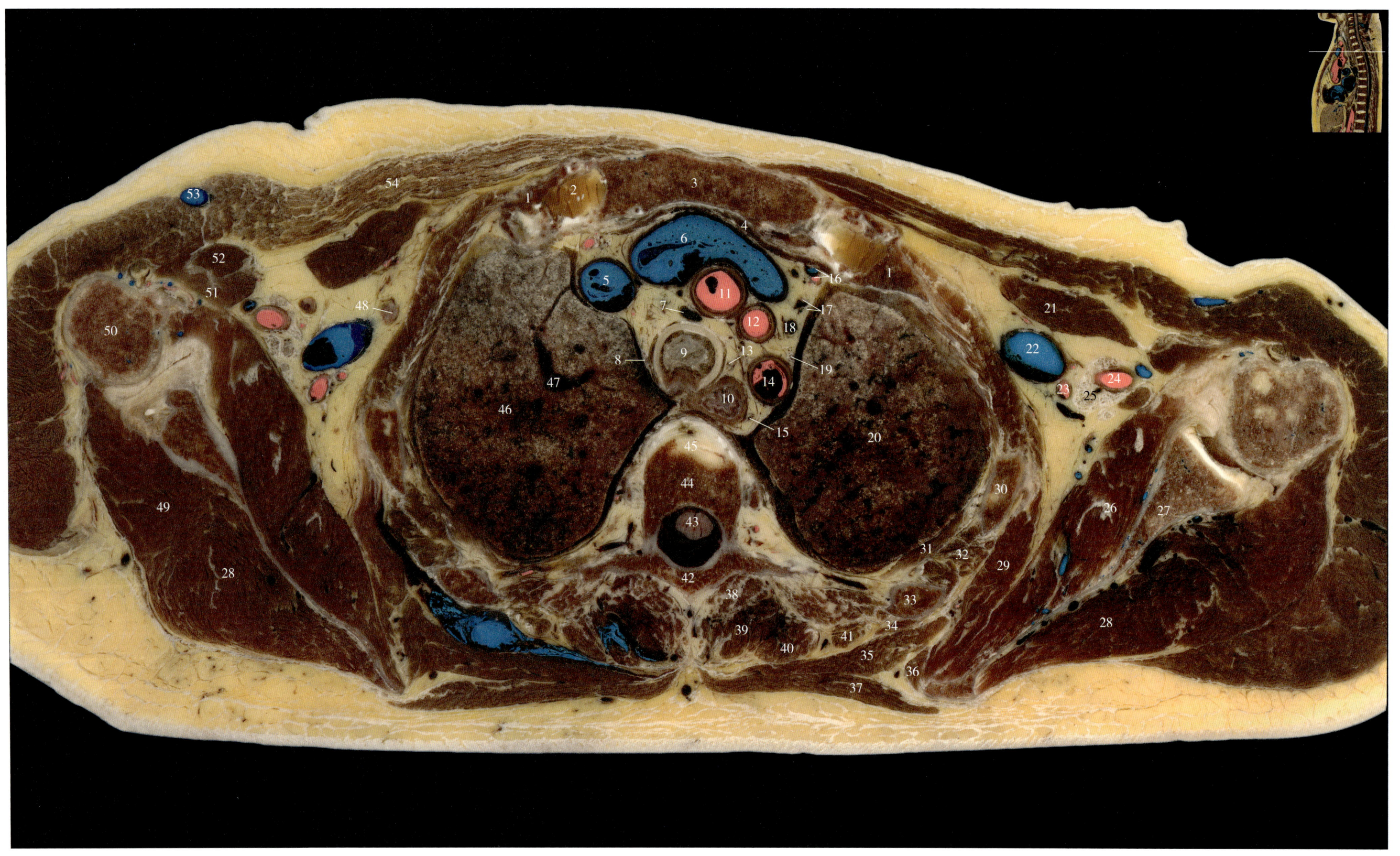

A. 断层标本图像

1. 第1肋骨 1st costal bone
2. 第1肋软骨 1st costal cartilage
3. 胸骨柄 manubrium sterni
4. 胸骨舌骨肌 sternohyoid
5. 右头臂静脉 right brachiocephalic vein
6. 左头臂静脉 left brachiocephalic vein
7. 右上气管旁淋巴结（2R）right upper paratracheal lymph nodes
8. 右迷走神经 right vagus nerve
9. 气管 trachea
10. 食管 esophagus
11. 头臂干 brachiocephalic trunk
12. 左颈总动脉 left common carotid artery
13. 左喉返神经 left recurrent laryngeal nerve
14. 左锁骨下动脉 left subclavian artery
15. 胸导管 thoracic duct
16. 胸廓内动、静脉 internal thoracic artery and vein
17. 膈神经和心包膈血管 phrenic nerve and pericardiacophrenic vessels
18. 左上气管旁淋巴结（2L）left upper paratracheal lymph nodes
19. 左迷走神经 left vagus nerve
20. 左肺上叶 superior lobe of left lung
21. 胸小肌 pectoralis minor
22. 腋静脉 axillary vein
23. 肩胛下动脉 subscapular artery
24. 腋动脉 axillary artery
25. 臂丛 brachial plexus
26. 肩胛下肌 subscapularis
27. 肩胛骨 scapula
28. 冈下肌 infraspinatus
29. 前锯肌 serratus anterior
30. 第2肋骨 2nd costal bone
30. 肋间最内肌 intercostales intimi
31. 肋间内、外肌 intercostales interni and externi
33. 第3肋骨 3rd costal bone
34. 上后锯肌 serratus posterior superior
35. 菱形肌 rhomboideus
36. 肩胛提肌 levator scapulae
37. 斜方肌 trapezius
38. 横突棘肌 transversospinales
39. 棘肌 spinales
40. 最长肌 longissimus
41. 髂肋肌 iliocostalis

42. 椎弓板 lamina of vertebral arch
43. 脊髓 spinal cord
44. 第3胸椎椎体 body of 3rd thoracic vertebra
45. T2-3椎间盘 T2-3 intervertebral disc
46. 右肺上叶 superior lobe of right lung
47. 尖段静脉尖支（V1）apical branch of apical segmental vein
48. 腋淋巴结 axillary lymph nodes
49. 小圆肌 teres minor
50. 肱骨 humerus
51. 喙肱肌 coracobrachialis
52. 肱二头肌短头 short head of biceps brachii
53. 头静脉 cephalic vein
54. 胸大肌 pectoralis major

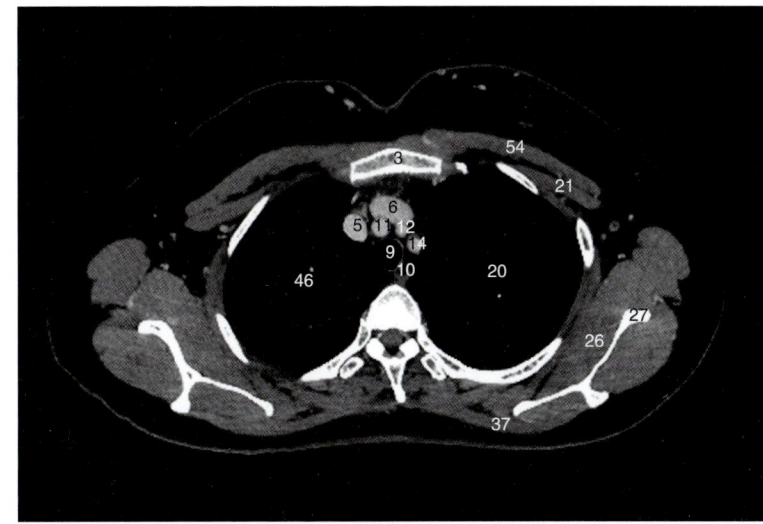

B. CT 纵隔窗增强图像

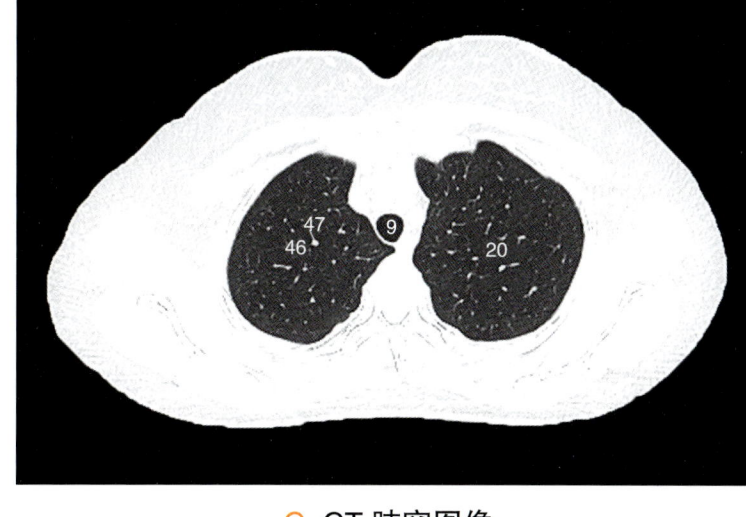

C. CT 肺窗图像

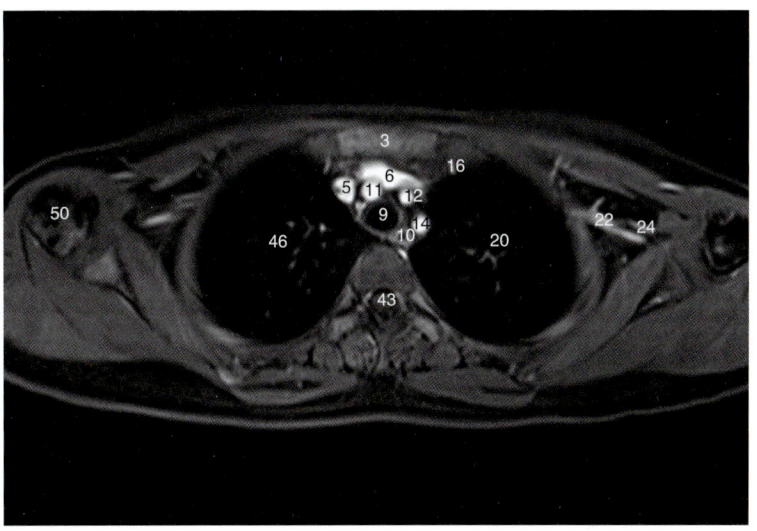

D. MR T1WI 增强图像

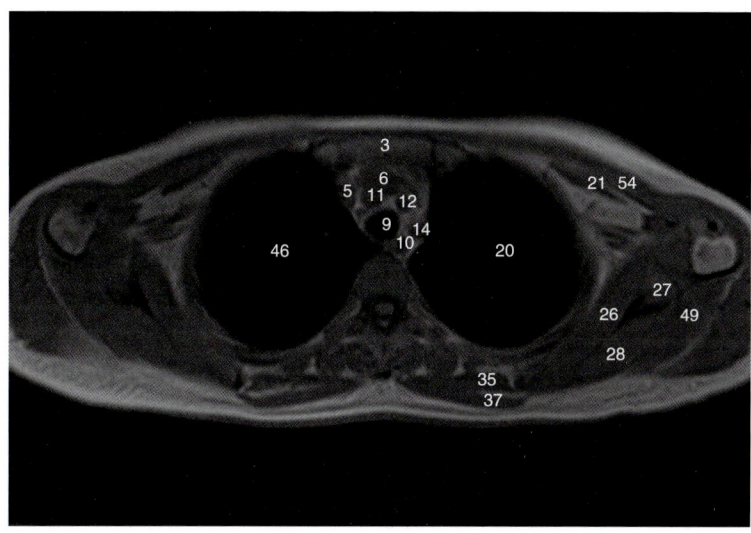

E. MR T1WI 平扫图像

关键结构：头臂静脉，气管前间隙。

此断面经第3胸椎椎体上份。

在第1胸肋关节的后方可见左头臂静脉进一步右移，其沿途的静脉属支有椎静脉、胸廓内静脉、肋间最上静脉和甲状腺下静脉等。在此断面中，头臂干、左颈总动脉和左锁骨下动脉三者的位置也更为靠近。IASLC 肺癌淋巴结分区中3区包含3a区与3p区，分别位于血管前方（前纵隔/血管前间隙）与气管后方（后纵隔）。在甲状腺癌中央区淋巴结清扫的过程中，有学者主张将3a区的淋巴结定为手术的清扫范围[16]。气管前间隙是由于颈段气管下段走行偏背侧，与带状肌及其附着韧带分离所形成的间隙，也是通向纵隔的潜在通道。舌骨下肌筋膜为其前壁，气管筋膜为后壁，上界为甲状软骨，下界为主动脉弓上缘。头臂静脉、甲状腺下静脉及淋巴结为该间隙的主要内容，该间隙主要由疏松脂肪结缔组织填充，成为气管切开和纵隔镜检查的标准通道[17]。正常情况下，分别来源于第三、四鳃囊的甲状腺、甲状旁腺和胸腺随胚胎发育而向下移位，最终分别定位于颈部和上纵隔，但甲状腺胚胎组织和甲状旁腺可部分随胸腺过度下降，并因其程度不同而最终定位于气管前间隙或上纵隔。与之相反，胸腺胚胎可以因下降不充分而在甲状腺区域或气管前遗有残迹。上述先天性异位之甲状腺、甲状旁腺或胸腺可以产生与正常部位相应器官病理类型和生物学特性完全相同的病变，如增生、腺瘤或恶性肿瘤等。

胸部连续横断层 18（FH.13150）

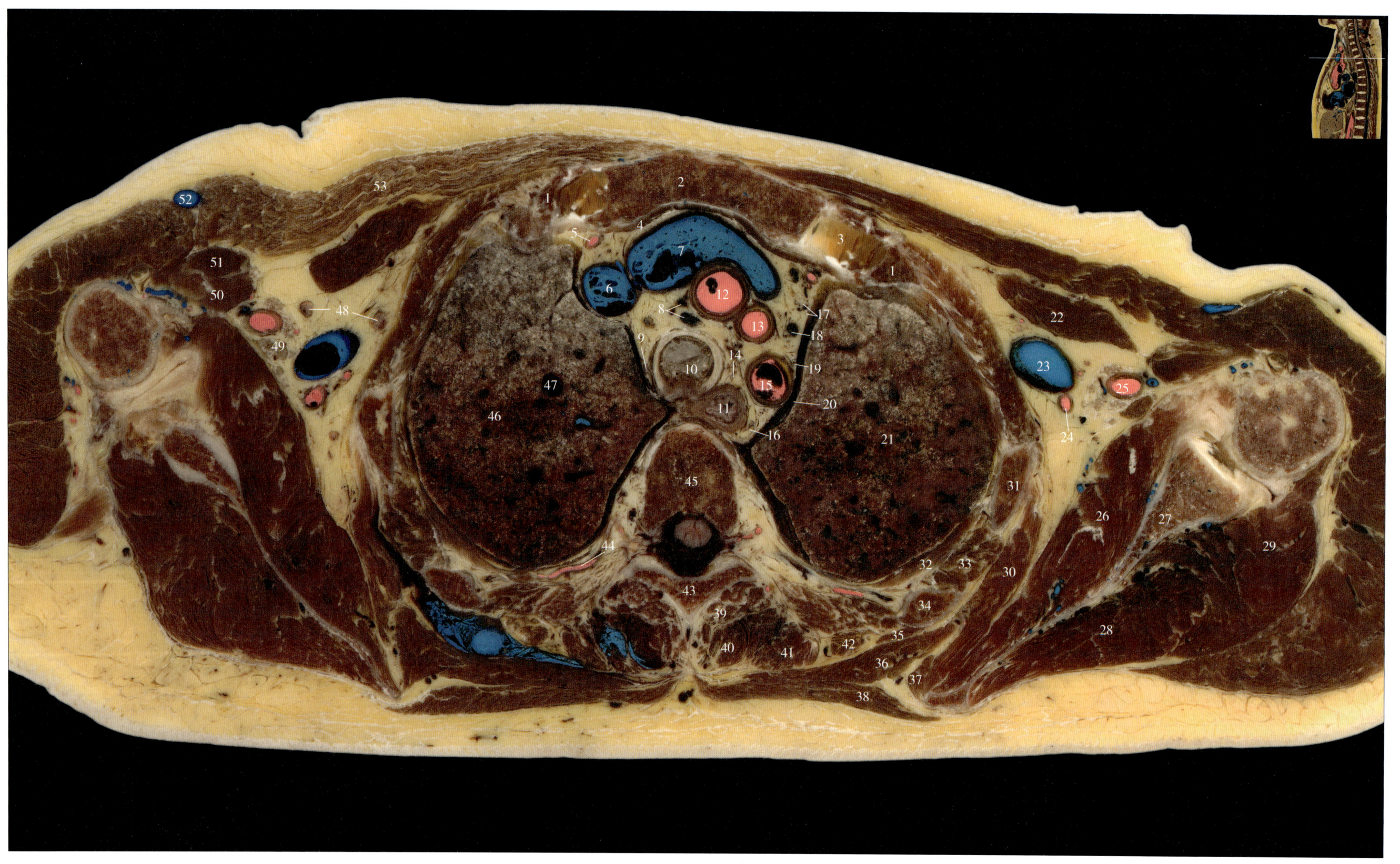

A. 断层标本图像

1. 第 1 肋骨 1st costal bone
2. 胸骨柄 manubrium sterni
3. 第 1 肋软骨 1st costal cartilage
4. 胸骨舌骨肌 sternohyoid
5. 胸廓内动脉 internal thoracic artery
6. 右头臂静脉 right brachiocephalic vein
7. 左头臂静脉 left brachiocephalic vein
8. 右上气管旁淋巴结（2R）right upper paratracheal lymph nodes
9. 右迷走神经 right vagus nerve
10. 气管 trachea
11. 食管 esophagus
12. 头臂干 brachiocephalic trunk
13. 左颈总动脉 left common carotid artery
14. 左喉返神经 left recurrent laryngeal nerve
15. 左锁骨下动脉 left subclavian artery
16. 胸导管 thoracic duct
17. 膈神经和心包膈血管 phrenic nerve and pericardiacophrenic vessels
18. 左上气管旁淋巴结（2L）left upper paratracheal lymph nodes
19. 左迷走神经 left vagus nerve
20. 胸膜腔 pleural cavity
21. 左肺上叶 superior lobe of left lung
22. 胸小肌 pectoralis minor
23. 腋静脉 axillary vein
24. 肩胛下动脉 subscapular artery
25. 腋动脉 axillary artery
26. 肩胛下肌 subscapularis
27. 肩胛骨 scapula
28. 冈下肌 infraspinatus
29. 小圆肌 teres minor
30. 前锯肌 serratus anterior
31. 第 2 肋骨 2nd costal bone
32. 肋间最内肌 intercostales intimi
33. 肋间内、外肌 intercostales interni and externi
34. 第 3 肋骨 3rd costal bone
35. 上后锯肌 serratus posterior superior
36. 菱形肌 rhomboideus
37. 肩胛提肌 levator scapulae
38. 斜方肌 trapezius
39. 横突棘肌 transversospinales
40. 棘肌 spinales
41. 最长肌 longissimus
42. 髂肋肌 iliocostalis
43. 椎弓板 lamina of vertebral arch
44. 肋间后动脉 posterior intercostal artery
45. 第 3 胸椎椎体 body of 3rd thoracic vertebra
46. 右肺上叶 superior lobe of right lung
47. 尖段静脉尖支（V1）apical branch of apical segmental vein
48. 腋淋巴结 axillary lymph nodes
49. 臂丛 brachial plexus
50. 喙肱肌 coracobrachialis
51. 肱二头肌短头 short head of biceps brachii
52. 头静脉 cephalic vein
53. 胸大肌 pectoralis major

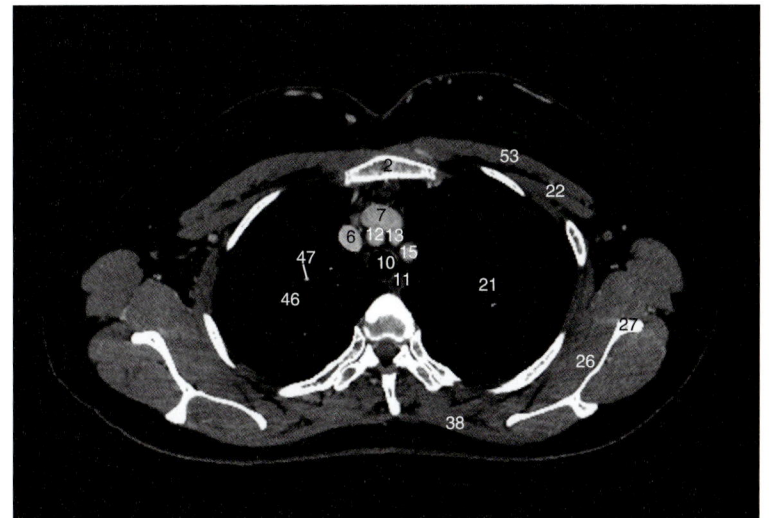

B. CT 纵隔窗增强图像

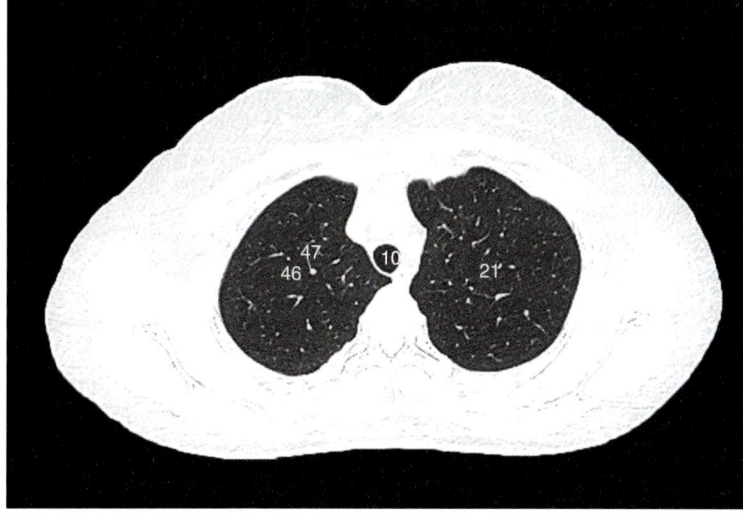

C. CT 肺窗图像

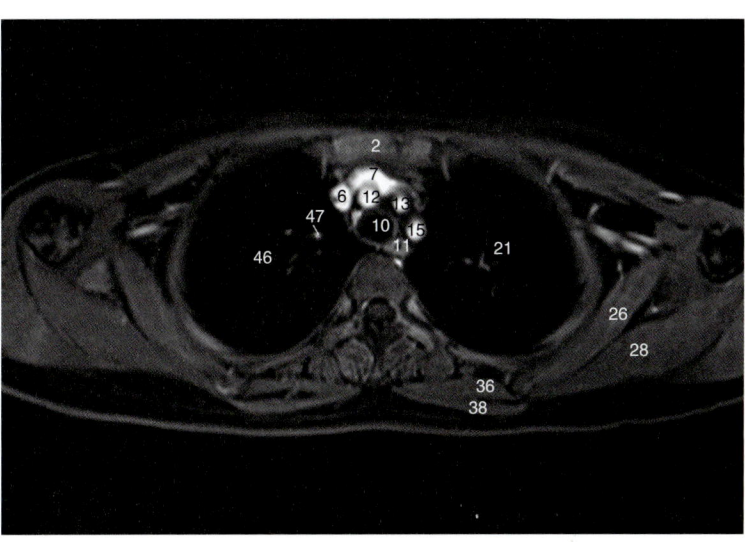

D. MR T1WI 增强图像

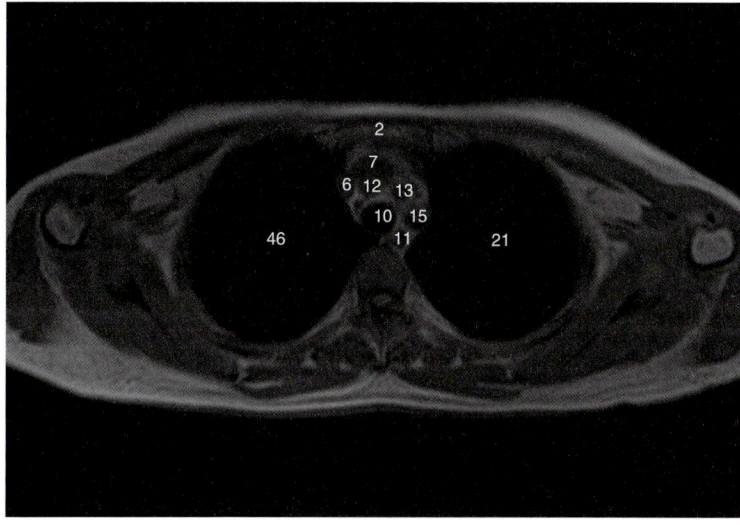

E. MR T1WI 平扫图像

关键结构：头臂静脉，主动脉弓 3 大分支。

此断面经第 3 胸椎椎体上份。

胸骨后左头臂静脉接近右头臂静脉，将要汇合成上腔静脉。上纵隔管道结构排列的特点是：气管居中，左侧是主动脉弓上发出的 3 大分支，由右向左依次为头臂干、左颈总动脉和左锁骨下动脉。从前向后，纵隔右侧面是右头臂静脉、气管、食管；纵隔左侧面是左头臂静脉及主动脉弓发出的 3 大分支。主动脉弓及其分支变异的不同种类可达 30 余种，分支则可有 1~6 支。目前，Williams 分型法将主动脉弓及主要分支的变异情况分为 A~H 8 种类型。临床及解剖上以 A、B、C 3 种分型最为常见，其他为少见的分型。A 型，即正常型，为最常见类型，即自主动脉弓凸面从右向左依次发出头臂干、左侧颈总动脉、左侧锁骨下动脉 3 大分支血管；B 型，共有 2 支分支血管从主动脉弓上发出，1 支为头臂干与左颈总动脉共干，另 1 支则为左锁骨下动脉；C 型，共有 4 支分支血管从主动脉弓上发出，从右向左依次为头臂干、左侧颈总动脉、左侧椎动脉及左侧锁骨下动脉。其中，A 型约占 84.3%，B 型约占 8.4%，C 型约占 3.5%，其他少见的类型（如混合变异型、右位主动脉弓型等）约占 3.8%。

胸部连续横断层 19（FH.13130）

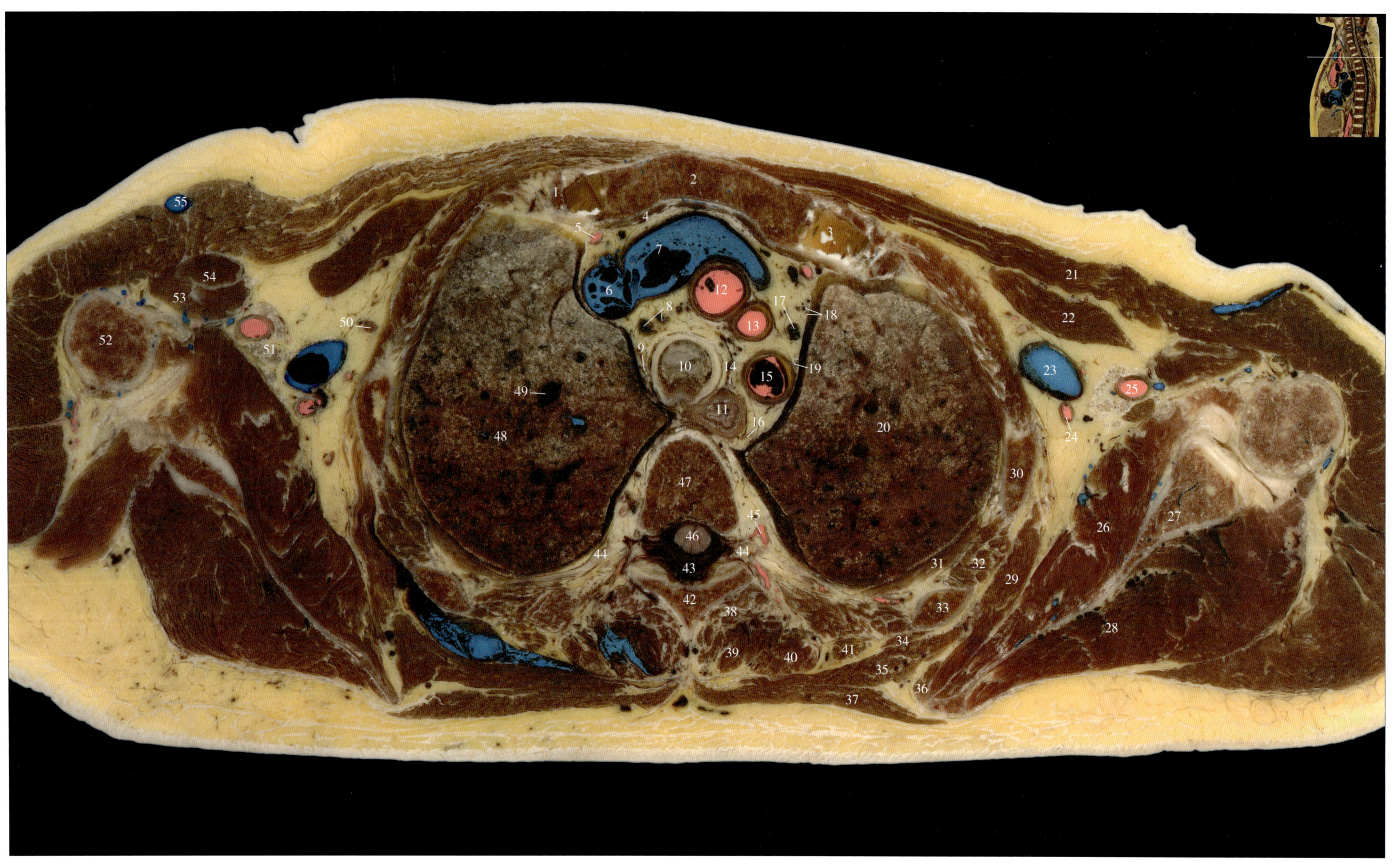

A. 断层标本图像

1. 第 1 肋骨 1st costal bone
2. 胸骨柄 manubrium sterni
3. 第 1 肋软骨 1st costal cartilage
4. 胸骨舌骨肌 sternohyoid
5. 胸廓内动脉 internal thoracic artery
6. 右头臂静脉 right brachiocephalic vein
7. 左头臂静脉 left brachiocephalic vein
8. 右下气管旁淋巴结（4R）right lower paratracheal lymph nodes
9. 右迷走神经 right vagus nerve
10. 气管 trachea
11. 食管 esophagus
12. 头臂干 brachiocephalic trunk
13. 左颈总动脉 left common carotid artery
14. 左喉返神经 left recurrent laryngeal nerve
15. 左锁骨下动脉 left subclavian artery
16. 胸导管 thoracic duct
17. 左上气管旁淋巴结（2L）left upper paratracheal lymph nodes
18. 膈神经和心包膈血管 phrenic nerve and pericardiacophrenic vessels
19. 左迷走神经 left vagus nerve
20. 左肺上叶 superior lobe of left lung
21. 胸大肌 pectoralis major
22. 胸小肌 pectoralis minor
23. 腋静脉 axillary vein
24. 肩胛下动脉 subscapular artery
25. 腋动脉 axillary artery
26. 肩胛下肌 subscapularis
27. 肩胛骨 scapula
28. 冈下肌 infraspinatus
29. 前锯肌 serratus anterior
30. 第 2 肋骨 2nd costal bone
31. 肋间最内肌 intercostales intimi
32. 肋间内、外肌 intercostales interni and externi
33. 第 3 肋骨 3rd costal bone
34. 上后锯肌 serratus posterior superior
35. 菱形肌 rhomboideus
36. 肩胛提肌 levator scapulae
37. 斜方肌 trapezius
38. 横突棘肌 transversospinales
39. 棘肌 spinales
40. 最长肌 longissimus
41. 髂肋肌 iliocostalis
42. 椎弓板 lamina of vertebral arch
43. 硬膜外隙 epidural space
44. 第 3 胸神经 3rd thoracic nerve
45. 肋间后动脉 posterior intercostal artery
46. 脊髓 spinal cord
47. 第 3 胸椎椎体 body of 3rd thoracic vertebra
48. 右肺上叶 superior lobe of right lung
49. 尖段静脉尖支（V1）apical branch of apical segmental vein
50. 腋淋巴结 axillary lymph nodes
51. 臂丛 brachial plexus
52. 肱骨 humerus
53. 喙肱肌 coracobrachialis
54. 肱二头肌短头 short head of biceps brachii
55. 头静脉 cephalic vein

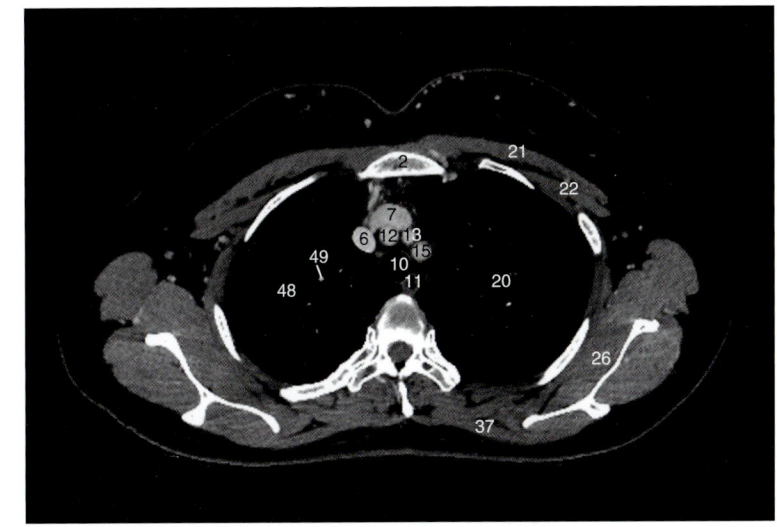

B. CT 纵隔窗增强图像

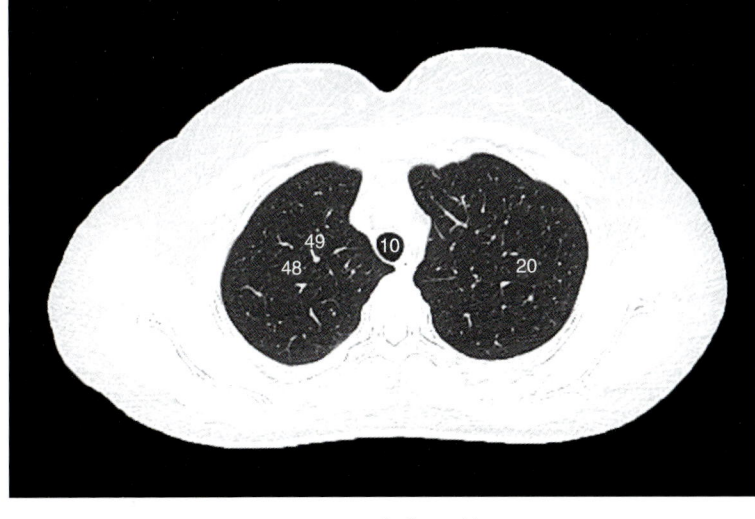

C. CT 肺窗图像

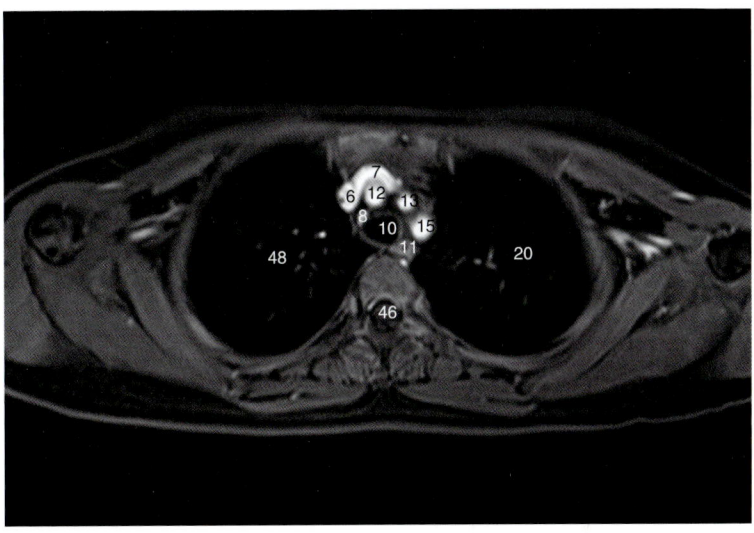

D. MR T1WI 增强图像

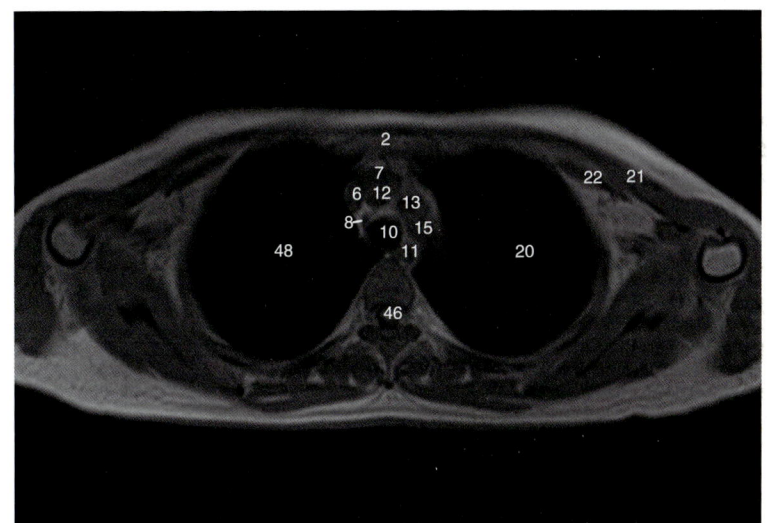

E. MR T1WI 平扫图像

关键结构：膈神经，心包膈血管，右下气管旁淋巴结，左上气管旁淋巴结。

此断面经第 3 胸椎椎体中份。

上纵隔内，左、右头臂静脉即将汇合成上腔静脉。膈神经由 C3~C5 前支组成，是颈丛中最重要的神经。膈神经在前斜角肌外侧缘上份形成主干，沿前斜角肌表面下行，在锁骨下动静脉间进入胸腔。它是混合性神经，其运动纤维支配膈肌，感觉纤维分布于胸膜、心包。右膈神经的感觉纤维还可分布到肝、胆囊和胆道系统。膈神经在胸腔内由两层胸膜包裹，覆盖膈神经的胸膜较疏松，易于分离。钝性分离即可游离整个胸段膈神经。膈神经损伤之后的主要表现为膈肌麻痹症状。患者无法自主呼吸，继而可能出现呼吸减弱[18]。膈神经受到刺激时会出现呃逆症状。胆囊的炎症可刺激分布于膈下中央部腹膜和胆囊的右膈神经末梢，此时患者可感到右侧肩部疼痛。心包膈血管位于纤维心包与纵隔胸膜之间，其中心包膈动脉发自胸廓内动脉上部，伴膈神经分布于膈、胸膜和心包。胸导管位于食管和左纵隔胸膜之间。此断面位于主动脉弓上缘与上腔静脉合成处之间，因此气管中线右侧的淋巴结为刚刚出现的右下气管旁淋巴结（4R）。主动脉弓 3 大分支与左头臂静脉之间的淋巴结为即将消失的左上气管旁淋巴结（2L）。

胸部连续横断层 20（FH.13110）

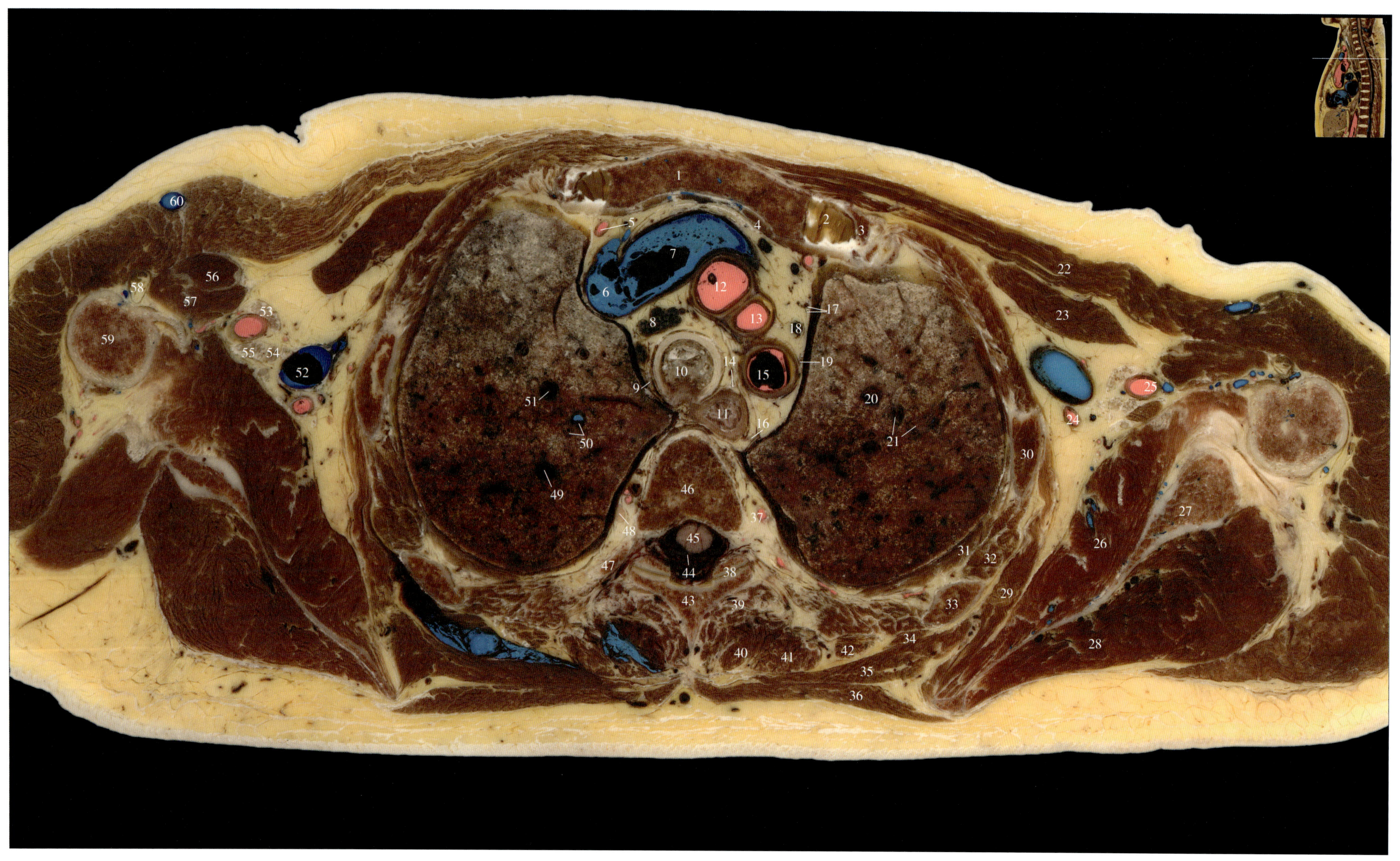

A. 断层标本图像

1. 胸骨柄 manubrium sterni
2. 第1肋软骨 1st costal cartilage
3. 第1肋骨 1st costal bone
4. 胸骨舌骨肌 sternohyoid
5. 胸廓内动脉 internal thoracic artery
6. 上腔静脉 superior vena cava
7. 左头臂静脉 left brachiocephalic vein
8. 右下气管旁淋巴结（4R）right lower paratracheal lymph nodes
9. 右迷走神经 right vagus nerve
10. 气管 trachea
11. 食管 esophagus
12. 头臂干 brachiocephalic trunk
13. 左颈总动脉 left common carotid artery
14. 左喉返神经 left recurrent laryngeal nerve
15. 左锁骨下动脉 left subclavian artery
16. 胸导管 thoracic duct
17. 膈神经和心包膈血管 phrenic nerve and pericardiacophrenic vessels
18. 左上气管旁淋巴结（2L）left upper paratracheal lymph nodes
19. 左迷走神经 left vagus nerve
20. 尖后段静脉（V1+2）apicoposterior segmental vein
21. 尖后段支气管（B1+2）和动脉（A1+2）apicoposterior segmental bronchus and artery
22. 胸大肌 pectoralis major
23. 胸小肌 pectoralis minor
24. 肩胛下动脉 subscapular artery
25. 腋动脉 axillary artery
26. 肩胛下肌 subscapularis
27. 肩胛骨 scapula
28. 冈下肌 infraspinatus
29. 前锯肌 serratus anterior
30. 第2肋骨 2nd costal bone
31. 肋间最内肌 intercostales intimi
32. 肋间内、外肌 intercostales interni and externi
33. 第3肋骨 3rd costal bone
34. 上后锯肌 serratus posterior superior
35. 菱形肌 rhomboideus
36. 斜方肌 trapezius
37. 肋间后动脉 posterior intercostal artery
38. 关节突关节 zygapophysial joint
39. 横突棘肌 transversospinales
40. 棘肌 spinales
41. 最长肌 longissimus
42. 髂肋肌 iliocostalis
43. 椎弓板 lamina of vertebral arch
44. 硬脊膜 spinal dura mater
45. 脊髓 spinal cord
46. 第3胸椎椎体 body of 3rd thoracic vertebra
47. 第4肋骨 4th costal bone
48. 胸交感神经节 thoracic sympathetic ganglion
49. 后段静脉（V2）posterior segmental vein
50. 尖段支气管（B1）和动脉（A1）apical segmental bronchus and artery
51. 尖段静脉尖支（V1）apical branch of apical segmental vein
52. 腋静脉 axillary vein
53. 臂丛外侧束 lateral cord of brachial plexus
54. 臂丛内侧束 medial cord of brachial plexus
55. 臂丛后束 posterior cord of brachial plexus
56. 肱二头肌短头 short head of biceps brachii
57. 喙肱肌 coracobrachialis
58. 肱二头肌长头 long head of biceps brachii
59. 肱骨 humerus
60. 头静脉 cephalic vein

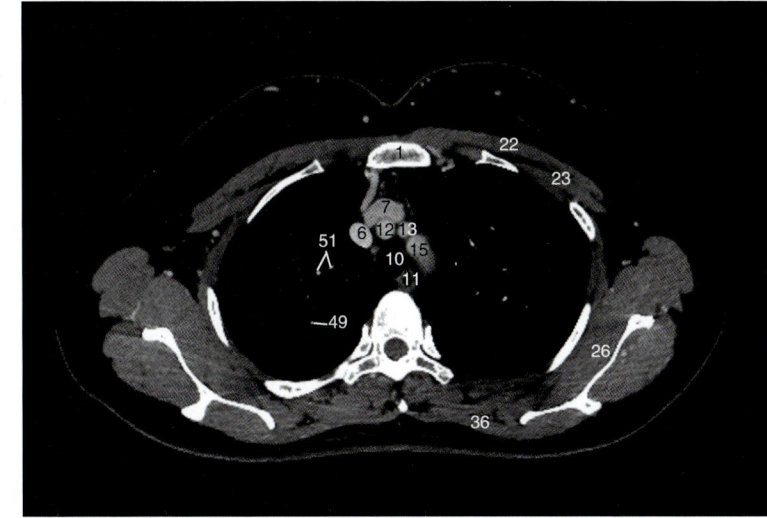

B. CT 纵隔窗增强图像

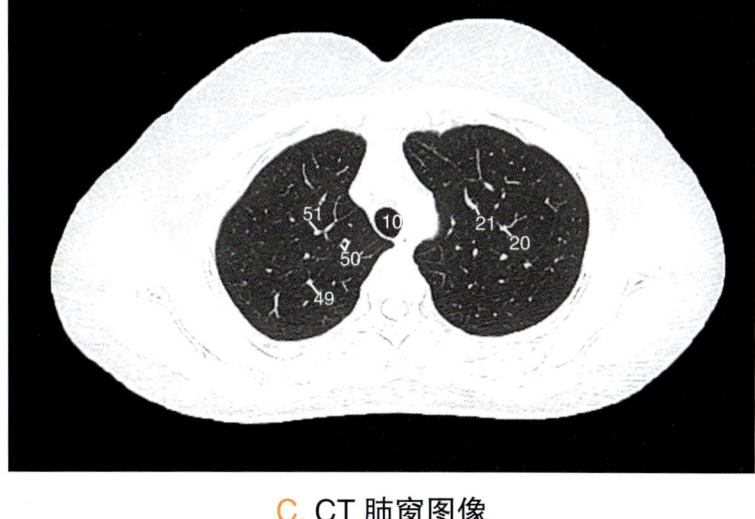

C. CT 肺窗图像

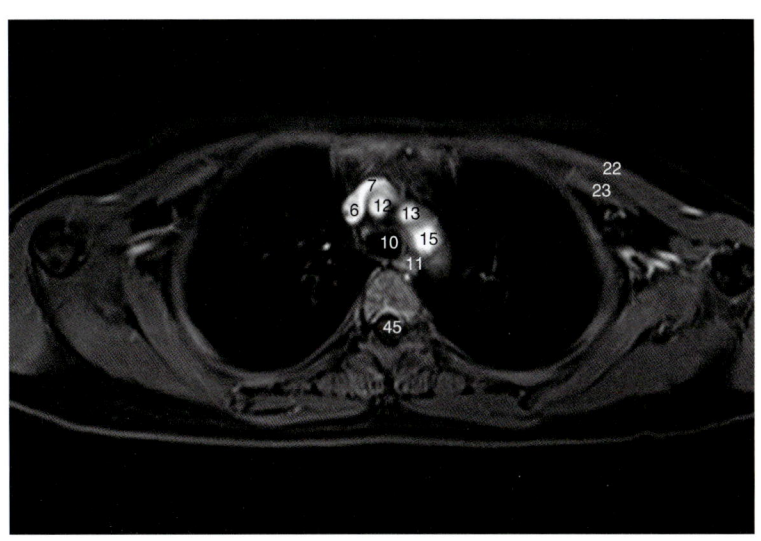

D. MR T1WI 增强图像

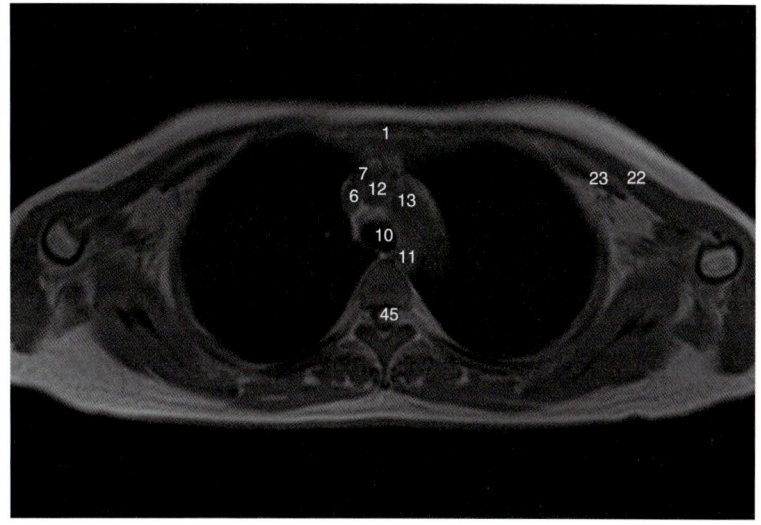

E. MR T1WI 平扫图像

关键结构：上腔静脉，胸大肌，胸小肌。

此断面经第3胸椎椎体中份。

胸大肌、胸小肌形成腋窝的前壁。在胸小肌后面，臂丛的3束（外侧束、内侧束、后束）分别从外、内、后三面包围腋动脉。胸骨后上纵隔内，左头臂静脉行向右与右头臂静脉汇合成上腔静脉。胸大肌在胸廓前上部浅层，起自锁骨部（锁骨内侧半）、胸肋部（胸骨和上位第5~6肋软骨）和腹部（腹直肌鞘的前壁），止于肱骨大结节嵴（锁骨部和腹部肌束上下交叉），肌腹呈扇形，向外上集中呈"U"形扁腱止于大结节嵴。胸大肌的血供有多个来源，其中以胸肩峰动脉的上、下胸肌支，腋动脉发出的胸肌支和胸廓内动脉的肋间前动脉和穿支较为重要，还有胸最上动脉的胸肌支等。

不同来源的血管，在肌内有丰富的吻合。支配神经主要为臂丛的胸外侧神经和胸内侧神经。胸小肌在胸大肌深面，为三角形扁肌，起自第3~5肋骨的前面及肋间肌表面的筋膜，止于肩胛骨的喙突。胸小肌拉肩胛骨向前下。肩胛骨固定时，胸小肌可上提肋骨，但在用力吸气时才有活动。胸小肌由胸内侧神经支配。胸小肌的动脉以胸肩峰动脉分支居多，较为恒定。胸小肌的静脉分布变异较大，未见明显伴行规律[19]。上腔静脉与气管之间可见2个右下气管旁淋巴结（4R），从纵隔淋巴结的数目来看，气管旁淋巴结右侧多于左侧。左颈总动脉起始处可见左上气管旁淋巴结（2L）。椎体两侧可见交感干神经节。

胸部连续横断层 21（FH.13090）

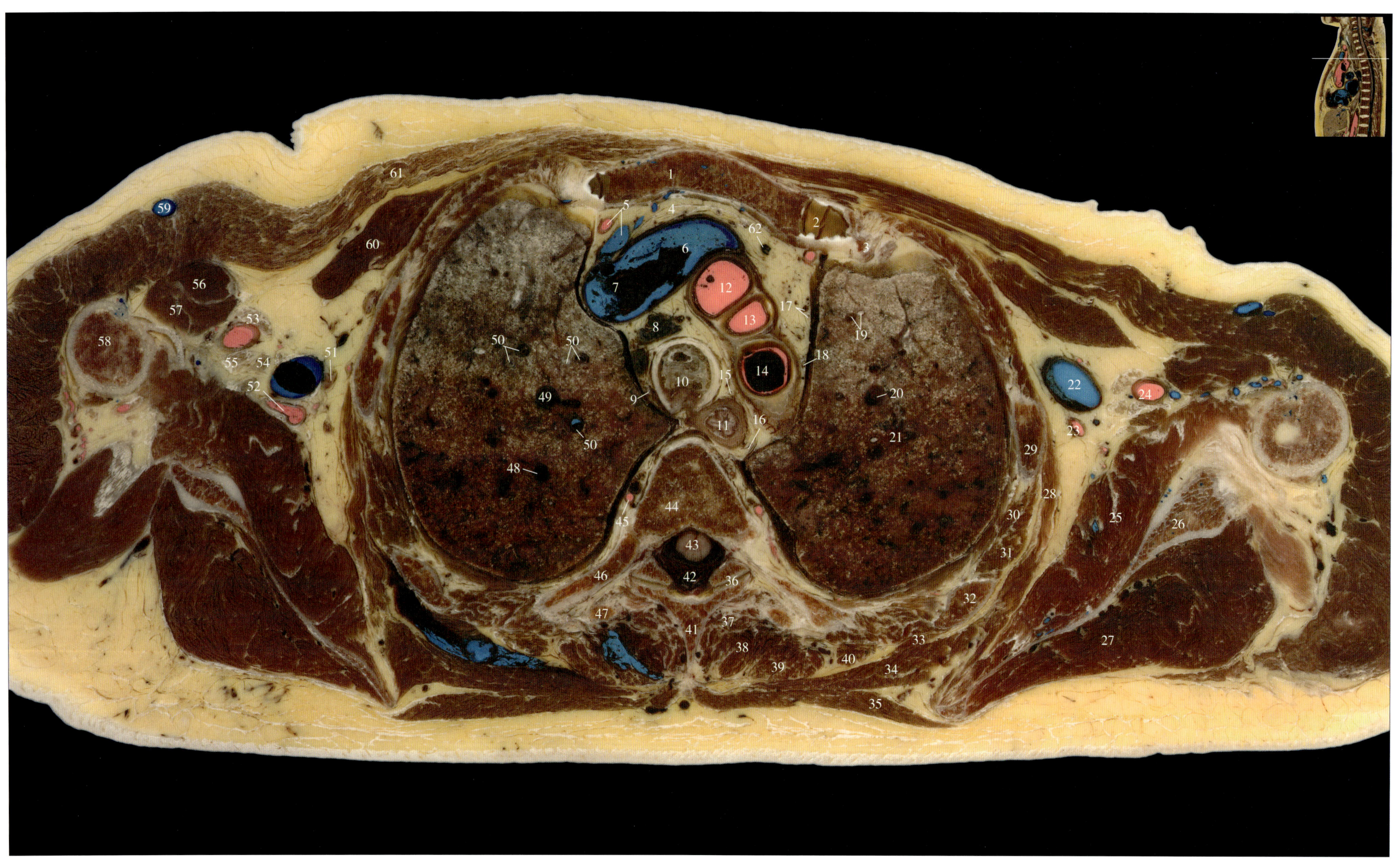

A. 断层标本图像

1. 胸骨柄 manubrium sterni
2. 第 1 肋软骨 1st costal cartilage
3. 第 1 肋骨 1st costal bone
4. 胸腺 thymus
5. 胸廓内动、静脉 internal thoracic artery and vein
6. 左头臂静脉 left brachiocephalic vein
7. 上腔静脉 superior vena cava
8. 右下气管旁淋巴结（4R）right lower paratracheal lymph nodes
9. 右迷走神经 right vagus nerve
10. 气管 trachea
11. 食管 esophagus
12. 头臂干 brachiocephalic trunk
13. 左颈总动脉 left common carotid artery
14. 左锁骨下动脉 left subclavian artery
15. 左喉返神经 left recurrent laryngeal nerve
16. 胸导管 thoracic duct
17. 膈神经和心包膈血管 phrenic nerve and pericardiacophrenic vessels
18. 左迷走神经 left vagus nerve
19. 前段支气管（B3）和动脉（A3）anterior segmental bronchus and artery
20. 尖后段静脉（V1+2）apicoposterior segmental vein
21. 尖后段支气管（B1+2）和动脉（A1+2）apicoposterior segmental bronchus and artery
22. 腋静脉 axillary vein
23. 肩胛下动脉 subscapular artery
24. 腋动脉 axillary artery
25. 肩胛下肌 subscapularis
26. 肩胛骨 scapula
27. 冈下肌 infraspinatus
28. 前锯肌 serratus anterior
29. 第 2 肋骨 2nd costal bone
30. 肋间内肌 intercostales interni
31. 肋间外肌 intercostales externi
32. 第 3 肋骨 3rd costal bone
33. 上后锯肌 serratus posterior superior
34. 菱形肌 rhomboideus
35. 斜方肌 trapezius
36. 关节突关节 zygapophysial joint
37. 横突棘肌 transversospinales
38. 棘肌 spinales
39. 最长肌 longissimus
40. 髂肋肌 iliocostalis
41. 棘突 spinous process
42. 硬膜外隙 epidural space
43. 脊髓 spinal cord
44. 第 3 胸椎椎体 body of 3rd thoracic vertebra
45. 肋间后动脉 posterior intercostal artery
46. 第 4 肋骨 4th costal bone
47. 横突 transverse process
48. 后段静脉（V2）posterior segmental vein
49. 尖段静脉尖支（V1）apical branch of apical segmental vein
50. 尖段支气管（B1）和动脉（A1）apical segmental bronchus and artery
51. 腋淋巴结 axillary lymph nodes
52. 旋肱后动脉 posterior circumflex humeral artery
53. 臂丛外侧束 lateral cord of brachial plexus
54. 臂丛内侧束 medial cord of brachial plexus
55. 臂丛后束 posterior cord of brachial plexus
56. 肱二头肌短头 short head of biceps brachii
57. 喙肱肌 coracobrachialis
58. 肱骨 humerus
59. 头静脉 cephalic vein
60. 胸小肌 pectoralis minor
61. 胸大肌 pectoralis major
62. 前纵隔淋巴结（3a）anterior mediastinal lymph nodes

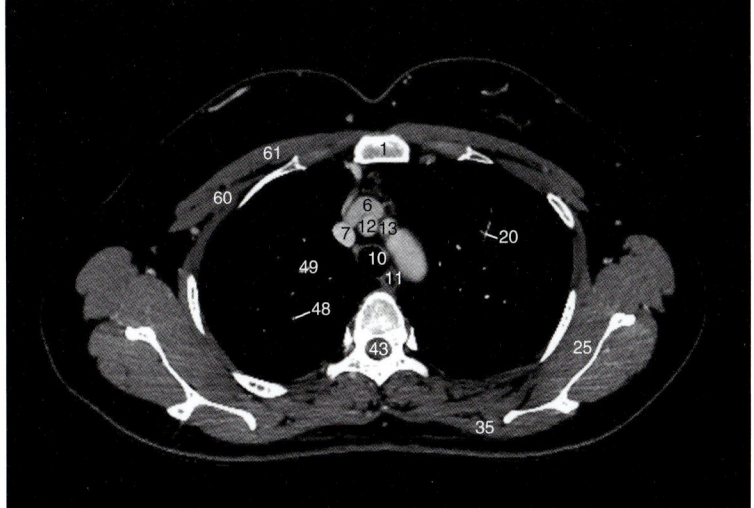

B. CT 纵隔窗增强图像

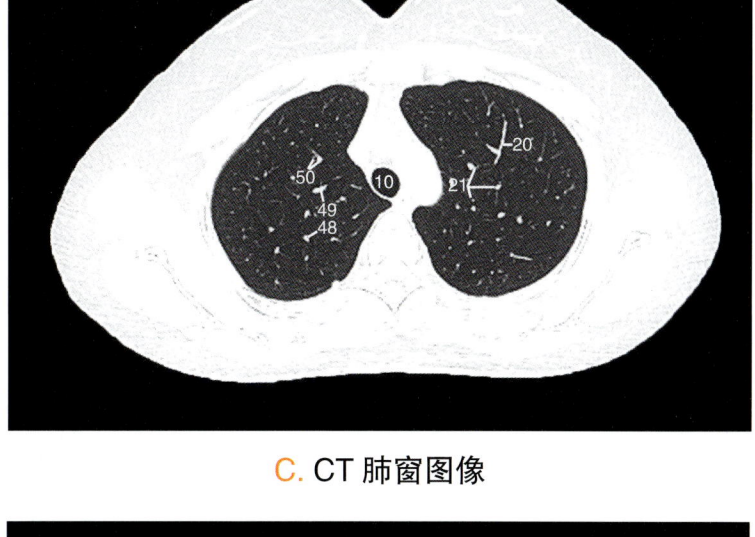

C. CT 肺窗图像

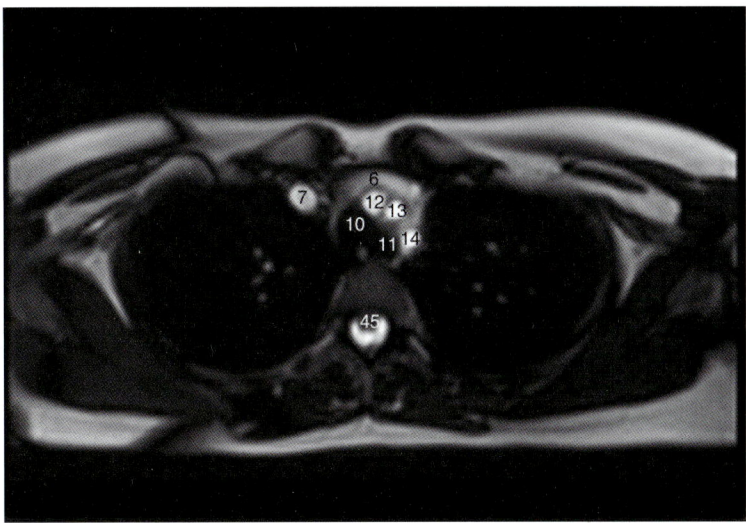

D. MR T2 WI 平扫图像

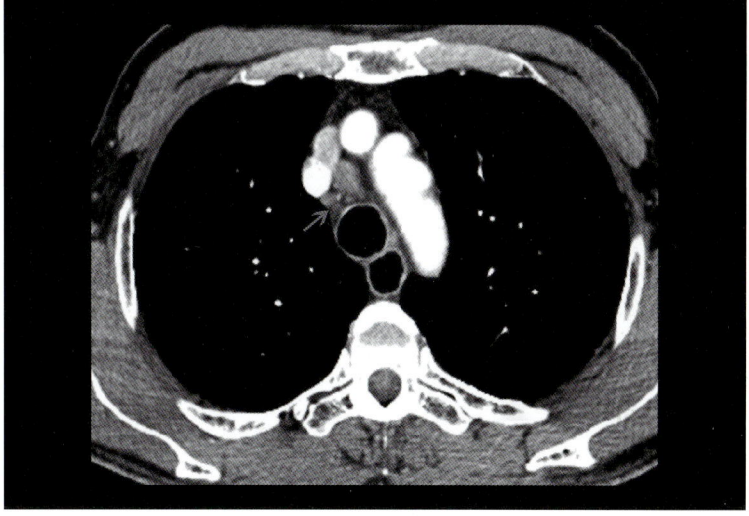

E. 4R 区淋巴结转移 CT 图像

关键结构：腋动脉，胸廓内动、静脉。

此断面经过第 3 胸椎椎体下份。

腋动脉来自锁骨下动脉，以胸小肌为标志分为三段。第一段：从第 1 肋外侧缘至胸小肌上缘，分支胸上动脉、胸肩峰动脉；第二段：被胸小肌覆盖，分支胸外侧动脉；第三段：胸小肌下缘至大圆肌下缘之间，分支肩胛下动脉、旋肱前动脉、旋肱后动脉。上纵隔前外侧可见两侧的胸廓内动、静脉。胸廓内动脉发自锁骨下动脉第一段的下壁，沿胸骨侧缘外侧 1~2 cm 处下行，居于上 6 肋软骨和肋间内肌的深面，胸横肌和胸内筋膜的浅面。至第 6 肋间隙处分为腹壁上动脉和肌膈动脉两终支。前者下行进入腹直肌鞘；后者在第 7~9 肋软骨后方斜向外下方，分支至心包下部和膈。在第 1 肋附近，从胸廓内动脉发出心包膈动脉，与膈神经伴行经肺根前方，在心包与纵隔胸膜之间下行至膈，沿途发出分支至心包和胸膜。冠状动脉旁路移植术中，用左胸廓内动脉建立到左冠状动脉前降支的旁路已成为"金标准"[20]。胸廓内静脉由腹壁上静脉和肌膈静脉汇合而成，初为 2 支，沿胸廓内动脉的两侧上升，至上端合并为 1 干，注入头臂静脉。大血管与气管之间的气管前间隙可见右下气管旁淋巴结（4R）。E 图所示为该区增大的转移淋巴结。

胸部连续横断层 22（FH.13070）

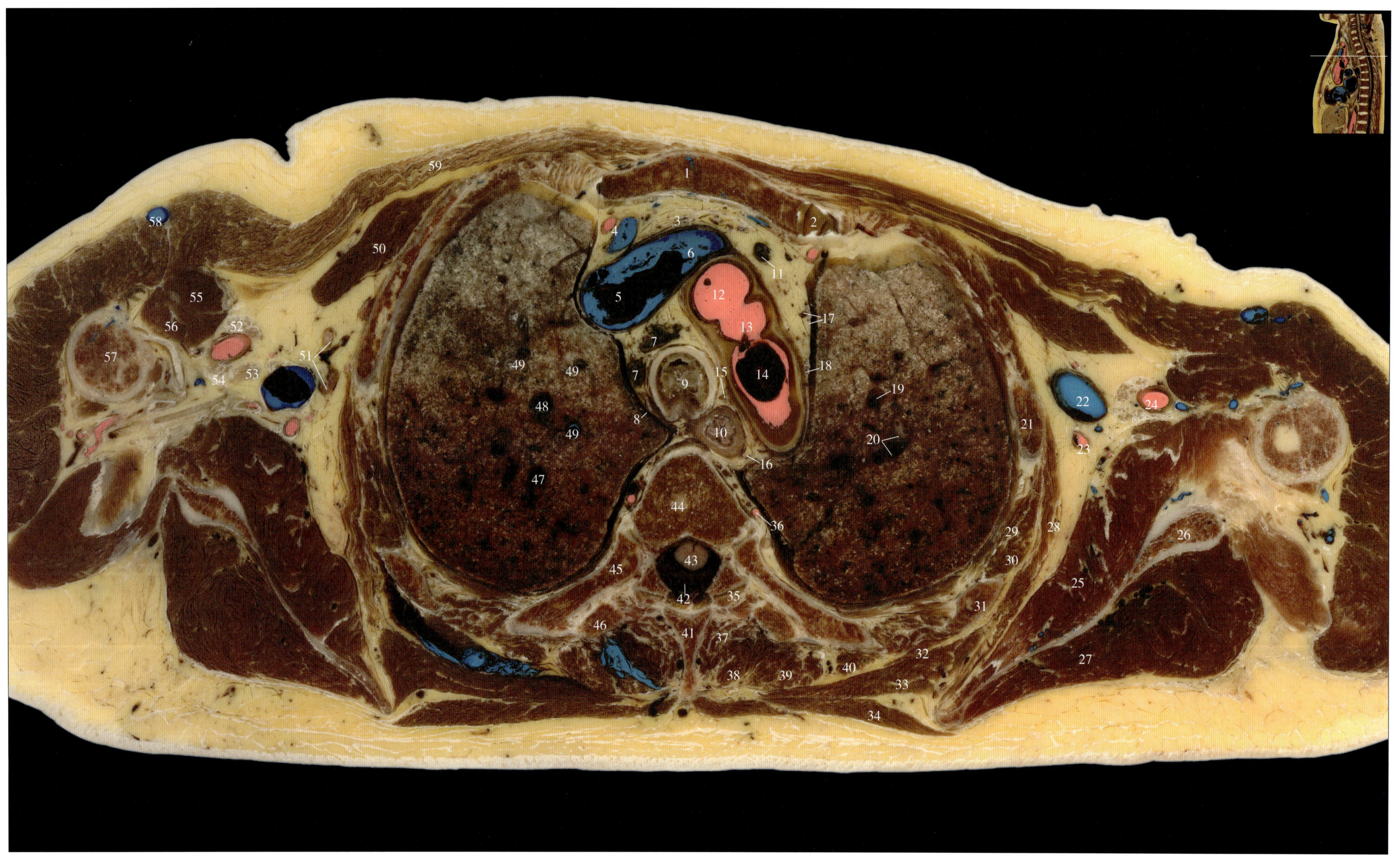

A. 断层标本图像

1. 胸骨柄 manubrium sterni
2. 第 1 肋软骨 1st costal cartilage
3. 胸腺 thymus
4. 胸廓内动、静脉 internal thoracic artery and vein
5. 上腔静脉 superior vena cava
6. 左头臂静脉 left brachiocephalic vein
7. 右下气管旁淋巴结（4R）right lower paratracheal lymph nodes
8. 右迷走神经 right vagus nerve
9. 气管 trachea
10. 食管 esophagus
11. 前纵隔淋巴结（3a）anterior mediastinal lymph nodes
12. 头臂干 brachiocephalic trunk
13. 左颈总动脉 left common carotid artery
14. 左锁骨下动脉 left subclavian artery
15. 左喉返神经 left recurrent laryngeal nerve
16. 胸导管 thoracic duct
17. 膈神经和心包膈血管 phrenic nerve and pericardiacophrenic vessels
18. 左迷走神经 left vagus nerve
19. 尖后段静脉（V1+2）apicoposterior segmental vein
20. 尖后段支气管（B1+2）和动脉（A1+2）apicoposterior segmental bronchus and artery
21. 第 2 肋骨 2nd costal bone
22. 腋静脉 axillary vein
23. 肩胛下动脉 subscapular artery
24. 腋动脉 axillary artery
25. 肩胛下肌 subscapularis
26. 肩胛骨 scapula
27. 冈下肌 infraspinatus
28. 前锯肌 serratus anterior
29. 肋间内肌 intercostales interni
30. 肋间外肌 intercostales externi
31. 第 3 肋骨 3rd costal bone
32. 上后锯肌 serratus posterior superior
33. 菱形肌 rhomboideus
34. 斜方肌 trapezius
35. 关节突关节 zygapophysial joint
36. 肋间后动脉 posterior intercostal artery
37. 横突棘肌 transversospinales
38. 棘肌 spinales
39. 最长肌 longissimus
40. 髂肋肌 iliocostalis
41. 棘突 spinous process
42. 硬脊膜 spinal dura mater
43. 脊髓 spinal cord
44. 第 3 胸椎椎体 body of 3rd thoracic vertebra
45. 第 4 肋骨 4th costal bone
46. 横突 transverse process
47. 后段静脉（V2）posterior segmental vein
48. 尖段静脉尖支（V1）apical branch of apical segmental vein
49. 尖段支气管（B1）和动脉（A1）apical segmental bronchus and artery
50. 胸小肌 pectoralis minor
51. 腋淋巴结 axillary lymph nodes
52. 臂丛外侧束 lateral cord of brachial plexus
53. 臂丛内侧束 medial cord of brachial plexus
54. 臂丛后束 posterior cord of brachial plexus
55. 肱二头肌短头 short head of biceps brachii
56. 喙肱肌 coracobrachialis
57. 肱骨 humerus
58. 头静脉 cephalic vein
59. 胸大肌 pectoralis major

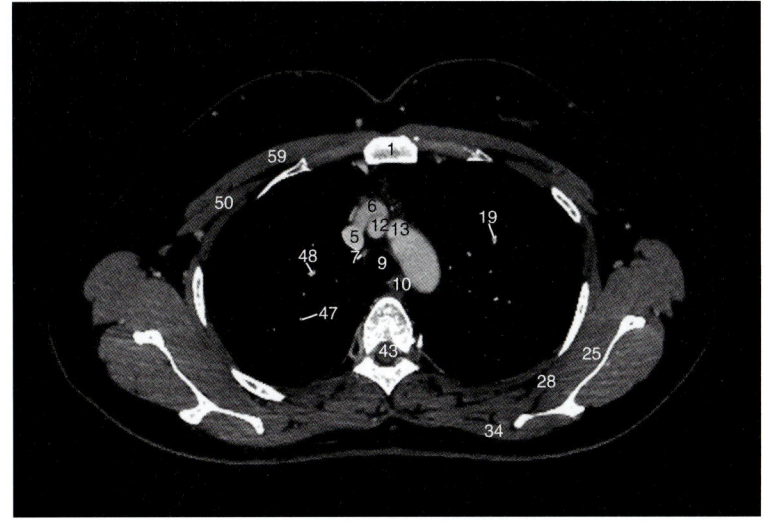

B. CT 纵隔窗增强图像

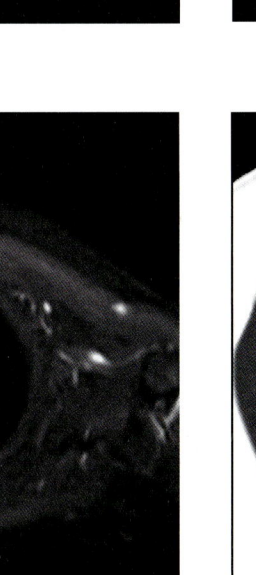

C. CT 肺窗图像

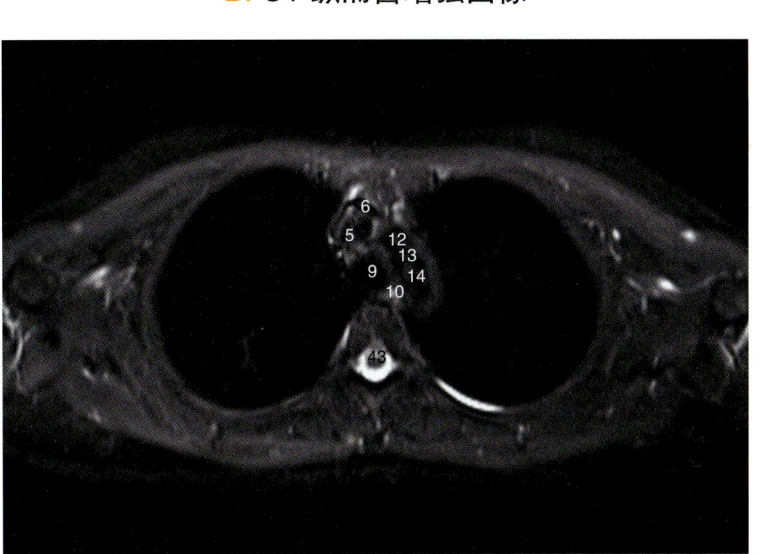

D. MR T2WI 抑脂图像

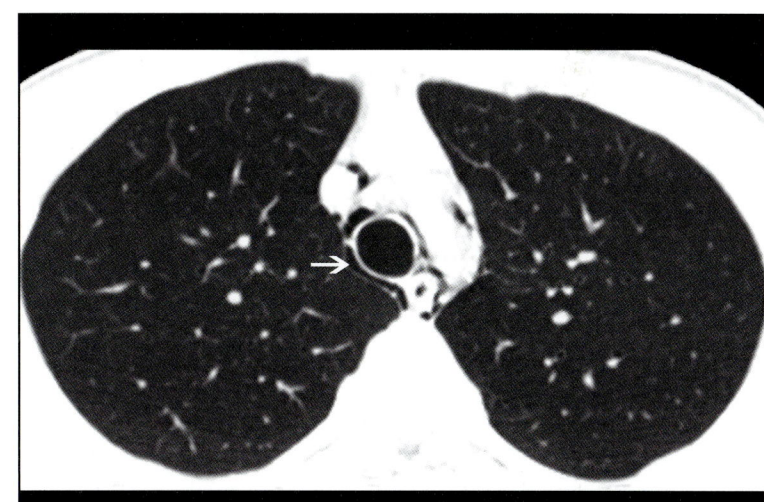

E. 纵隔气肿 CT 图像

关键结构：前纵隔淋巴结，腋淋巴结。

断面经第 3 胸椎椎体下份。

接近主动脉弓三大分支的起始处。部分主动脉弓被切及，其在影像上清楚易辨，常作为识别邻近结构的标志。两侧胸膜前返折线和肺的前缘向中线靠近，肺的横断面呈牛角形。气管前间隙内可见 2 个淋巴结，因为此处为上腔静脉合成处，此区淋巴结为右下气管旁淋巴结（4R）。血管前间隙内可见前纵隔淋巴结（3a）。腋淋巴结约 20~30 个，可分为 5 群：①外侧群，沿腋静脉远侧段排列，收纳上肢大部分淋巴管。手和前臂感染时首先侵及此群。②前群，位于前锯肌的表面，循胸外侧血管分布，收纳乳房、胸前外侧壁、脐平面以上腹前壁的淋巴管。乳腺癌时首先侵及此群。③后群，位于肩胛下血管周围，收纳背上部、颈后部、肩关节及胸后壁的淋巴。④中央群，位于腋腔底部中央的结缔组织中，收纳上述三群淋巴结的输出管。⑤腋尖群，又称锁骨下群，位于胸小肌上部、锁胸筋膜深面，沿腋动脉近侧段排列，收纳乳房上部及中央群的淋巴。乳腺癌改良根治术中腋窝淋巴结清扫是不可或缺的步骤。腋窝淋巴结清扫及病理学检查是判断乳腺癌患者腋窝淋巴结状态最可靠的方法。腋窝淋巴结分期对评估患者预后和制订治疗方案具有重要参考价值[21]。此断面中，上纵隔大血管于 CT 上观察清晰，因为血管周围衬有脂肪，且被低密度的肺组织包绕，具备较好的对比。E 图所示为纵隔气肿病例，可见纵隔大血管周围游离的低密度气体影（箭头所示）。

胸部连续横断层 23（FH.13050）

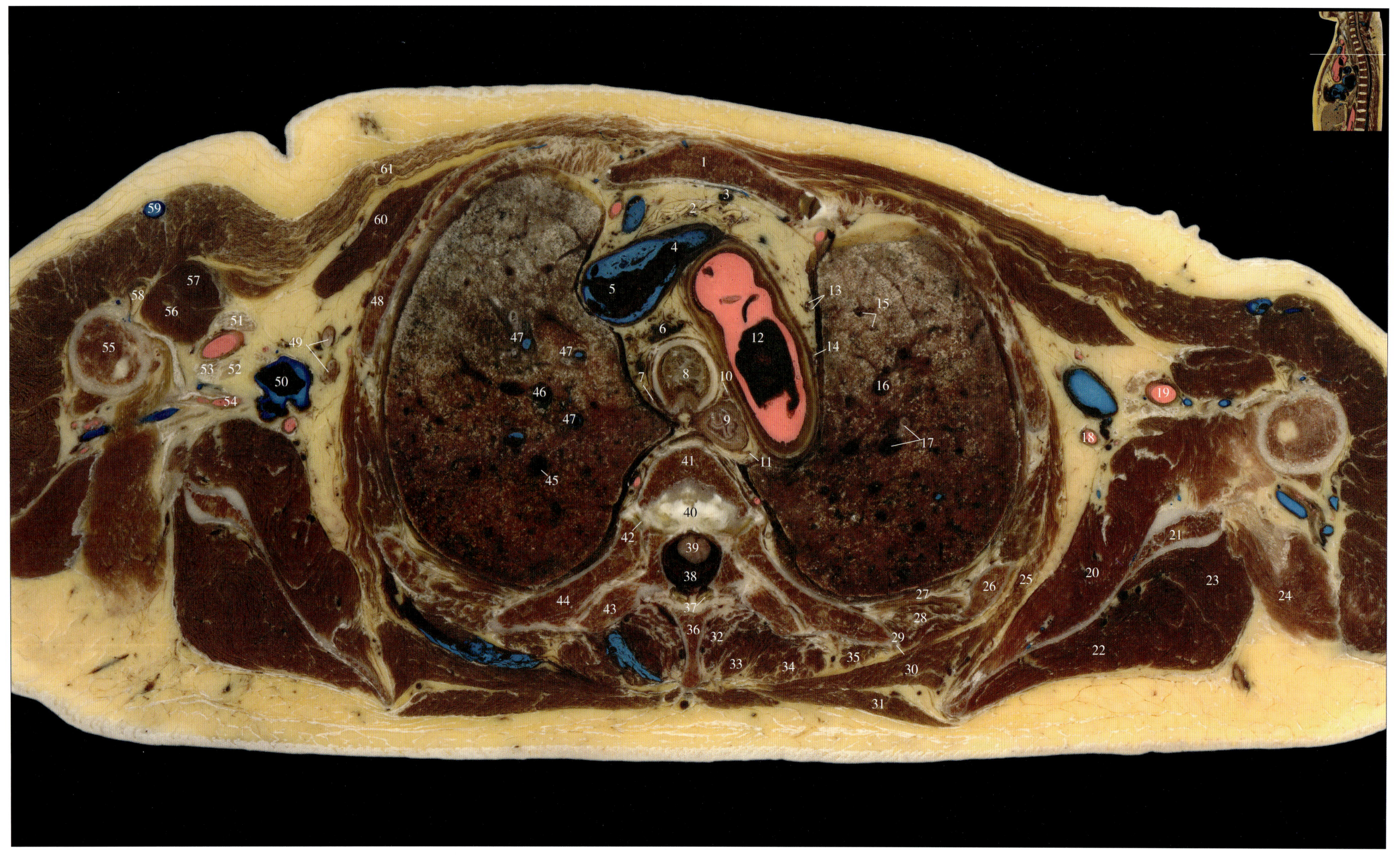

A. 断层标本图像

1. 胸骨柄 manubrium sterni
2. 胸腺 thymus
3. 前纵隔淋巴结（3a）anterior mediastinal lymph nodes
4. 左头臂静脉 left brachiocephalic vein
5. 上腔静脉 superior vena cava
6. 右下气管旁淋巴结（4R）right lower paratracheal lymph nodes
7. 右迷走神经 right vagus nerve
8. 气管 trachea
9. 食管 esophagus
10. 左喉返神经 left recurrent laryngeal nerve
11. 胸导管 thoracic duct
12. 主动脉弓 aortic arch
13. 膈神经和心包膈血管 phrenic nerve and pericardiacophrenic vessels
14. 左迷走神经 left vagus nerve
15. 前段支气管（B3）和动脉（A3）anterior segmental bronchus and artery
16. 尖后段静脉（V1+2）apicoposterior segmental vein
17. 尖后段支气管（B1+2）和动脉（A1+2）apicoposterior segmental bronchus and artery
18. 肩胛下动脉 subscapular artery
19. 腋动脉 axillary artery
20. 肩胛下肌 subscapularis
21. 肩胛骨 scapula
22. 冈下肌 infraspinatus
23. 小圆肌 teres minor
24. 肱三头肌 triceps brachii
25. 前锯肌 serratus anterior
26. 第 3 肋骨 3rd costal bone
27. 肋间最内肌 intercostales intimi
28. 肋间内、外肌 intercostales interni and externi
29. 上后锯肌 serratus posterior superior
30. 菱形肌 rhomboideus
31. 斜方肌 trapezius
32. 横突棘肌 transversospinales
33. 棘肌 spinales
34. 最长肌 longissimus
35. 髂肋肌 iliocostalis
36. 棘突 spinous process
37. 黄韧带 ligamenta flava
38. 硬膜外隙 epidural space
39. 脊髓 spinal cord
40. T3-4 椎间盘 T3-4 intervertebral disc
41. 第 3 胸椎椎体 body of 3rd thoracic vertebra
42. 肋头关节 joint of costal head
43. 横突 transverse process
44. 第 4 肋骨 4th costal bone
45. 后段静脉（V2）posterior segmental vein
46. 尖段静脉尖支（V1）apical branch of apical segmental vein
47. 尖段支气管（B1）和动脉（A1）apical segmental bronchus and artery
48. 第 2 肋骨 2nd costal bone
49. 腋淋巴结 axillary lymph nodes
50. 腋静脉 axillary vein
51. 臂丛外侧束 lateral cord of brachial plexus
52. 臂丛内侧束 medial cord of brachial plexus
53. 臂丛后束 posterior cord of brachial plexus
54. 旋肱后动脉 posterior humeral circumflex artery
55. 肱骨 humerus
56. 喙肱肌 coracobrachialis
57. 肱二头肌短头 short head of biceps brachii
58. 肱二头肌长头 long head of biceps brachii
59. 头静脉 cephalic vein
60. 胸小肌 pectoralis minor
61. 胸大肌 pectoralis major

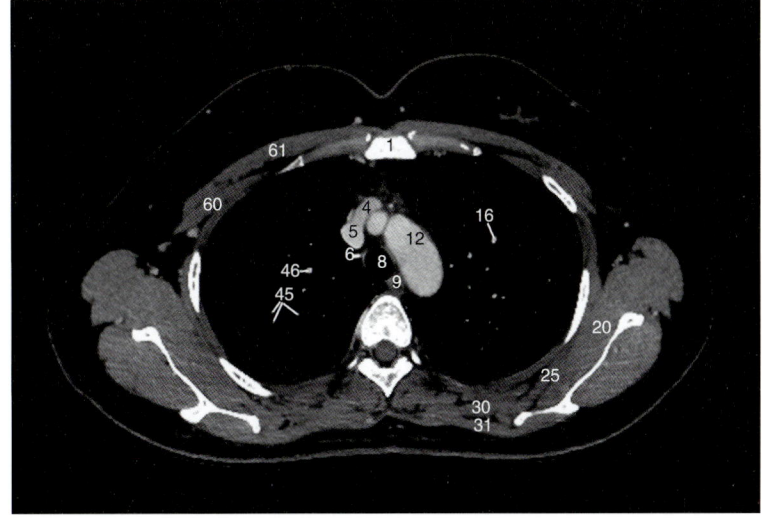

B. CT 纵隔窗增强图像

C. CT 肺窗图像

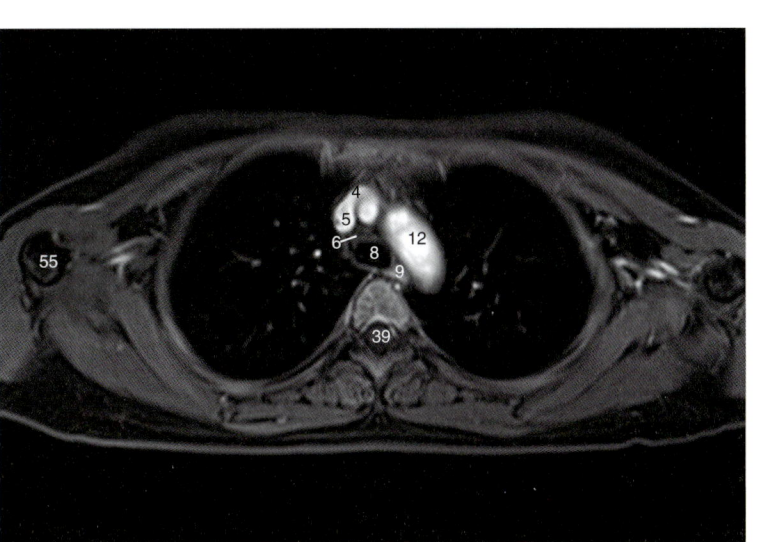

D. MR T1WI 增强图像

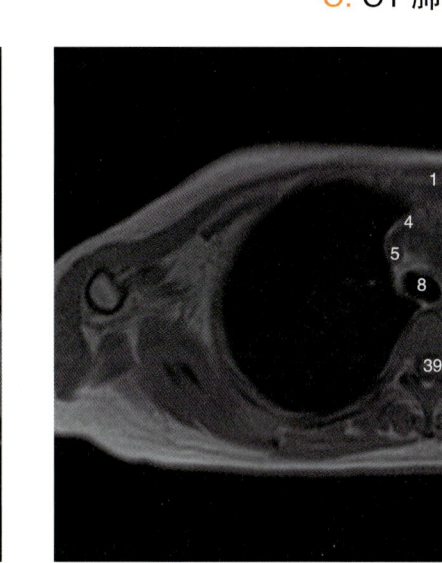

E. MR T1WI 平扫图像

关键结构：主动脉弓。

此断面经 T3-4 椎间盘上份。

主动脉弓位于上纵隔，平胸骨角平面（或第 4 胸椎）以上水平，于右侧第 2 胸肋关节水平从右前方走行至左后方，主动脉弓凸面最常见自右向左依次发出以下 3 支分支血管：头臂干、左颈总动脉和左锁骨下动脉。主动脉弓分型的主要依据是头臂干开口、左颈总动脉及左锁骨下动脉（主动脉弓顶部）之间的关系，主动脉弓分支分型：A 型，主动脉弓顶切线到头臂干起始部的距离等于或小于头臂干宽度；B 型，主动脉弓顶切线到头臂干起始部的距离等于 2 倍头臂干的宽度；C 型，主动脉弓顶切线到头臂干起始部的距离等于 3 倍或以上头臂干宽度，此分型的部分意义在于其影响包括冠状动脉支架术、颈动脉支架术在内的介入治疗的操作难度。主动脉弓部疾病包括累及主动脉弓部的动脉瘤、假性动脉瘤、主动脉夹层、主动脉溃疡和壁间血肿等病变。主要病因包括动脉的老化、动脉硬化、高血压、遗传性疾病（马凡综合征等）及自身免疫性疾病等[22]。主动脉弓的右前方为胸腺。左心包膈血管、左膈神经、左迷走神经位于主动脉弓的外侧。主动脉弓的内侧从前向后依次是上腔静脉、气管、食管。气管食管沟与主动脉弓之间有左喉返神经。食管、主动脉弓、椎体之间有胸导管。前纵隔淋巴结（3a）依然可见，位于胸腺的左前方。在上腔静脉与气管之间，可见 2 个右下气管旁淋巴结（4R）。

胸部连续横断层 24（FH.13030）

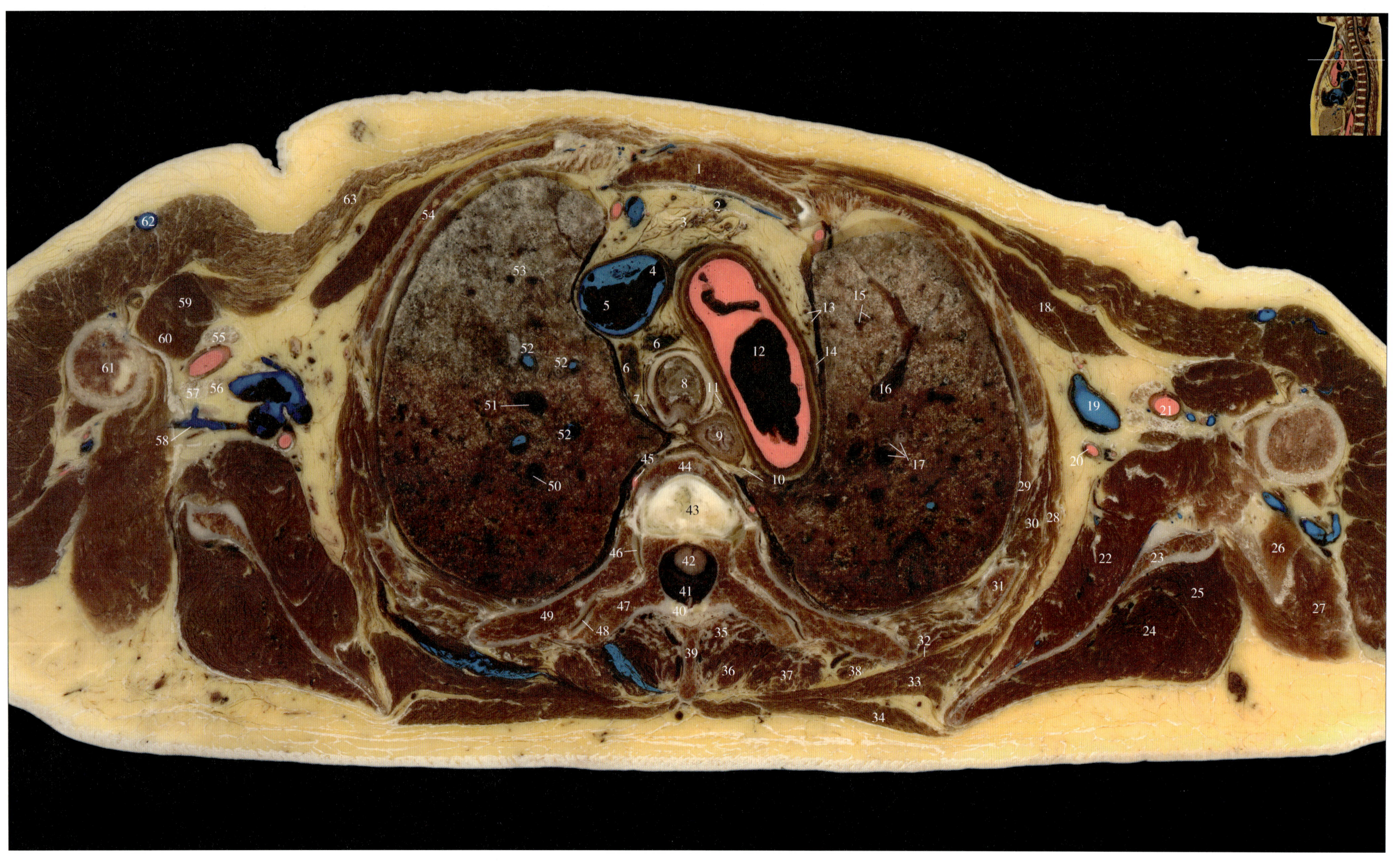

A. 断层标本图像

1. 胸骨柄 manubrium sterni
2. 前纵隔淋巴结（3a）anterior mediastinal lymph nodes
3. 胸腺 thymus
4. 左头臂静脉 left brachiocephalic vein
5. 上腔静脉 superior vena cava
6. 右下气管旁淋巴结（4R）right lower paratracheal lymph nodes
7. 右迷走神经 right vagus nerve
8. 气管 trachea
9. 食管 esophagus
10. 胸导管 thoracic duct
11. 左喉返神经 left recurrent laryngeal nerve
12. 主动脉弓 aortic arch
13. 膈神经和心包膈血管 phrenic nerve and pericardiacophrenic vessels
14. 左迷走神经 left vagus nerve
15. 前段支气管（B3）和动脉（A3）anterior segmental bronchus and artery
16. 尖后段静脉（V1+2）apicoposterior segmental vein
17. 尖后段支气管（B1+2）和动脉（A1+2）apicoposterior segmental bronchus and artery
18. 胸小肌 pectoralis minor
19. 腋静脉 axillary vein
20. 肩胛下动脉 subscapular artery
21. 腋动脉 axillary artery
22. 肩胛下肌 subscapularis
23. 肩胛骨 scapula
24. 冈下肌 infraspinatus
25. 小圆肌 teres minor
26. 大圆肌 teres major
27. 肱三头肌 triceps brachii
28. 前锯肌 serratus anterior
29. 肋间最内肌 intercostales intimi
30. 肋间内、外肌 intercostales interni and externi
31. 第3肋骨 3rd costal bone
32. 上后锯肌 serratus posterior superior
33. 菱形肌 rhomboideus
34. 斜方肌 trapezius
35. 横突棘肌 transversospinales
36. 棘肌 spinales
37. 最长肌 longissimus
38. 髂肋肌 iliocostalis
39. 棘突 spinous process
40. 黄韧带 ligamenta flava
41. 硬膜外隙 epidural space
42. 脊髓 spinal cord
43. T3-4椎间盘 T3-4 intervertebral disc
44. 第3胸椎椎体 body of 3rd thoracic vertebra
45. 肋间后动脉 posterior intercostal artery
46. 肋头关节 joint of costal head
47. 横突 transverse process
48. 肋横突关节 costotransverse joint
49. 第4肋骨 4th costal bone
50. 后段静脉（V2）posterior segmental vein
51. 尖段静脉尖支（V1）apical branch of apical segmental vein
52. 尖段支气管（B1）和动脉（A1）apical segmental bronchus and artery
53. 尖段静脉（V1）apical segmental vein
54. 第2肋骨 2nd costal bone
55. 臂丛外侧束 lateral cord of brachial plexus
56. 臂丛内侧束 medial cord of brachial plexus
57. 臂丛后束 posterior cord of brachial plexus
58. 旋肱后静脉 posterior humeral circumflex vein
59. 肱二头肌短头 short head of biceps brachii
60. 喙肱肌 coracobrachialis
61. 肱骨 humerus
62. 头静脉 cephalic vein
63. 胸大肌 pectoralis major

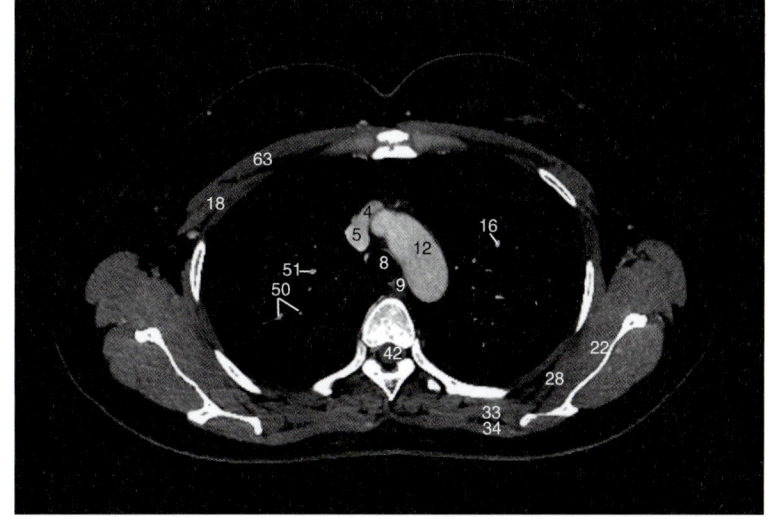

B. CT 纵隔窗增强图像

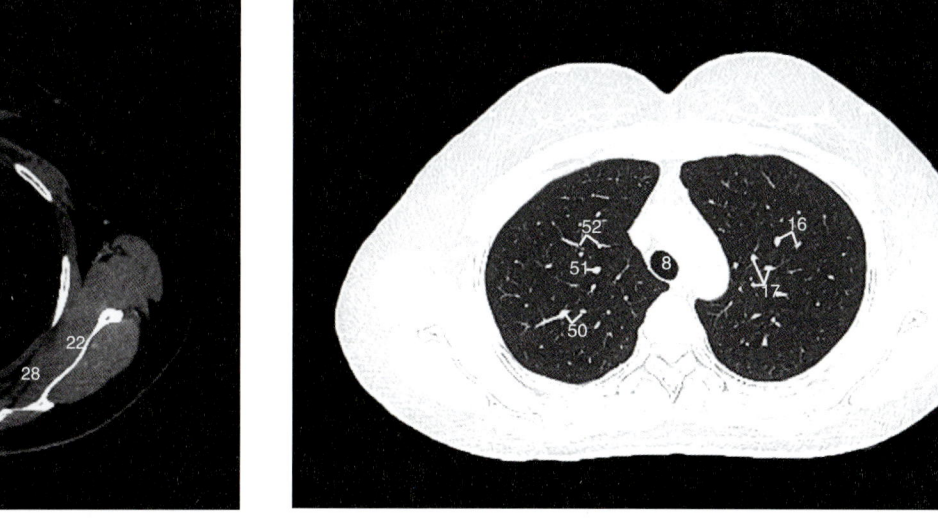

C. CT 肺窗图像

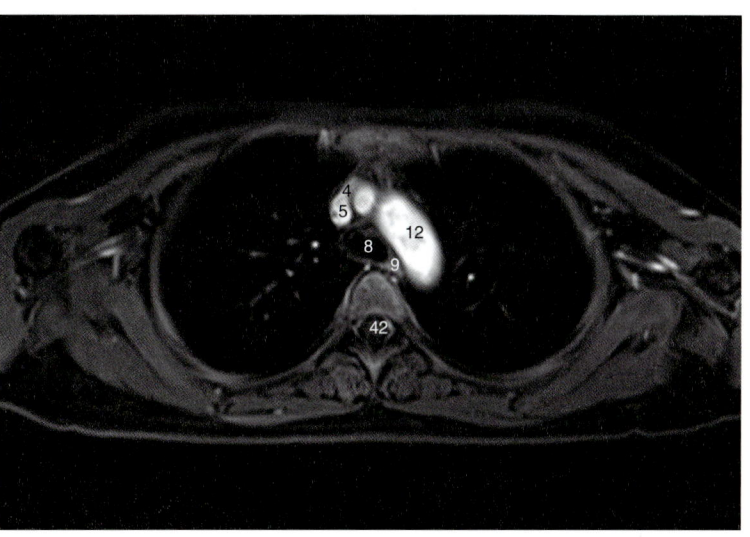

D. MR T1WI 增强图像

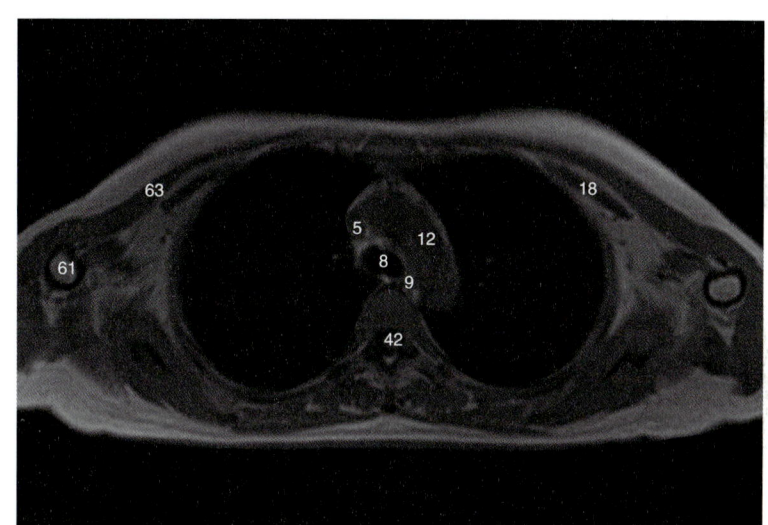

E. MR T1WI 平扫图像

关键结构：气管前间隙，右下气管旁淋巴结。

断面经 T3-4 椎间盘中份。

位于大血管和气管之间的为气管前间隙。此间隙向上经胸廓上口与颈部的气管前间隙相续连，向下达气管隆嵴平面。此断面内，胸骨与胸腺之间可见前纵隔淋巴结（3a）。上腔静脉由左、右头臂静脉在右侧第1胸肋结合处汇合而成，下行至第2胸肋关节后方穿纤维心包，平第3胸肋关节下缘注入右心房。在穿纤维心包之前，有奇静脉注入。上腔静脉前方有胸腺和肺，后方有气管和迷走神经，左侧有升主动脉和主动脉弓，右侧有膈神经和心包膈血管。上纵隔管道结构常见的另一变异是左上腔静脉，左上腔静脉常在主动脉三大分支的外侧，沿纵隔左缘下行注入右心房。永存左上腔静脉是一种先天性心血管畸形，是由胎儿期左前主静脉与左 Cuiver 管不闭合形成，多引流入冠状静脉窦，该畸形多合并其他先天性畸形[23]。超声心动图可探及扩张的冠状静脉窦，右心导管检查时如果导管进入畸形的左上腔静脉或心血管造影时显示该静脉则可确诊。单纯的双永存上腔静脉无须治疗，但如果该静脉引流入左房而引起发绀，则需外科结扎，如合并其他畸形且这些畸形需要手术纠正者，手术时也需阻断左侧上腔静脉。在上腔静脉与气管之间可见2个右下气管旁淋巴结（4R）。在 CT 图像上，上腔静脉后方和气管之间为一低密度三角区，称气管前间隙或气管前腔静脉后间隙，该间隙内常见直径 <7 mm 的 4 区淋巴结。

胸部连续横断层 25 (FH.13010)

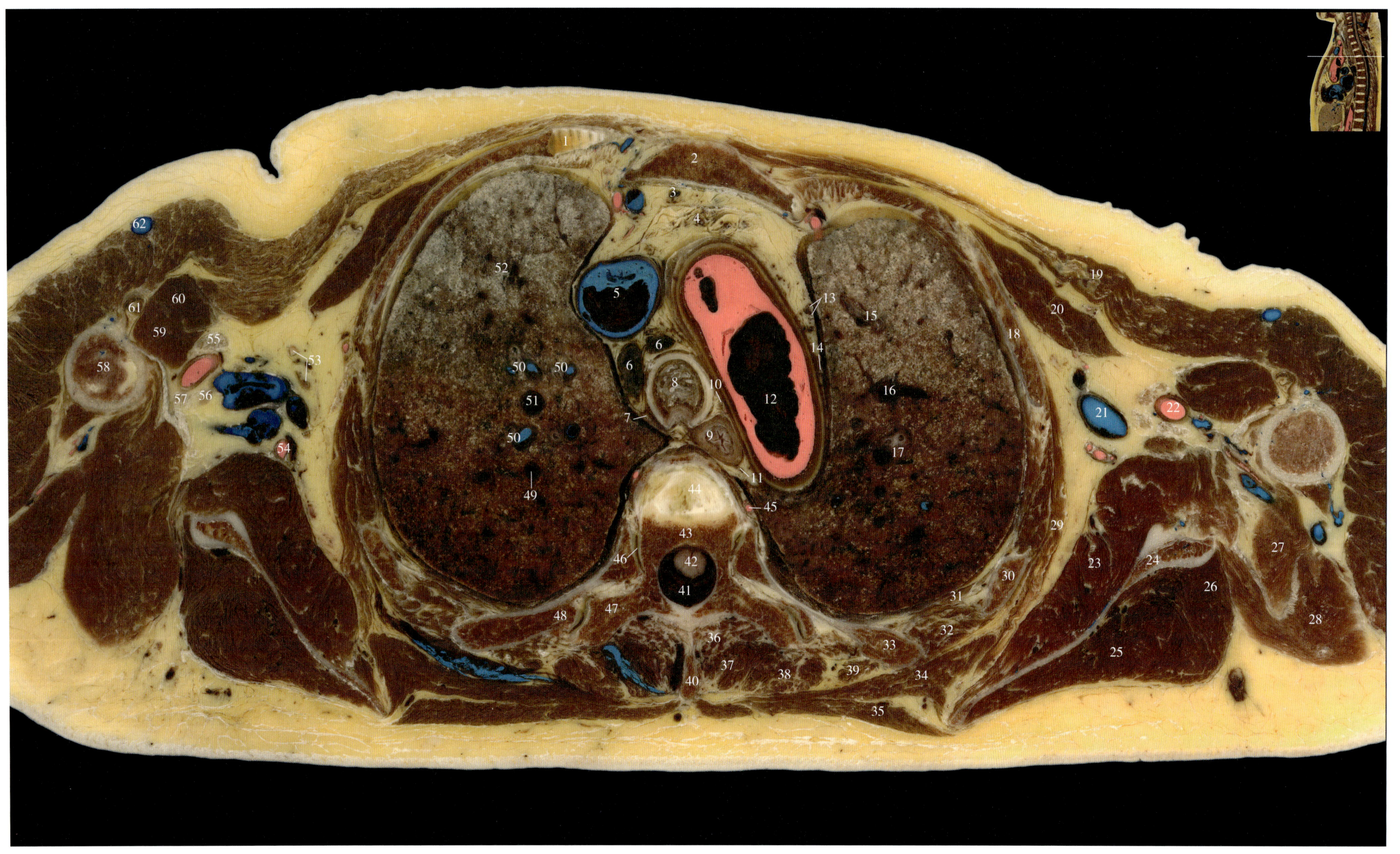

A. 断层标本图像

1. 第 2 肋软骨 2nd costal cartilage
2. 胸骨柄 manubrium sterni
3. 前纵隔淋巴结（3a）anterior mediastinal lymph nodes
4. 胸腺 thymus
5. 上腔静脉 superior vena cava
6. 右下气管旁淋巴结（4R）right lower paratracheal lymph nodes
7. 右迷走神经 right vagus nerve
8. 气管 trachea
9. 食管 esophagus
10. 左喉返神经 left recurrent laryngeal nerve
11. 胸导管 thoracic duct
12. 主动脉弓 aortic arch
13. 膈神经和心包膈血管 phrenic nerve and pericardiacophrenic vessels
14. 左迷走神经 left vagus nerve
15. 前段支气管（B3）和动脉（A3）anterior segmental bronchus and artery
16. 尖后段静脉（V1+2）apicoposterior segmental vein
17. 尖后段支气管（B1+2）和动脉（A1+2）apicoposterior segmental bronchus and artery
18. 第 2 肋骨 2nd costal bone
19. 胸大肌 pectoralis major
20. 胸小肌 pectoralis minor
21. 腋静脉 axillary vein
22. 腋动脉 axillary artery
23. 肩胛下肌 subscapularis
24. 肩胛骨 scapula
25. 冈下肌 infraspinatus
26. 小圆肌 teres minor
27. 大圆肌 teres major
28. 肱三头肌 triceps brachii
29. 前锯肌 serratus anterior
30. 第 3 肋骨 3rd costal bone
31. 肋间最内肌 intercostales intimi
32. 肋间内、外肌 intercostales interni and externi
33. 第 4 肋骨 4th costal bone
34. 菱形肌 rhomboideus
35. 斜方肌 trapezius
36. 横突棘肌 transversospinales
37. 棘肌 spinales
38. 最长肌 longissimus
39. 髂肋肌 iliocostalis
40. 棘突 spinous process
41. 硬膜外隙 epidural space
42. 脊髓 spinal cord
43. 第 4 胸椎椎体 body of 4th thoracic vertebra
44. T3-4 椎间盘 T3-4 intervertebral disc
45. 肋间后动脉 posterior intercostal artery
46. 肋头关节 joint of costal head
47. 横突 transverse process
48. 肋横突关节 costotransverse joint
49. 后段静脉（V2）posterior segmental vein
50. 尖段支气管（B1）和动脉（A1）apical segmental bronchus and artery
51. 尖段静脉尖支（V1）apical branch of apical segmental vein
52. 尖段静脉（V1）apical segmental vein
53. 腋淋巴结 axillary lymph nodes
54. 肩胛下动脉 subscapular artery
55. 臂丛外侧束 lateral cord of brachial plexus
56. 臂丛内侧束 medial cord of brachial plexus
57. 臂丛后束 posterior cord of brachial plexus
58. 肱骨 humerus
59. 喙肱肌 coracobrachialis
60. 肱二头肌短头 short head of biceps brachii
61. 肱二头肌长头 long head of biceps brachii
62. 头静脉 cephalic vein

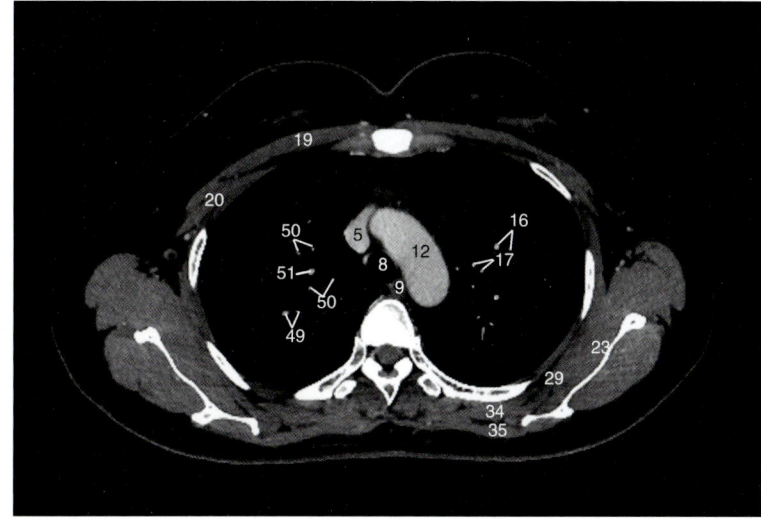

B. CT 纵隔窗增强图像

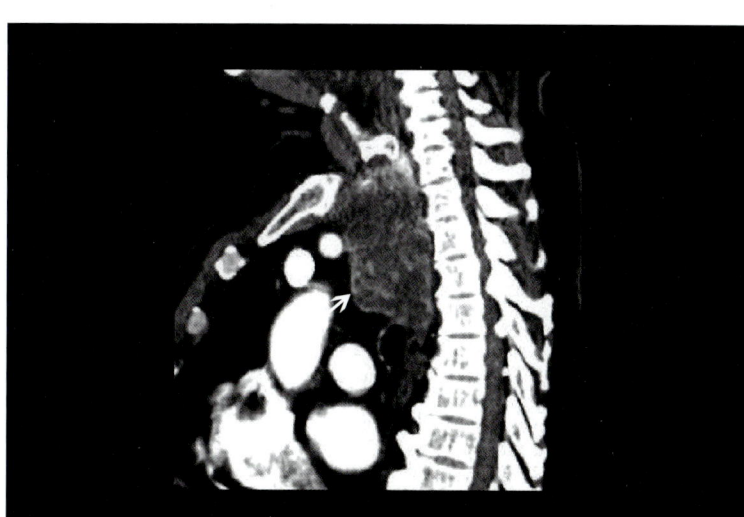

C. CT 肺窗图像

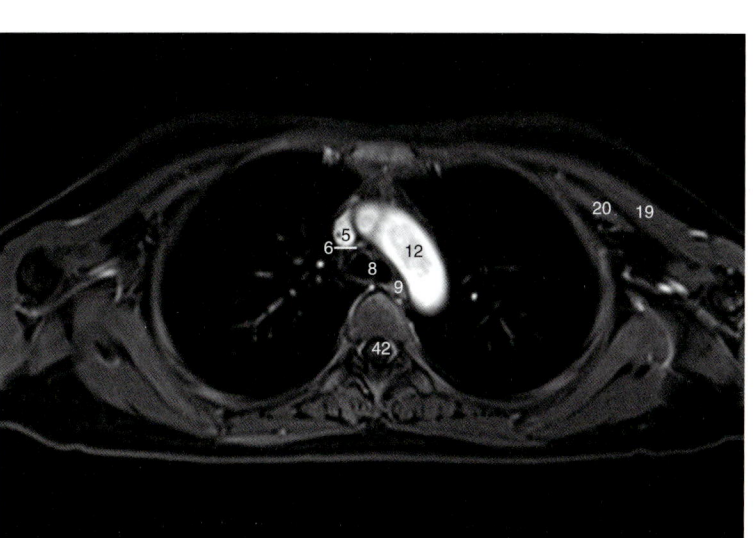

D. MR T1WI 增强图像

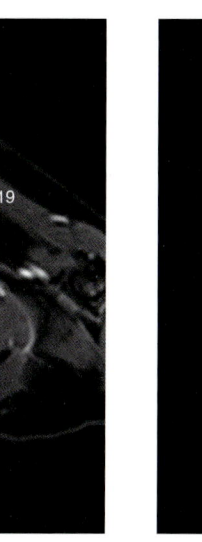

E. 胸骨后甲状腺肿矢状位 CT 图像

关键结构：上腔静脉，胸骨后间隙。

此断面经 T3-4 椎间盘下份。

上腔静脉于本断面完全合成。左迷走神经紧贴主动脉弓外侧，右迷走神经紧贴气管右侧。该标本右肺上叶尖段静脉分为尖支、上支和下支。其中尖支向下注入后段静脉，上支和下支汇入尖段静脉。沿尖段静脉、后段静脉走行方向连线，可将右肺上叶尖段与其外侧的后段、前段划分开来；沿后段静脉走行方向划线，可将后段与前方的前段、尖段划分开来。左肺上叶由前向后依次可见前段和尖后段，可依尖后段静脉走行方向划线将上述二者划分开来。此断面上，尖后段较大。胸骨后间隙位于胸骨后方，胸内筋膜前方，向下至膈。该间隙的炎症可向纵隔蔓延，甚而穿破膈肌扩散至腹膜外脂肪层。胸骨后甲状腺肿是上纵隔的常见病变，占纵隔肿瘤的 5.7%，其发病率国内报道占甲状腺疾病的 9%~16%；国外统计该病的发病率为 2.6%~30.4%，占所有甲状腺手术的 3%~20%。胸骨后甲状腺肿以 40 岁以上女性居多，其生长缓慢，患者就诊时体积多已较大，故病程长，如胸骨后甲状腺肿矢状位 CT 图像中箭头所示。胸骨后甲状腺肿良性病变居多，恶性病变占发病率的 3%~10%。胸骨后甲状腺肿一般分为 3 种类型：Ⅰ型为不完全型，甲状腺肿部分或大部分延伸于胸骨后，与颈部甲状腺组织相连接；Ⅱ型为完全型胸骨后甲状腺肿，甲状腺肿沿气管延伸完全坠入胸骨后，仅存小血管、纤维锁带与颈部甲状腺组织相连；Ⅲ型为胸内迷走甲状腺肿，可出现在舌至膈之间的任何部位[24]。

胸部连续横断层 26（FH.12990）

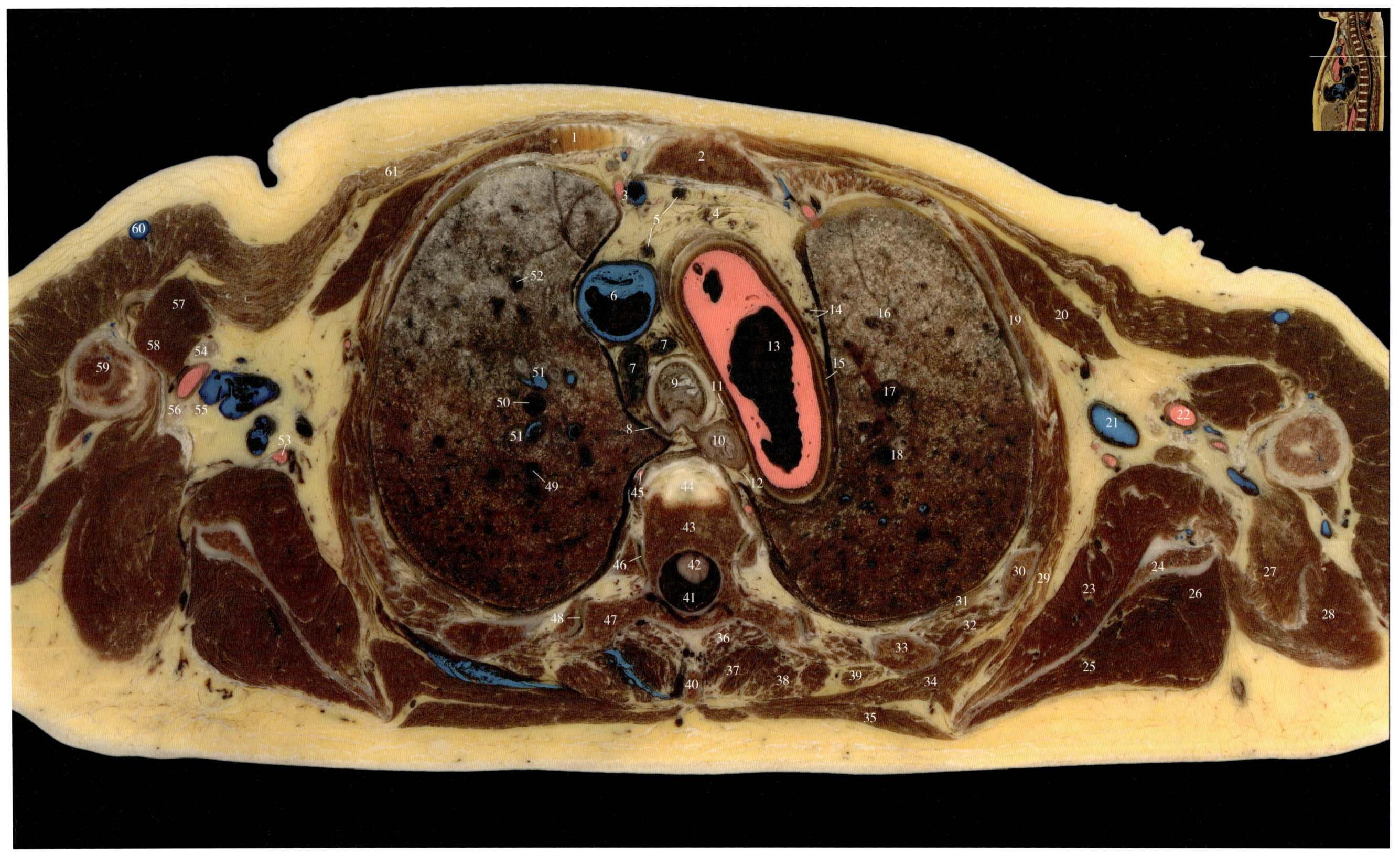

A. 断层标本图像

1. 第2肋软骨 2nd costal cartilage
2. 胸骨柄 manubrium sterni
3. 胸廓内动、静脉 internal thoracic artery and vein
4. 胸腺 thymus
5. 前纵隔淋巴结（3a）anterior mediastinal lymph nodes
6. 上腔静脉 superior vena cava
7. 右下气管旁淋巴结（4R）right lower paratracheal lymph nodes
8. 右迷走神经 right vagus nerve
9. 气管 trachea
10. 食管 esophagus
11. 左喉返神经 left recurrent laryngeal nerve
12. 胸导管 thoracic duct
13. 主动脉弓 aortic arch
14. 膈神经和心包膈血管 phrenic nerve and pericardiacophrenic vessels
15. 左迷走神经 left vagus nerve
16. 前段支气管（B3）和动脉（A3）anterior segmental bronchus and artery
17. 尖后段静脉（V1+2）apicoposterior segmental vein
18. 尖后段支气管（B1+2）和动脉（A1+2）apicoposterior segmental bronchus and artery
19. 第2肋骨 2nd costal bone
20. 胸小肌 pectoralis minor
21. 腋静脉 axillary vein
22. 腋动脉 axillary artery
23. 肩胛下肌 subscapularis
24. 肩胛骨 scapula
25. 冈下肌 infraspinatus
26. 小圆肌 teres minor
27. 大圆肌 teres major
28. 肱三头肌 triceps brachii
29. 前锯肌 serratus anterior
30. 第3肋骨 3rd costal bone
31. 肋间最内肌 intercostales intimi
32. 肋间内、外肌 intercostales interni and externi
33. 第4肋骨 4th costal bone
34. 菱形肌 rhomboideus
35. 斜方肌 trapezius
36. 横突棘肌 transversospinales
37. 棘肌 spinales
38. 最长肌 longissimus
39. 髂肋肌 iliocostalis
40. 棘突 spinous process
41. 硬膜外隙 epidural space
42. 脊髓 spinal cord
43. 第4胸椎椎体 body of 4th thoracic vertebra
44. T3-4椎间盘 T3-4 intervertebral disc
45. 肋间后动脉 posterior intercostal artery
46. 肋头关节 joint of costal head
47. 横突 transverse process
48. 肋横突关节 costotransverse joint
49. 后段静脉（V2）posterior segmental vein
50. 尖段静脉尖支（V1）apical branch of apical segmental vein
51. 尖段支气管（B1）和动脉（A1）apical segmental bronchus and artery
52. 尖段静脉（V1）apical segmental vein
53. 肩胛下动脉 subscapular artery
54. 臂丛外侧束 lateral cord of brachial plexus
55. 臂丛内侧束 medial cord of brachial plexus
56. 臂丛后束 posterior cord of brachial plexus
57. 肱二头肌短头 short head of biceps brachii
58. 喙肱肌 coracobrachialis
59. 肱骨 humerus
60. 头静脉 cephalic vein
61. 胸大肌 pectoralis major

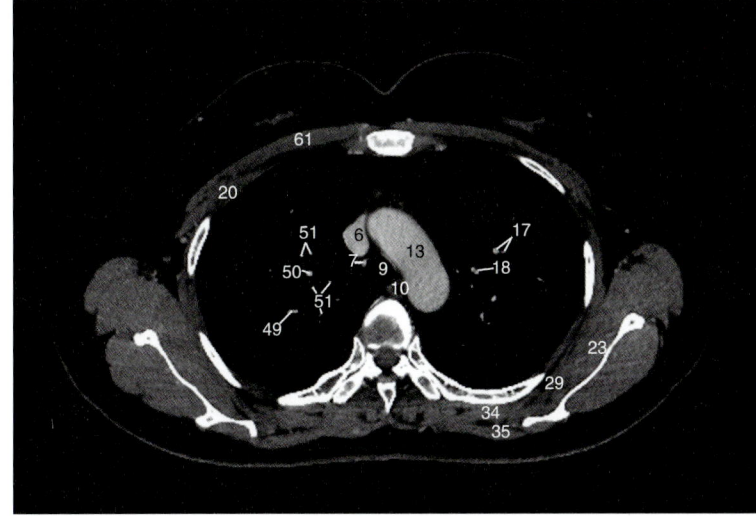

B. CT 纵隔窗增强图像

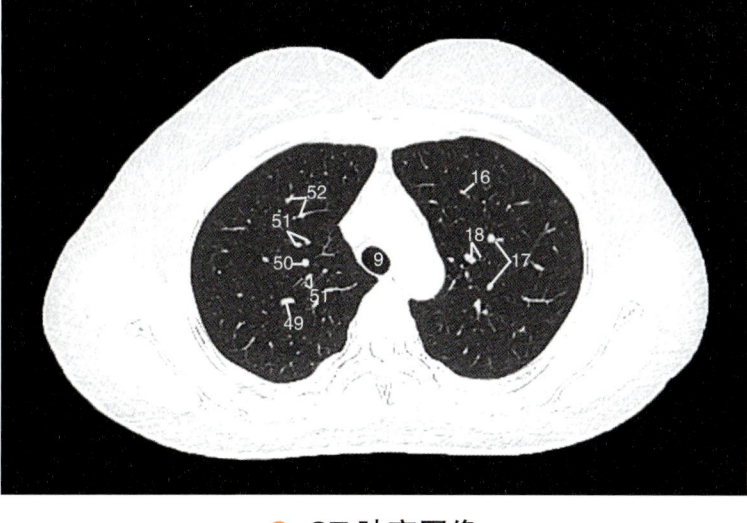

C. CT 肺窗图像

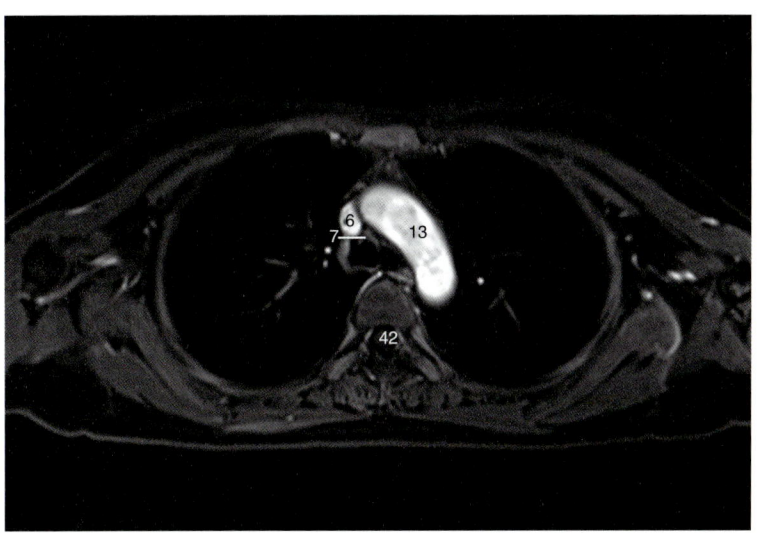

D. MR T1WI 增强图像

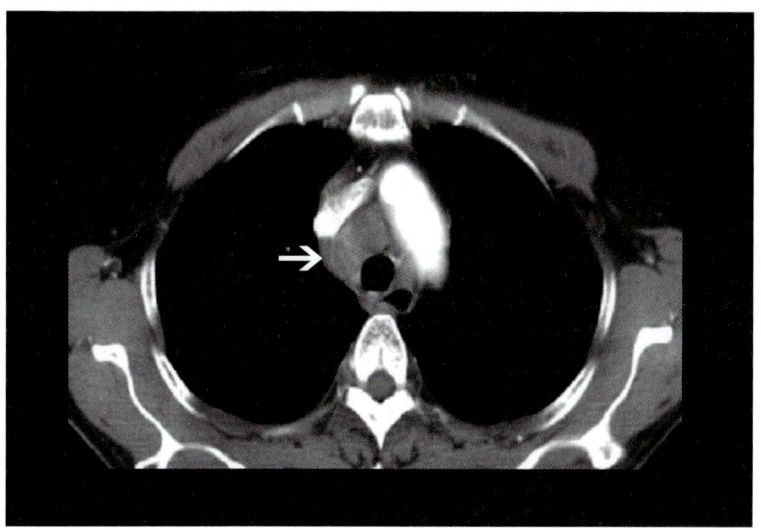

E. 4R 区淋巴结转移 CT 图像

关键结构：前纵隔淋巴结，奇静脉弓淋巴结。

此断面经第4胸椎椎体上份。

在两侧纵隔胸膜、胸骨柄和脊柱之间为上纵隔。在上纵隔内可见主动脉弓成腊肠样贴近纵隔左缘，弓的左缘微凸，右缘微凹，并由前斜向左后方。主动脉弓的内侧从前向后依次是上腔静脉、气管、食管。前纵隔淋巴结（3a）出现在血管前间隙，可见2枚。在主动脉弓右侧、上腔静脉后方和气管前方之间充满疏松结缔组织和脂肪组织的区域，称气管前间隙。此间隙向上经胸廓上口与颈部的气管前间隙相续连，向下达气管隆嵴平面。间隙内有气管前淋巴结（奇静脉弓淋巴结）和心包上隐窝。该断层气管前间隙内有2个奇静脉弓淋巴结，其属于右下气管旁淋巴结（4R），出现率为100%[25]。E图箭头所示为肺癌伴该区域淋巴结转移。气管旁淋巴结以气管左缘为界，分为左、右两组（4L、4R）。4L位于气管左侧缘和动脉韧带之间，上界为主动脉弓上缘，下界为左肺动脉干上缘（气管隆嵴水平）；4R包括右侧气管旁和气管前淋巴结，上界为头臂静脉与气管交叉处下缘，下界为奇静脉弓下缘（气管隆嵴水平）。

胸部连续横断层 27（FH.12970）

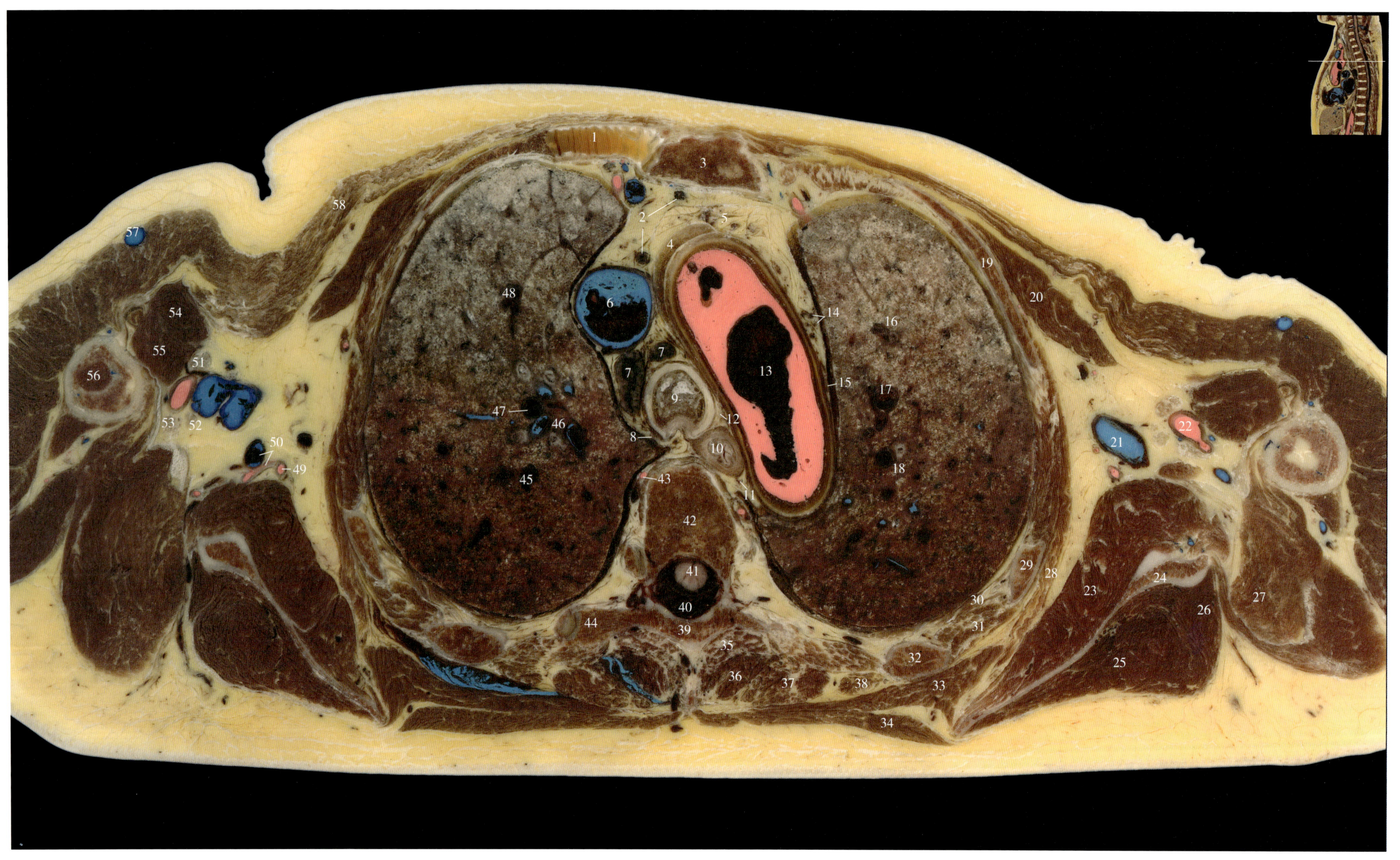

A. 断层标本图像

1. 第 2 肋软骨 2nd costal cartilage
2. 前纵隔淋巴结（3a）anterior mediastinal lymph nodes
3. 胸骨柄 manubrium sterni
4. 心包上隐窝 superior recess of pericardium
5. 胸腺 thymus
6. 上腔静脉 superior vena cava
7. 右下气管旁淋巴结（4R）right lower paratracheal lymph nodes
8. 右迷走神经 right vagus nerve
9. 气管 trachea
10. 食管 esophagus
11. 胸导管 thoracic duct
12. 左喉返神经 left recurrent laryngeal nerve
13. 主动脉弓 aortic arch
14. 膈神经和心包膈血管 phrenic nerve and pericardiacophrenic vessels
15. 左迷走神经 left vagus nerve
16. 前段支气管（B3）和动脉（A3）anterior segmental bronchus and artery
17. 尖后段静脉（V1+2）apicoposterior segmental vein
18. 尖后段支气管（B1+2）和动脉（A1+2）apicoposterior segmental bronchus and artery
19. 第 2 肋骨 2nd costal bone
20. 胸小肌 pectoralis minor
21. 腋静脉 axillary vein
22. 腋动脉 axillary artery
23. 肩胛下肌 subscapularis
24. 肩胛骨 scapula
25. 冈下肌 infraspinatus
26. 小圆肌 teres minor
27. 大圆肌 teres major
28. 前锯肌 serratus anterior
29. 第 3 肋骨 3rd costal bone
30. 肋间最内肌 intercostales intimi
31. 肋间内、外肌 intercostales interni and externi
32. 第 4 肋骨 4th costal bone
33. 菱形肌 rhomboideus
34. 斜方肌 trapezius
35. 横突棘肌 transversospinales
36. 棘肌 spinales
37. 最长肌 longissimus
38. 髂肋肌 iliocostalis
39. 椎弓板 lamina of vertebral arch
40. 硬膜外隙 epidural space
41. 脊髓 spinal cord
42. 第 4 胸椎椎体 body of 4th thoracic vertebra
43. 肋间后动脉 posterior intercostal artery
44. 横突 transverse process
45. 后段静脉（V2）posterior segmental vein
46. 尖段支气管（B1）和动脉（A1）apical segmental bronchus and artery
47. 尖段静脉尖支（V1）apical branch of apical segmental vein
48. 尖段静脉（V1）apical segmental vein
49. 胸背动脉 thoracodorsal artery
50. 旋肩胛动、静脉 circumflex scapular artery and vein
51. 臂丛外侧束 lateral cord of brachial plexus
52. 臂丛内侧束 medial cord of brachial plexus
53. 臂丛后束 posterior cord of brachial plexus
54. 肱二头肌短头 short head of biceps brachii
55. 喙肱肌 coracobrachialis
56. 肱骨 humerus
57. 头静脉 cephalic vein
58. 胸大肌 pectoralis major

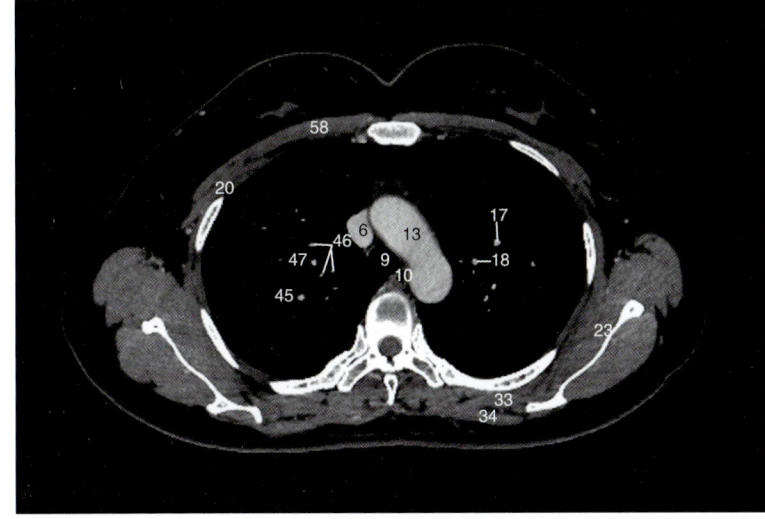

B. CT 纵隔窗增强图像

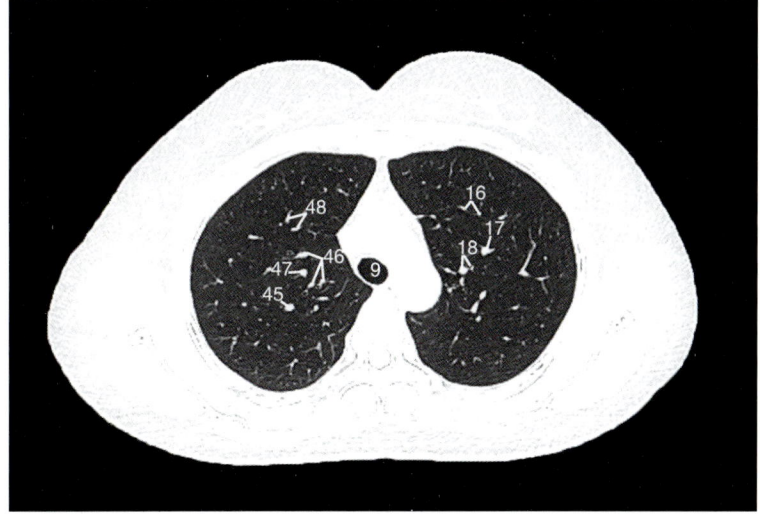

C. CT 肺窗图像

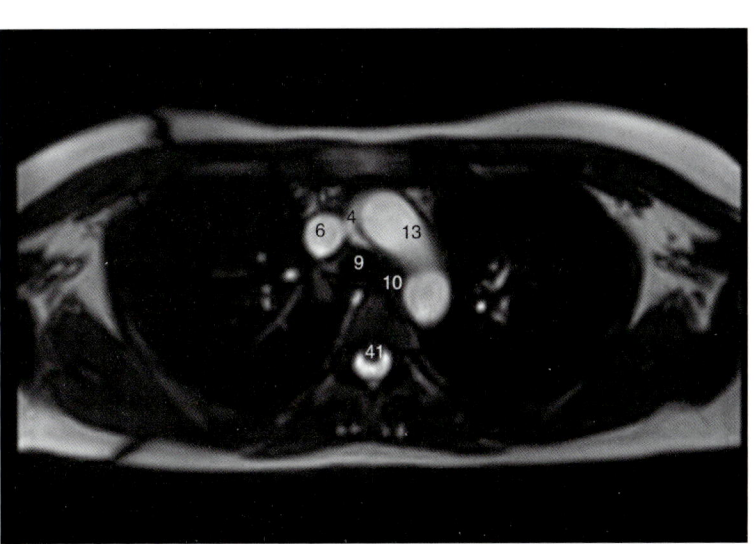

D. MR T2WI 平扫图像

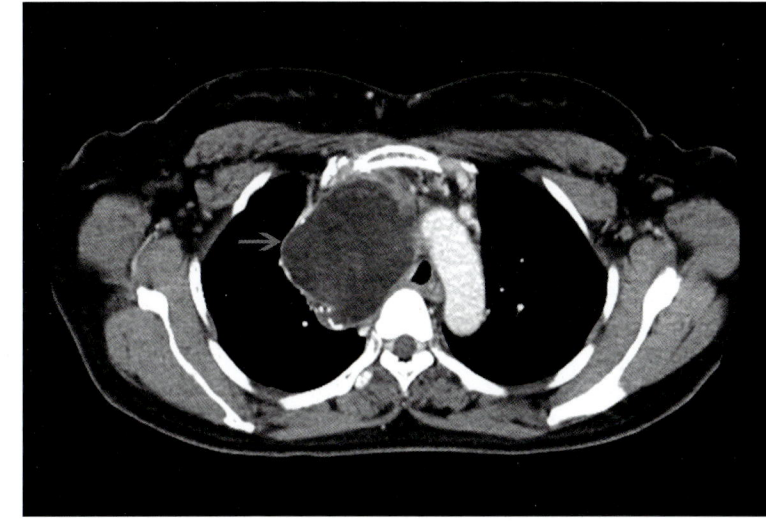

E. 畸胎瘤 CT 图像

关键结构：心包上隐窝，背肌，背阔肌。

此断面经第 4 胸椎椎体上份。

肺的横断面呈牛角状。心包上隐窝呈弯月状，位于主动脉弓的右前方，前方为胸腺。左心包膈血管、左膈神经、左迷走神经位于主动脉弓的外侧。主动脉弓的内侧从前向后依次是上腔静脉、气管、食管。气管食管间沟与主动脉弓之间有左喉返神经。食管、主动脉弓、椎体之间有胸导管。E 图箭头所示为畸胎瘤，该瘤以前、中纵隔最多见，较大者肿块可突向中、后纵隔。畸胎类肿瘤分为囊性畸胎瘤（皮样囊肿）和实性畸胎瘤（畸胎瘤）。多数肿块呈类圆形，边缘清晰光滑，可有分叶。囊性畸胎瘤呈均匀囊性密度，囊壁常见蛋壳样钙化。实性畸胎瘤呈混杂密度，内可见软组织密度、脂肪密度、水样密度钙化等成分。肿块内脂液平面具有一定特征性。肿瘤内骨化及牙齿影是畸胎类肿瘤的特征性表现。增强扫描后肿瘤的囊壁及实质部分可见轻至中度强化。囊性畸胎瘤有自发破裂的倾向，可导致胸膜腔积液、肺部感染等[26]。背肌分为浅、中、深 3 层。浅层包括斜方肌、背阔肌、肩胛提肌和菱形肌。背阔肌皮瓣是临床最常用的肌皮瓣之一，因部位隐蔽、血运丰富、切取范围大、抗感染能力强，是理想的肌皮瓣选择，常被用于修复上肢、颈部、面部及胸部大面积缺损[27]。背肌中层为上、下后锯肌，较薄，为呼吸肌。背深层肌为竖脊肌（包括髂肋肌、最长肌、棘肌）和横突棘肌（可分为半棘肌、多裂肌、回旋肌）及一些小的短肌。

胸部连续横断层 28 (FH.12950)

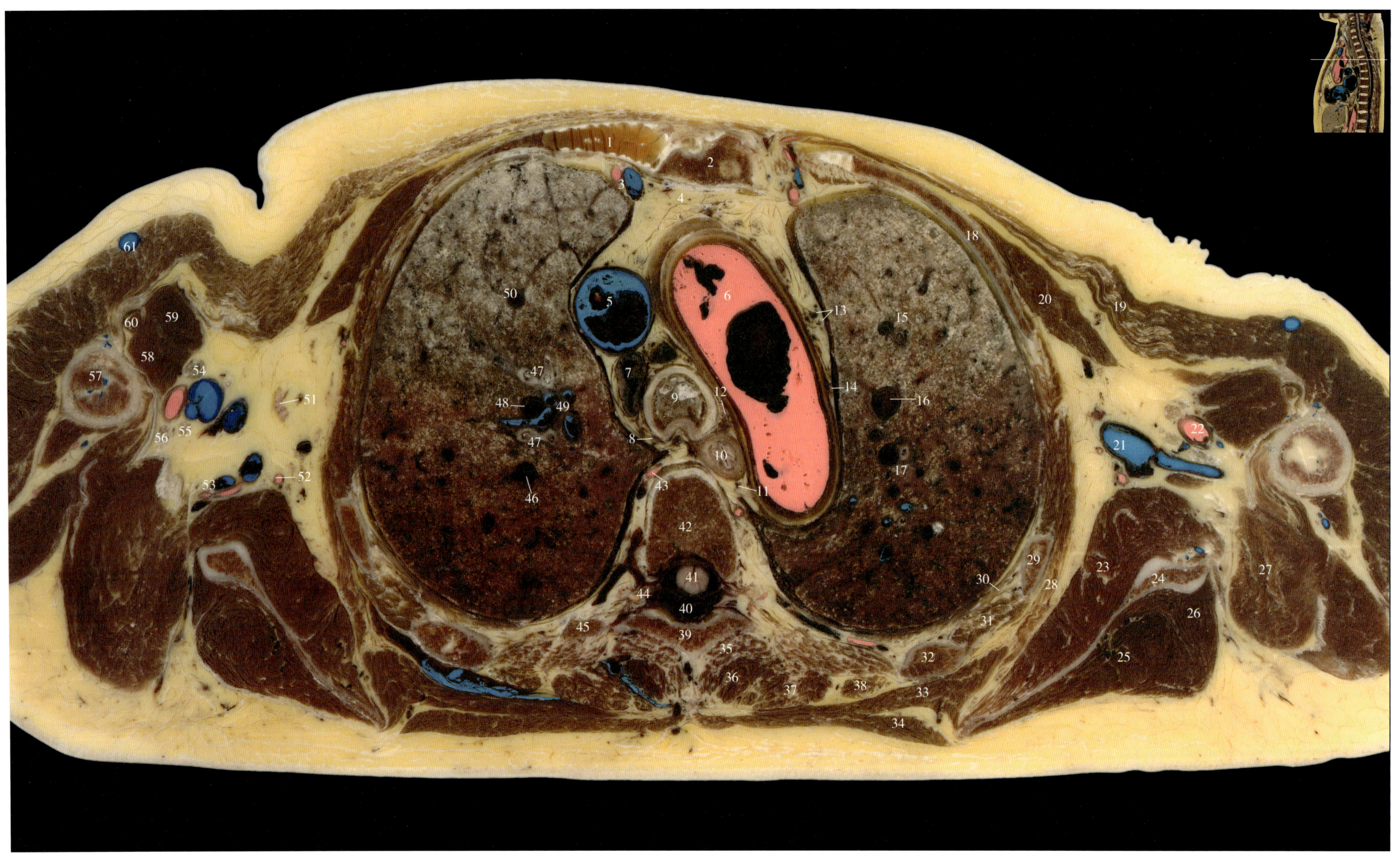

A. 断层标本图像

1. 第2肋软骨 2nd costal cartilage
2. 胸骨柄 manubrium sterni
3. 胸廓内动、静脉 internal thoracic artery and vein
4. 胸腺 thymus
5. 上腔静脉 superior vena cava
6. 主动脉弓 aortic arch
7. 右下气管旁淋巴结（4R）right lower paratracheal lymph nodes
8. 右迷走神经 right vagus nerve
9. 气管 trachea
10. 食管 esophagus
11. 胸导管 thoracic duct
12. 左喉返神经 left recurrent laryngeal nerve
13. 膈神经和心包膈血管 phrenic nerve and pericardiacophrenic vessels
14. 左迷走神经 left vagus nerve
15. 前段支气管（B3）和动脉（A3）anterior segmental bronchus and artery
16. 尖后段静脉（V1+2）apicoposterior segmental vein
17. 尖后段支气管（B1+2）和动脉（A1+2）apicoposterior segmental bronchus and artery
18. 第2肋骨 2nd costal bone
19. 胸大肌 pectoralis major
20. 胸小肌 pectoralis minor
21. 腋静脉 axillary vein
22. 腋动脉 axillary artery
23. 肩胛下肌 subscapularis
24. 肩胛骨 scapula
25. 冈下肌 infraspinatus
26. 小圆肌 teres minor
27. 大圆肌 teres major
28. 前锯肌 serratus anterior
29. 第3肋骨 3rd costal bone
30. 肋间最内肌 intercostales intimi
31. 肋间内、外肌 intercostales interni and externi
32. 第4肋骨 4th costal bone
33. 菱形肌 rhomboideus
34. 斜方肌 trapezius
35. 横突棘肌 transversospinales
36. 棘肌 spinales
37. 最长肌 longissimus
38. 髂肋肌 iliocostalis
39. 椎弓板 lamina of vertebral arch
40. 硬膜外隙 epidural space
41. 脊髓 spinal cord
42. 第4胸椎椎体 body of 4th thoracic vertebra
43. 肋间后动脉 posterior intercostal artery
44. 第4胸神经 4th thoracic nerve
45. 横突 transverse process
46. 后段静脉（V2）posterior segmental vein
47. 尖段支气管（B1）apical segmental bronchus
48. 尖段静脉尖支（V1）apical branch of apical segmental vein
49. 尖段动脉（A1）apical segmental artery
50. 尖段静脉（V1）apical segmental vein
51. 腋淋巴结 axillary lymph nodes
52. 胸背动脉 thoracodorsal artery
53. 旋肩胛动、静脉 circumflex scapular artery and vein
54. 臂丛外侧束 lateral cord of brachial plexus
55. 臂丛内侧束 medial cord of brachial plexus
56. 臂丛后束 posterior cord of brachial plexus
57. 肱骨 humerus
58. 喙肱肌 coracobrachialis
59. 肱二头肌短头 short head of biceps brachii
60. 肱二头肌长头 long head of biceps brachii
61. 头静脉 cephalic vein

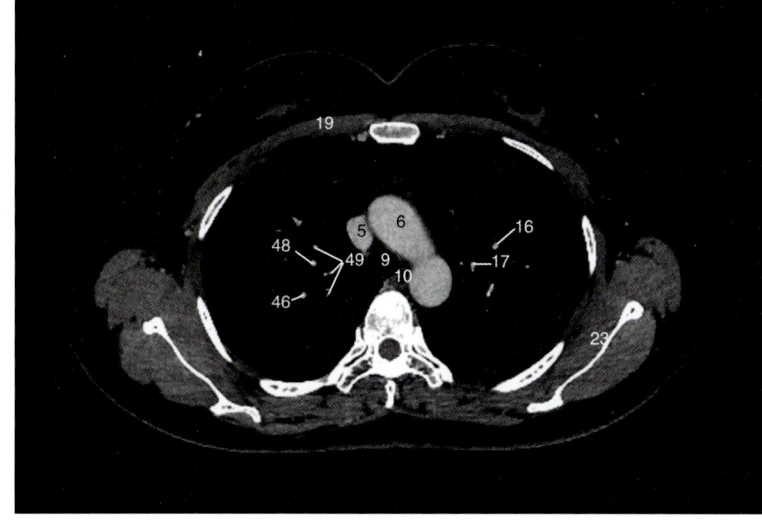

B. CT 纵隔窗增强图像

C. CT 肺窗图像

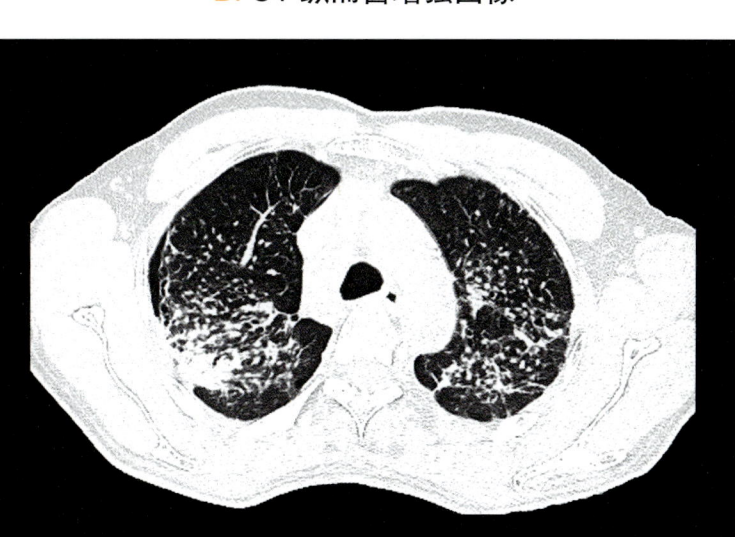

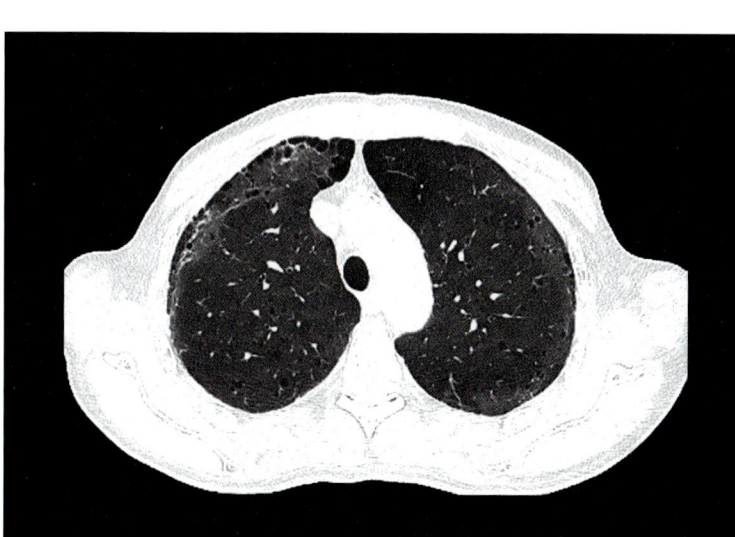

D. 肺结核合并右侧气胸 CT 图像

E. 间质性肺炎合并肺气肿 CT 图像

关键结构：肺上叶，胸廓内动、静脉。

此断面经第4胸椎椎体上份。

胸廓内动脉在胸膜顶前方、正对椎动脉起始处发自锁骨下动脉下壁，于锁骨下静脉后方、胸膜顶前方下降入胸腔，与胸廓内静脉伴行。双肺断面逐渐扩大，左肺上叶从前向后为前段和尖后段；右肺上叶为前段、尖段和后段。双肺上叶为结核的好发部位，如图 D 所示，影像学表现为双肺多发团片状、结节状高密度影，分布不均匀，部分小叶间隔增厚，右侧胸腔同时见弧形气体密度影。图 E 所示为双肺上叶间质性肺炎，影像学表现为双肺胸膜下絮状、弧形高密度影，局部呈网格样改变，小叶间隔增厚；双肺亦可见类圆形乏肺纹理透光区，提示肺气肿表现。右下气管旁淋巴结（4R）显示清晰，包括右气管旁淋巴结和气管前淋巴结。应用成人尸体解剖乳胶填充剂行胸部淋巴结灌注后，游离各区淋巴结发现，纵隔淋巴结以隆嵴下淋巴结和右下气管旁淋巴结为最多，其次为右气管支气管旁、左支气管旁和主-肺动脉窗区淋巴结。纵隔各区以隆嵴下区（7区）淋巴结最大，其次是右气管支气管旁（10R）淋巴结。气管旁淋巴结自上而下直至隆嵴下淋巴结逐渐增大，并且右侧大于左侧，即下大于上，右大于左[28]。隆嵴下淋巴结最大，平均短径为 6.4 mm ± 3.1 mm，长径为 7.6 mm ± 4.1 mm，其余各级短径平均为 3.4~5.5 mm，长径平均为 4.1~6.4 mm；每组的 CT 测量值与解剖测量值有着密切的对应关系[29]。

胸部连续横断层29（FH.12930）

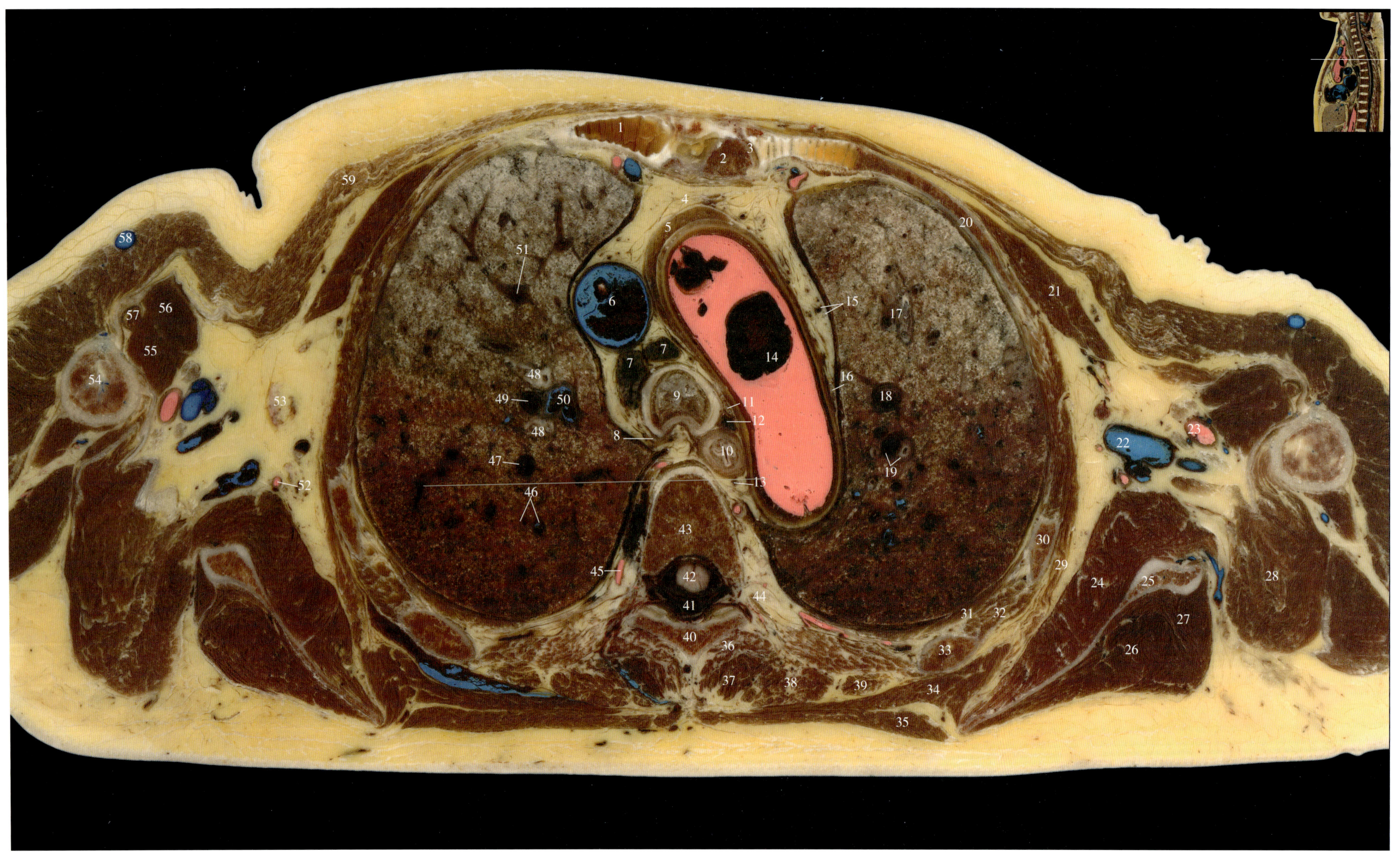

A. 断层标本图像

1. 第 2 肋软骨 2nd costal cartilage
2. 胸骨柄 manubrium sterni
3. 第 2 胸肋关节 2nd sternocostal joint
4. 胸腺 thymus
5. 心包上隐窝 superior recess of pericardium
6. 上腔静脉 superior vena cava
7. 右下气管旁淋巴结（4R）right lower paratracheal lymph nodes
8. 右迷走神经 right vagus nerve
9. 气管 trachea
10. 食管 esophagus
11. 左喉返神经 left recurrent laryngeal nerve
12. 左下气管旁淋巴结（4L）left lower paratracheal lymph nodes
13. 胸导管 thoracic duct
14. 主动脉弓 aortic arch
15. 膈神经和心包膈血管 phrenic nerve and pericardiacophrenic vessels
16. 左迷走神经 left vagus nerve
17. 前段支气管（B3）和动脉（A3）anterior segmental bronchus and artery
18. 尖后段静脉（V1+2）apicoposterior segmental vein
19. 尖后段支气管（B1+2）和动脉（A1+2）apicoposterior segmental bronchus and artery
20. 第 2 肋骨 2nd costal bone
21. 胸小肌 pectoralis minor
22. 腋静脉 axillary vein
23. 腋动脉 axillary artery
24. 肩胛下肌 subscapularis
25. 肩胛骨 scapula
26. 冈下肌 infraspinatus
27. 小圆肌 teres minor
28. 大圆肌 teres major
29. 前锯肌 serratus anterior
30. 第 3 肋骨 3rd costal bone
31. 肋间最内肌 intercostales intimi
32. 肋间内、外肌 intercostales interni and externi
33. 第 4 肋骨 4th costal bone
34. 菱形肌 rhomboideus
35. 斜方肌 trapezius
36. 横突棘肌 transversospinales
37. 棘肌 spinales
38. 最长肌 longissimus
39. 髂肋肌 iliocostalis
40. 椎弓板 lamina of vertebral arch
41. 硬膜外隙 epidural space
42. 脊髓 spinal cord
43. 第 4 胸椎椎体 body of 4th thoracic vertebra
44. 第 4 胸神经 4th thoracic nerve
45. 肋间后动脉 posterior intercostal artery
46. 后段支气管（B2）和动脉（A2）posterior segmental bronchus and artery
47. 后段静脉（V2）posterior segmental vein
48. 尖段支气管（B1）apical segmental bronchus
49. 尖段静脉尖支（V1）apical branch of apical segmental vein
50. 尖段动脉（A1）apical segmental artery
51. 尖段静脉（V1）apical segmental vein
52. 胸背动脉 thoracodorsal artery
53. 腋淋巴结 axillary lymph nodes
54. 肱骨 humerus
55. 喙肱肌 coracobrachialis
56. 肱二头肌短头 short head of biceps brachii
57. 肱二头肌长头 long head of biceps brachii
58. 头静脉 cephalic vein
59. 胸大肌 pectoralis major

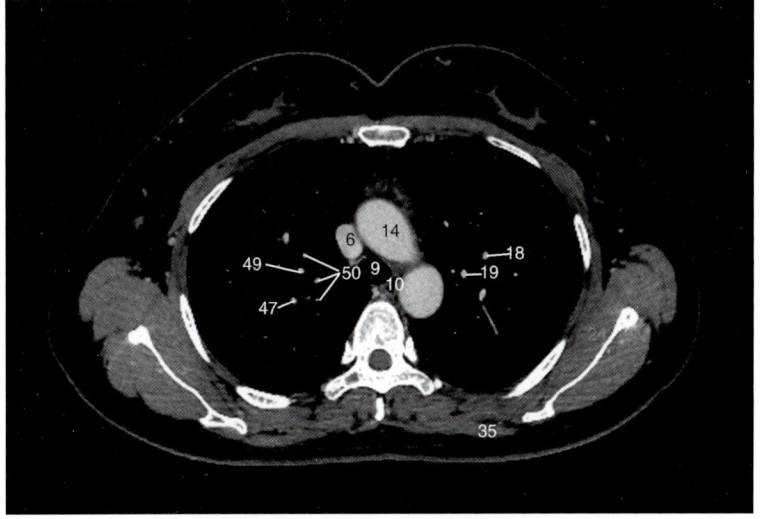

B. CT 纵隔窗增强图像

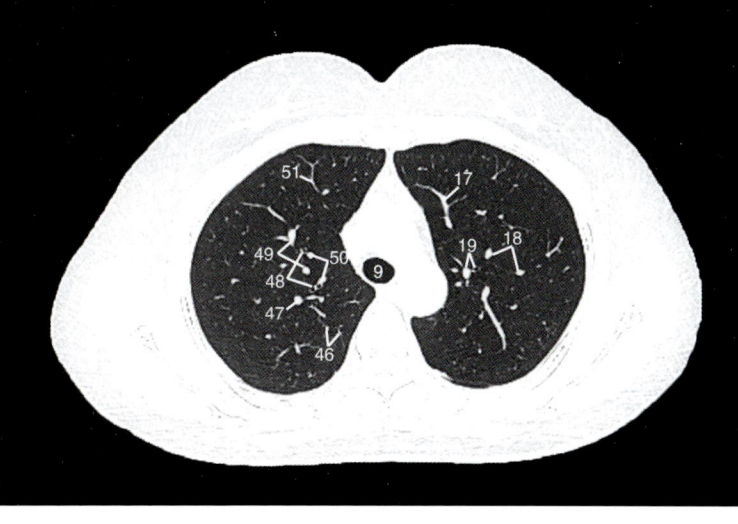

C. CT 肺窗图像

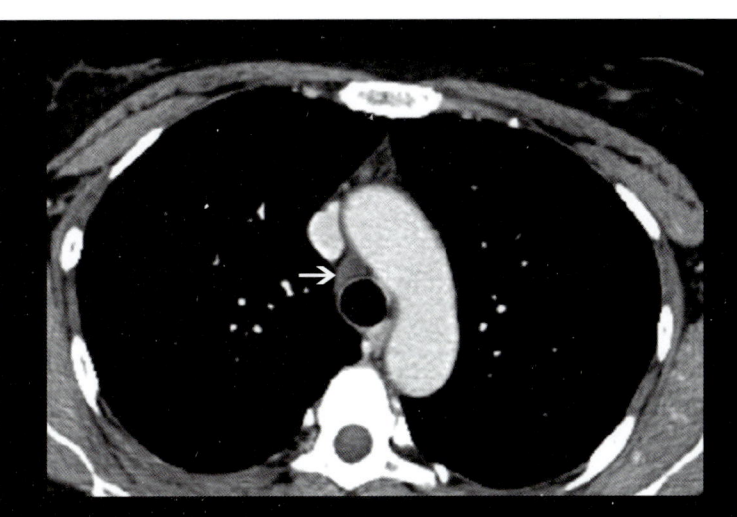

D. 正常心包上隐窝 CT 图像

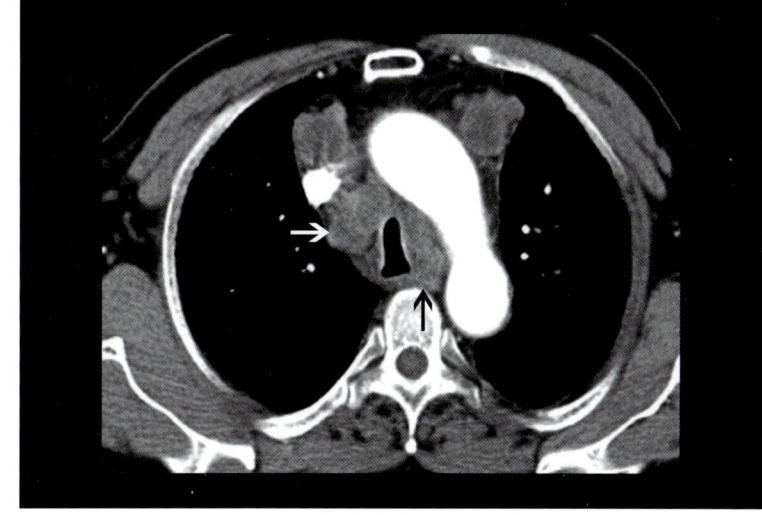

E. 4R、4L 区淋巴结转移 CT 图像

关键结构：心包上隐窝，右下气管旁淋巴结，左下气管旁淋巴结。

此断面经第 4 胸椎椎体中份。

心包上隐窝呈弯月状，位于主动脉弓的右前方，前方为胸腺。其在 CT 检查时，心包上隐窝的积液可能会被误诊为冠状动脉、主动脉夹层、肿大淋巴结，或是右肺小的转移病灶，增强扫描具有一定的鉴别意义。心包上隐窝亦称心包上窦或主动脉上隐窝，它构成心包返折的上界。在气管分叉水平，心包上隐窝围绕升主动脉的前、右、后面和肺动脉干前方，直至肺动脉干与左肺动脉交角处。横轴位 CT 图像上，心包上隐窝通常表现为紧邻升主动脉后壁的半月形水样密度结构，影像学表现变异较大。心包上隐窝有时位置较高，表现为高骑跨的心包上隐窝[30,31]，即正常部位的心包上隐窝沿主动脉向上延伸至右侧气管旁区、头臂血管和气管之间。CT 图像上表现为边缘锐利、均匀的水样密度结构，无壁可见，其尾侧与升主动脉后方常见部位的心包上隐窝相连续。D 图箭头所示为正常心包上隐窝。上腔静脉与气管之间可见右下气管旁淋巴结（4R）。气管食管与主动脉弓之间可见左下气管旁淋巴结（4L）。4R、4L 区淋巴结转移 CT 图像中箭头所示为增大的转移淋巴结。

胸部连续横断层 30（FH.12910）

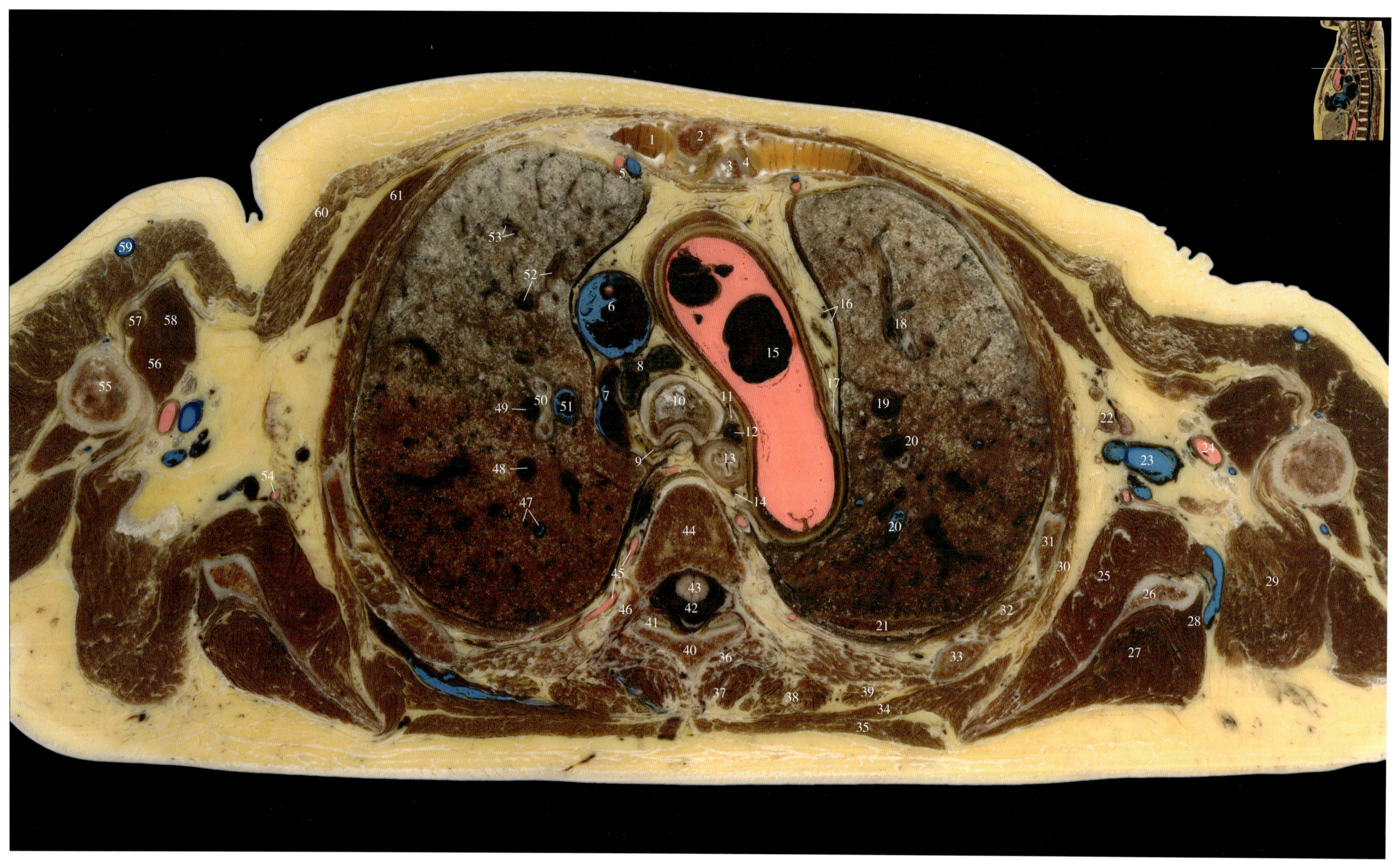

A. 断层标本图像

1. 第2肋软骨 2nd costal cartilage
2. 胸骨体 body of sternum
3. 胸骨柄 manubrium sterni
4. 第2胸肋关节 2nd sternocostal joint
5. 胸廓内动、静脉 internal thoracic artery and vein
6. 上腔静脉 superior vena cava
7. 奇静脉弓 arch of azygos vein
8. 右下气管旁淋巴结（4R）right lower paratracheal lymph nodes
9. 右迷走神经 right vagus nerve
10. 气管 trachea
11. 左喉返神经 left recurrent laryngeal nerve
12. 左下气管旁淋巴结（4L）left lower paratracheal lymph nodes
13. 食管 esophagus
14. 胸导管 thoracic duct
15. 主动脉弓 aortic arch
16. 膈神经和心包膈血管 phrenic nerve and pericardiacophrenic vessels
17. 左迷走神经 left vagus nerve
18. 左肺前段支气管（B3）和动脉（A3）left anterior segmental bronchus and artery
19. 尖后段静脉（V1+2）apicoposterior segmental vein
20. 尖后段支气管（B1+2）和动脉（A1+2）apicoposterior segmental bronchus and artery
21. 左肺斜裂 oblique fissure of left lung
22. 腋淋巴结 axillary lymph nodes
23. 腋静脉 axillary vein
24. 腋动脉 axillary artery
25. 肩胛下肌 subscapularis
26. 肩胛骨 scapula
27. 冈下肌 infraspinatus
28. 小圆肌 teres minor
29. 大圆肌 teres major
30. 前锯肌 serratus anterior
31. 第3肋骨 3rd costal bone
32. 肋间内、外肌 intercostales interni and externi
33. 第4肋骨 4th costal bone
34. 菱形肌 rhomboideus
35. 斜方肌 trapezius
36. 横突棘肌 transversospinales
37. 棘肌 spinales
38. 最长肌 longissimus
39. 髂肋肌 iliocostalis
40. 椎弓板 lamina of vertebral arch
41. 关节突关节 zygapophysial joint
42. 硬膜外隙 epidural space
43. 脊髓 spinal cord
44. 第4胸椎椎体 body of 4th thoracic vertebra
45. 肋间后动脉 posterior intercostal artery
46. 第5肋骨 5th costal bone
47. 后段支气管（B2）和动脉（A2）posterior segmental bronchus and artery
48. 后段静脉（V2）posterior segmental vein
49. 尖段静脉尖支（V1）apical branch of apical segmental vein
50. 尖段支气管（B1）apical segmental bronchus
51. 尖段动脉（A1）apical segmental artery
52. 尖段静脉（V1）apical segmental vein
53. 右肺前段支气管（B3）和动脉（A3）rigth anterior segmental bronchus and artery
54. 胸背动脉 thoracodorsal artery
55. 肱骨 humerus
56. 喙肱肌 coracobrachialis
57. 肱二头肌长头 long head of biceps brachii
58. 肱二头肌短头 short head of biceps brachii
59. 头静脉 cephalic vein
60. 胸大肌 pectoralis major
61. 胸小肌 pectoralis minor

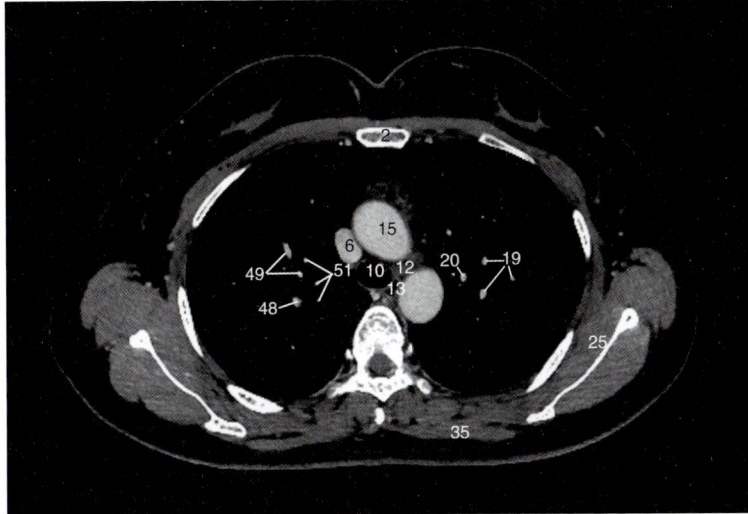

B. CT 纵隔窗增强图像

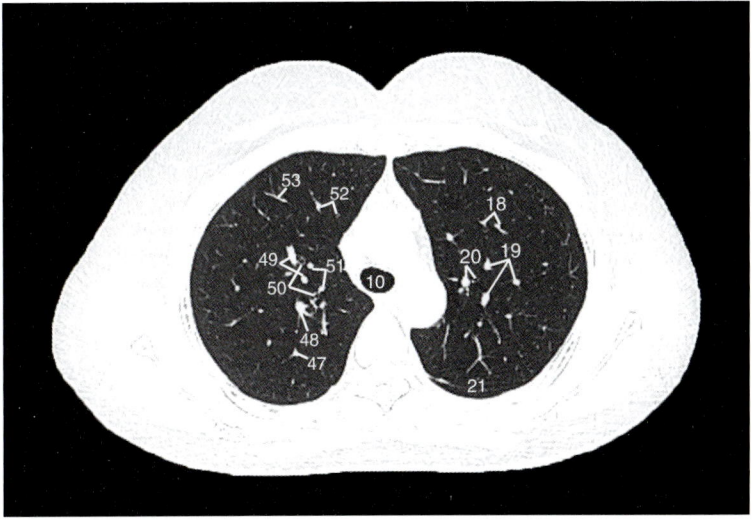

C. CT 肺窗图像

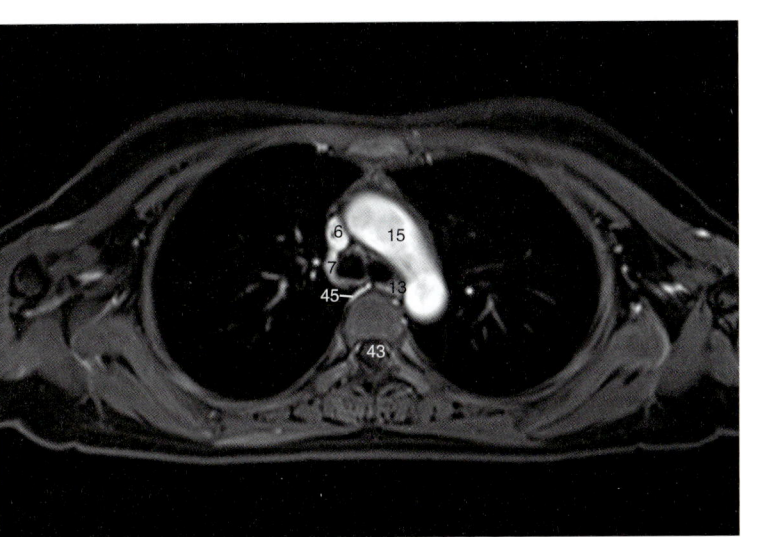

D. MR T1WI 增强图像

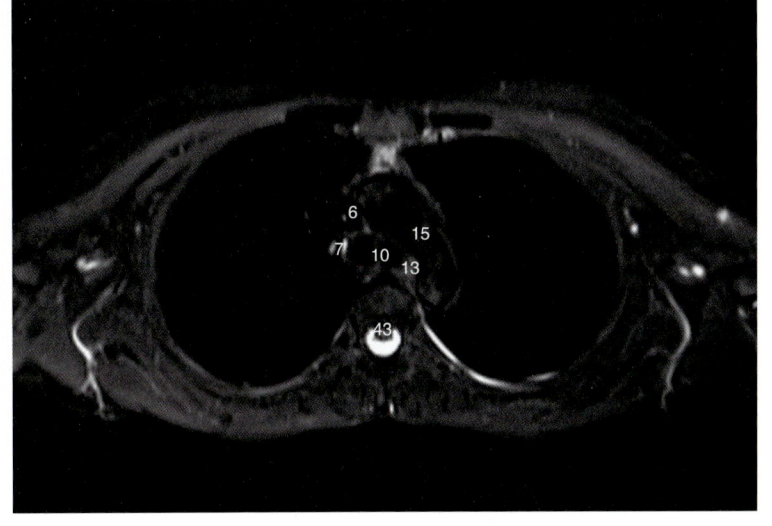

E. MR T2WI 抑脂图像

关键结构：胸骨角，奇静脉弓，第4胸椎椎体。

断面经第4胸椎椎体中份。

前方为胸骨角，亦称"Louis角"，是胸骨柄和胸骨体的连接处，向前微突成角，由软骨连接形成柄胸结合，两侧分别与第2肋软骨形成胸肋关节。交接处的稍微隆起，成为前胸壁计数肋骨的重要标志。胸骨角部位又相当于左、右主支气管分叉处，主动脉弓下缘水平、心房上缘、上下纵隔交界部，后方平对T4-5椎间盘。奇静脉于第4胸椎高度形成奇静脉弓，位于纵隔右侧，从后方行向前，形成平滑向外的隆凸，注入上腔静脉。奇静脉弓勾绕了右肺门，因此其可以视为右肺门出现的标志。当奇静脉发育异常自右肺尖向下走行、陷入肺内则形成奇裂，分隔右上肺叶的内侧部为奇叶[32]。奇裂包括4层胸膜，即脏胸膜与壁胸膜各2层。X线检查发现率约为0.5%，呈右上肺野内带弧形线状或带状影，终止于右肺门上方2~4 cm处，终止处呈逗点状，此即为副裂内奇静脉。CT则可直接显示副裂的全程。轴位图像上为右上叶内侧弧形密度影，上部呈线状，下部为带状。矢状位或斜矢状位重组可显示奇静脉及其连接的右上肋间后静脉、上腔静脉。增强扫描可清楚显示奇裂内奇静脉强化；重组图像可观察异常走行奇静脉的全程。100%出现的奇静脉弓旁淋巴结（4R）和心包上隐窝位于升主动脉、上腔静脉、奇静脉弓和气管围成的气管前间隙内。左肺可见斜裂出现，斜裂后方为左肺下叶背段，又称上段。

胸部连续横断层 31（FH.12890）

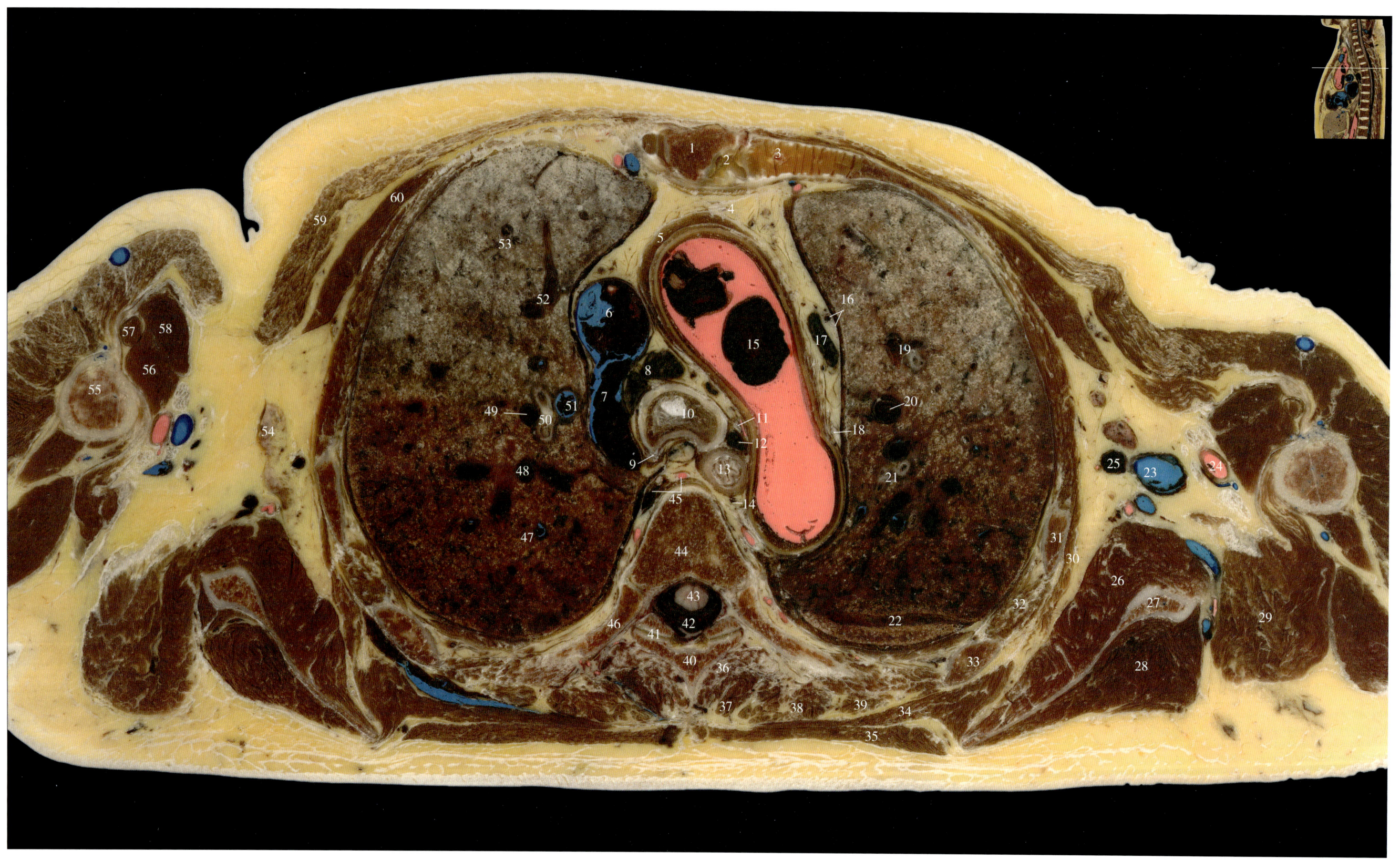

A. 断层标本图像

1. 胸骨体 body of sternum
2. 第 2 胸肋关节 2nd sternocostal joint
3. 第 2 肋软骨 2nd costal cartilage
4. 胸腺 thymus
5. 心包上隐窝 superior recess of pericardium
6. 上腔静脉 superior vena cava
7. 奇静脉弓 arch of azygos vein
8. 右下气管旁淋巴结（4R）right lower paratracheal lymph nodes
9. 右迷走神经 right vagus nerve
10. 气管 trachea
11. 左喉返神经 left recurrent laryngeal nerve
12. 左下气管旁淋巴结（4L）left lower paratracheal lymph nodes
13. 食管 esophagus
14. 胸导管 thoracic duct
15. 主动脉弓 aortic arch
16. 膈神经和心包膈血管 phrenic nerve and pericardiacophrenic vessels
17. 主动脉弓旁淋巴结（6 区）paraaortic lymph nodes
18. 左迷走神经 left vagus nerve
19. 左肺前段支气管（B3）和动脉（A3）left anterior segmental bronchus and artery
20. 尖后段静脉（V1+2）apicoposterior segmental vein
21. 尖后段支气管（B1+2）和动脉（A1+2）apicoposterior segmental bronchus and artery
22. 左肺斜裂 oblique fissure of left lung
23. 腋静脉 axillary vein
24. 腋动脉 axillary artery
25. 胸外侧静脉 lateral thoracic vein
26. 肩胛下肌 subscapularis
27. 肩胛骨 scapula
28. 冈下肌 infraspinatus
29. 大圆肌 teres major
30. 前锯肌 serratus anterior
31. 第 3 肋骨 3rd costal bone
32. 肋间内、外肌 intercostales interni and externi
33. 第 4 肋骨 4th costal bone
34. 菱形肌 rhomboideus
35. 斜方肌 trapezius
36. 横突棘肌 transversospinales
37. 棘肌 spinales
38. 最长肌 longissimus
39. 髂肋肌 iliocostalis
40. 椎弓板 lamina of vertebral arch
41. 关节突关节 zygapophysial joint
42. 硬膜外隙 epidural space
43. 脊髓 spinal cord
44. 第 4 胸椎椎体 body of 4th thoracic vertebra
45. 肋间后动、静脉 posterior intercostal artery and vein
46. 第 5 肋骨 5th costal bone
47. 后段支气管（B2）和动脉（A2）posterior segmental bronchus and artery
48. 后段静脉（V2）posterior segmental vein
49. 尖段静脉尖支（V1）apical branch of apical segmental vein
50. 尖段支气管（B1）apical segmental bronchus
51. 尖段动脉（A1）apical segmental artery
52. 尖段静脉（V1）apical segmental vein
53. 右肺前段支气管（B3）和动脉（A3）right anterior segmental bronchus and artery
54. 腋淋巴结 axillary lymph nodes
55. 肱骨 humerus
56. 喙肱肌 coracobrachialis
57. 肱二头肌长头 long head of biceps brachii
58. 肱二头肌短头 short head of biceps brachii
59. 胸大肌 pectoralis major
60. 胸小肌 pectoralis minor

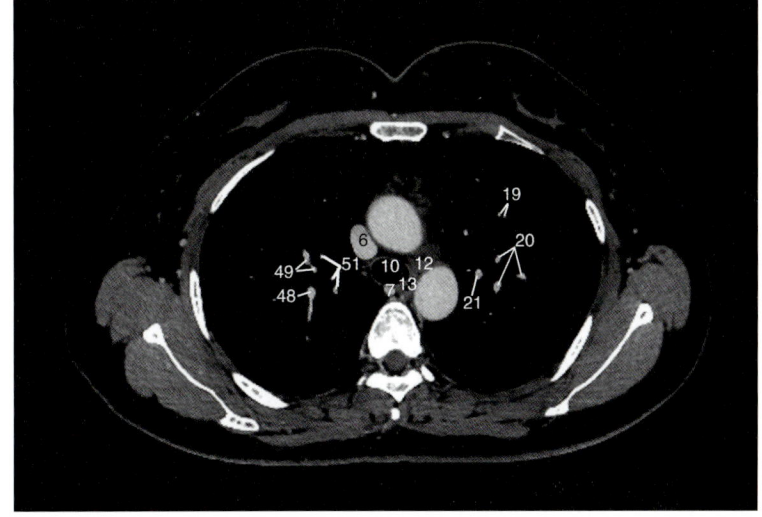

B. CT 纵隔窗增强图像

C. CT 肺窗图像

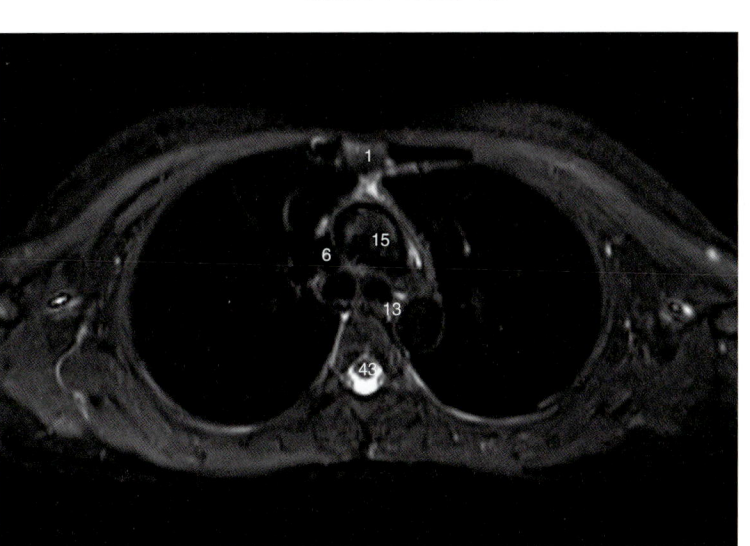

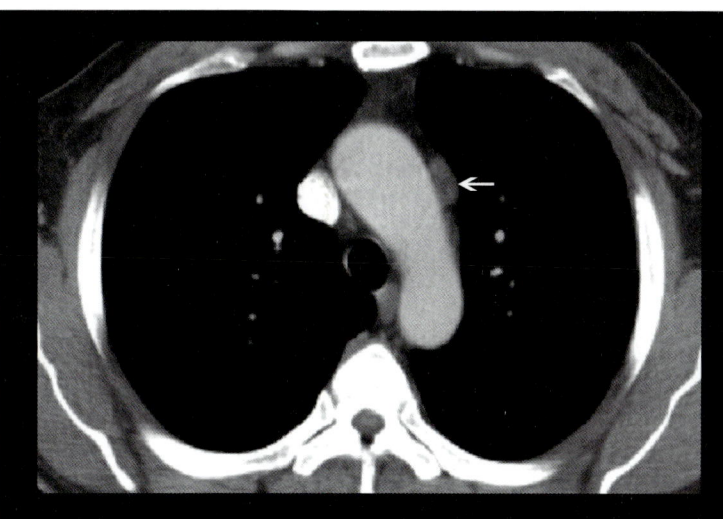

D. MR T2WI 抑脂图像

E. 6 区淋巴结转移 CT 图像

关键结构：胸外侧静脉，主动脉弓旁淋巴结。

断面经第 4 胸椎椎体下份。

胸壁外侧见胸外侧静脉注入腋静脉。奇静脉弓、下腔静脉与气管之间可见右下气管旁淋巴结（4R），主动脉弓与气管之间可见左下气管旁淋巴结（4L），主动脉弓外侧与左肺之间可见主动脉弓旁淋巴结（6 区）。左肺因出现斜裂，分为上叶与下叶。主动脉弓旁淋巴结（6 区）位于升主动脉和主动脉弓前方或外侧，其上缘为与主动脉弓上缘的切线，下缘即主动脉弓下缘。研究表明，纵隔淋巴结是否发生转移与患者性别、年龄、吸烟、病理、胸膜是否凹陷、是否毛刺等资料无显著关联性，而与原发灶大小、分化程度显著相关。原发病灶体积越大、分化程度越低越容易出现淋巴结转移。因此，在临床工作中，对于病灶体积较大而分化程度较低的肿瘤应高度关注。纵隔淋巴结转移最常见的病因是肺癌[33]。食管癌患者纵隔淋巴结转移的位置取决于原发肿瘤的位置。胸段纵隔淋巴结受累于上胸段食管癌的所占比例较小；中、下胸段食管癌的比例较大。胸部淋巴结肿大的另一个原因是淋巴瘤。纵隔淋巴瘤多位于纵隔的上中部，常为双侧病变，病变多呈多发结节状，部分淋巴瘤容易融合呈分叶状团块，增强扫描呈轻中度强化，易包绕血管。6 区淋巴结转移 CT 图像中的箭头所示为主动脉弓旁增大淋巴结。

胸部连续横断层 32 (FH.12870)

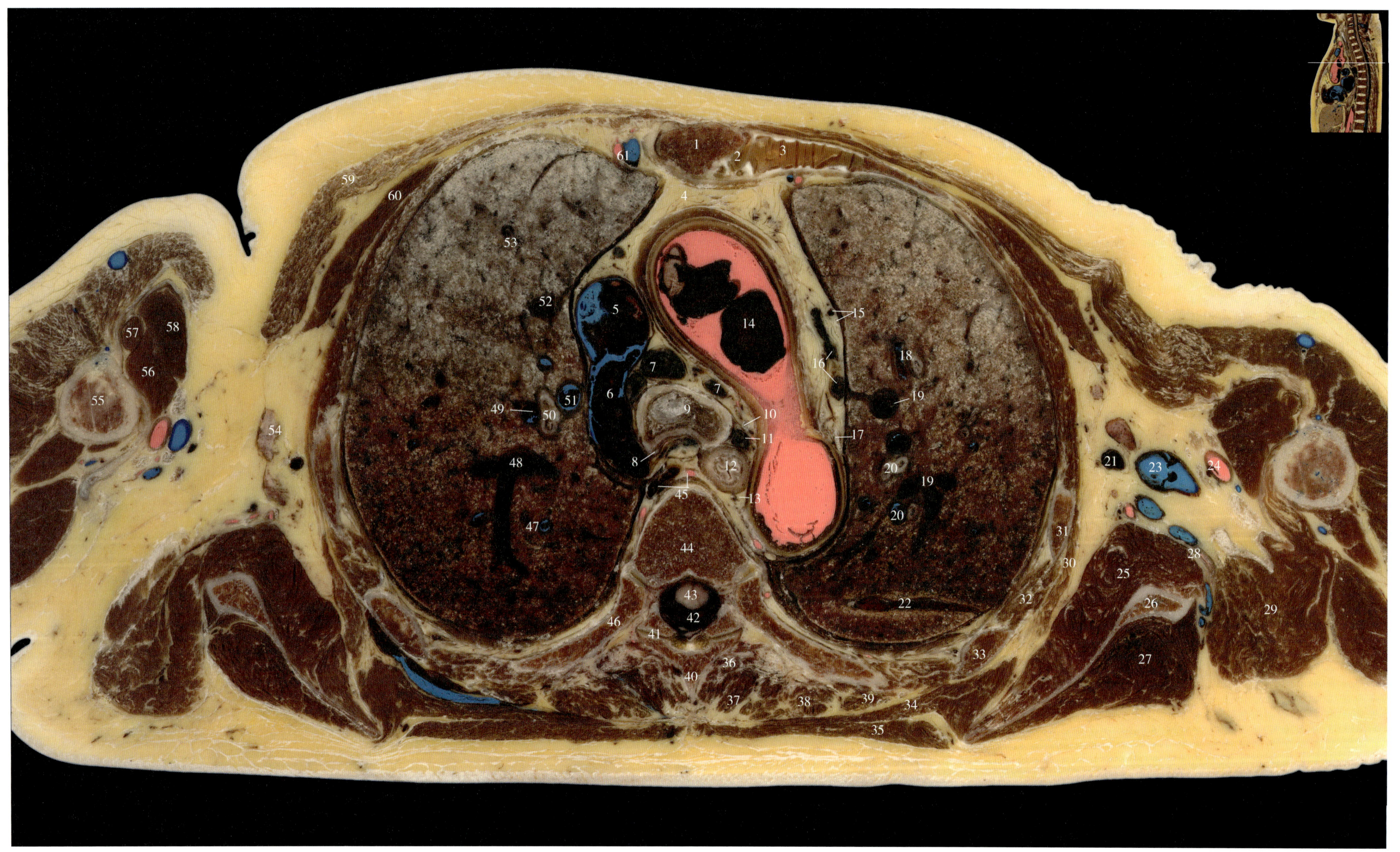

A. 断层标本图像

1. 胸骨体 body of sternum
2. 第 2 胸肋关节 2nd sternocostal joint
3. 第 2 肋软骨 2nd costal cartilage
4. 胸腺 thymus
5. 上腔静脉 superior vena cava
6. 奇静脉弓 arch of azygos vein
7. 右下气管旁淋巴结（4R） right lower paratracheal lymph nodes
8. 右迷走神经 right vagus nerve
9. 气管 trachea
10. 左喉返神经 left recurrent laryngeal nerve
11. 左下气管旁淋巴结（4L） left lower paratracheal lymph nodes
12. 食管 esophagus
13. 胸导管 thoracic duct
14. 主动脉弓 aortic arch
15. 膈神经和心包膈血管 phrenic nerve and pericardiacophrenic vessels
16. 主动脉弓旁淋巴结（6 区） paraaortic lymph nodes
17. 左迷走神经 left vagus nerve
18. 左肺前段支气管（B3）和动脉（A3） left anterior segmental bronchus and artery
19. 尖后段静脉（V1+2） apicoposterior segmental vein
20. 尖后段支气管（B1+2）与动脉（A1+2） apicoposterior segmental bronchus and artery
21. 胸外侧静脉 lateral thoracic vein
22. 斜裂 oblique fissure
23. 腋静脉 axillary vein
24. 腋动脉 axillary artery
25. 肩胛下肌 subscapularis
26. 肩胛骨 scapula
27. 冈下肌 infraspinatus
28. 旋肩胛动、静脉 circumflex scapular artery and vein
29. 大圆肌 teres major
30. 前锯肌 serratus anterior
31. 第 3 肋骨 3rd costal bone
32. 肋间内、外肌 intercostales interni and externi
33. 第 4 肋骨 4th costal bone
34. 菱形肌 rhomboideus
35. 斜方肌 trapezius
36. 横突棘肌 transversospinales
37. 棘肌 spinales
38. 最长肌 longissimus
39. 髂肋肌 iliocostalis
40. 棘突 spinous process
41. 关节突关节 zygapophysial joint
42. 硬膜外隙 epidural space
43. 脊髓 spinal cord
44. 第 4 胸椎椎体 body of 4th thoracic vertebra
45. 肋间后动、静脉 posterior intercostal artery and vein
46. 第 5 肋骨 5th costal bone
47. 后段支气管（B2）和动脉（A2） posterior segmental bronchus and artery
48. 后段静脉（V2） posterior segmental vein
49. 尖段静脉尖支（V1） apical branch of apical segmental vein
50. 尖段支气管（B1） apical segmental bronchus
51. 尖段动脉（A1） apical segmental artery
52. 尖段静脉（V1） apical segmental vein
53. 右肺前段支气管（B3）和动脉（A3） right anterior segmental bronchus and artery
54. 腋淋巴结 axillary lymph nodes
55. 肱骨 humerus
56. 喙肱肌 coracobrachialis
57. 肱二头肌长头 long head of biceps brachii
58. 肱二头肌短头 short head of biceps brachii
59. 胸大肌 pectoralis major
60. 胸小肌 pectoralis minor
61. 胸廓内动、静脉 internal thoracic artery and vein

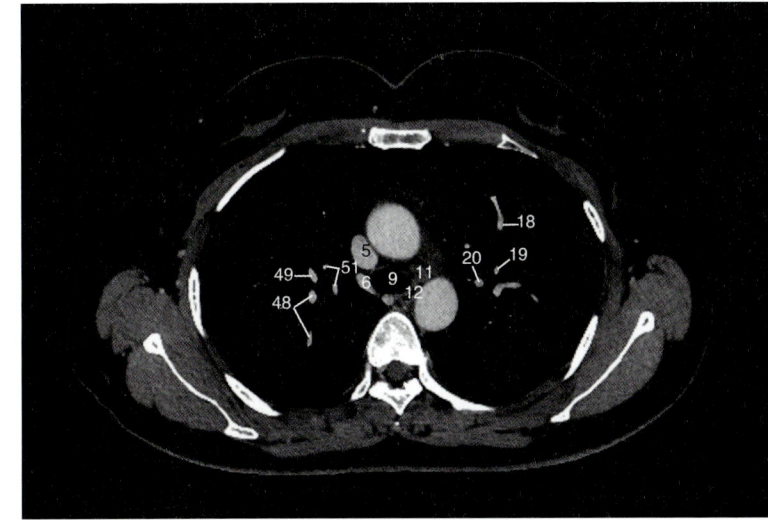

B. CT 纵隔窗增强图像

C. CT 肺窗图像

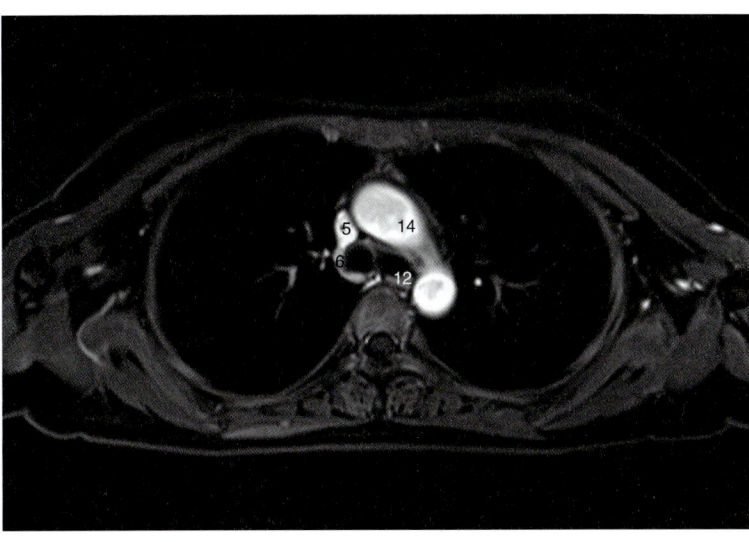

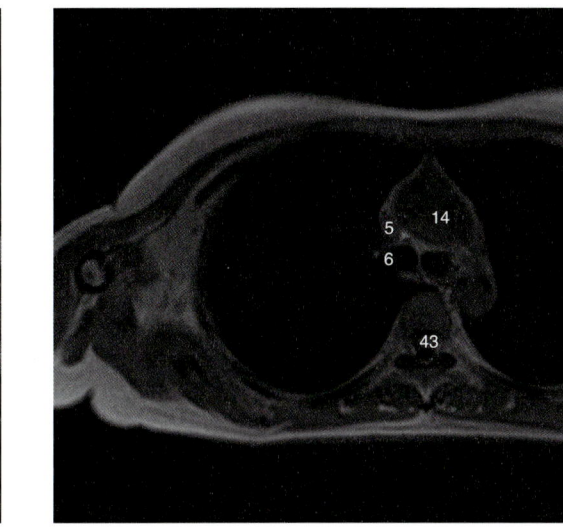

D. MR T1WI 增强图像

E. MR T1WI 平扫图像

关键结构：奇静脉弓，迷走神经，肺上叶。

此断面经第 4 胸椎椎体下份。

双肺上叶断面扩大，右肺上叶尖段静脉、后段静脉之间弧形连线的内侧为尖段，外侧为后段与前段，二者可依据后段静脉走行方向划分开来。左肺上叶可沿尖后段静脉走行方向，将位于后方的尖后段与前方的前段分割开来。斜裂后方为下叶上段。纵隔内，奇静脉弓、上腔静脉及主动脉弓下缘被切及。右迷走神经比较恒定的位于气管、食管和奇静脉之间的三角间隙内；左迷走神经位于主动脉右前方，膈神经右后方。迷走神经为混合神经，含有躯体运动、内脏运动、内脏感觉、躯体感觉 4 种纤维。迷走神经支气管支与交感神经共同构成肺丛，发出细支支配支气管与肺。

迷走神经末梢释放乙酰胆碱与气道表面的上皮和分泌细胞 M 型胆碱能受体结合，引起纤毛摆动频率增加和气道黏液分泌增加，与支气管平滑肌的 M 型胆碱能受体结合，引起支气管平滑肌痉挛、支气管收缩、气道张力增加。在肺部，迷走神经参与肺扩张反射，当肺扩张时牵拉呼吸道，使呼吸道扩张，刺激牵张感受器，沿迷走神经传入冲动进入延髓，加速吸气过程转换为呼气过程，使呼吸频率增加。此外，主动脉体内化学感受器在动脉血氧分压降低、动脉二氧化碳分压或氢离子浓度升高时受到刺激，感觉信号经迷走神经传入神经中枢，反射性地引起呼吸加深加快。

65

胸部连续横断层 33（FH.12850）

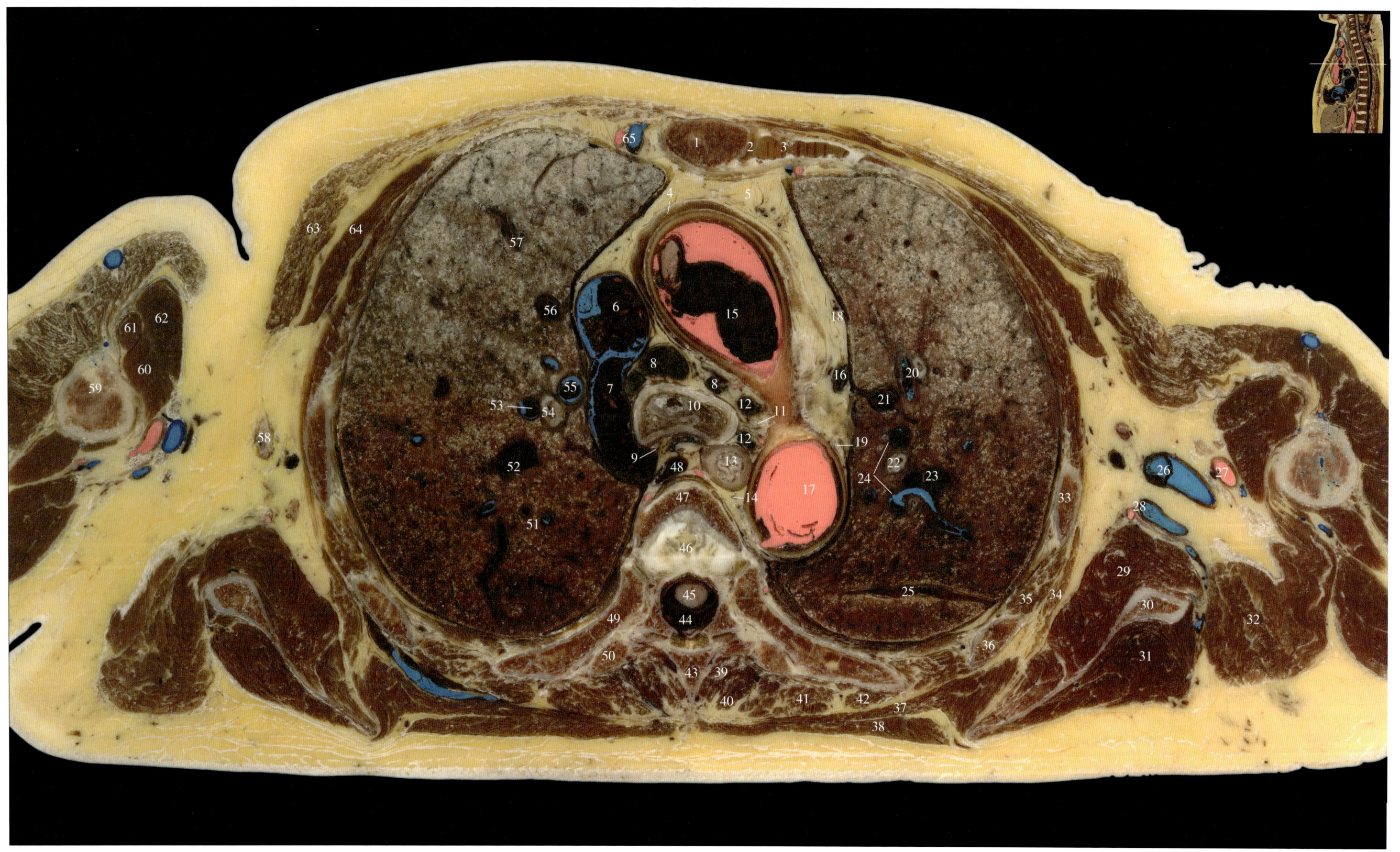

A. 断层标本图像

1. 胸骨角 sternal angle
2. 第 2 胸肋关节 2nd sternocostal joint
3. 第 2 肋软骨 2nd costal cartilage
4. 心包上隐窝 superior recess of pericardium
5. 胸腺 thymus
6. 上腔静脉 superior vena cava
7. 奇静脉弓 arch of azygos vein
8. 右下气管旁淋巴结（4R）right lower paratracheal lymph nodes
9. 右迷走神经 right vagus nerve
10. 气管 trachea
11. 左喉返神经 left recurrent laryngeal nerve
12. 左下气管旁淋巴结（4L）left lower paratracheal lymph nodes
13. 食管 esophagus
14. 胸导管 thoracic duct
15. 升主动脉 ascending aorta
16. 主动脉弓旁淋巴结（6 区）paraaortic lymph nodes
17. 降主动脉 descending aorta
18. 膈神经和心包膈血管 phrenic nerve and pericardiacophrenic vessels
19. 左迷走神经 left vagus nerve
20. 左肺前段支气管（B3）和动脉（A3）left anterior segmental bronchus and artery
21. 尖后段静脉段间支（V1+2）intersegmental ramus of apicoposterior segmental vein
22. 尖后段支气管（B1+2）apicoposterior segmental bronchus
23. 尖后段静脉段内支（V1+2）intrasegmental ramus of apicoposterior segmental vein
24. 尖后段动脉（A1+2）apicoposterior segmental artery
25. 斜裂 oblique fissure
26. 腋静脉 axillary vein
27. 腋动脉 axillary artery
28. 旋肩胛动、静脉 circumflex scapular artery and vein
29. 肩胛下肌 subscapularis
30. 肩胛骨 scapula
31. 冈下肌 infraspinatus
32. 大圆肌 teres major
33. 第 3 肋骨 3rd costal bone
34. 前锯肌 serratus anterior
35. 肋间内、外肌 intercostales interni and externi
36. 第 4 肋骨 4th costal bone
37. 菱形肌 rhomboideus
38. 斜方肌 trapezius
39. 横突棘肌 transversospinales
40. 棘肌 spinales
41. 最长肌 longissimus
42. 髂肋肌 iliocostalis
43. 棘突 spinous process
44. 硬膜外隙 epidural space
45. 脊髓 spinal cord
46. T4-5 椎间盘 T4-5 intervertebral disc
47. 第 4 胸椎椎体 body of 4th thoracic vertebra
48. 奇静脉 azygos vein
49. 第 5 肋骨 5th costal bone
50. 横突 transverse process
51. 右肺后段支气管（B2）和动脉（A2）right posterior segmental bronchus and artery
52. 后段静脉（V2）posterior segmental vein
53. 尖段静脉尖支（V1）apical branch of apical segmental vein
54. 尖段支气管（B1）apical segmental bronchus
55. 尖段动脉（A1）apical segmental artery
56. 尖段静脉（V1）apical segmental vein
57. 右肺前段支气管（B3）和动脉（A3）right anterior segmental bronchus and artery
58. 腋淋巴结 axillary lymph nodes
59. 肱骨 humerus
60. 喙肱肌 coracobrachialis
61. 肱二头肌长头 long head of biceps brachii
62. 肱二头肌短头 short head of biceps brachii
63. 胸大肌 pectoralis major
64. 胸小肌 pectoralis minor
65. 胸廓内动、静脉 internal thoracic artery and vein

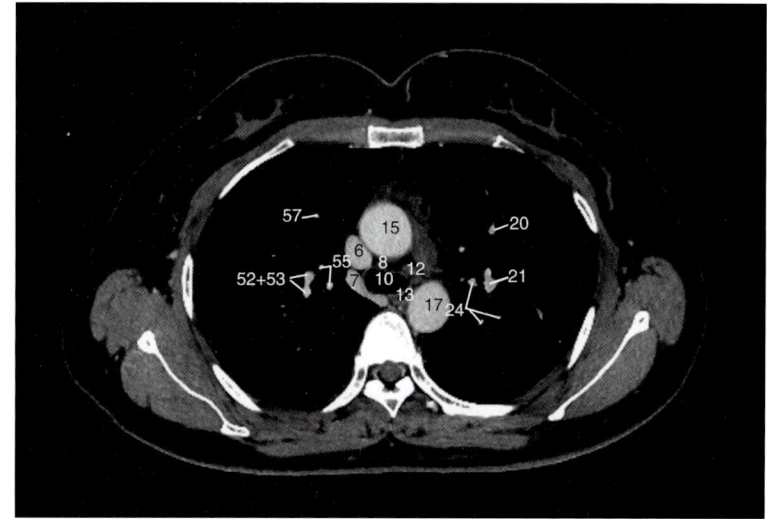

B. CT 纵隔窗增强图像

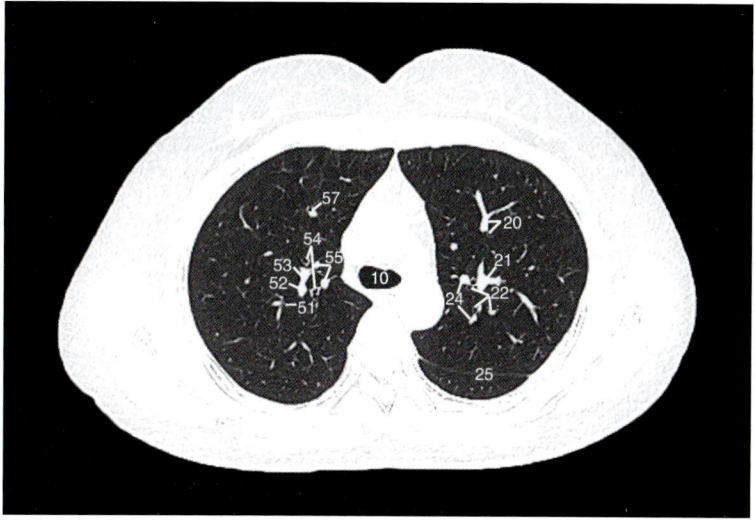

C. CT 肺窗图像

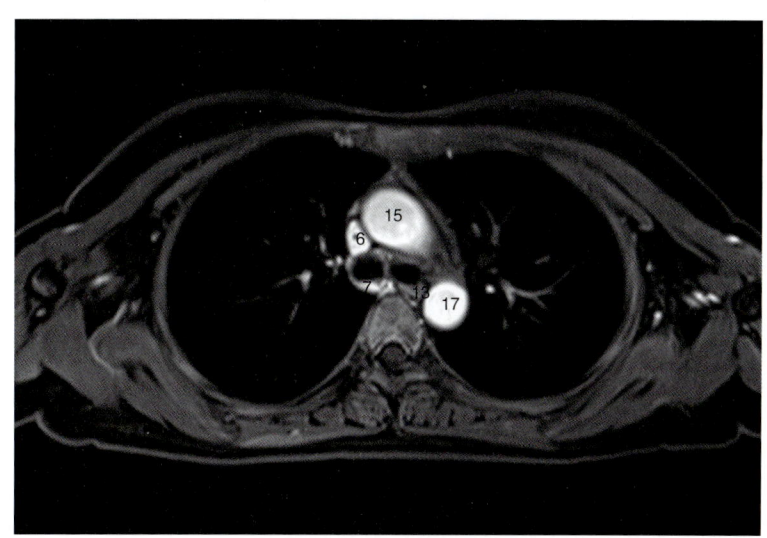

D. MR T1WI 增强图像

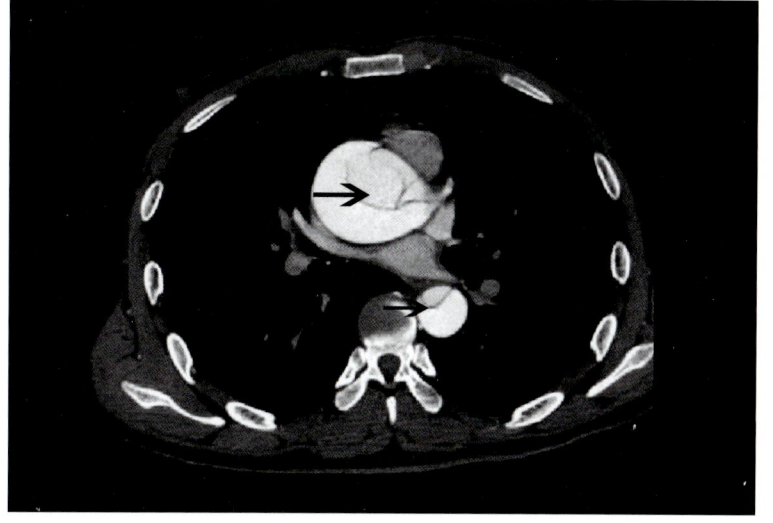

E. Stanford A 型主动脉夹层 CT 图像

关键结构：胸骨角，升主动脉，胸主动脉。

此断面经 T4-5 椎间盘上份。

此为胸骨角平面，可见前后稍扁呈卵圆形的气管杈、主动脉弓起止端、奇静脉弓。此平面以胸骨角和第 4 胸椎椎体下缘为界，将纵隔分为上、下纵隔。下纵隔又以心包的前、后壁为界，分为前纵隔、中纵隔和后纵隔。升主动脉在胸骨左缘后方，平对第 3 肋间隙处起自左心室，向前右上方斜行，达右侧第 2 胸肋关节处，续于主动脉弓。降主动脉又分为胸主动脉和腹主动脉。胸主动脉位于后纵隔内，起自第 4 胸椎下缘的左侧，下降到第 12 胸椎前方，穿膈的主动脉裂孔入腹腔，移行为腹主动脉。主动脉夹层是较常见也是最复杂、最危险的心血管疾病之一，发病率为（5~10）/100 万[34]。主动脉夹层诊断分型标准：（1）Stanford 型，①A 型，升主动脉、主动脉弓或近胸降主动脉内膜撕裂，剥离主要累及升主动脉弓部，也可延及降主动脉及腹主动脉；②B 型，主动脉峡部内膜撕裂，剥离仅累及降主动脉或延伸至腹主动脉，但不累及升主动脉，很少累及主动脉弓。（2）Debakey 分型，①Ⅰ型，升主动脉内膜撕裂，但剥离可扩展于整个主动脉，包括腹主动脉甚至双髂动脉；②Ⅱ型，升主动脉内膜撕裂，剥离也仅限于升主动脉；③Ⅲ型，主动脉峡部内膜撕裂，剥离仅累及降主动脉者为Ⅲa 型，剥离达腹主动脉者为Ⅲb 型。E 图箭头所示为主动脉夹层内撕裂的内膜。

胸部连续横断层 34 (FH.12830)

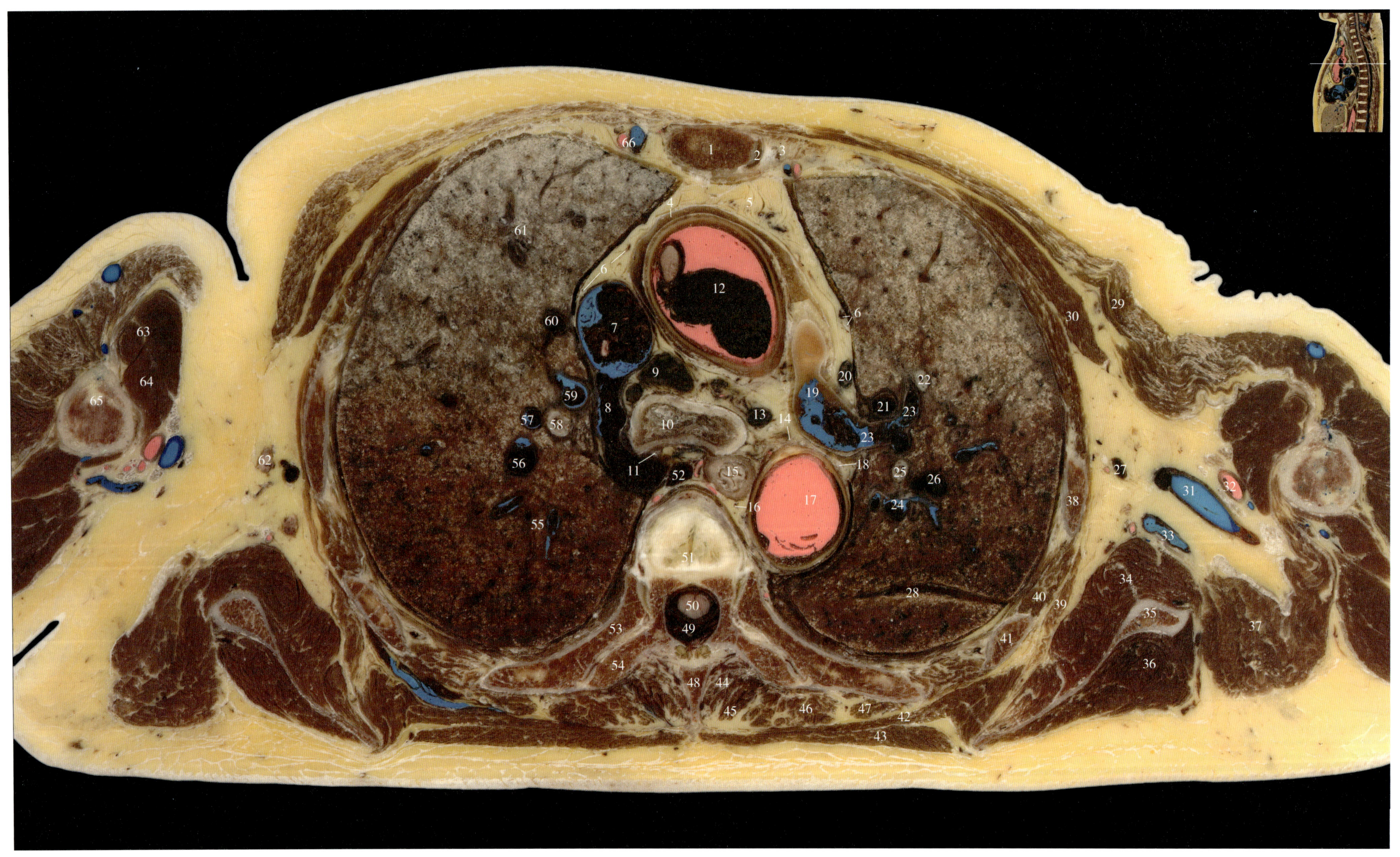

A. 断层标本图像

1. 胸骨体 body of sternum
2. 第2胸肋关节 2nd sternocostal joint
3. 第2肋软骨 2nd costal cartilage
4. 心包上隐窝 superior recess of pericardium
5. 胸腺 thymus
6. 膈神经和心包膈血管 phrenic nerve and pericardiacophrenic vessels
7. 上腔静脉 superior vena cava
8. 奇静脉弓 arch of azygos vein
9. 右下气管旁淋巴结（4R）right lower paratracheal lymph nodes
10. 气管 trachea
11. 右迷走神经 right vagus nerve
12. 升主动脉 ascending aorta
13. 主动脉弓下淋巴结（5区）subaortic lymph nodes
14. 左喉返神经 left recurrent laryngeal nerve
15. 食管 esophagus
16. 胸导管 thoracic duct
17. 降主动脉 descending aorta
18. 左迷走神经 left vagus nerve
19. 左肺动脉 left pulmonary artery
20. 主动脉弓下淋巴结（5区）subaortic lymph nodes
21. 尖后段静脉段间支（V1+2）intersegmental ramus of apicoposterior segmental vein
22. 左肺前段支气管（B3）left anterior segmental bronchus
23. 左肺前段动脉（A3）left anterior segmental artery
24. 尖后段动脉（A1+2）apicoposterior segmental artery
25. 尖后段支气管（B1+2）apicoposterior segmental bronchus
26. 尖后段静脉段内支（V1+2）intrasegmental ramus of apicoposterior segmental vein
27. 胸外侧静脉 lateral thoracic vein
28. 斜裂 oblique fissure
29. 胸大肌 pectoralis major
30. 胸小肌 pectoralis minor
31. 腋静脉 axillary vein
32. 腋动脉 axillary artery
33. 旋肩胛静脉 circumflex scapular vein
34. 肩胛下肌 subscapularis
35. 肩胛骨 scapula
36. 冈下肌 infraspinatus
37. 大圆肌 teres major
38. 第3肋骨 3rd costal bone
39. 前锯肌 serratus anterior
40. 肋间内、外肌 intercostales interni and externi
41. 第4肋骨 4th costal bone
42. 菱形肌 rhomboideus
43. 斜方肌 trapezius
44. 横突棘肌 transversospinales
45. 棘肌 spinales
46. 最长肌 longissimus
47. 髂肋肌 iliocostalis
48. 棘突 spinous process
49. 硬膜外隙 epidural space
50. 脊髓 spinal cord
51. T4-5椎间盘 T4-5 intervertebral disc
52. 奇静脉 azygos vein
53. 第5肋骨 5th costal bone
54. 横突 transverse process
55. 后段支气管（B2）和动脉（A2）posterior segmental bronchus and artery
56. 后段静脉（V2）posterior segmental vein
57. 尖段静脉尖支（V1）apical branch of apical segmental vein
58. 尖段支气管（B1）apical segmental bronchus
59. 尖段动脉（A1）apical segmental artery
60. 尖段静脉（V1）apical segmental vein
61. 右肺前段支气管（B3）和动脉（A3）right anterior segmental bronchus and artery
62. 腋淋巴结 axillary lymph nodes
63. 肱二头肌长、短头 long and short heads of biceps brachii
64. 喙肱肌 coracobrachialis
65. 肱骨 humerus
66. 胸廓内动、静脉 internal thoracic artery and vein

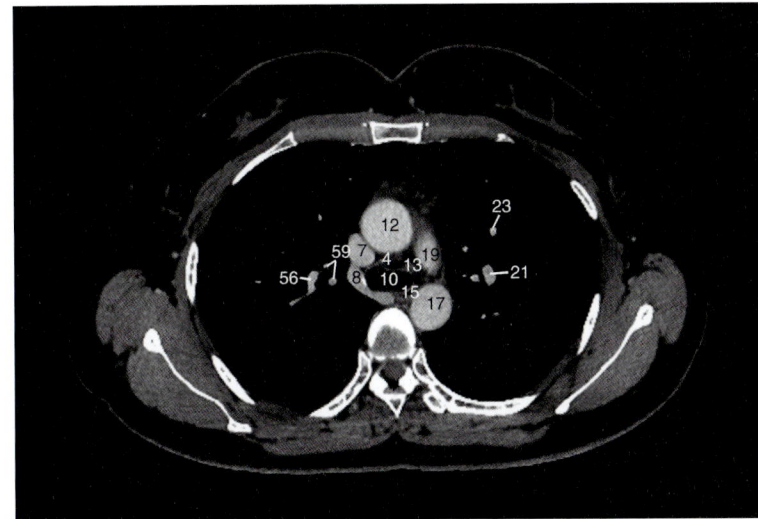

B. CT 纵隔窗增强图像

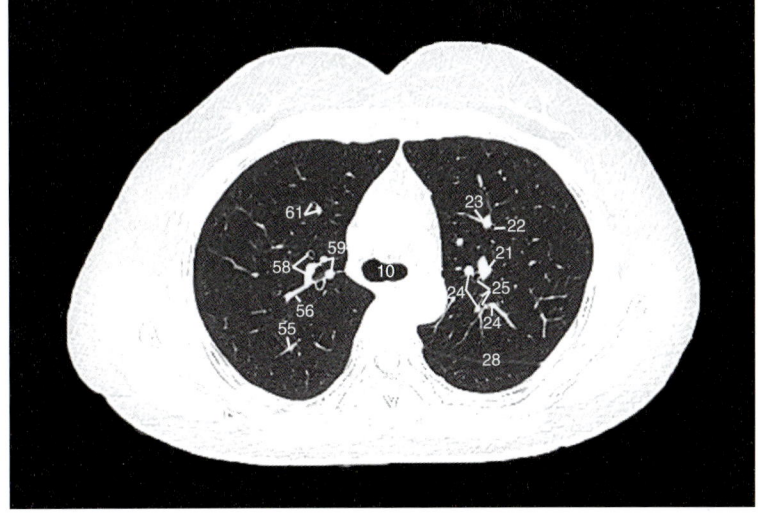

C. CT 肺窗图像

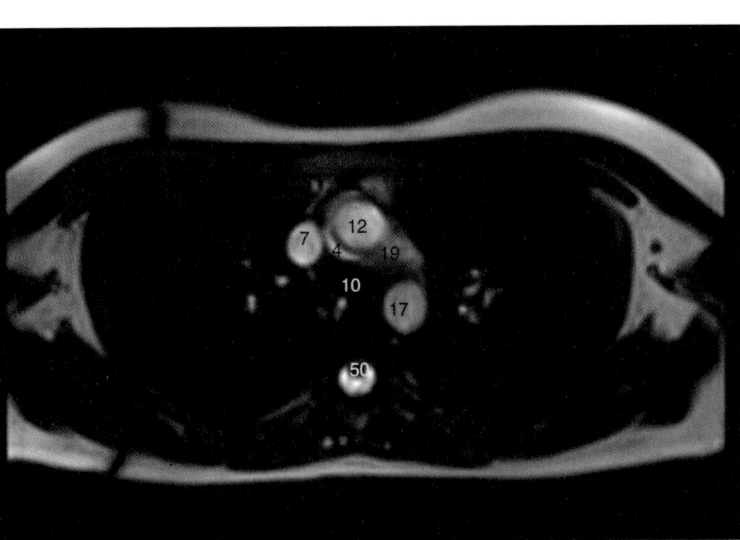

D. MR T2WI 平扫图像

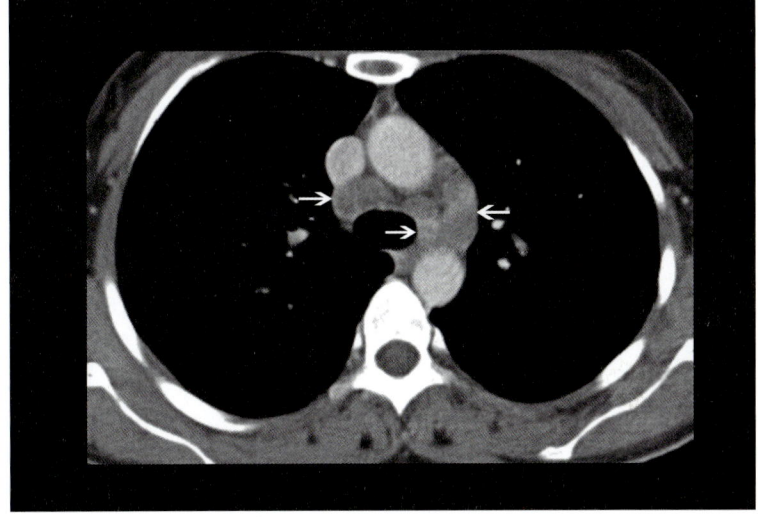

E. 4区、5区淋巴结转移 CT 图像

关键结构：主动脉肺动脉窗，左喉返神经，主动脉弓下淋巴结。

此断面经T4-5椎间盘中份。

纵隔内，左肺动脉刚刚被切及，主动脉弓消失，延续为升主动脉和胸主动脉。于升主动脉与胸主动脉之间至纵隔左缘，为充满疏松结缔组织和脂肪组织的区域，称为主动脉肺动脉窗。其范围是主动脉弓下缘和肺动脉权上缘之间1~2cm的小区域，其左外侧界为纵隔胸膜，内侧界为气管，前方为主动脉升部，后方为食管和主动脉降部。此区含有动脉韧带、左喉返神经和主动脉弓下淋巴结（5区）。CT可以显示该区淋巴结。肺癌转移至此区域淋巴结时，可引起声音嘶哑，提示直接的纵隔侵犯或转移淋巴结增大压迫喉返神经并致声带麻痹。此症状常突然发生、进展迅速，有时甚至完全失声，同时大多数患者伴有胸痛等症状，经休息和抗炎对症治疗2周以上仍无效果。因此，声音嘶哑可能是肺癌的重要临床表抑或患者就诊时的首发症状。此断面正好切及左迷走神经勾绕主动脉弓下面，返折形成左喉返神经。主动脉肺动脉窗可视为左肺门出现的标志。肺门区结构将肺内侧面分为纵隔部、肺门区与脊柱部3个部分，将肺与纵隔之间的胸膜腔分为前、后两部。在左肺门区，可见以短干发自左肺动脉的前段动脉及前方的尖后段静脉段间支。4区、5区淋巴结转移CT图像中的肿大的淋巴结，且部分融合，如箭头所示。

胸部连续横断层 35（FH.12810）

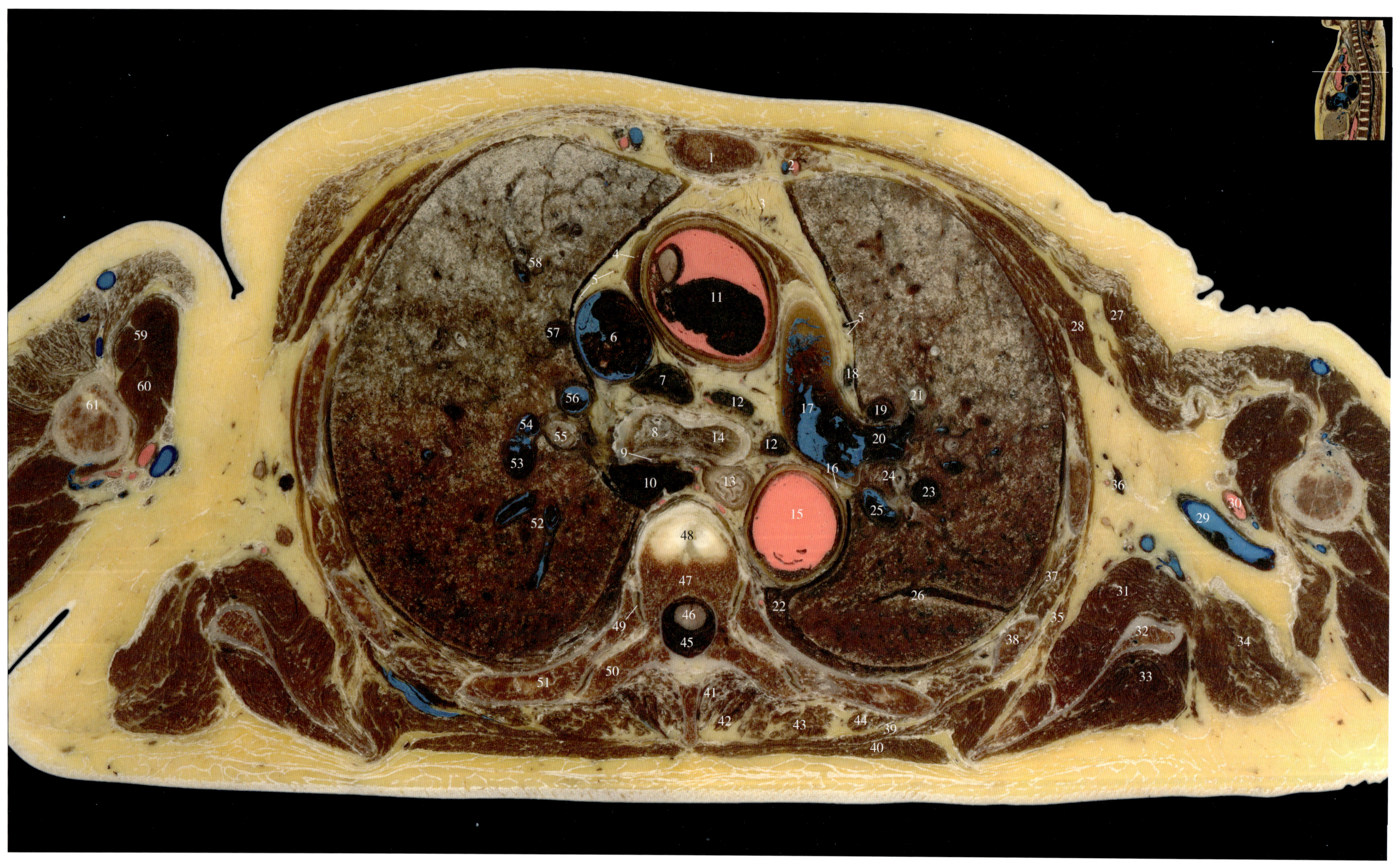

A. 断层标本图像

1. 胸骨体 body of sternum
2. 胸廓内动、静脉 internal thoracic artery and vein
3. 胸腺 thymus
4. 心包上隐窝 superior recess of pericardium
5. 膈神经和心包膈血管 phrenic nerve and pericardiacophrenic vessels
6. 上腔静脉 superior vena cava
7. 右下气管旁淋巴结（4R）right lower paratracheal lymph nodes
8. 右主支气管 right principal bronchus
9. 右迷走神经 right vagus nerve
10. 奇静脉 azygos vein
11. 升主动脉 ascending aorta
12. 主动脉弓下淋巴结（5区）subaortic lymph nodes
13. 食管 esophagus
14. 左主支气管 left principal bronchus
15. 降主动脉 descending aorta
16. 左迷走神经 left vagus nerve
17. 左肺动脉 left pulmonary artery
18. 主动脉弓下淋巴结（5区）subaortic lymph nodes
19. 尖后段静脉段间支（V1+2）intersegmental ramus of apicoposterior segmental vein
20. 左肺前段动脉（A3）left anterior segmental artery
21. 左肺前段支气管（B3）left anterior segmental bronchus
22. 胸膜腔 pleural cavity
23. 尖后段静脉段内支（V1+2）intrasegmental ramus of apicoposterior segmental vein
24. 尖后段支气管（B1+2）apicoposterior segmental bronchus
25. 尖后段动脉（A1+2）apicoposterior segmental artery
26. 斜裂 oblique fissure
27. 胸大肌 pectoralis major
28. 胸小肌 pectoralis minor
29. 腋静脉 axillary vein
30. 腋动脉 axillary artery
31. 肩胛下肌 subscapularis
32. 肩胛骨 scapula
33. 冈下肌 infraspinatus
34. 大圆肌 teres major
35. 前锯肌 serratus anterior
36. 胸外侧静脉 lateral thoracic vein
37. 肋间内、外肌 intercostales interni and externi
38. 第4肋骨 4th costal bone
39. 菱形肌 rhomboideus
40. 斜方肌 trapezius
41. 横突棘肌 transversospinales
42. 棘肌 spinales
43. 最长肌 longissimus
44. 髂肋肌 iliocostalis
45. 硬膜外腔 epidural space
46. 脊髓 spinal cord
47. 第5胸椎椎体 body of 5th thoracic vertebra
48. T4-5 椎间盘 T4-5 intervertebral disc
49. 肋头关节 joint of costal head
50. 横突 transverse process
51. 第5肋骨 5th costal bone
52. 后段支气管（B2）和动脉（A2）posterior segmental bronchus and artery
53. 后段静脉（V2）posterior segmental vein
54. 尖段静脉尖支（V1）apical branch of apical segmental vein
55. 尖段支气管（B1）apical segmental bronchus
56. 尖段动脉（A1）apical segmental artery
57. 尖段静脉（V1）apical segmental vein
58. 右肺前段支气管（B3）和动脉（A3）anterior segmental bronchus and artery
59. 肱二头肌长、短头 long and short heads of biceps brachii
60. 喙肱肌 coracobrachialis
61. 肱骨 humerus

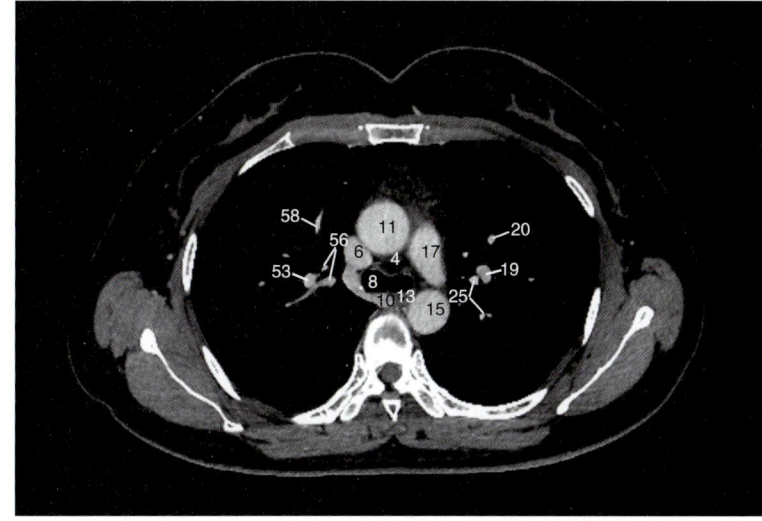

B. CT 纵隔窗增强图像

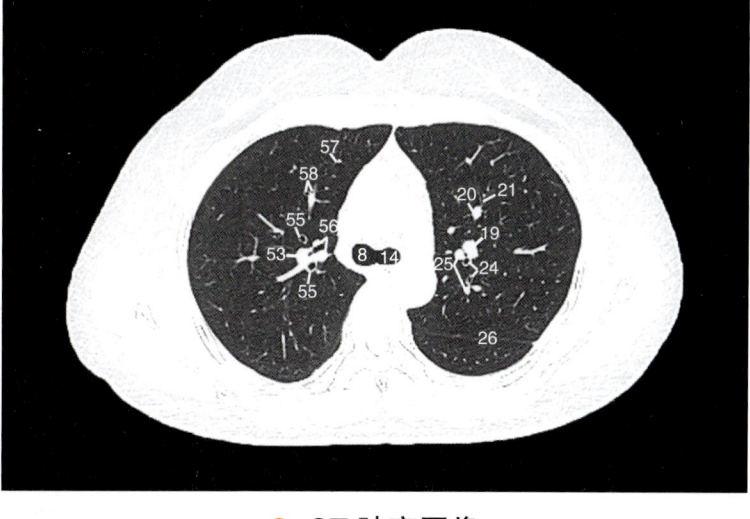

C. CT 肺窗图像

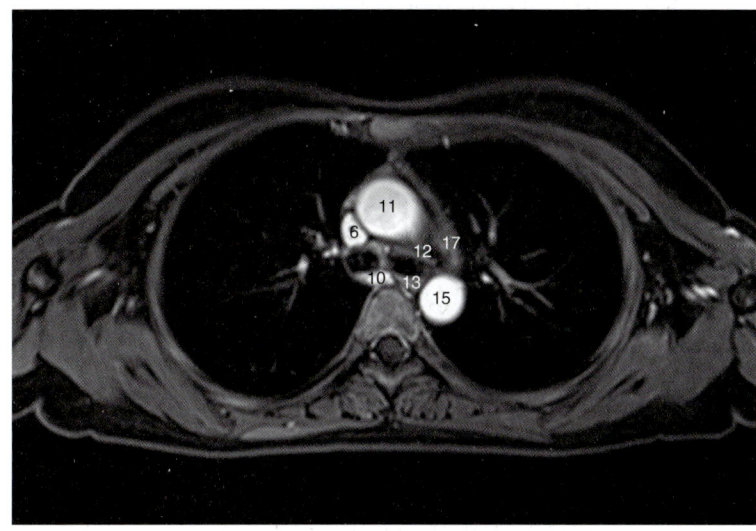

D. MR T1WI 增强图像

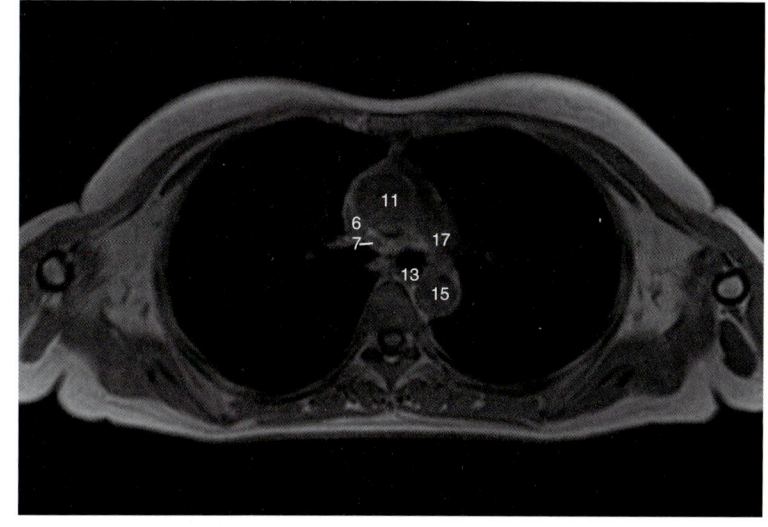

E. MR T1WI 平扫图像

关键结构：气管杈，食管。

此断面经 T4-5 椎间盘下份。

气管在胸骨角平面分为左、右主支气管，分叉处称为气管杈。其内面有一向上凸出的半月状嵴，称为气管隆嵴。成人气管杈的位置高低变化较大，约 58% 平对第 5 胸椎椎体，10% 平对 T4-5 椎间盘，12% 平对 T5-6 椎间盘。成人气管平均长度：男性为 10.6 cm，女性为 9.8 cm。小儿气管细小，位置深，活动度大。相邻气管软骨间以弹性纤维形成的环状韧带（又称气管韧带）连结。气管有软骨作为支架，可使管腔保持于开放状态，保证呼吸功能的正常进行，气管后方的膜壁具有一定的舒缩性，有利于食管扩张，易于食团顺利下行入胃。由于气管的横断面形态变化很大，同一标本的不同断面，其形态亦不同，但以马蹄形为多，亦可呈三角形、卵圆形或梨形。儿童气管的横断面多呈卵圆形，少数为马蹄形。气管的某些断面形态可与疾病有关，如"刀鞘"气管，即断面上矢径大于冠状径 1 倍以上的气管，与慢性呼吸道阻塞性肺部疾病有关。气管在不同的平面其毗邻亦不相同，而它的后面恒定的与食管相邻，大多数人的食管不在气管的正后方，而是居其左后方，胸段食管在 CT 图像上易于识别。食管的管径及管壁依气体的多少和管壁的收缩状态而有变化，管壁厚度超过 3 mm 应支持食管造影对食管疾病的诊断。

胸部连续横断层 36（FH.12790）

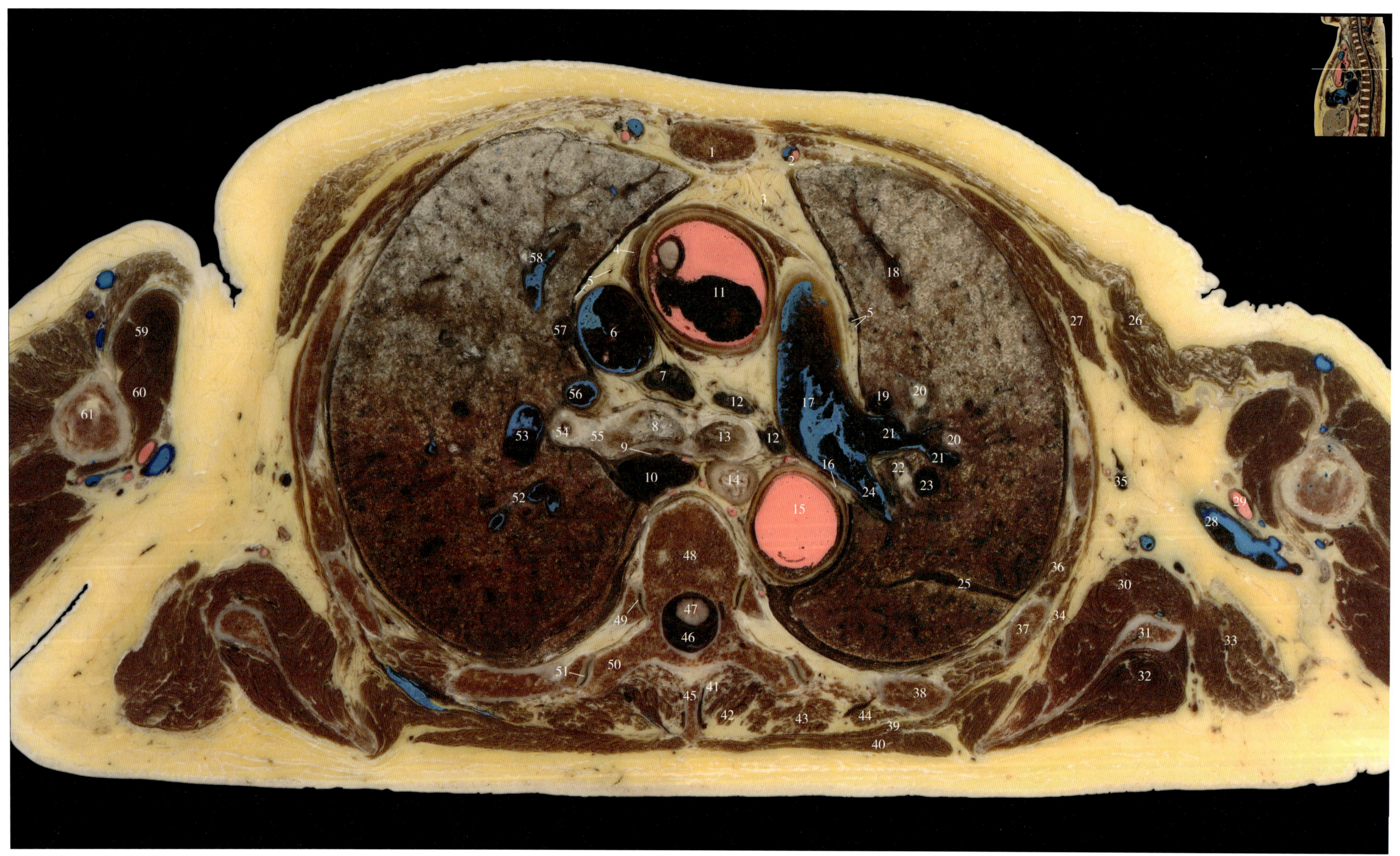

A. 断层标本图像

1. 胸骨体 body of sternum
2. 胸廓内动、静脉 internal thoracic artery and vein
3. 胸腺 thymus
4. 心包上隐窝 superior recess of pericardium
5. 膈神经和心包膈血管 phrenic nerve and pericardiacophrenic vessels
6. 上腔静脉 superior vena cava
7. 右下气管旁淋巴结（4R）right lower paratracheal lymph nodes
8. 右主支气管 right principal bronchus
9. 右迷走神经 right vagus nerve
10. 奇静脉 azygos vein
11. 升主动脉 ascending aorta
12. 主动脉弓下淋巴结（5区）subaortic lymph nodes
13. 左主支气管 left principal bronchus
14. 食管 esophagus
15. 胸主动脉 thoracic aorta
16. 左迷走神经 left vagus nerve
17. 左肺动脉 left pulmonary artery
18. 前段静脉（V3）anterior segmental artery
19. 尖后段静脉段间支（V1+2）intersegmental ramus of apicoposterior segmental vein
20. 左肺前段支气管（B3）left anterior segmental bronchus
21. 左肺前段动脉（A3）left anterior segmental artery
22. 尖后段支气管（B1+2）apicoposterior segmental bronchus
23. 尖后段静脉段内支（V1+2）intrasegmental ramus of apicoposterior segmental vein
24. 尖后段动脉（A1+2）apicoposterior segmental artery
25. 斜裂 oblique fissure
26. 胸大肌 pectoralis major
27. 胸小肌 pectoralis minor
28. 腋静脉 axillary vein
29. 腋动脉 axillary artery
30. 肩胛下肌 subscapularis
31. 肩胛骨 scapula
32. 冈下肌 infraspinatus
33. 大圆肌 teres major
34. 前锯肌 serratus anterior
35. 胸外侧静脉 lateral thoracic vein
36. 肋间内、外肌 intercostales interni and externi
37. 第4肋骨 4th costal bone
38. 第5肋骨 5th costal bone
39. 菱形肌 rhomboideus
40. 斜方肌 trapezius
41. 横突棘肌 transversospinales
42. 棘肌 spinales
43. 最长肌 longissimus
44. 髂肋肌 iliocostalis
45. 棘突 spinous process
46. 硬膜外隙 epidural space
47. 脊髓 spinal cord
48. 第5胸椎椎体 body of 5th thoracic vertebra
49. 肋头关节 joint of costal head
50. 横突 transverse process
51. 肋横突关节 costotransverse joint
52. 后段支气管（B2）和动脉（A2）posterior segmental bronchus and artery
53. 后段静脉（V2）posterior segmental vein
54. 尖段支气管（B1）apical segmental bronchus
55. 右肺上叶支气管 superior lobar bronchus of right lung
56. 尖段动脉（A1）apical segmental artery
57. 尖段静脉（V1）apical segmental vein
58. 右肺前段支气管（B3）和动脉（A3）right anterior segmental bronchus and artery
59. 肱二头肌长、短头 long and short heads of biceps brachii
60. 喙肱肌 coracobrachialis
61. 肱骨 humerus

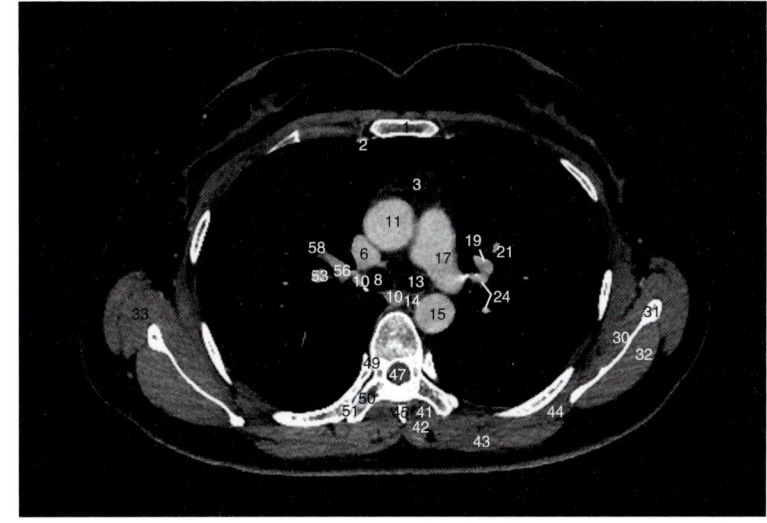

B. CT 纵隔窗增强图像

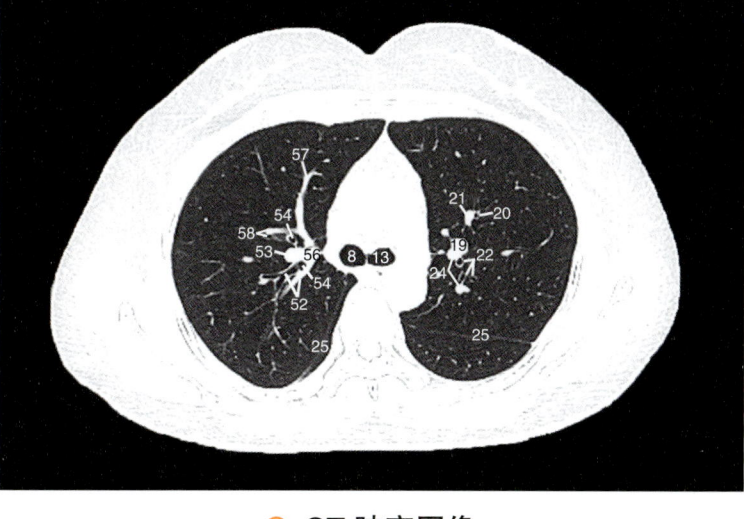

C. CT 肺窗图像

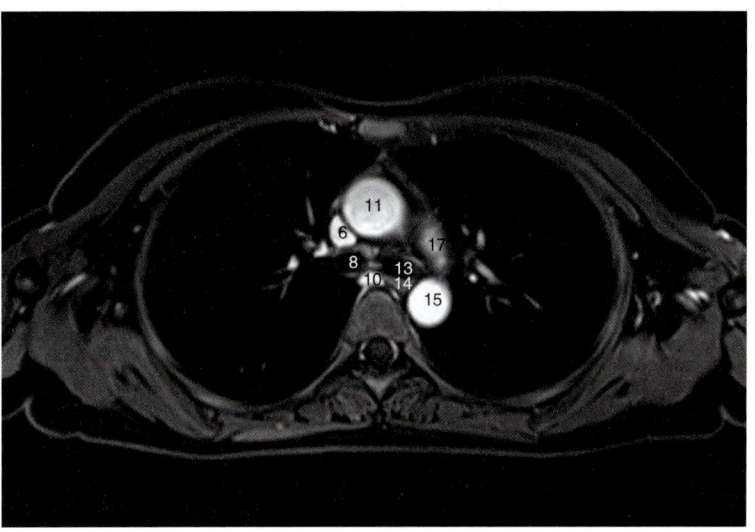

D. MR T1WI 增强图像

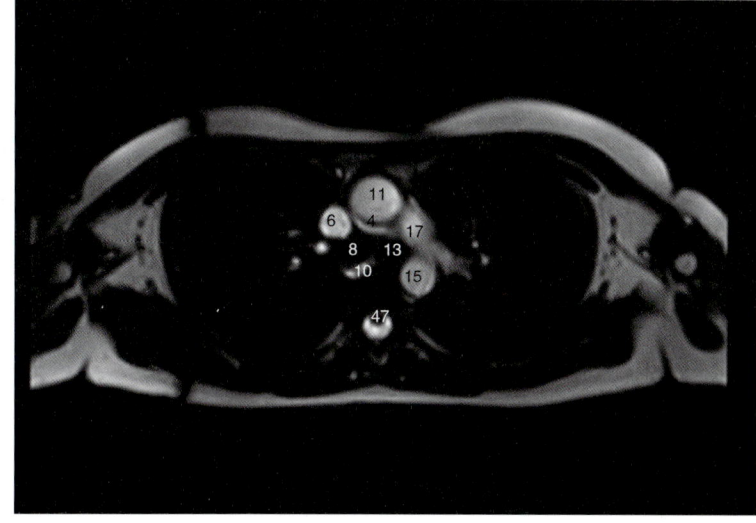

E. MR T2WI 平扫图像

关键结构：左主支气管，右主支气管。

此断面经过第5胸椎椎体上份。

于纵隔内见气管分叉为左、右主支气管。在气管权下方层面左、右主支气管逐渐分离，分别进入左、右肺门。主支气管管壁构造与气管类似，由软骨环、平滑肌纤维及结缔组织构成。但软骨环相对较小，膜壁相对较大。软骨环的数量一般是左主支气管7~8个，右主支气管3~4个。CT测量男性左、右主支气管的长度分别为 50.3 mm ± 4.7 mm 和 19.7 mm ± 5.2 mm，女性左、右主支气管的长度分别为 46.3 mm ± 4.5 mm 和 18.2 mm ± 4.1 mm，左主支气管的长度是右主支气管长度的3~4倍[35]。故在横断面中，右主支气管出现层面明显较左主支气管少。由于右主支气管较短，在气管分叉后很快见右主支气管发出右肺上叶支气管。男性左、右主支气管开口处内径分别为 14.3 mm ± 1.5 mm 和 15.7 mm ± 1.6 mm，女性左、右主支气管开口处内径分别为 12.8 mm ± 1.6 mm 和 14.1 mm ± 1.4 mm[35]。由于右主支气管较左主支气管短、宽、走向更陡直，因而吸入性气管异物易落入右主支气管。右肺特别是下叶感染或脓肿的发病率也较左肺高。

胸部连续横断层 37（FH.12770）

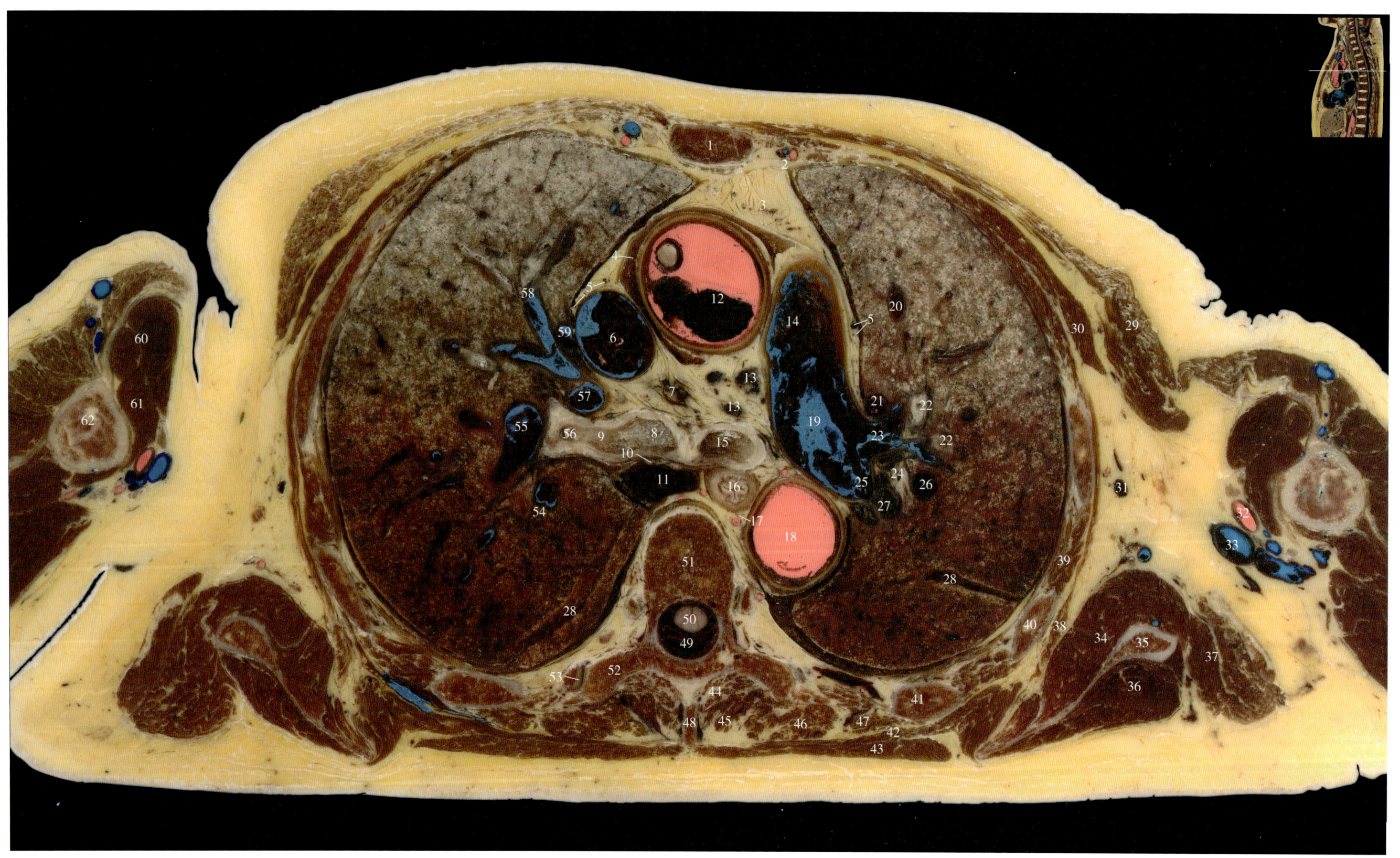

A. 断层标本图像

1. 胸骨体 body of sternum
2. 胸廓内动、静脉 internal thoracic artery and vein
3. 胸腺 thymus
4. 心包上隐窝 superior recess of pericardium
5. 膈神经和心包膈血管 phrenic nerve and pericardiacophrenic vessels
6. 上腔静脉 superior vena cava
7. 右下气管旁淋巴结（4R）right lower paratracheal lymph nodes
8. 右主支气管 right principal bronchus
9. 右肺上叶支气管 superior lobar bronchus of right lung
10. 右迷走神经 right vagus nerve
11. 奇静脉 azygos vein
12. 升主动脉 ascending aorta
13. 主动脉弓下淋巴结（5区）subaortic lymph nodes
14. 肺动脉干 pulmonary trunk
15. 左主支气管 left principal bronchus
16. 食管 esophagus
17. 胸导管 thoracic duct
18. 胸主动脉 thoracic aorta
19. 左肺动脉 left pulmonary artery
20. 左肺前段静脉（V3）left anterior segmental vein
21. 尖后段静脉段间支（V1+2）intersegmental ramus of apicoposterior segmental vein
22. 左肺前段支气管（B3）left anterior segmental bronchus
23. 左肺前段动脉（A3）left anterior segmental artery
24. 尖后段支气管（B1+2）apicoposterior segmental bronchus
25. 尖后段动脉（A1+2）apicoposterior segmental artery
26. 尖后段静脉段内支（V1+2）intrasegmental ramus of apicoposterior segmental vein
27. 左肺叶淋巴结（12L）left lobar lymph nodes
28. 斜裂 oblique fissure
29. 胸大肌 pectoralis major
30. 胸小肌 pectoralis minor
31. 胸外侧静脉 lateral thoracic vein
32. 腋动脉 axillary artery
33. 腋静脉 axillary vein
34. 肩胛下肌 subscapularis
35. 肩胛骨 scapula
36. 冈下肌 infraspinatus
37. 大圆肌 teres major
38. 前锯肌 serratus anterior
39. 肋间内、外肌 intercostales interni and externi
40. 第4肋骨 4th costal bone
41. 第5肋骨 5th costal bone
42. 菱形肌 rhomboideus
43. 斜方肌 trapezius
44. 横突棘肌 transversospinales
45. 棘肌 spinales
46. 最长肌 longissimus
47. 髂肋肌 iliocostalis
48. 棘突 spinous process
49. 硬膜外隙 epidural space
50. 脊髓 spinal cord
51. 第5胸椎椎体 body of 5th thoracic vertebra
52. 横突 transverse process
53. 肋横突关节 costotransverse joint
54. 后段支气管（B2）和动脉（A2）posterior segmental bronchus and artery
55. 后段静脉（V2）posterior segmental vein
56. 尖段支气管（B1）apical segmental bronchus
57. 尖段动脉（A1）apical segmental artery
58. 右肺前段支气管（B3）和动脉（A3）right anterior segmental bronchus and artery
59. 尖段静脉（V1）apical segmental vein
60. 肱二头肌长、短头 long and short heads of biceps brachii
61. 喙肱肌 coracobrachialis
62. 肱骨 humerus

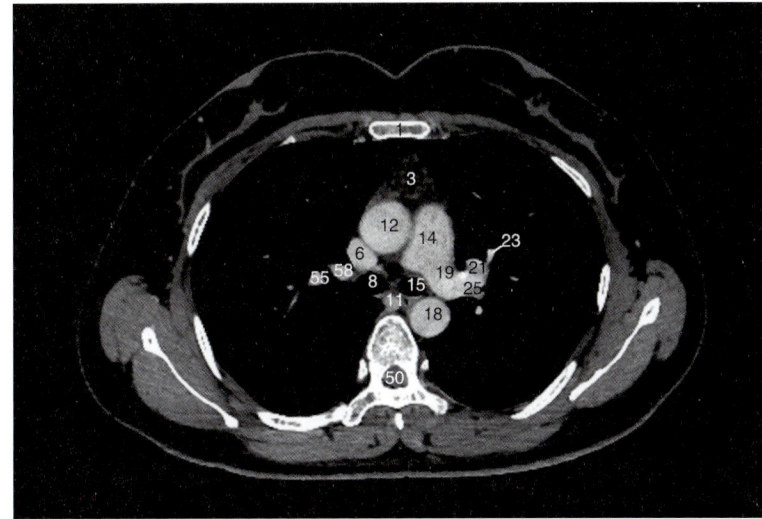

B. CT 纵隔窗增强图像

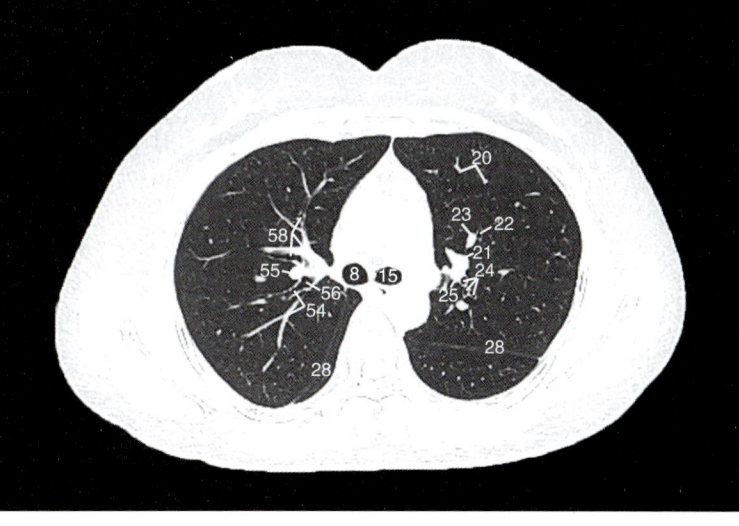

C. CT 肺窗图像

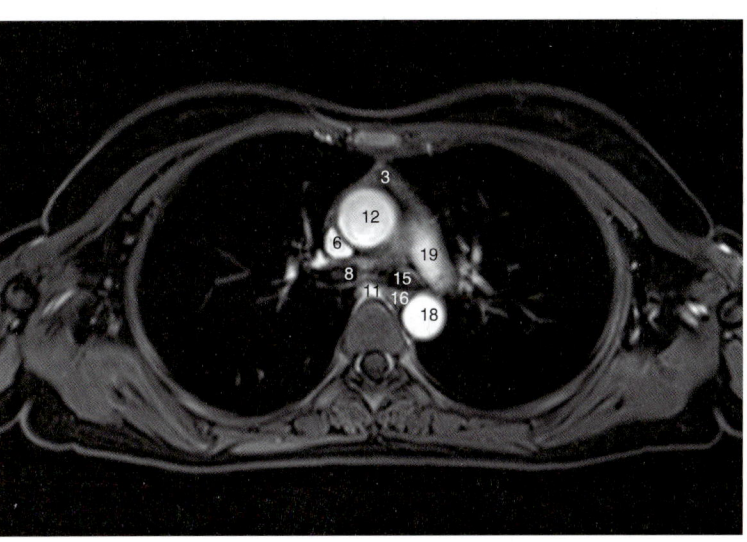

D. MR T1WI 增强图像

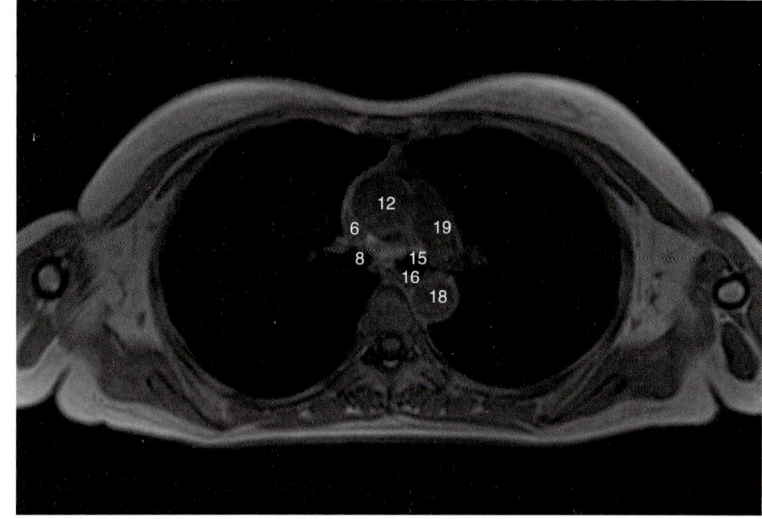

E. MR T1WI 平扫图像

关键结构：右肺上叶支气管，左肺前段动脉。

断面经第5胸椎椎体上份。

在紧邻气管杈下方的层面，由于右主支气管较短，故很快见右主支气管向外侧发出右肺上叶支气管，该分支短而水平，为进入右肺门层面的标志。右肺上叶支气管长度 0.8 cm ± 0.2 cm，外横径 1.1 cm ± 0.1 cm[36]，分支进入上叶的尖段、后段和前段。尖段支气管发出后垂直上行，断面表现常为圆管状，紧靠肺门；前段支气管和后段支气管起始部较为水平，前段支气管行向前下，后段支气管继续行向后上，上叶支气管平面通常为尖段消失平面。左主支气管的外侧见急拐入左肺门的左肺动脉，是左肺门出现的标志。左肺动脉进入左肺上叶后，通常不发出上叶动脉，而是在左肺动脉远端向前、后分别发出前段动脉和后段动脉，主干下行变为左肺下叶动脉，靠近斜裂。在左肺上叶支气管以上平面，主要出现前段和尖后段的结构。横断面左肺门典型表现为左肺动脉及其发出的前段动脉，尖后段动脉位于肺门较中心的部位，在它们外侧由前向后是与肺动脉相伴行的前段支气管和尖后段支气管。左肺动脉与前段动脉一起形成"鱼钩样"外观，钩绕尖后段静脉（段间支）。

胸部连续横断层 38（FH.12750）

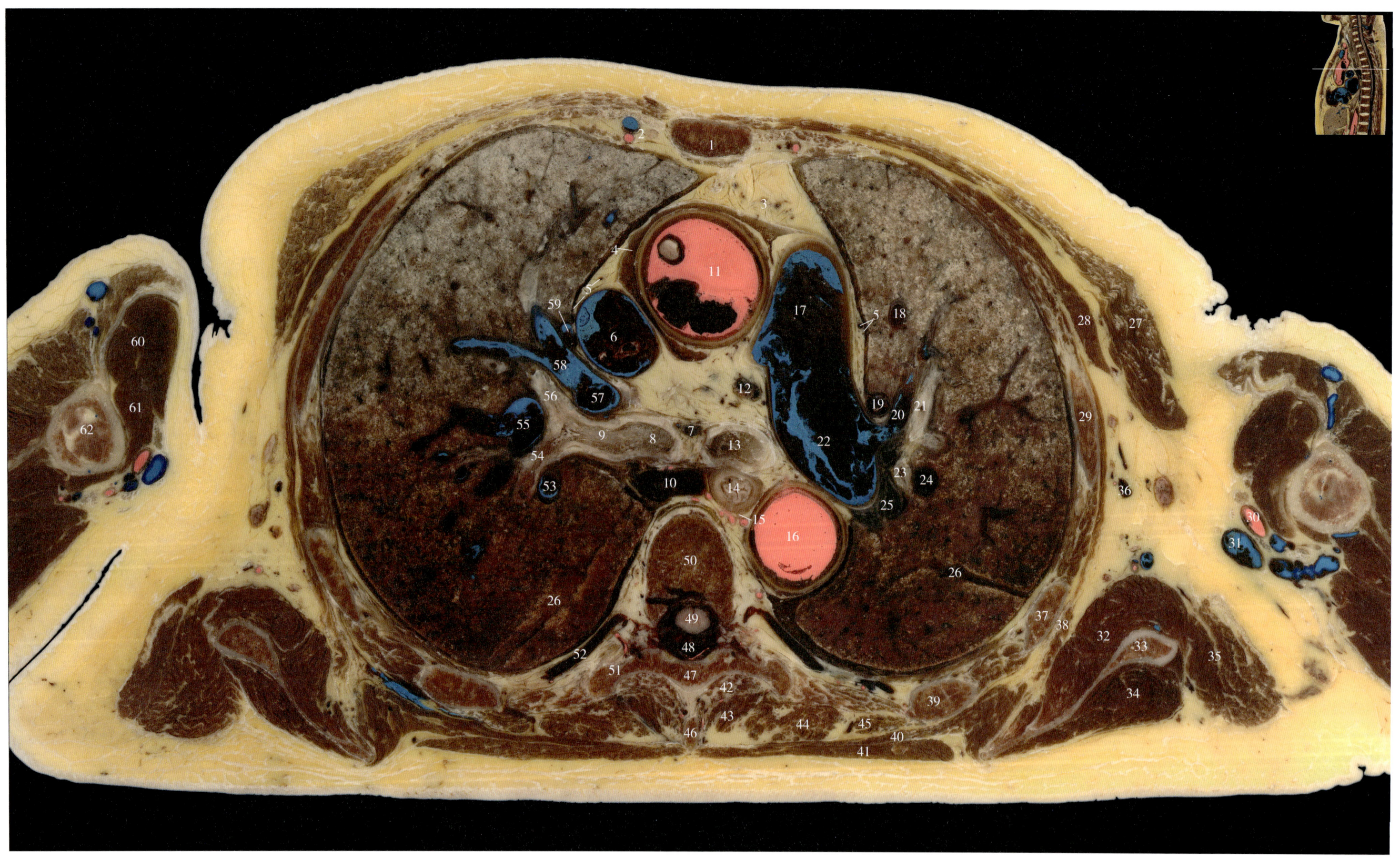

A. 断层标本图像

1. 胸骨体 body of sternum
2. 胸廓内动、静脉 internal thoracic artery and vein
3. 胸腺 thymus
4. 心包上隐窝 superior recess of pericardium
5. 膈神经和心包膈血管 phrenic nerve and pericardiacophrenic vessels
6. 上腔静脉 superior vena cava
7. 隆嵴下淋巴结（7区）subcarinal lymph nodes
8. 右主支气管 right principal bronchus
9. 右肺上叶支气管 superior lobar bronchus of right lung
10. 奇静脉 azygos vein
11. 升主动脉 ascending aorta
12. 主动脉弓下淋巴结（5区）subaortic lymph nodes
13. 左主支气管 left principal bronchus
14. 食管 esophagus
15. 胸导管 thoracic duct
16. 胸主动脉 thoracic aorta
17. 肺动脉干 pulmonary trunk
18. 左肺前段静脉（V3）left anterior segmental vein
19. 尖后段静脉段间支（V1+2）intersegmental ramus of apicoposterior segmental vein
20. 左肺前段动脉（A3）left anterior segmental artery
21. 左肺前段支气管（B3）left anterior segmental bronchus
22. 左肺动脉 left pulmonary artery
23. 尖后段支气管（B1+2）apicoposterior segmental bronchus
24. 尖后段静脉段内支（V1+2）intrasegmental ramus of apicoposterior segmental vein
25. 左肺叶淋巴结（12L）left lobar lymph nodes
26. 斜裂 oblique fissure
27. 胸大肌 pectoralis major
28. 胸小肌 pectoralis minor
29. 第3肋骨 3rd costal bone
30. 腋动脉 axillary artery
31. 腋静脉 axillary vein
32. 肩胛下肌 subscapularis
33. 肩胛骨 scapula
34. 冈下肌 infraspinatus
35. 大圆肌 teres major
36. 胸外侧静脉 lateral thoracic vein
37. 第4肋骨 4th costal bone
38. 前锯肌 serratus anterior
39. 第5肋骨 5th costal bone
40. 菱形肌 rhomboideus
41. 斜方肌 trapezius
42. 横突棘肌 transversospinales
43. 棘肌 spinales
44. 最长肌 longissimus
45. 髂肋肌 iliocostalis
46. 棘突 spinous process
47. 椎弓板 lamina of vertebral arch
48. 硬膜外隙 epidural space
49. 脊髓 spinal cord
50. 第5胸椎椎体 body of 5th thoracic vertebra
51. 横突 transverse process
52. 肋间后静脉 posterior intercostal vein
53. 后段动脉（A2）posterior segmental artery
54. 后段支气管（B2）posterior segmental bronchus
55. 后段静脉（V2）posterior segmental vein
56. 右肺前段支气管（B3）right anterior segmental bronchus
57. 右肺上叶动脉 right superior lobar artery
58. 右肺前段动脉（A3）right anterior segmental artery
59. 尖段静脉（V1）apical segmental vein
60. 肱二头肌长、短头 long and short heads of biceps brachii
61. 喙肱肌 coracobrachialis
62. 肱骨 humerus

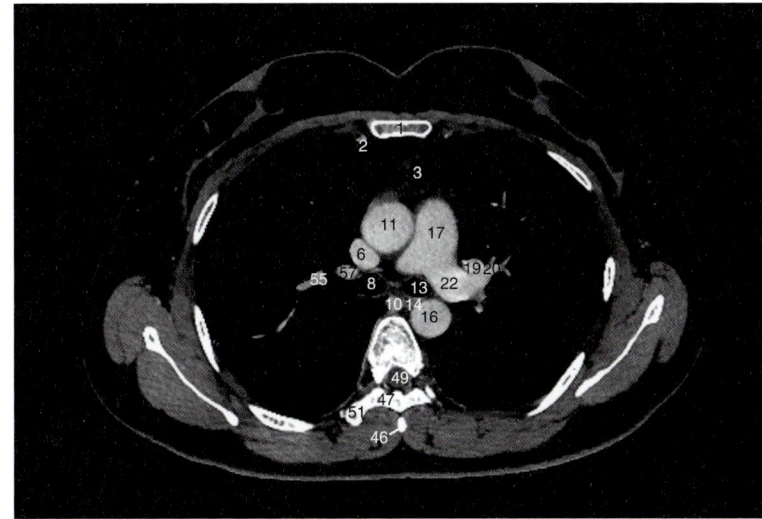

B. CT 纵隔窗增强图像

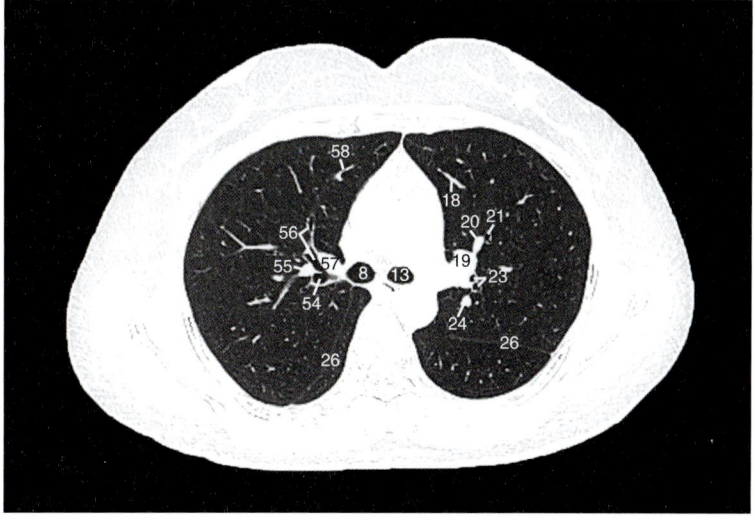

C. CT 肺窗图像

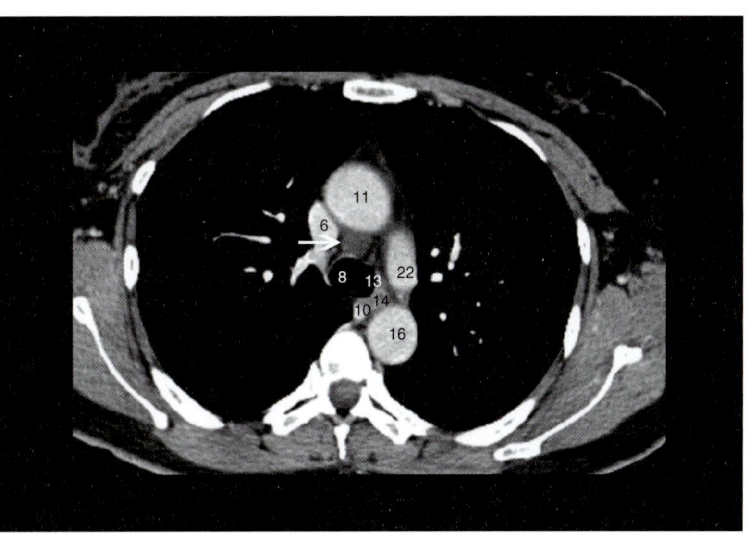

D. 正常心包上隐窝 CT 图像

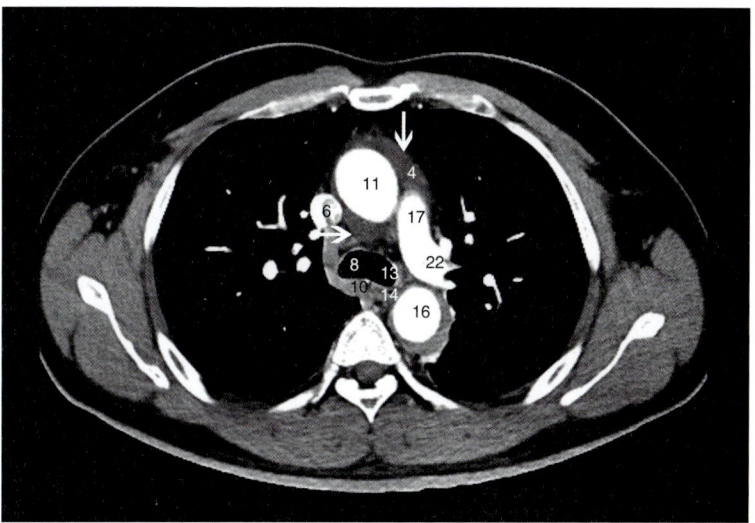

E. 心包上隐窝积液 CT 图像

关键结构：左肺前段支气管和动脉，右肺上叶动脉，心包上隐窝。

断面经第5胸椎椎体中份。

自右肺上叶支气管进入上叶至右肺上叶静脉离开上叶层面，右肺门处主要出现的是右肺上叶门。右肺上叶支气管和上叶动脉伴行，在较高的位置进入上叶门。上叶动脉的分支类型中，"前干 + 后升动脉"型是最常见，占54%，其次为"前干 + 前升动脉 + 后升动脉"型及"上前干 + 下前干 + 后升动脉"型，分别占12.9%和12.1%[37]。上叶静脉收集三支静脉，在较低的位置出上叶门。此断面及相邻断面居于右肺上叶门较高的位置，故见右肺上叶支气管继续水平地进入右肺，右肺上叶动脉伴行于其前内侧。上叶支气管远端前、后分别发出前段支气管和后段支气管。

85%的后段静脉位于前、后段支气管二者的夹角内，为段间支，位置较为恒定，其向外侧延长线分隔前、后两段。右主支气管和上叶支气管的后壁均与肺组织相贴，在CT图像上境界清晰，若模糊或增强是肺门后肿块的可靠指征。左肺门处结构仍为近左肺门中心位置的左肺动脉及其发出的前段动脉、前段支气管、尖后段支气管和动脉等结构。心包上隐窝于此断面中显示清晰，环形围绕与升主动脉周围。D图箭头示正常的心包上隐窝的图像。心包上隐窝积液CT图像中箭头示心包积液时心包上隐窝区域增大并可见积液影，可较好地显示心包上隐窝的范围。

77

胸部连续横断层 39（FH.12730）

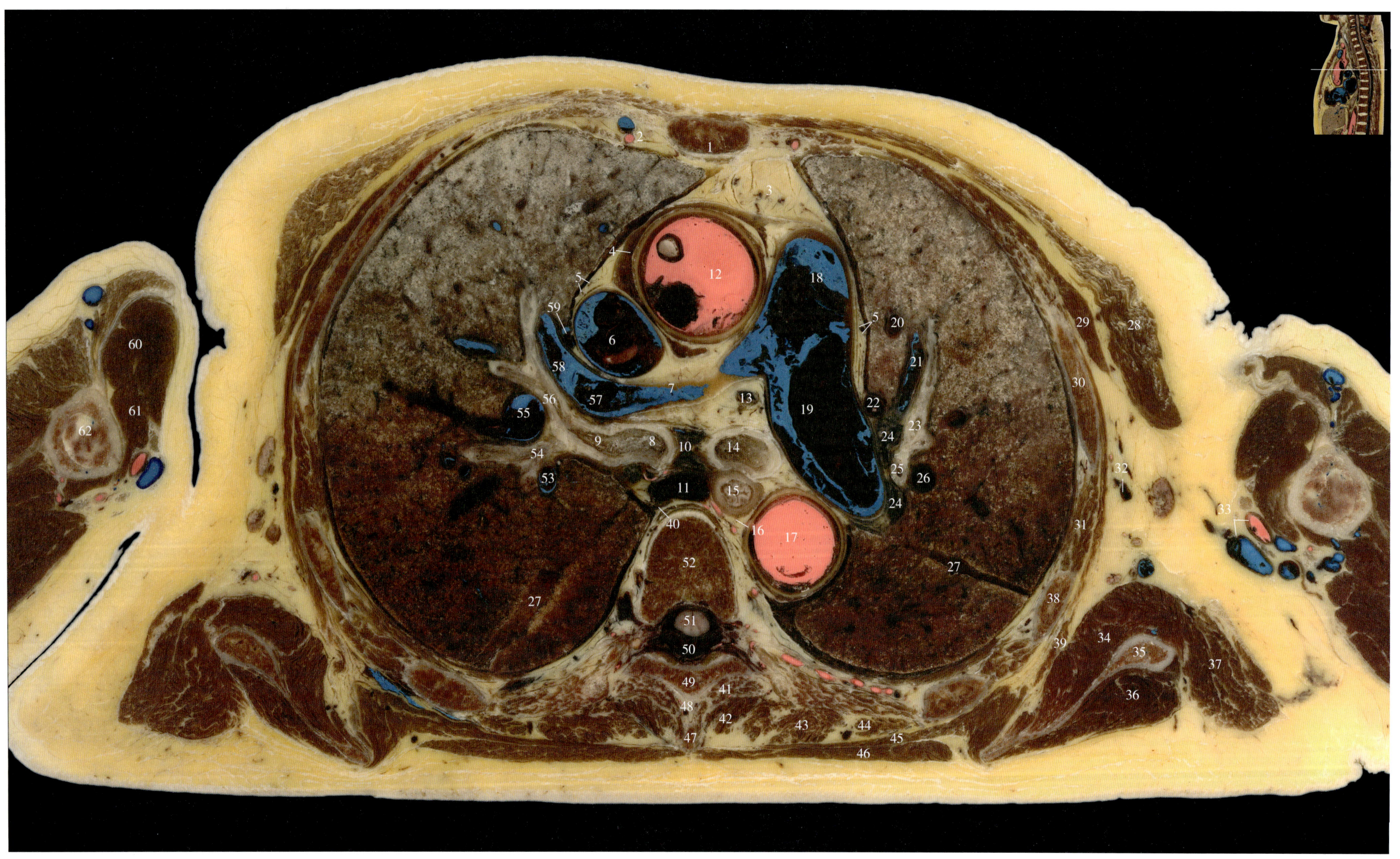

A. 断层标本图像

1. 胸骨体 body of sternum
2. 胸廓内动、静脉 internal thoracic artery and vein
3. 胸腺 thymus
4. 心包上隐窝 superior recess of pericardium
5. 膈神经和心包膈血管 phrenic nerve and pericardiacophrenic vessels
6. 上腔静脉 superior vena cava
7. 右肺动脉 right pulmonary artery
8. 右主支气管 right principal bronchus
9. 右肺上叶支气管 superior lobar bronchus of right lung
10. 隆嵴下淋巴结（7区）subcarinal lymph nodes
11. 奇静脉 azygos vein
12. 升主动脉 ascending aorta
13. 主动脉弓下淋巴结（5区）subaortic lymph nodes
14. 左主支气管 left principal bronchus
15. 食管 esophagus
16. 胸导管 thoracic duct
17. 胸主动脉 thoracic aorta
18. 肺动脉干 pulmonary trunk
19. 左肺动脉 left pulmonary artery
20. 左肺前段静脉（V3）left anterior segmental vein
21. 左肺前段动脉（A3）left anterior segmental artery
22. 尖后段静脉段间支（V1+2）intersegmental ramus of apicoposterior segmental vein
23. 左肺前段支气管（B3）left anterior segmental bronchus
24. 左肺叶淋巴结（12L）left lobar lymph nodes
25. 尖后段支气管（B1+2）apicoposterior segmental bronchus
26. 尖后段静脉段内支（V1+2）intrasegmental ramus of apicoposterior segmental vein
27. 斜裂 oblique fissure
28. 胸大肌 pectoralis major
29. 胸小肌 pectoralis minor
30. 第3肋骨 3rd costal bone
31. 肋间内、外肌 intercostales interni and externi
32. 胸外侧静脉 lateral thoracic vein
33. 腋动、静脉 axillary artery and vein
34. 肩胛下肌 subscapularis
35. 肩胛骨 scapula
36. 冈下肌 infraspinatus
37. 大圆肌 teres major
38. 第4肋骨 4th costal bone
39. 前锯肌 serratus anterior
40. 奇静脉食管隐窝 azygoesophageal recess
41. 横突棘肌 transversospinales
42. 棘肌 spinales
43. 最长肌 longissimus
44. 髂肋肌 iliocostalis
45. 菱形肌 rhomboideus
46. 斜方肌 trapezius
47. 棘突 spinous process
48. 棘间韧带 interspinous ligament
49. 椎弓板 lamina of vertebral arch
50. 硬膜外隙 epidural space
51. 脊髓 spinal cord
52. 第5胸椎椎体 body of 5th thoracic vertebra
53. 右肺后段动脉（A2）right posterior segmental artery
54. 右肺后段支气管（B2）right posterior segmental bronchus
55. 右肺后段静脉（V2）right posterior segmental vein
56. 右肺前段支气管（B3）right anterior segmental bronchus
57. 右肺上叶动脉 right superior lobar artery
58. 右肺前段动脉（A3）right anterior segmental artery
59. 右肺尖段静脉（V1）right apical segmental vein
60. 肱二头肌长、短头 long and short heads of biceps brachii
61. 喙肱肌 coracobrachialis
62. 肱骨 humerus

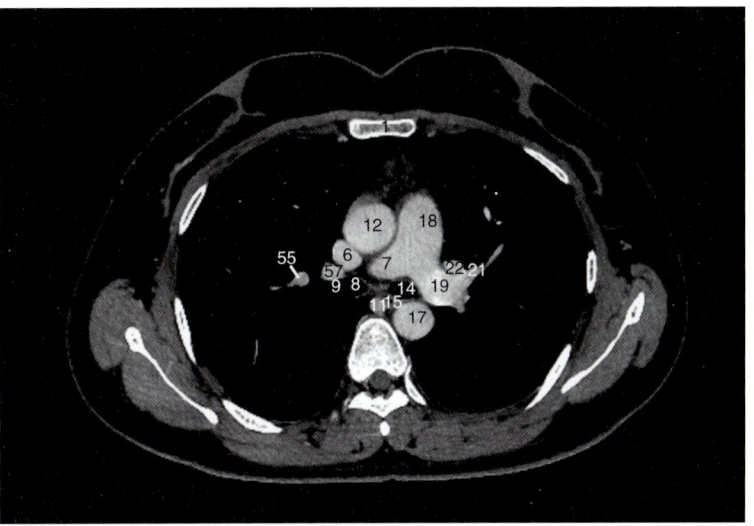

B. CT 纵隔窗增强图像

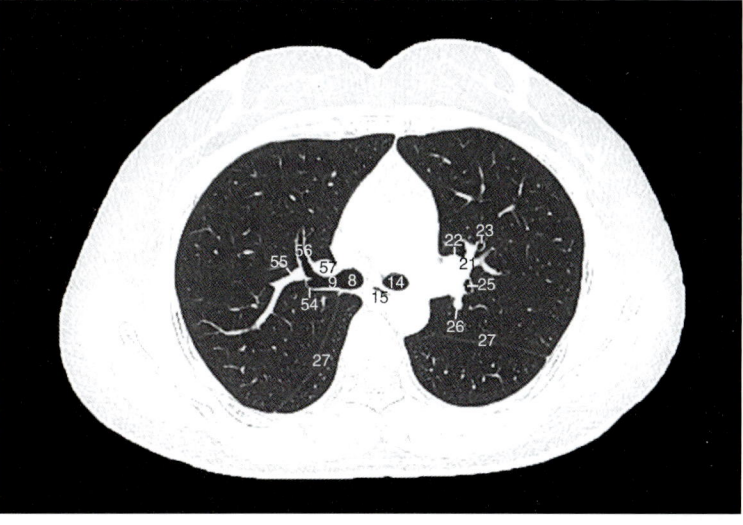

C. CT 肺窗图像

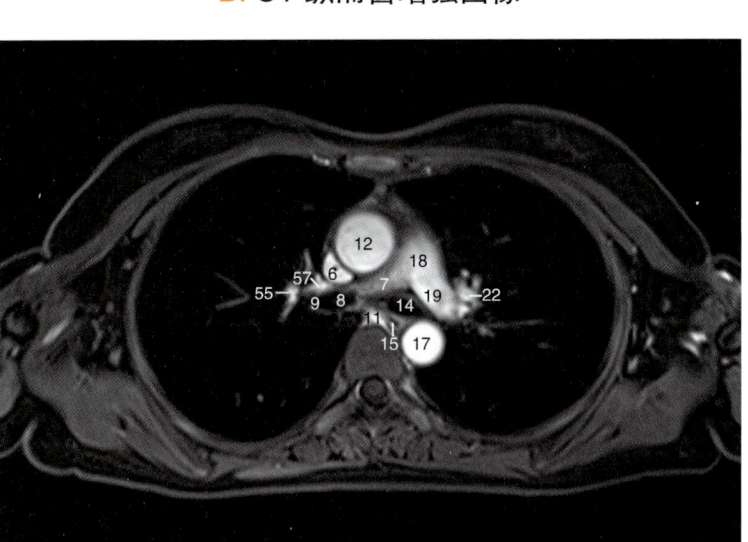

D. MR T1WI 增强图像

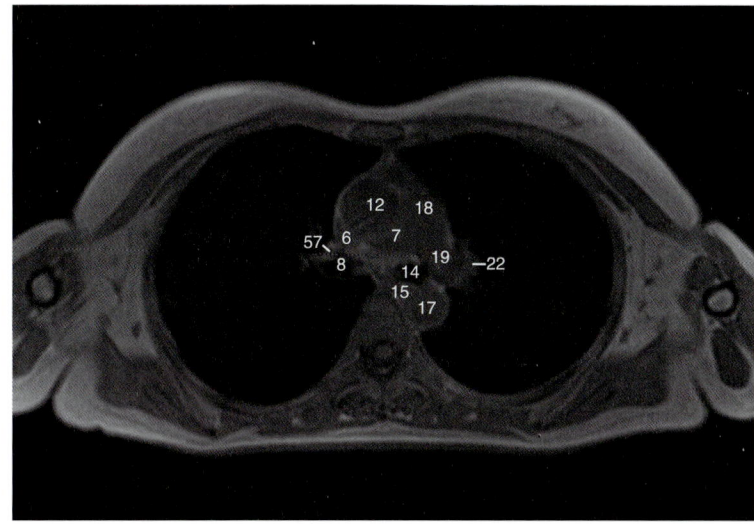

E. MR T1WI 平扫图像

关键结构：右肺尖段静脉，右肺后段支气管，右肺后段动脉，后段静脉。

此断面经第5胸椎椎体中份。

右肺门内主要出现右肺上叶门上部的结构，从前内侧向后外侧管道依次排列分别为尖段静脉、前段动脉、前段支气管、后段静脉和后段支气管。尖段静脉分为前支和尖支，位于胸膜下的为浅静脉，位于深处靠近支气管的为深静脉，94%的前支为浅静脉，6%的为深支；66%的尖支为浅静脉，34%的尖支为深静脉[38]。上叶支气管向前外侧和后外侧分别发出前段支气管和后段支气管，前段支气管有前段动脉伴行，动脉位于支气管前内侧，共同行向前外侧下方；后段支气管长1.3（0.8~2.2）cm[36]，起始部水平，后逐渐行向后上，后段动脉常伴行于支气管的后内侧。后段静脉段间支位置较为固定，68.2%的前、后段支气管在同一平面发出，这种情况下后段静脉出现在前、后段支气管外侧的夹角处；当前、后段支气管不在同一平面发出时，占31.8%，后段静脉出现在前段支气管的后方或后段支气管的前方[39]，后段静脉及其属支（或延长线）可作为区分前、后段的解剖标志。故从尖段支气管至上叶支气管下缘层面的CT图像上，右肺门前缘是由尖段静脉和尖段动脉，后缘（由外至内）由后段支气管、上叶支气管和中间支气管构成，而后段静脉构成右肺门外侧缘。

胸部连续横断层 40（FH.12710）

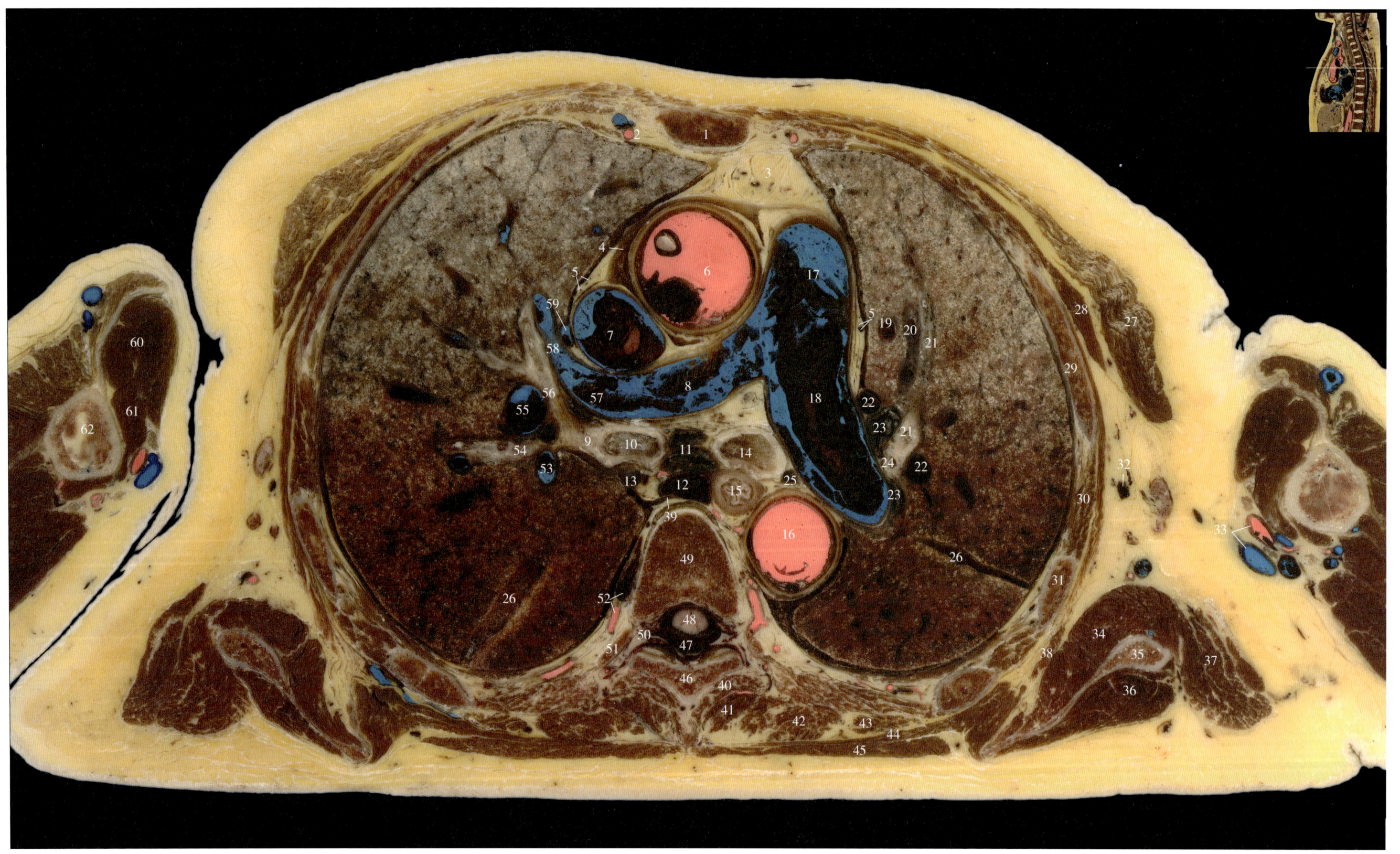

A. 断层标本图像

1. 胸骨体 body of sternum
2. 胸廓内动、静脉 internal thoracic artery and vein
3. 胸腺 thymus
4. 心包上隐窝 superior recess of pericardium
5. 膈神经和心包膈血管 phrenic nerve and pericardiacophrenic vessels
6. 升主动脉 ascending aorta
7. 上腔静脉 superior vena cava
8. 右肺动脉 right pulmonary artery
9. 右肺上叶支气管 superior lobar bronchus of right lung
10. 中间支气管 intermediate bronchus
11. 隆嵴下淋巴结（7区）subcarinal lymph nodes
12. 奇静脉 azygos vein
13. 右肺门淋巴结（10R）right hilar lymph nodes
14. 左主支气管 left principal bronchus
15. 食管 esophagus
16. 胸主动脉 thoracic aorta
17. 肺动脉干 pulmonary trunk
18. 左肺动脉 left pulmonary artery
19. 左肺前段静脉（V3）left anterior segmental vein
20. 左肺前段动脉（A3）left anterior segmental artery
21. 左肺前段支气管（B3）left anterior segmental bronchus
22. 尖后段静脉（V1+2）apicoposterior segmental vein
23. 左肺叶淋巴结（12L）left lobar lymph nodes
24. 尖后段支气管（B1+2）apicoposterior segmental bronchus
25. 左肺门淋巴结（10L）left hilar lymph nodes
26. 斜裂 oblique fissure
27. 胸大肌 pectoralis major
28. 胸小肌 pectoralis minor
29. 第3肋骨 3rd costal bone
30. 肋间内、外肌 intercostales interni and externi
31. 第4肋骨 4th costal bone
32. 胸外侧静脉 lateral thoracic vein
33. 腋动、静脉 axillary artery and vein
34. 肩胛下肌 subscapularis
35. 肩胛骨 scapula
36. 冈下肌 infraspinatus
37. 大圆肌 teres major
38. 前锯肌 serratus anterior
39. 奇静脉食管隐窝 azygoesophageal recess
40. 横突棘肌 transversospinales
41. 棘肌 spinales
42. 最长肌 longissimus
43. 髂肋肌 iliocostalis
44. 菱形肌 rhomboideus
45. 斜方肌 trapezius
46. 椎弓板 lamina of vertebral arch
47. 硬膜外隙 epidural space
48. 脊髓 spinal cord
49. 第5胸椎椎体 body of 5th thoracic vertebra
50. 椎间孔 intervertebral foramen
51. 第6肋骨 6th costal bone
52. 肋间后动、静脉 posterior intercostal artery and vein
53. 右肺后段动脉（A2）right posterior segmental artery
54. 右肺后段支气管（B2）right posterior segmental bronchus
55. 右肺后段静脉（V2）right posterior segmental vein
56. 右肺前段支气管（B3）right anterior segmental bronchus
57. 右肺上叶动脉 right superior lobar artery
58. 右肺前段动脉（A3）right anterior segmental artery
59. 右肺尖段静脉（V1）right apical segmental vein
60. 肱二头肌长、短头 long and short heads of biceps brachii
61. 喙肱肌 coracobrachialis
62. 肱骨 humerus

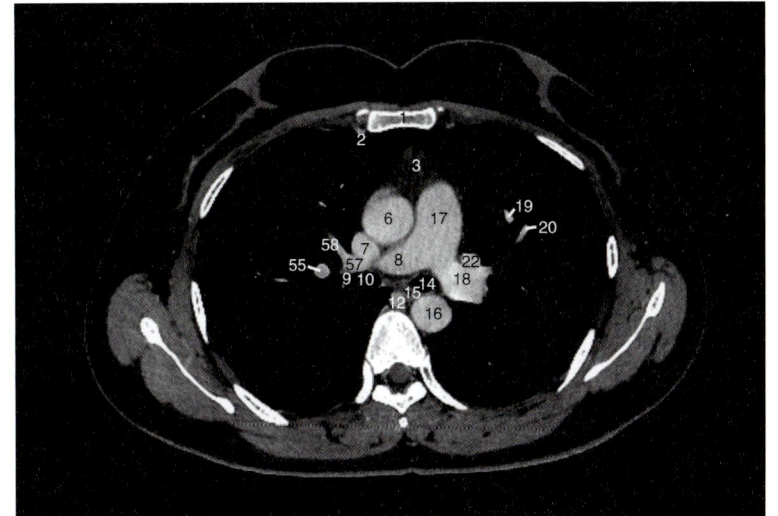

B. CT 纵隔窗增强图像

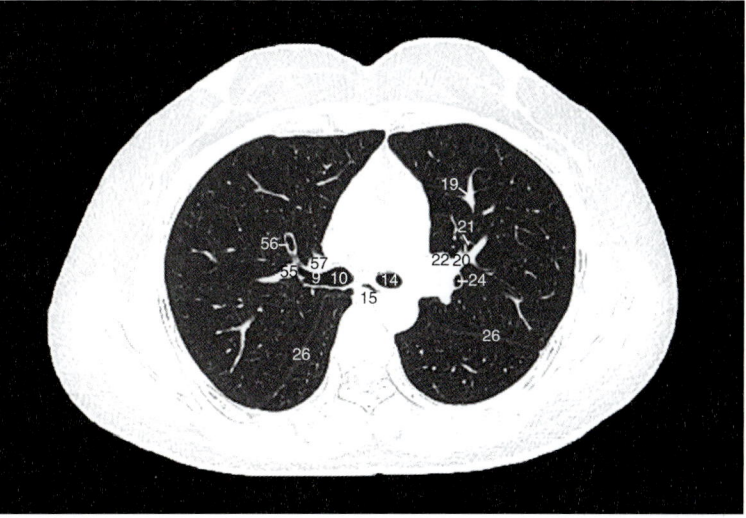

C. CT 肺窗图像

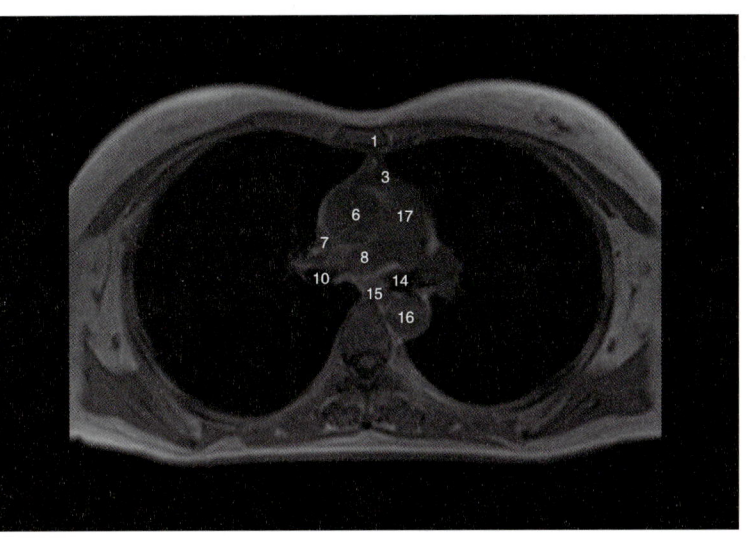

D. MR T1WI 平扫图像

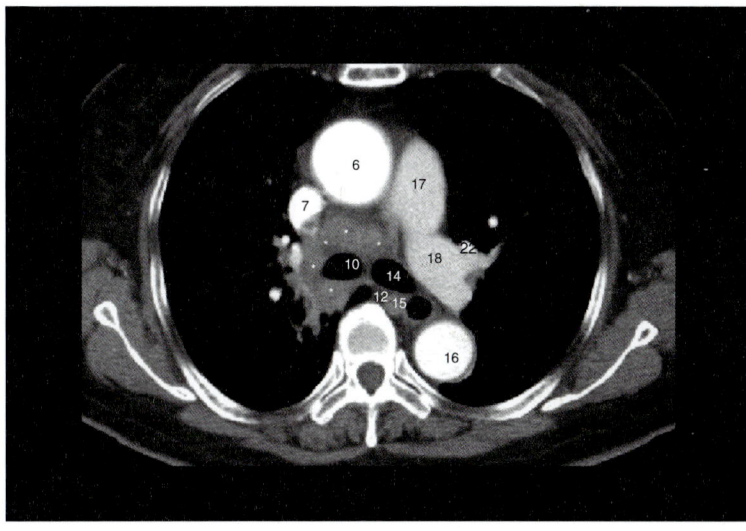

E. 10区淋巴结转移图像

关键结构：隆嵴下间隙，隆嵴下淋巴结，中间支气管。

此断面经第5胸椎椎体中份。

从主动脉弓到肺动脉杈层面，纵隔内结构由前至后可分为4层：第1层为血管前间隙和胸腺；第2层从右向左依次为上腔静脉、升主动脉和心包上隐窝、左肺动脉或肺动脉杈；第3层为气管杈或左、右主支气管、隆嵴下间隙；第4层为奇静脉、食管、胸导管和胸主动脉。此断面在纵隔第3层内见左、右主支气管逐渐分开，隆嵴下间隙逐渐变大。该间隙上通气管前间隙，可认为是气管前间隙的延续。在横断面中，隆嵴下间隙的前界是肺动脉杈和右肺动脉的后壁，两侧为左、右主支气管，后界为食管前壁。在胸骨角平面及以下2 cm范围内均可显示隆嵴下间隙，从气管杈下缘至右肺动脉下缘，该间隙的高度为18.6 mm ± 3.3 mm；

在正中矢状切面，从肺动脉后壁至食管前壁，该间隙的厚度为12.1 mm ± 1.4 mm。该间隙内隆嵴下淋巴结出现率为100%，以2~3个为多见，且多融合成三角形或新月形，CT测量其最大短横径为6.4 mm ± 3.1 mm[40]。右主支气管发出上叶支气管后，进一步向外下方发出中间支气管，该支气管发出后始终位于右肺门后部，横断面呈椭圆形，横径大于前后径，外横径为1.3 cm ± 0.2 cm，长度为1.8 cm ± 0.3 cm[36]。左肺上叶门处，随着层面下移并逐渐低于尖后段动脉和前段动脉起始部，尖后段支气管和前段支气管的伴行动脉逐渐消失，同时两支气管逐渐靠拢并即将合并。在10区淋巴结转移图像中可发现左、右主支气管周围的肿大淋巴结，分别位于10R和10L区。

胸部连续横断层 41（FH.12690）

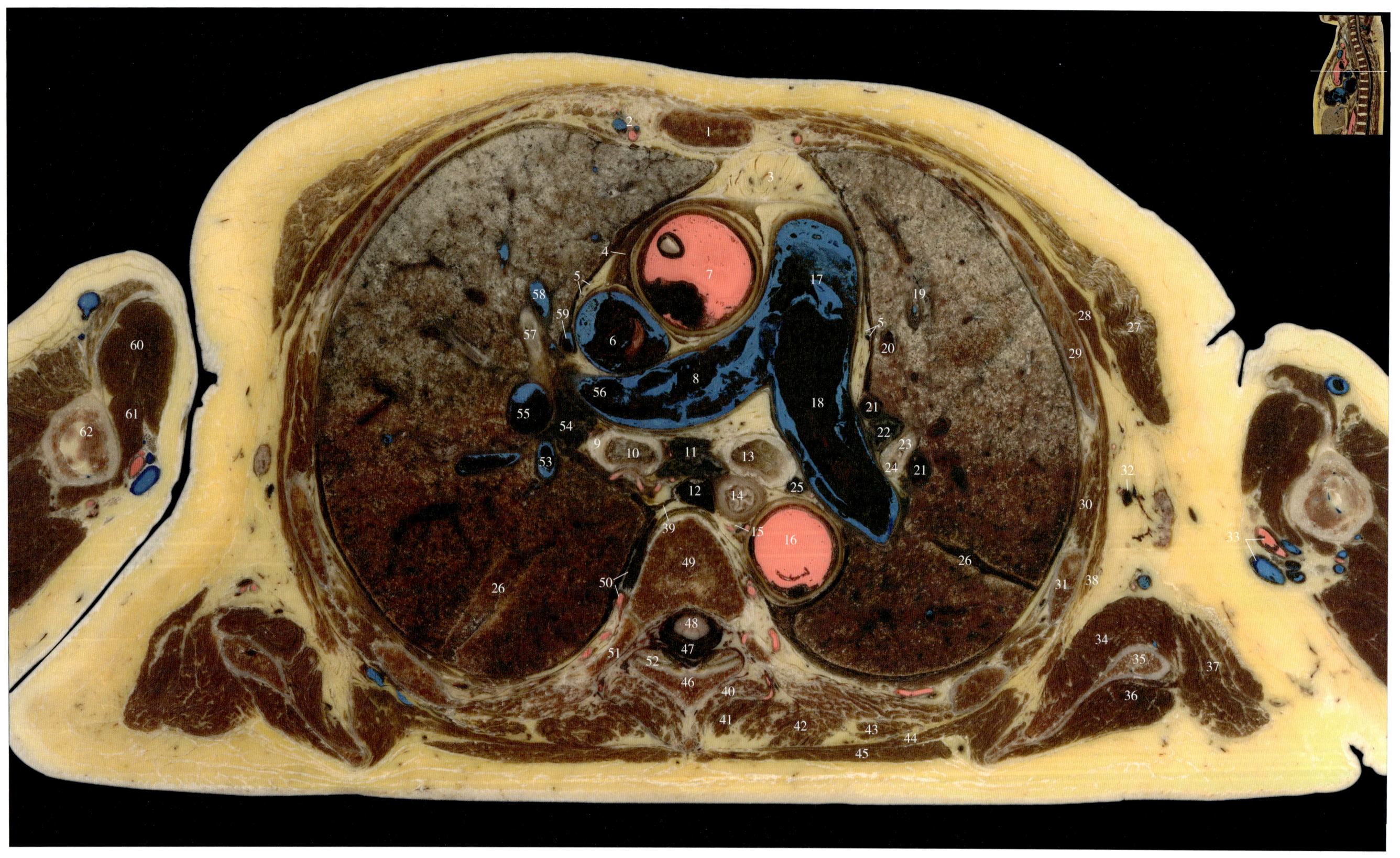

A. 断层标本图像

1. 胸骨体 body of sternum
2. 胸廓内动、静脉 internal thoracic artery and vein
3. 胸腺 thymus
4. 心包上隐窝 superior recess of pericardium
5. 膈神经和心包膈血管 phrenic nerve and pericardiacophrenic vessels
6. 上腔静脉 superior vena cava
7. 升主动脉 ascending aorta
8. 右肺动脉 right pulmonary artery
9. 右肺上叶支气管 superior lobar bronchus of right lung
10. 中间支气管 intermediate bronchus
11. 隆嵴下淋巴结（7区）subcarinal lymph nodes
12. 奇静脉 azygos vein
13. 左主支气管 left principal bronchus
14. 食管 esophagus
15. 胸导管 thoracic duct
16. 胸主动脉 thoracic aorta
17. 肺动脉干 pulmonary trunk
18. 左肺动脉 left pulmonary artery
19. 左肺前段支气管（B3）和动脉（A3）left anterior segmental bronchus and artery
20. 左肺前段静脉（V3）left anterior segmental vein
21. 尖后段静脉（V1+2）apicoposterior segmental vein
22. 左肺叶淋巴结（12L）left lobar lymph nodes
23. 左肺前段支气管（B3）left anterior segmental bronchus
24. 尖后段支气管（B1+2）apicoposterior segmental bronchus
25. 左肺门淋巴结（10L）left hilar lymph nodes
26. 斜裂 oblique fissure
27. 胸大肌 pectoralis major
28. 胸小肌 pectoralis minor
29. 第3肋骨 3rd costal bone
30. 肋间内、外肌 intercostales interni and externi
31. 第4肋骨 4th costal bone
32. 胸外侧静脉 lateral thoracic vein
33. 腋动、静脉 axillary artery and vein
34. 肩胛下肌 subscapularis
35. 肩胛骨 scapula

36. 冈下肌 infraspinatus
37. 大圆肌 teres major
38. 前锯肌 serratus anterior
39. 奇静脉食管隐窝 azygoesophageal recess
40. 横突棘肌 transversospinales
41. 棘肌 spinales
42. 最长肌 longissimus
43. 髂肋肌 iliocostalis
44. 菱形肌 rhomboideus
45. 斜方肌 trapezius
46. 椎弓板 lamina of vertebral arch
47. 硬膜外隙 epidural space
48. 脊髓 spinal cord
49. 第5胸椎椎体 body of 5th thoracic vertebra
50. 肋间后动、静脉 posterior intercostal artery and vein
51. 第6肋骨 6th costal bone
52. 关节突关节 zygapophysial joint
53. 右肺后段动脉（A2）right posterior segmental artery
54. 右叶间淋巴结（11R）right interlobar lymph nodes
55. 右肺后段静脉（V2）right posterior segmental vein
56. 右肺上叶动脉 right superior lobar artery
57. 右肺前段支气管（B3）right anterior segmental bronchus
58. 右肺前段动脉（A3）right anterior segmental artery
59. 右肺尖段静脉（V1）right apical segmental vein
60. 肱二头肌长、短头 long and short heads of biceps brachii
61. 喙肱肌 coracobrachialis
62. 肱骨 humerus

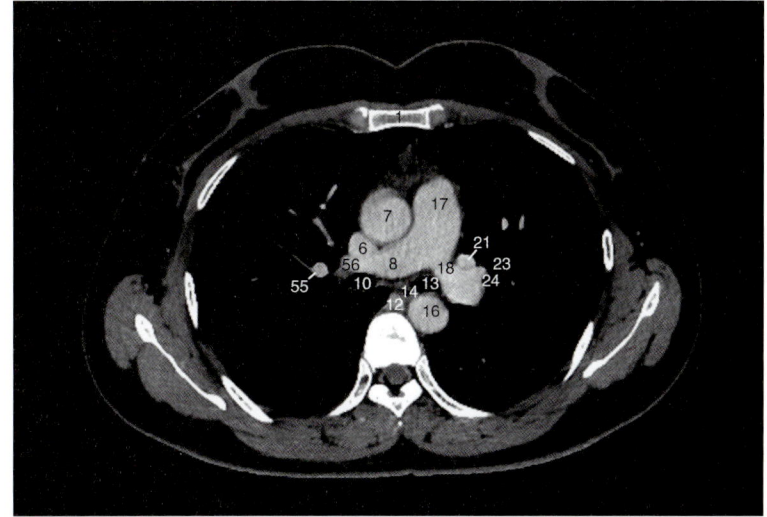

B. CT 纵隔窗增强图像

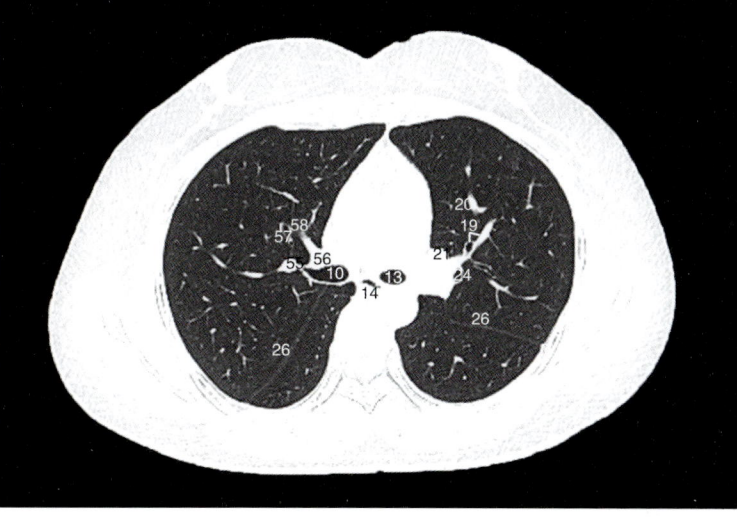

C. CT 肺窗图像

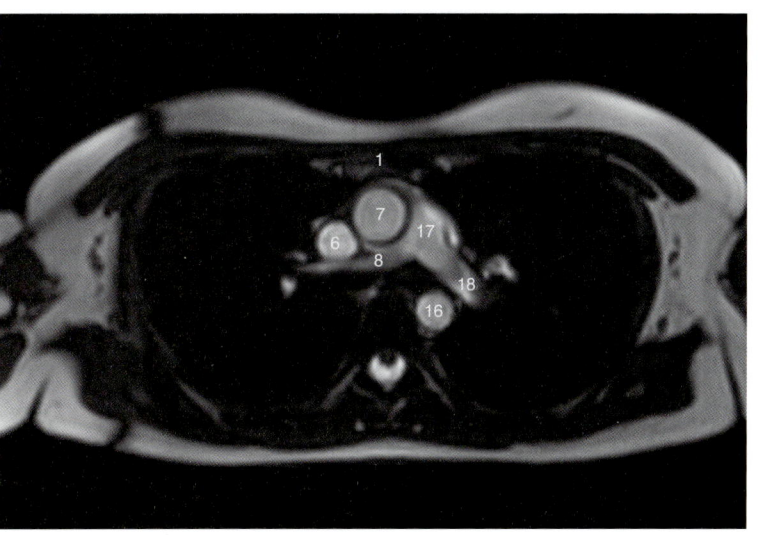

D. MR T2WI 平扫图像

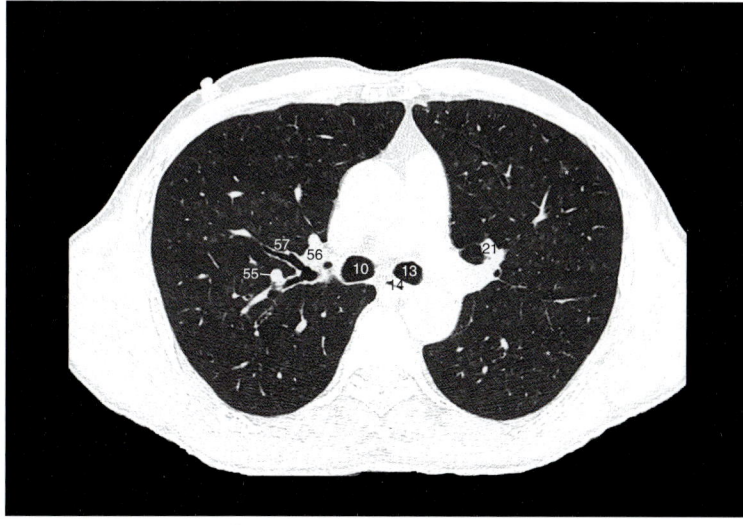

E. 细支气管炎 CT 图像

关键结构：右肺叶间淋巴结，左肺支气管上干。

此断面经第5胸椎椎体下份。

左肺上叶门结构紧靠上叶支气管上方，由尖后段支气管和前段支气管合并形成的上干出现在左肺门中心位置，其前方及外侧主要出现静脉（常为尖后段静脉的段间支和段内支），后方及内侧为左肺动脉及其延续的左肺下叶动脉。上干较短，长度为 0.8 cm ± 0.2 cm，垂直上行，断面表现为圆管状，其他纵行的支气管还包括：右肺尖段支气管和左肺尖后段支气管，它们在横断面均表现为圆管状断面。左肺上干有3种分支类型，64%分支为尖后段和前段支气管，23%分支为尖段、后段和前段支气管，另 10%分支为尖前段支气管和后段支气管[36]。此断面在纵隔及两肺门处见多组淋巴结：右肺上叶支气管和中间支气管之间，见右叶间淋巴结（11R）；隆嵴下间隙内见隆嵴下淋巴结（7区）；左肺上干支气管周围见左肺叶淋巴结（12L）；左侧肺门区见左肺门淋巴结（10L）。E 图示肺内细支气管炎的 CT 表现。细支气管炎为小呼吸道病变的总称，可分为感染性、吸入性及非感染性3类。表现为肺内弥漫性或局限性边界模糊的小叶中心结节、树芽征，可合并细支气管或气管扩张，小叶性、节段性实变或磨玻璃病变。

胸部连续横断层 42（FH.12670）

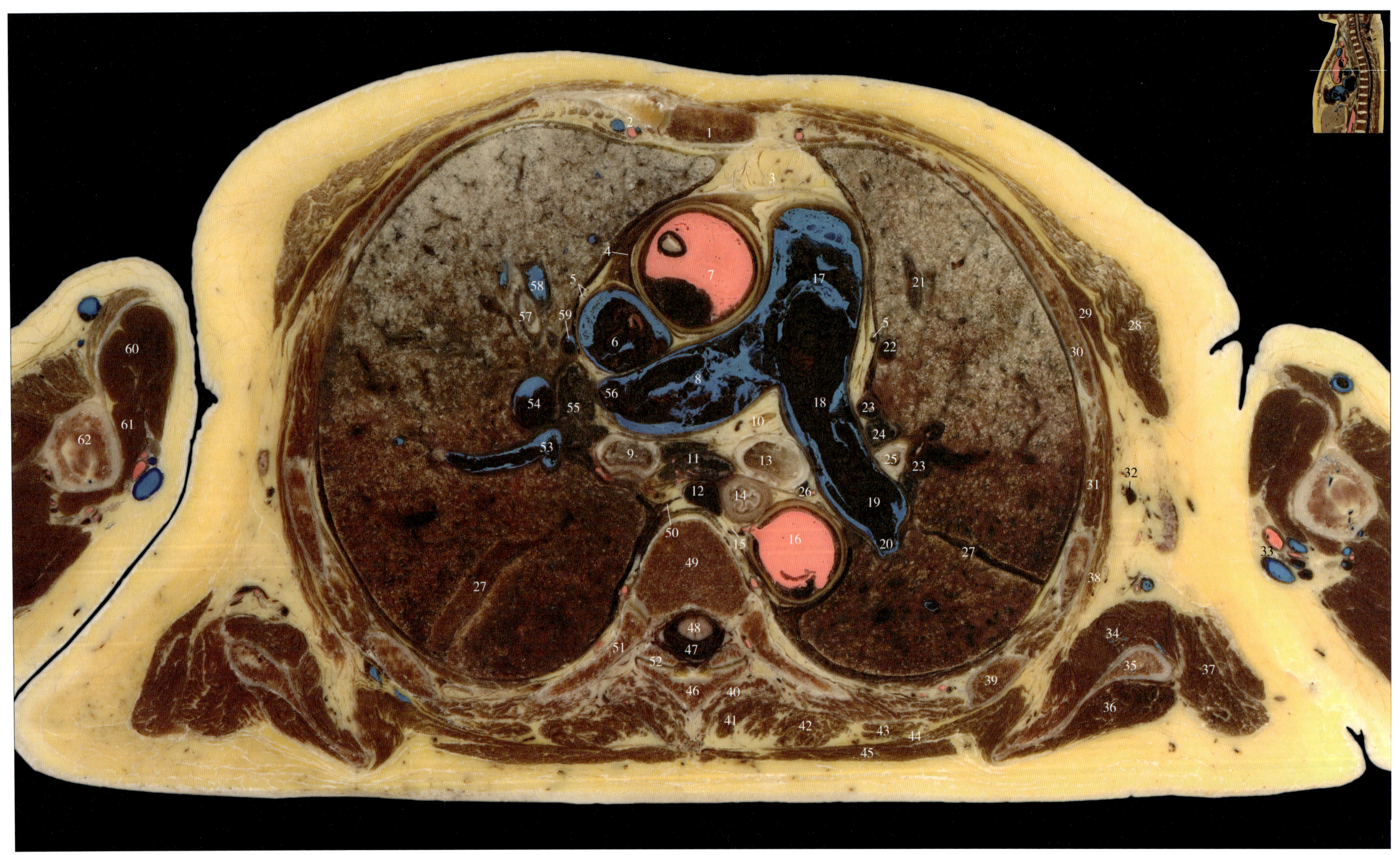

A. 断层标本图像

1. 胸骨体 body of sternum
2. 胸廓内动、静脉 internal thoracic artery and vein
3. 胸腺 thymus
4. 心包上隐窝 superior recess of pericardium
5. 膈神经和心包膈血管 phrenic nerve and pericardiacophrenic vessels
6. 上腔静脉 superior vena cava
7. 升主动脉 ascending aorta
8. 右肺动脉 right pulmonary artery
9. 中间支气管 intermediate bronchus
10. 左心耳 left auricle
11. 隆嵴下淋巴结（7区）subcarinal lymph nodes
12. 奇静脉 azygos vein
13. 左主支气管 left principal bronchus
14. 食管 esophagus
15. 胸导管 thoracic duct
16. 胸主动脉 thoracic aorta
17. 肺动脉干 pulmonary trunk
18. 左肺动脉 left pulmonary artery
19. 左肺下叶动脉 left inferior lobar artery
20. 左肺上段动脉（A6）left superior segmental artery
21. 左肺前段支气管（B3）和动脉（A3）left anterior segmental bronchus and artery
22. 左肺前段静脉（V3）left anterior segmental vein
23. 尖后段静脉（V1+2）apicoposterior segmental vein
24. 左肺叶淋巴结（12L）left lobar lymph nodes
25. 左肺上叶支气管上干 superior trunk of left superior lobar bronchus
26. 左肺门淋巴结（10L）left hilar lymph nodes
27. 斜裂 oblique fissure
28. 胸大肌 pectoralis major
29. 胸小肌 pectoralis minor
30. 第3肋骨 3rd costal bone
31. 肋间内、外肌 intercostales interni and externi
32. 胸外侧静脉 lateral thoracic vein
33. 腋动、静脉 axillary artery and vein
34. 肩胛下肌 subscapularis
35. 肩胛骨 scapula
36. 冈下肌 infraspinatus
37. 大圆肌 teres major
38. 前锯肌 serratus anterior
39. 第5肋骨 5th costal bone
40. 横突棘肌 transversospinales
41. 棘肌 spinales
42. 最长肌 longissimus
43. 髂肋肌 iliocostalis
44. 菱形肌 rhomboideus
45. 斜方肌 trapezius
46. 椎弓板 lamina of vertebral arch
47. 硬膜外隙 epidural space
48. 脊髓 spinal cord
49. 第5胸椎椎体 body of 5th thoracic vertebra
50. 奇静脉食管隐窝 azygoesophageal recess
51. 第6肋骨 6th costal bone
52. 关节突关节 zygapophysial joint
53. 右肺后段动脉（A2）right posterior segmental artery
54. 右肺后段静脉（V2）right posterior segmental vein
55. 右肺叶间淋巴结（11R）right interlobar lymph nodes
56. 右肺上叶动脉 right superior lobar artery
57. 右肺前段支气管（B3）right anterior segmental bronchus
58. 右肺前段动脉（A3）right anterior segmental artery
59. 尖段静脉（V1）apical segmental vein
60. 肱二头肌长、短头 long and short heads of biceps brachii
61. 喙肱肌 coracobrachialis
62. 肱骨 humerus
63. 尖后段支气管（B1+2）apicoposterior segmental bronchus

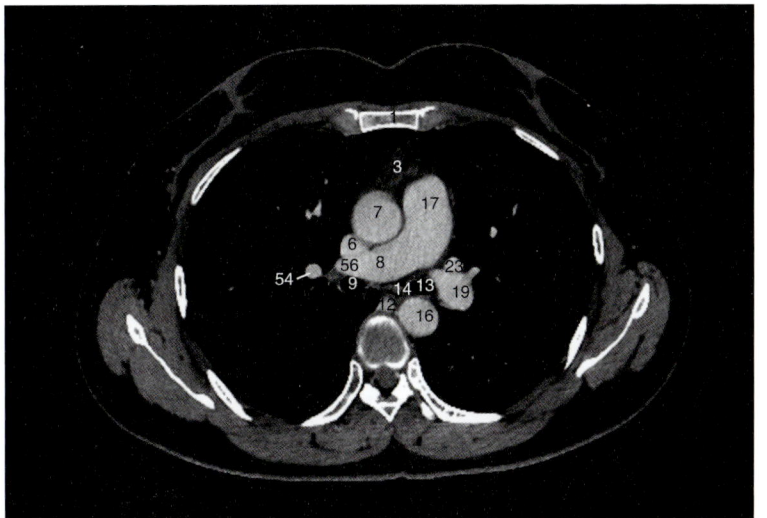

B. CT 纵隔窗增强图像

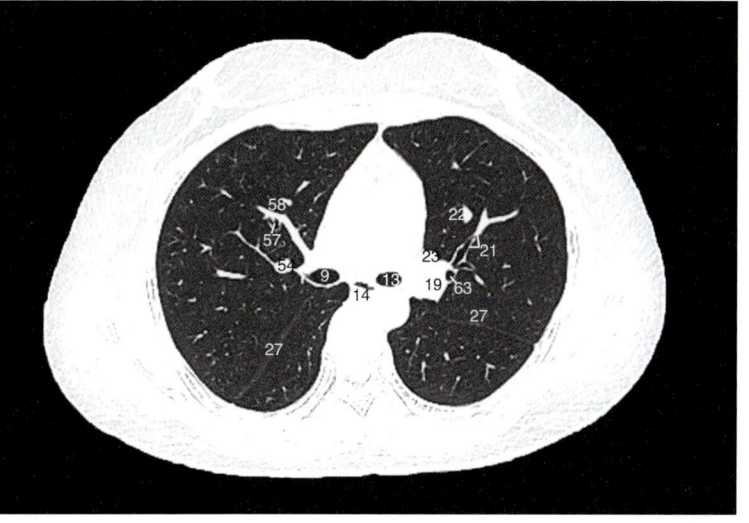

C. CT 肺窗图像

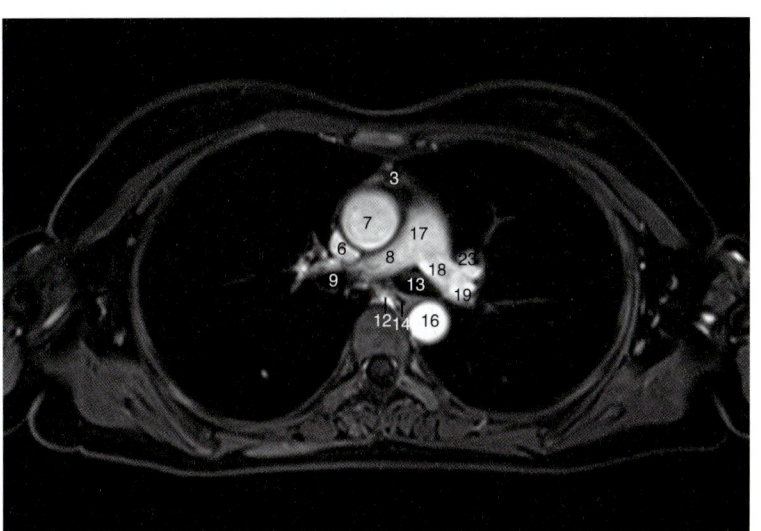

D. MR T1WI 增强图像

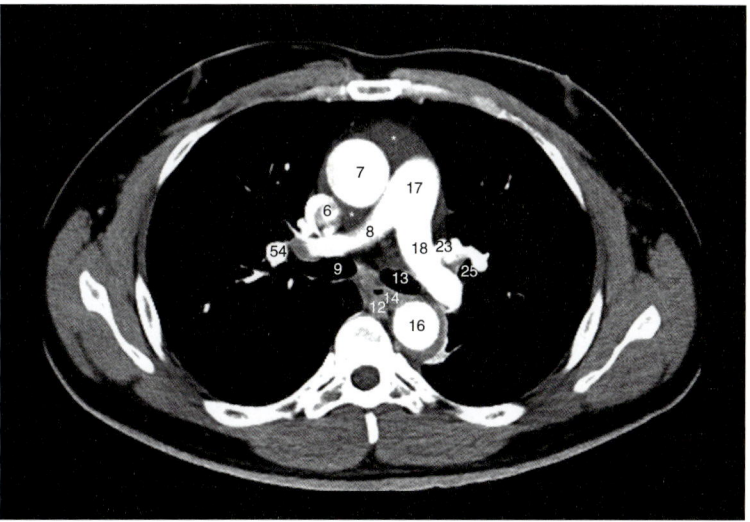

E. 心包积液 CT 图像

关键结构：肺动脉杈，左肺动脉，右肺动脉。

此断面经第5胸椎椎体下份。

在纵隔第二层内见肺动脉干分为左肺动脉和右肺动脉，形成"三叶草状"肺动脉杈。肺动脉杈前部为肺动脉干，位于心底的大血管最左侧，向下方断面可追踪至右心室流出道。肺动脉干全长位于心包内，长度为 4.5 cm ± 0.8 cm，直径为 3.0 cm ± 0.5 cm。其分支包括右肺动脉和左肺动脉，有35%的左肺动脉高于右肺动脉，左、右肺动脉，以及肺动脉干高度相同的情况约占65%[36]。右肺动脉长而水平，全长的4/5在心包内，前方被上腔静脉和升主动脉遮盖，MRI测量显示右肺动脉直径为 16.9 mm ± 2.6 mm。左肺动脉相对较短，同时只有1/2在心包内，左肺动脉直径为 16.3 mm ± 1.8 mm。

MRI测量显示一个心动周期内，右肺动脉和左肺动脉的血流量分别为 38.9 mL ± 4.5 mL 和 33.7 mL ± 3.2 mL，右肺动脉血流量明显大于左肺动脉[41]。右肺动脉以此平面为标准，在其远端向上叶门发出右肺上叶动脉，主干逐渐行向外下，演变为叶间动脉，并逐渐分支为中叶和下叶动脉；左肺动脉进入左肺门后，即逐渐发出前段动脉和尖后段动脉进入上叶，左肺动脉绕上叶支气管下行至其外侧，靠近斜裂，变为下叶动脉[42]。图E所示为心包积液，病因可有结核、化脓、病毒、风湿等，多为渗出性液体。影像学表现为心包厚度>4 mm，可见沿心脏轮廓、大血管根部分布的环形异常密度影，多为低密度，出血时为高密度。

胸部连续横断层 43（FH.12650）

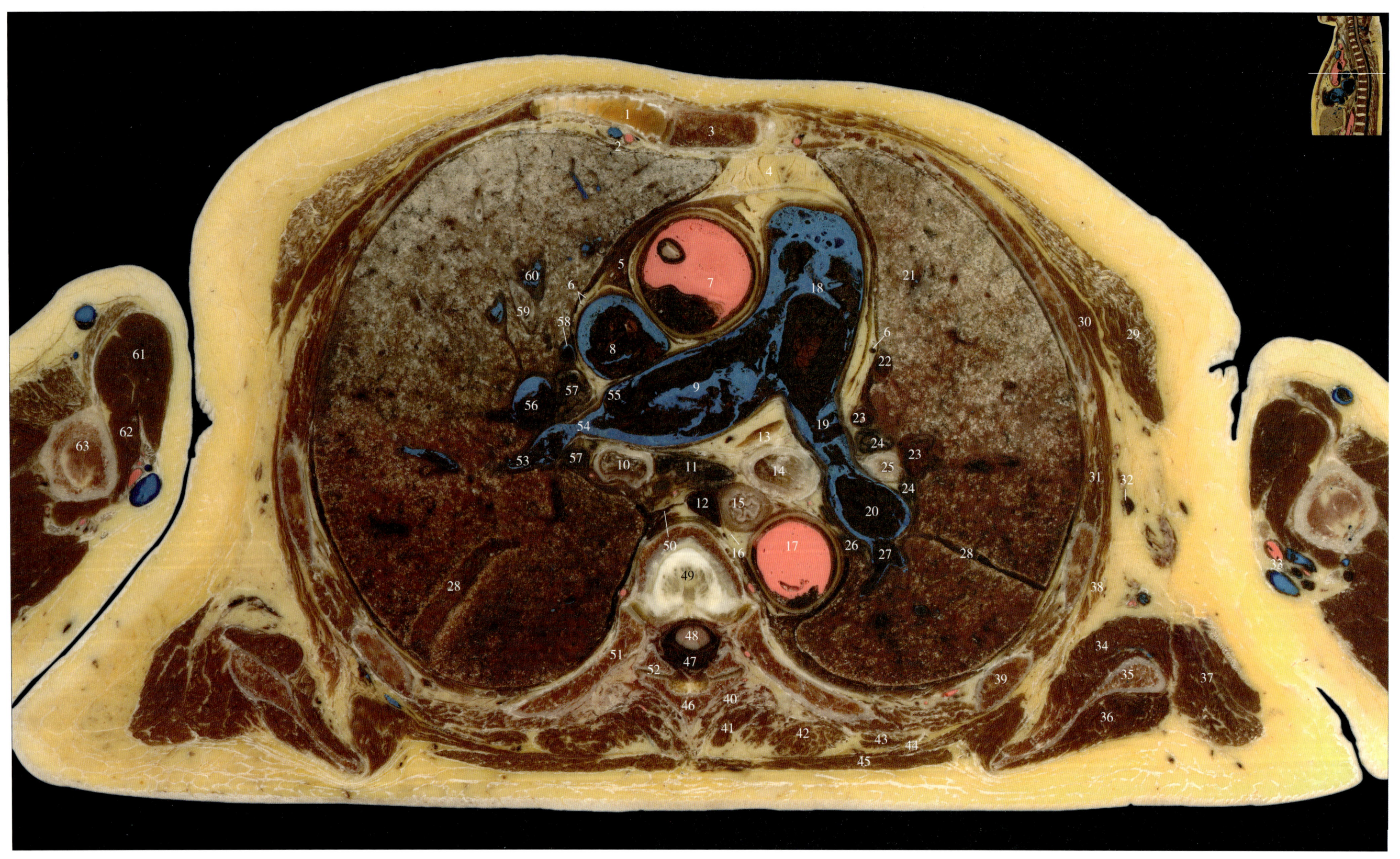

A. 断层标本图像

1. 第3肋软骨 3rd costal cartilage
2. 胸廓内动、静脉 internal thoracic artery and vein
3. 胸骨体 body of sternum
4. 胸腺 thymus
5. 心包上隐窝 superior recess of pericardium
6. 膈神经和心包膈血管 phrenic nerve and pericardiacophrenic vessels
7. 升主动脉 ascending aorta
8. 上腔静脉 superior vena cava
9. 右肺动脉 right pulmonary artery
10. 中间支气管 intermediate bronchus
11. 隆嵴下淋巴结（7区）subcarinal lymph nodes
12. 奇静脉 azygos vein
13. 左心耳 left auricle
14. 左主支气管 left principal bronchus
15. 食管 esophagus
16. 胸导管 thoracic duct
17. 胸主动脉 thoracic aorta
18. 肺动脉干 pulmonary trunk
19. 左肺动脉 left pulmonary artery
20. 左肺下叶动脉 left inferior lobar artery
21. 左肺前段支气管（B3）和动脉（A3）left anterior segmental bronchus and artery
22. 左肺前段静脉（V3）left anterior segmental vein
23. 尖后段静脉（V1+2）apicoposterior segmental vein
24. 左肺叶淋巴结（12L）left lobar lymph nodes
25. 左肺上叶支气管上干 superior trunk of left superior lobar bronchus
26. 左肺叶间淋巴结（11L）left interlobar lymph nodes
27. 左肺上段动脉（A6）left superior segmental artery
28. 斜裂 oblique fissure
29. 胸大肌 pectoralis major
30. 胸小肌 pectoralis minor
31. 肋间内、外肌 intercostales interni and externi
32. 胸外侧静脉 lateral thoracic vein
33. 腋动、静脉 axillary artery and vein
34. 肩胛下肌 subscapularis
35. 肩胛骨 scapula
36. 冈下肌 infraspinatus
37. 大圆肌 teres major
38. 前锯肌 serratus anterior
39. 第5肋骨 5th costal bone
40. 横突棘肌 transversospinales
41. 棘肌 spinales
42. 最长肌 longissimus
43. 髂肋肌 iliocostalis
44. 菱形肌 rhomboideus
45. 斜方肌 trapezius
46. 棘突 spinous process
47. 硬膜外隙 epidural space
48. 脊髓 spinal cord
49. T5-6 椎间盘 T5-6 intervertebral disc
50. 奇静脉食管隐窝 azygoesophageal recess
51. 第6肋骨 6th costal bone
52. 关节突关节 zygapophysial joint
53. 右肺后段动脉（A2）right posterior segmental artery
54. 右肺叶间动脉 right interlobar artery
55. 右肺上叶动脉 right superior lobar artery
56. 右肺后段静脉（V2）right posterior segmental vein
57. 右肺叶间淋巴结（11R）right interlobar lymph nodes
58. 右肺尖段静脉（V1）right apical segmental vein
59. 右肺前段支气管（B3）right anterior segmental bronchus
60. 右肺前段动脉（A3）right anterior segmental artery
61. 肱二头肌 biceps brachii
62. 喙肱肌 coracobrachialis
63. 肱骨 humerus
64. 尖后段支气管（B1+2）apicoposterior segmental bronchus
65. 右肺前段静脉（V3）right anterior segmental vein

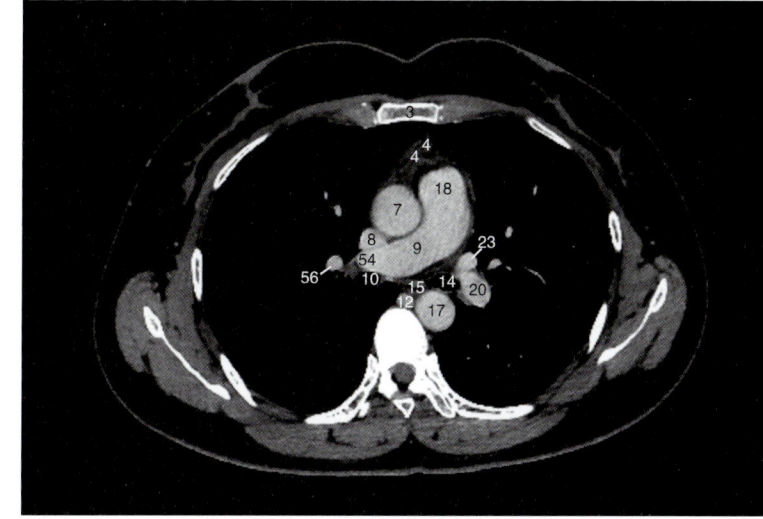

B. CT 纵隔窗增强图像

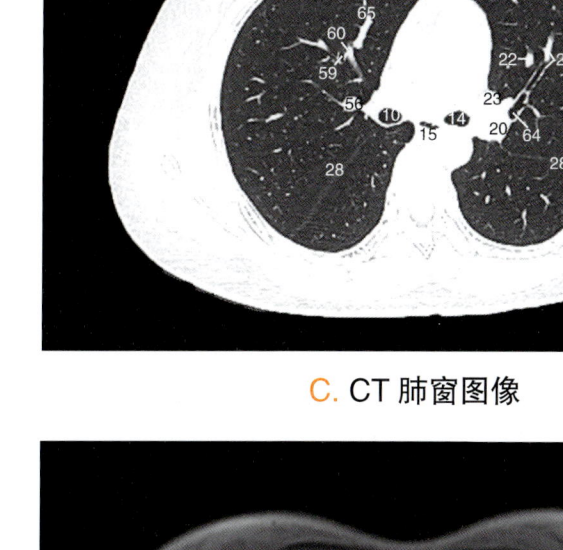

C. CT 肺窗图像

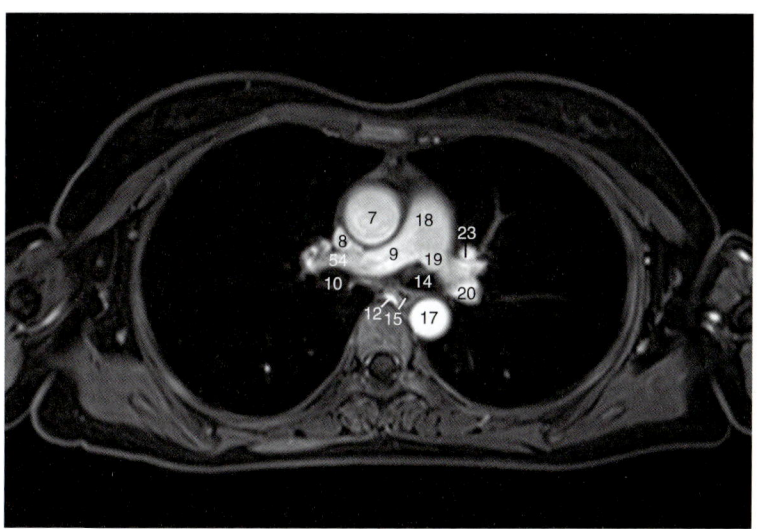

D. MR T1WI 增强图像

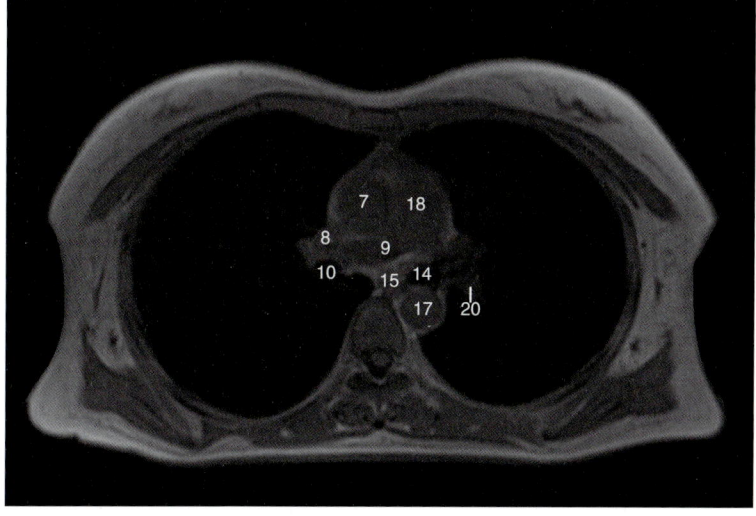

E. MR T1WI 平扫图像

关键结构：右肺叶间动脉，上段动脉。

此断面经 T5-6 椎间盘上份。

右肺叶间动脉在右肺门管道中位置最靠外侧，CT 上构成右肺门向外侧的最凸起部，靠近斜裂，较为明显。右肺动脉发出上叶动脉后，经上腔静脉和中间支气管之间行至肺门处，连于斜裂，移行为右肺叶间动脉，右肺叶间动脉的直径为 12.0 mm ± 1.6 mm，位置关系较为恒定，是 CT 测量右肺动脉心包段的理想部位[43]。叶间动脉继续下行，在斜裂处进一步分为中叶动脉和下叶动脉。叶间动脉亦可发出一支或两支动脉至右肺上叶，分布于前、后段者称为升动脉；分布于后段者称为后升动脉；分布于前段者称为前升动脉。以一支型多见，占 75.8%，其中又以后升动脉居多，为 66.1%，升动脉及前升动脉分别为 8.1% 和 1.6%；两支型，即"前升动脉 + 后升动脉"仅占 12.9%；还有 11.3% 的右肺上叶动脉未出现叶间支[37]。斜裂后方为下叶上段，左、右两侧下叶上段内，上段动脉先于支气管进入段内，左肺上段动脉以单干多见，占 76.1% ± 3.1%，在舌动脉干稍上方自下叶动脉后壁水平发出；右肺上段动脉也以单干多见，占 73.3% ± 3.6%，发自叶间动脉后壁[36]。

胸部连续横断层 44（FH.12630）

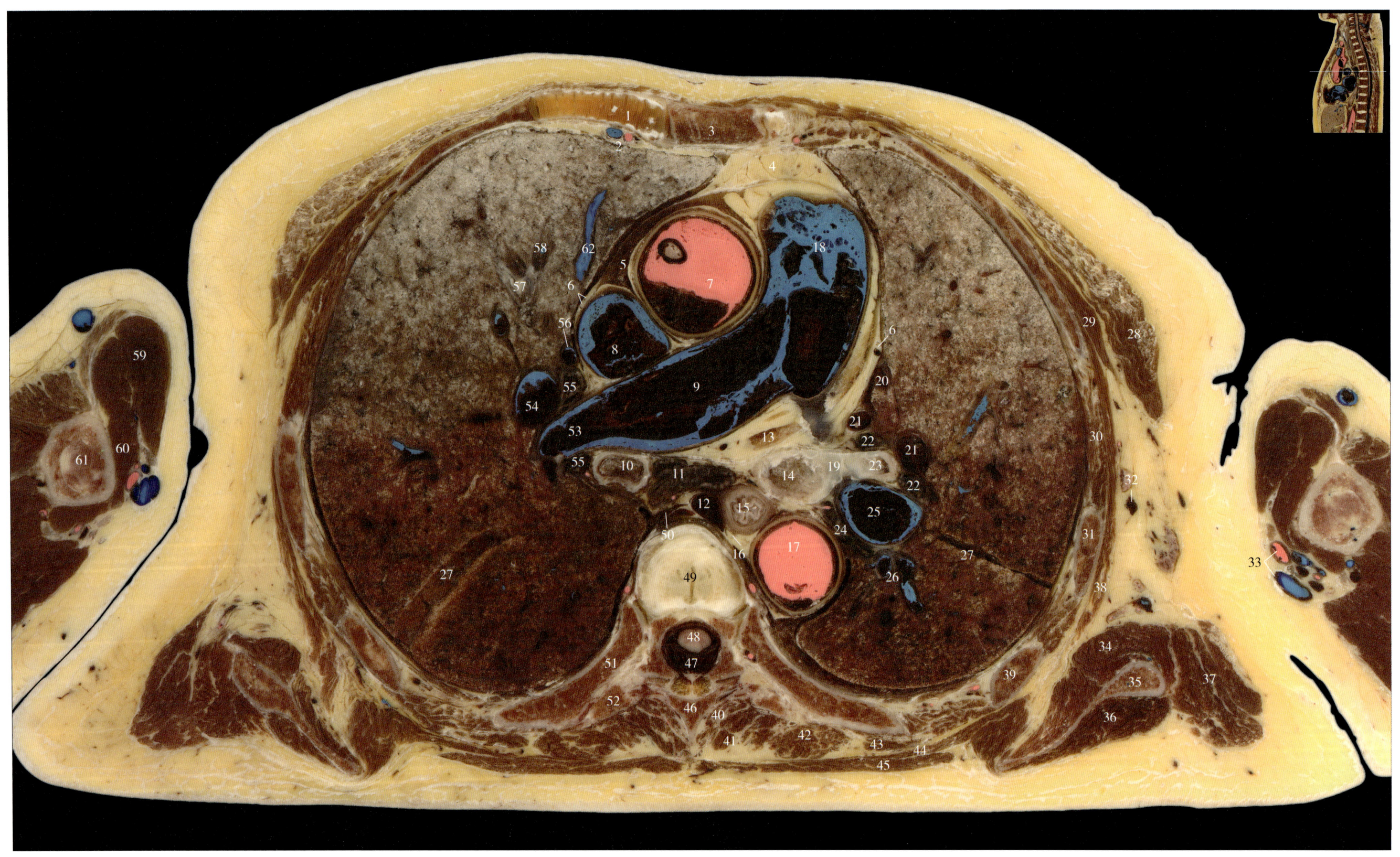

A. 断层标本图像

1. 第3肋软骨 3rd costal cartilage
2. 胸廓内动、静脉 internal thoracic artery and vein
3. 胸骨体 body of sternum
4. 胸腺 thymus
5. 心包上隐窝 superior recess of pericardium
6. 膈神经和心包膈血管 phrenic nerve and pericardiacophrenic vessels
7. 升主动脉 ascending aorta
8. 上腔静脉 superior vena cava
9. 右肺动脉 right pulmonary artery
10. 中间支气管 intermediate bronchus
11. 隆嵴下淋巴结（7区）subcarinal lymph nodes
12. 奇静脉 azygos vein
13. 左心耳 left auricle
14. 左主支气管 left principal bronchus
15. 食管 esophagus
16. 胸导管 thoracic duct
17. 胸主动脉 thoracic aorta
18. 肺动脉干 pulmonary trunk
19. 上叶支气管 superior lobar bronchus of left lung
20. 左肺前段静脉（V3）left anterior segmental vein
21. 尖后段静脉（V1+2）apicoposterior segmental vein
22. 左肺叶淋巴结（12L）left lobar lymph nodes
23. 左肺上叶支气管上干 superior trunk of left superior lobar bronchus
24. 左叶间淋巴结（11L）left interlobar lymph nodes
25. 左肺下叶动脉 left inferior lobar artery
26. 左肺上段动脉（A6）left superior segmental artery
27. 斜裂 oblique fissure
28. 胸大肌 pectoralis major
29. 胸小肌 pectoralis minor
30. 肋间内、外肌 intercostales interni and externi
31. 第4肋骨 4th costal bone
32. 胸外侧静脉 lateral thoracic vein
33. 腋动、静脉 axillary artery and vein
34. 肩胛下肌 subscapularis
35. 肩胛骨 scapula
36. 冈下肌 infraspinatus
37. 大圆肌 teres major
38. 前锯肌 serratus anterior
39. 第5肋骨 5th costal bone
40. 横突棘肌 transversospinales
41. 棘肌 spinales
42. 最长肌 longissimus
43. 髂肋肌 iliocostalis
44. 菱形肌 rhomboideus
45. 斜方肌 trapezius
46. 棘突 spinous process
47. 硬膜外隙 epidural space
48. 脊髓 spinal cord
49. T5-6椎间盘 T5-6 intervertebral disc
50. 奇静脉食管隐窝 azygoesophageal recess
51. 第6肋骨 6th costal bone
52. 横突 transverse process
53. 右肺叶间动脉 right interlobar artery
54. 右肺后段静脉（V2）right posterior segmental vein
55. 右叶间淋巴结（11R）right interlobar lymph nodes
56. 右肺尖段静脉（V1）right apical segmental vein
57. 右肺前段支气管（B3）right anterior segmental bronchus
58. 右肺前段动脉（A3）right anterior segmental artery
59. 肱二头肌 biceps brachii
60. 喙肱肌 coracobrachialis
61. 肱骨 humerus
62. 右肺前段静脉（V3）right anterior segmental vein
63. 左肺前段支气管（B3）和动脉（A3）left anterior segmental bronchus and artery

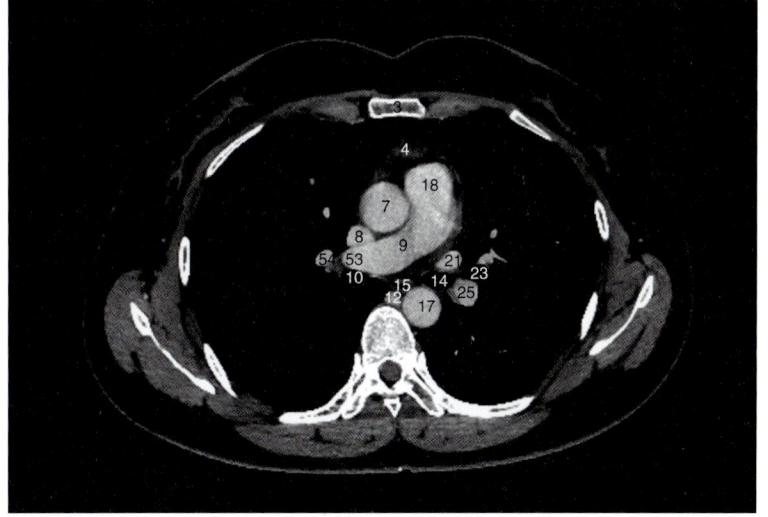

B. CT 纵隔窗增强图像

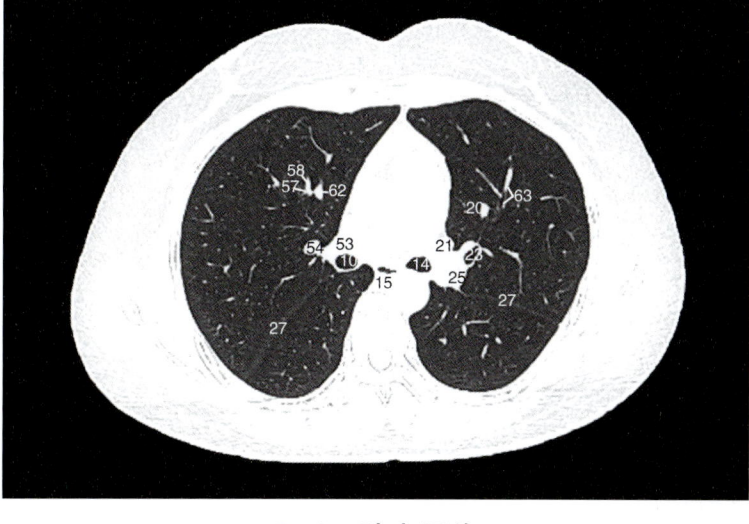

C. CT 肺窗图像

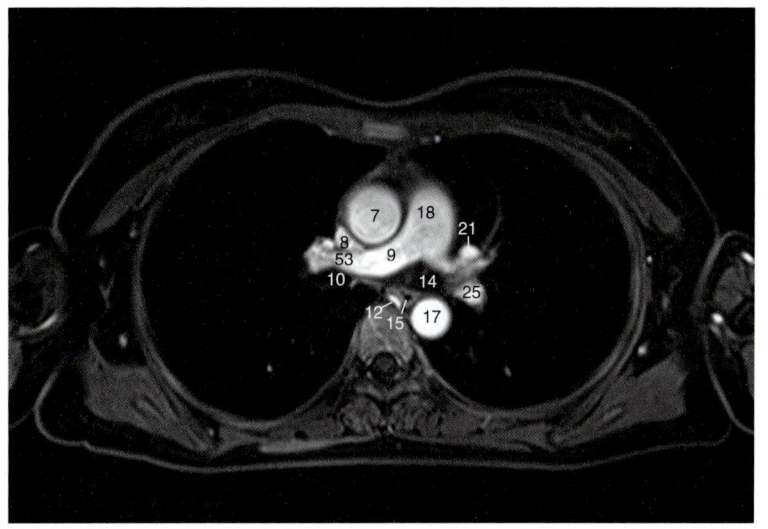

D. MR T1WI 增强图像

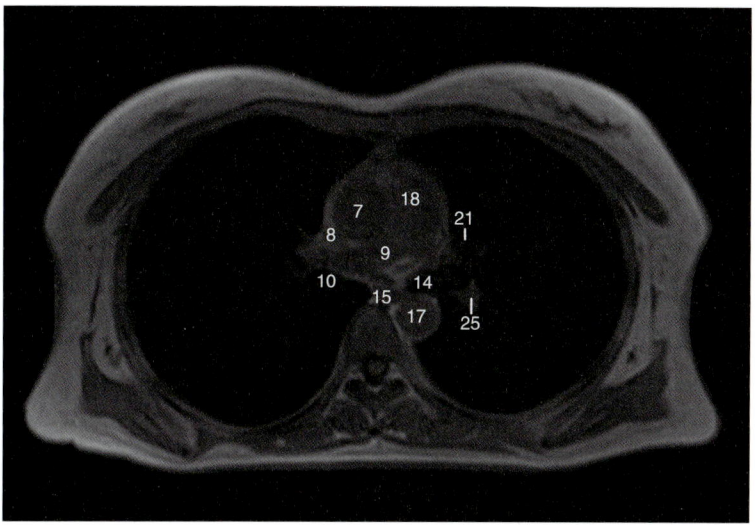

E. MR T1WI 平扫图像

关键结构：左肺上叶支气管，左肺上叶支气管上干。

此断面经过 T5-6 椎间盘中份。

纵隔内肺动脉杈"三叶草"状分叉结构因左肺动脉消失而打破。纵隔前部由右向左依次可见上腔静脉、升主动脉和肺动脉干。两肺斜裂前移，肺下叶变大，上叶变小。左主支气管水平发出上叶支气管后，左肺门处的主要结构变为左肺上叶支气管和下叶动脉，上叶支气管构成左肺门前缘，下叶动脉构成左肺门后缘。上叶支气管长度为 0.9 cm ± 0.2 cm，外横径为 1.3 cm ± 0.2 cm。86.6% ± 1.3% 的上叶支气管进一步分为上干和下干[36]，上干断面表现为圆管，垂直上行，位于左肺动脉外侧，进一步分为尖后段支气管和前段支气管；下干行向前外侧下方，进一步分为上、下舌段支气管。此断面的左肺下叶内，位于胸主动脉与左肺下叶动脉之间，有小舌样肺组织抵至左主支气管后壁，这一现象在 CT 图像上常可见到，有时也见肿大淋巴结将舌状肺组织被推出两大血管之外，提示肺门或左肺下叶有病变。

胸部连续横断层 45 （FH.12610）

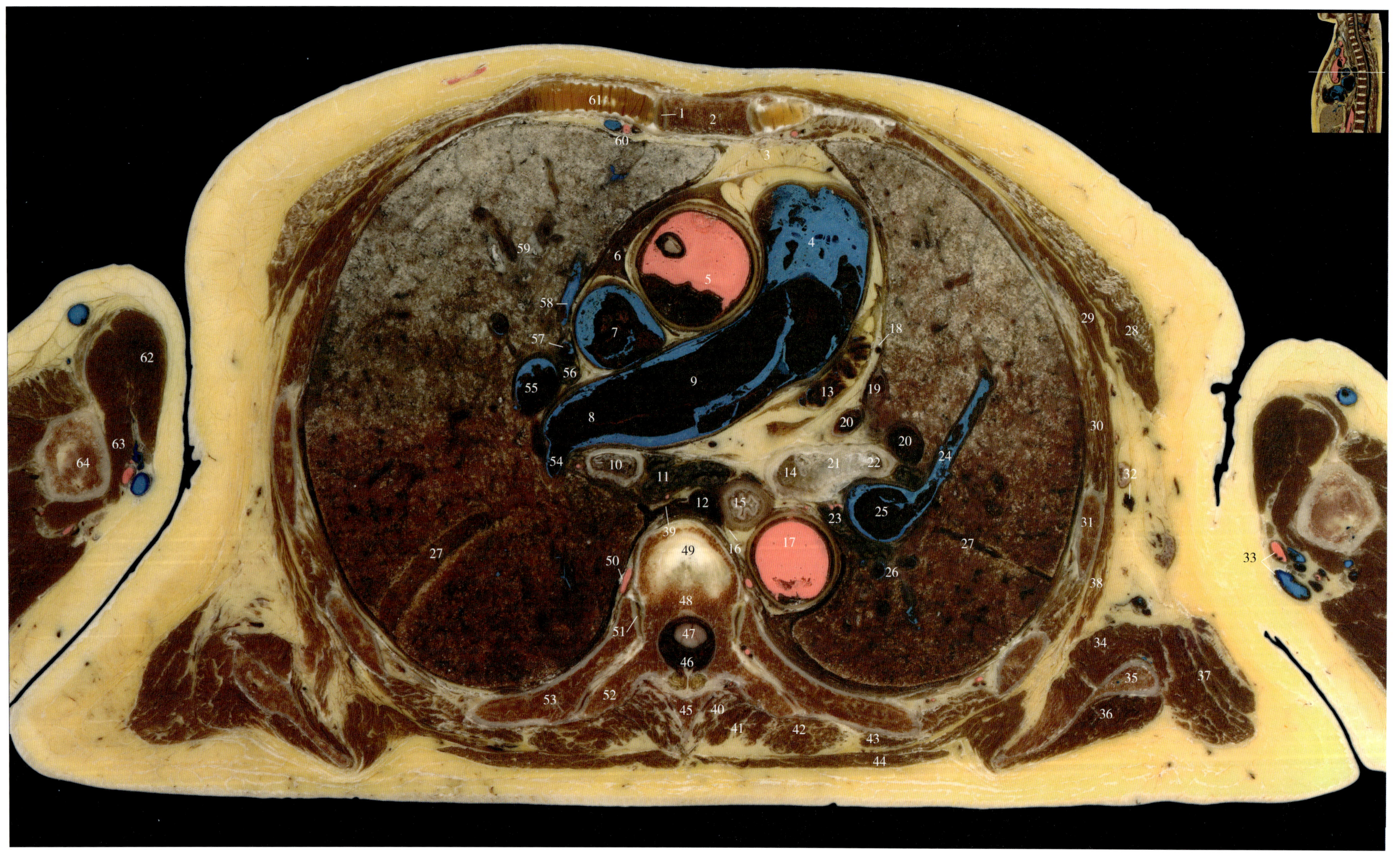

A. 断层标本图像

1. 第3胸肋关节 3rd sternocostal joint
2. 胸骨体 body of sternum
3. 胸腺 thymus
4. 肺动脉干 pulmonary trunk
5. 升主动脉 ascending aorta
6. 心包上隐窝 superior recess of pericardium
7. 上腔静脉 superior vena cava
8. 右肺叶间动脉 right interlobar artery
9. 右肺动脉 right pulmonary artery
10. 中间支气管 intermediate bronchus
11. 隆嵴下淋巴结（7区）subcarinal lymph nodes
12. 奇静脉 azygos vein
13. 左心耳 left auricle
14. 左主支气管 left principal bronchus
15. 食管 esophagus
16. 胸导管 thoracic duct
17. 胸主动脉 thoracic aorta
18. 膈神经和心包膈血管 phrenic nerve and pericardiacophrenic vessels
19. 左肺前段静脉（V3）left anterior segmental vein
20. 尖后段静脉（V1+2）apicoposterior segmental vein
21. 左肺上叶支气管 superior lobar bronchus of left lung
22. 左肺上叶支气管上干 superior trunk of left superior lobar bronchus
23. 左肺叶间淋巴结（11L）left interlobar lymph nodes
24. 上舌段动脉（A4）superior lingular segmental artery
25. 左肺下动脉 left inferior lobar artery
26. 左肺上段动脉（A6）left superior segmental artery
27. 斜裂 oblique fissure
28. 胸大肌 pectoralis major
29. 胸小肌 pectoralis minor
30. 肋间内、外肌 intercostales interni and externi
31. 第4肋骨 4th costal bone
32. 胸外侧静脉 lateral thoracic vein
33. 腋动、静脉 axillary artery and vein
34. 肩胛下肌 subscapularis
35. 肩胛骨 scapula
36. 冈下肌 infraspinatus
37. 大圆肌 teres major
38. 前锯肌 serratus anterior
39. 奇静脉食管隐窝 azygoesophageal recess
40. 横突棘肌 transversospinales
41. 棘肌 spinales
42. 最长肌 longissimus
43. 髂肋肌 iliocostalis
44. 斜方肌 trapezius
45. 棘突 spinous process
46. 硬膜外隙 epidural space
47. 脊髓 spinal cord
48. 第6胸椎椎体 body of 6th thoracic vertebra
49. T5-6椎间盘 T5-6 intervertebral disc
50. 肋间后动脉 posterior intercostal artery
51. 肋头关节 joint of costal head
52. 横突 transverse process
53. 第6肋骨 6th costal bone
54. 右肺上段动脉（A6）right superior segmental artery
55. 右肺后段静脉（V2）right posterior segmental vein
56. 右肺叶间淋巴结（11R）right interlobar lymph nodes
57. 右肺尖段静脉（V1）right apical segmental vein
58. 右肺前段静脉（V3）right anterior segmental vein
59. 右肺前段支气管（B3）和动脉（A3）right anterior segmental bronchus and artery
60. 胸廓内动、静脉 internal thoracic artery and vein
61. 第3肋软骨 3rd costal cartilage
62. 肱二头肌 biceps brachii
63. 喙肱肌 coracobrachialis
64. 肱骨 humerus

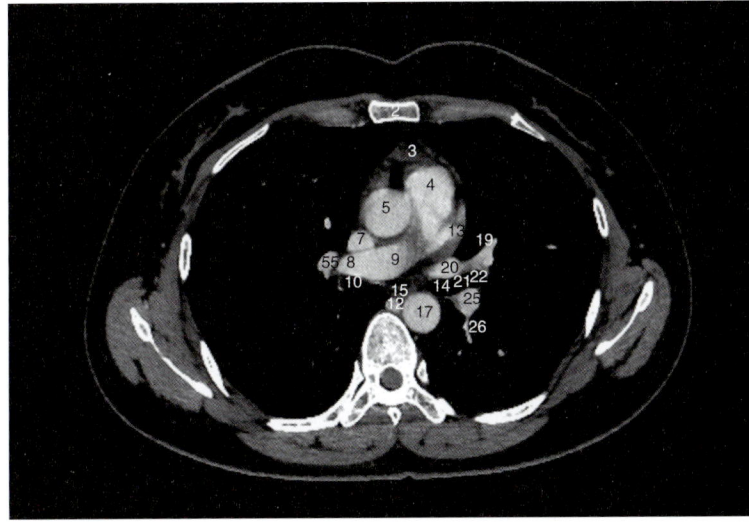

B. CT 纵隔窗增强图像

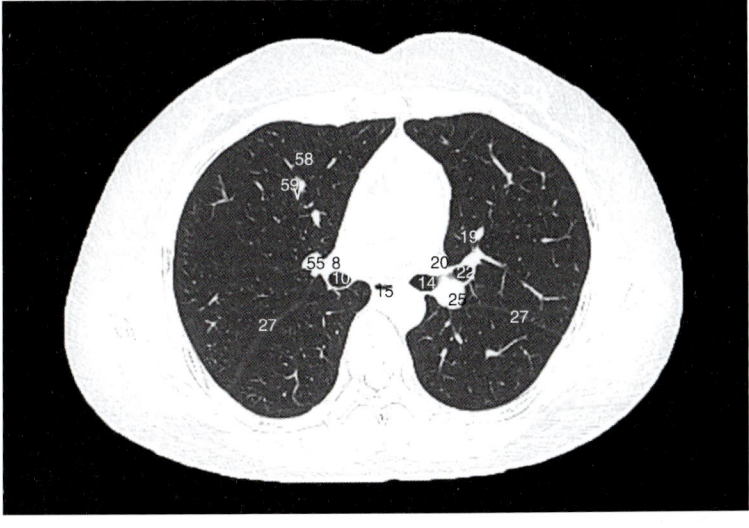

C. CT 肺窗图像

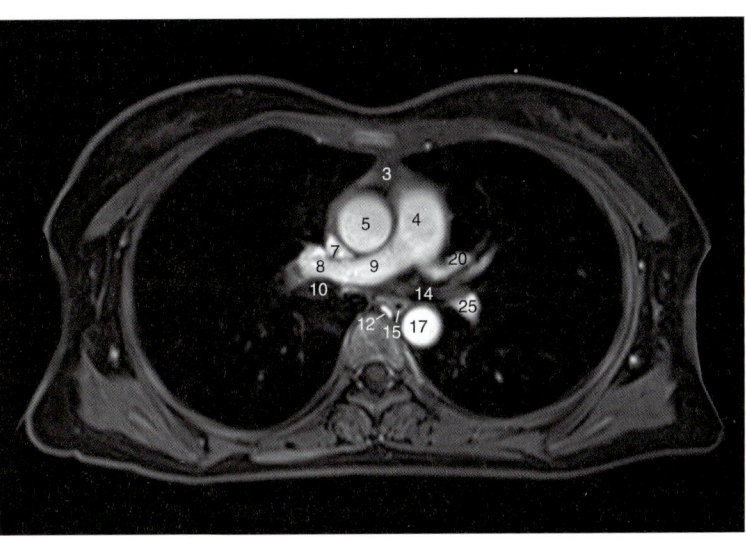

D. MR T1WI 增强图像

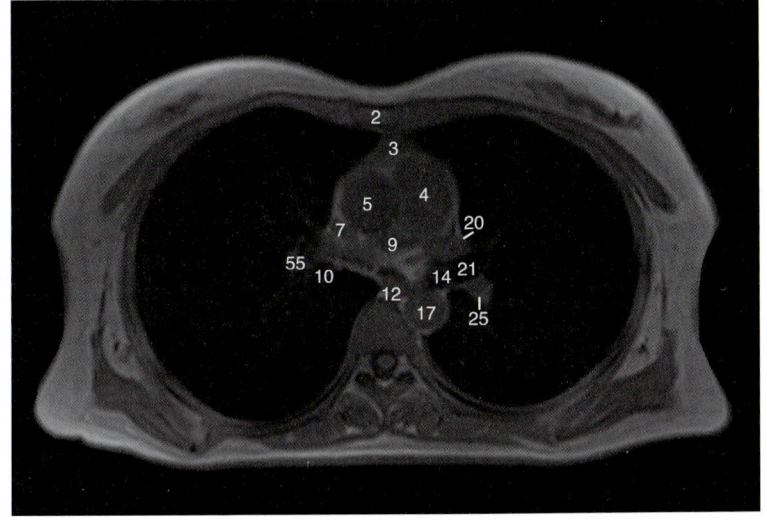

E. MR T1WI 平扫图像

关键结构：左肺尖后段静脉，左肺下叶动脉。

此断面经过T5-6椎间盘下份。

斜裂前方为左肺上叶门，在左肺上叶支气管以上平面，上叶门主要显示尖后段和前段的结构。段支气管、段动脉和段静脉这3套肺内管道中，在此断面仅在左肺门上叶门前部出现段静脉的属支，表现为尖后段静脉和前段静脉的逐渐汇合。尖后段静脉的变异较大，尖段静脉与后段静脉（高位型）可以共干形成尖后段静脉，出现率约为71.25%，汇合高度多介于左肺动脉上、下缘层面之间；尖段静脉不与后段静脉（低位型）共干时，后段静脉较低，向后外下移位，与前段静脉汇合形成后前段静脉，出现率28.75%，再汇入左肺上静脉[41]。尖后段静脉干是划分尖后段和前段的标志，合成后常位于左肺门前部，紧贴左肺纵隔面中部，尖后段静脉的段内支则绕上干或上叶支气管前方或前外侧向尖后段静脉干汇合。左肺动脉在进入左肺门后，呈弓形（左肺动脉弓）从左主支气管的前上方绕至上叶支气管的后下方，移行为下叶动脉，直径为 $11.3\ mm \pm 1.4\ mm$ [41]。由于其绕上叶支气管进入下叶门，其位置只能位于下叶支气管的外侧，故典型表现为下叶支气管（或基底干支气管）位于内侧，下叶动脉（或其分支）围绕于外侧，左肺下叶动脉通常并在斜裂内向前外侧发出舌段动脉进入上、下舌段（占 $47.7\% \pm 5.2\%$）[34]。

胸部连续横断层 46（FH.12590）

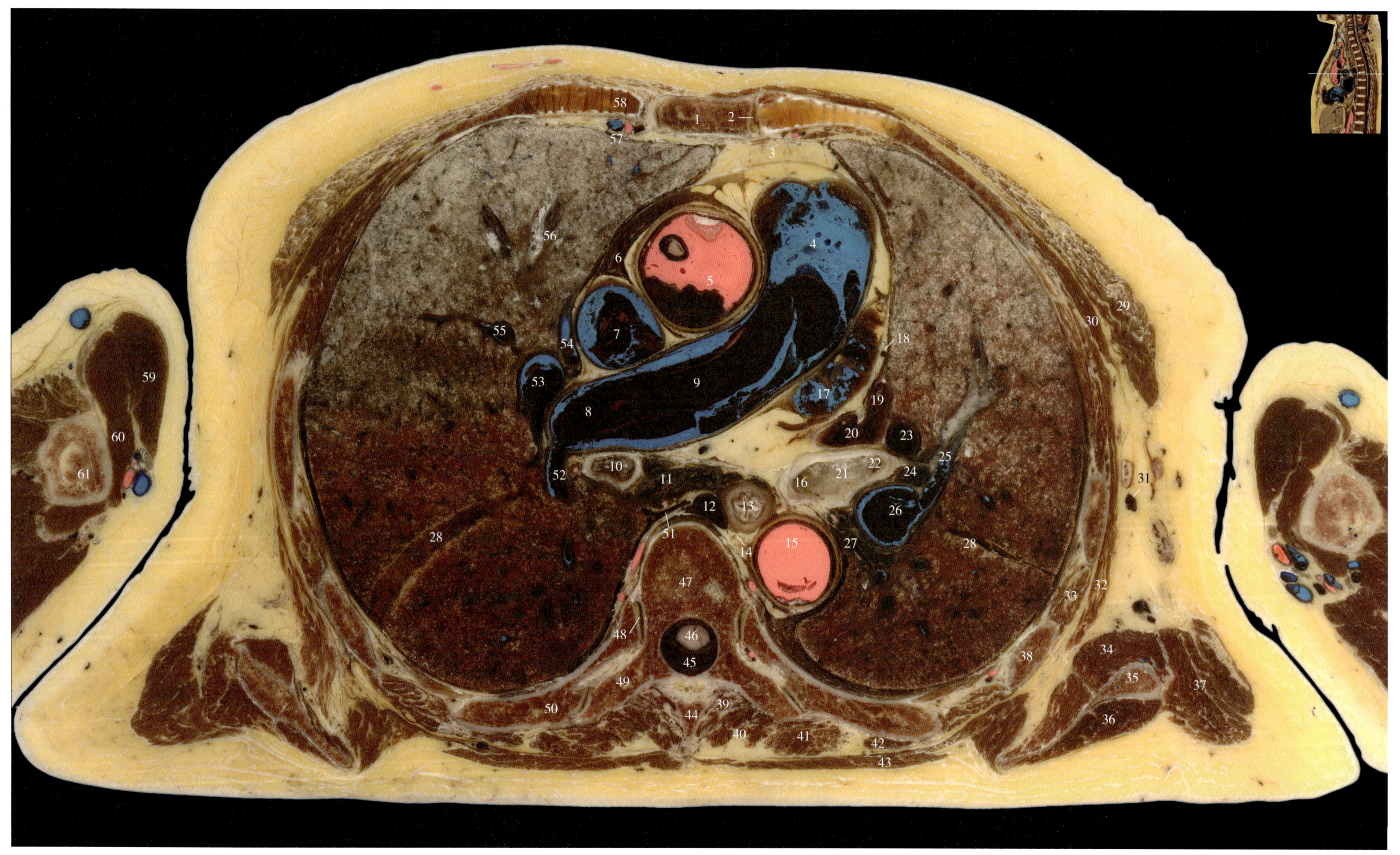

A. 断层标本图像

1. 胸骨体 body of sternum
2. 第 3 胸肋关节 3rd sternocostal joint
3. 胸腺 thymus
4. 肺动脉干 pulmonary trunk
5. 升主动脉 ascending aorta
6. 心包上隐窝 superior recess of pericardium
7. 上腔静脉 superior vena cava
8. 右肺叶间动脉 right interlobar artery
9. 右肺动脉 right pulmonary artery
10. 中间支气管 intermediate bronchus
11. 隆嵴下淋巴结（7区）subcarinal lymph nodes
12. 奇静脉 azygos vein
13. 食管 esophagus
14. 胸导管 thoracic duct
15. 胸主动脉 thoracic aorta
16. 左主支气管 left principal bronchus
17. 左心耳 left auricle
18. 膈神经和心包膈血管 phrenic nerve and pericardiacophrenic vessels
19. 左肺前段静脉（V3）left anterior segmental vein
20. 左上肺静脉 left superior pulmonary vein
21. 左肺上叶支气管 superior lobar bronchus of left lung
22. 左肺上叶支气管上干 superior trunk of left superior lobar bronchus
23. 尖后段静脉（V1+2）apicoposterior segmental vein
24. 左肺叶淋巴结（12L）left lobar lymph nodes
25. 上舌段支气管（B4）和动脉（A4）superior lingular segmental bronchus and artery
26. 左肺下叶动脉 left inferior lobar artery
27. 左肺叶间淋巴结（11L）left interlobar lymph nodes
28. 斜裂 oblique fissure
29. 胸大肌 pectoralis major
30. 胸小肌 pectoralis minor
31. 胸外侧静脉 lateral thoracic vein
32. 前锯肌 serratus anterior
33. 肋间内、外肌 intercostales interni and externi
34. 肩胛下肌 subscapularis
35. 肩胛骨 scapula
36. 冈下肌 infraspinatus
37. 大圆肌 teres major
38. 第 5 肋骨 5th costal bone
39. 横突棘肌 transversospinales
40. 棘肌 spinales
41. 最长肌 longissimus
42. 髂肋肌 iliocostalis
43. 斜方肌 trapezius
44. 棘突 spinous process
45. 硬膜外隙 epidural space
46. 脊髓 spinal cord
47. 第 6 胸椎椎体 body of 6th thoracic vertebra
48. 肋头关节 joint of costal head
49. 横突 transverse process
50. 第 6 肋骨 6th costal bone
51. 奇静脉食管隐窝 azygoesophageal recess
52. 右肺上段静脉（A6）right superior segmental artery
53. 右肺后段静脉（V2）right posterior segmental vein
54. 右肺尖前段静脉（V1+3）right apicoanterior segmental vein
55. 右肺前段静脉（V3）right anterior segmental vein
56. 右肺前段动脉（A3）和支气管（B3）right anterior segmental artery and bronchus
57. 胸廓内动、静脉 internal thoracic artery and vein
58. 第 3 肋软骨 3rd costal cartilage
59. 肱二头肌 biceps brachii
60. 喙肱肌 coracobrachialis
61. 肱骨 humerus
62. 左肺上段动脉（A6）left superior segmental artery

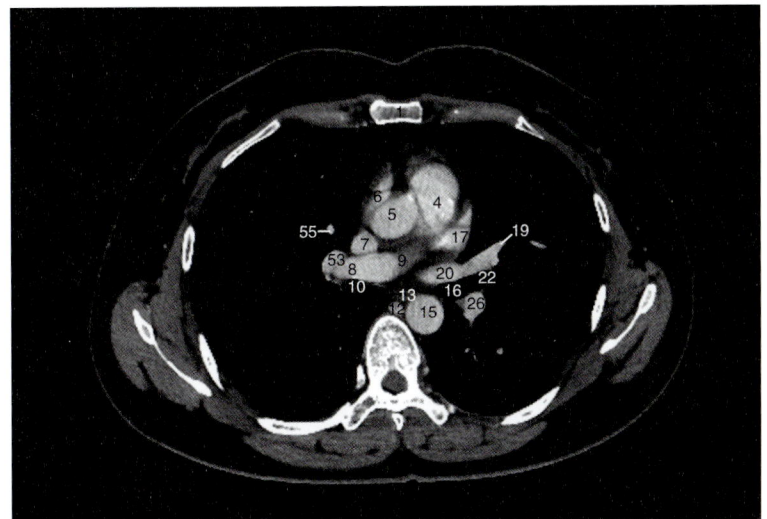

B. CT 纵隔窗增强图像

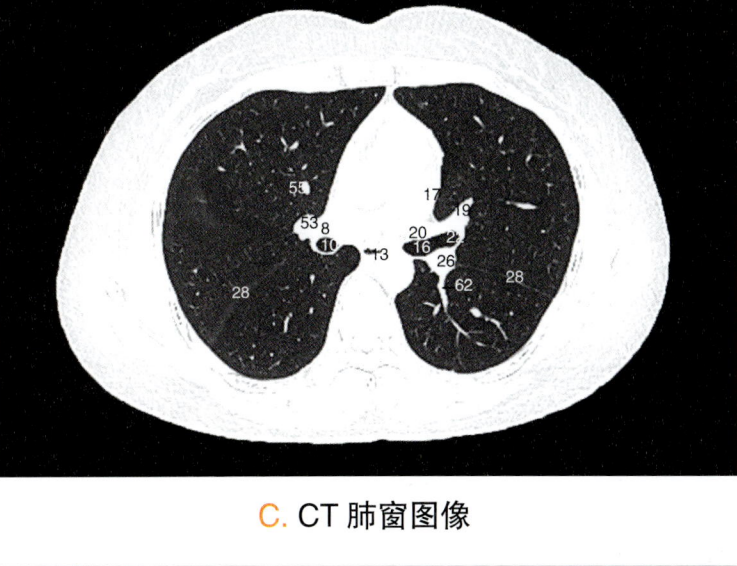

C. CT 肺窗图像

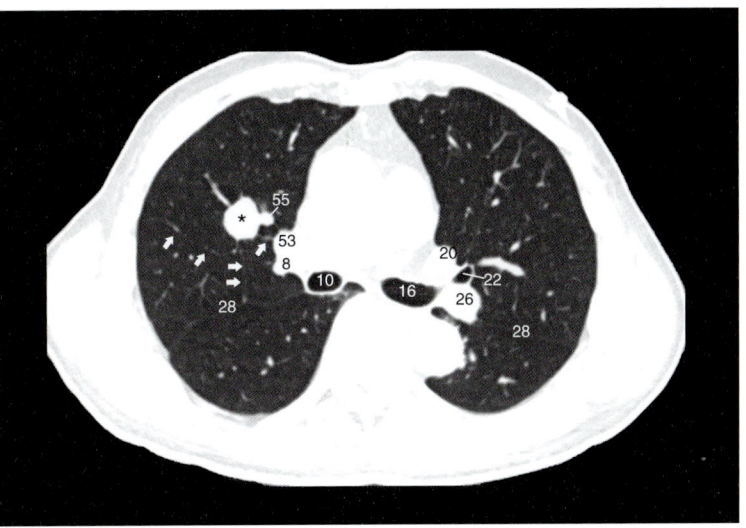

D. 右肺上叶转移瘤 CT 图像

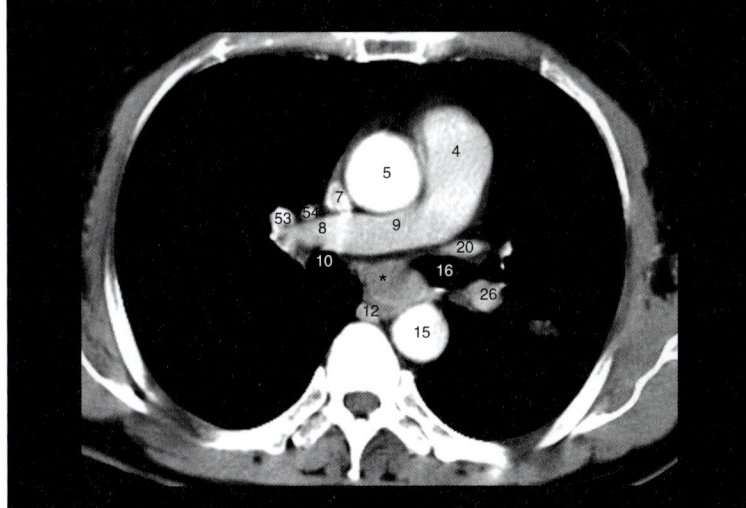

E. 7 区淋巴结转移 CT 图像

关键结构：左心耳，隆嵴下淋巴结。

断面经第 6 胸椎椎体上份。

肺动脉的后方为左心耳，左心耳是心脏内血栓容易形成的部位，脑卒中 80% 来源于左心耳血栓栓塞，研究左心耳的解剖结构特点对临床左心耳血栓形成和预防血栓栓塞有重要意义[44]。左心耳位于左心房前上方、左心室上方、肺动脉及升主动脉左侧、左上肺静脉的前方，因而左心耳形态的形成与这些结构有着明显的关系。左心耳外观通常呈锯齿形，下缘有 1~6 个不等的切迹，而上缘也可能有切迹出现，内壁有梳状肌而粗糙，断面中常出现在肺动脉干与左上肺静脉之间，行向后内侧。标本测量，左心耳深度为 20.5 mm ± 6.4 mm，长径为 15.8 mm ± 5.7 mm，短径为 10.4 mm ± 4.9 mm。左心耳口位于左心耳的后内侧，其与左上肺静脉口距离为 4.8 mm ± 1.9 mm，与左下肺静脉口距离为 7.8 mm ± 2.3 mm，距二尖瓣环距离为 10.3 mm ± 3.4 mm[45]。CT 测量表明，左心耳口位置可高于左上肺静脉平面（2.4%）、与左上肺静脉位于同一平面（86.2%），低于左上肺静脉平面（11.4%）。在左心耳和左上肺静脉开口之间均有一皱襞[46]。在左心耳内形成血栓前和形成血栓后，左心耳都明显增大，左心耳功能明显降低，发现心耳过大，应考虑是否已有血栓形成，或即将形成血栓的可能。此断面仍可见隆嵴下淋巴结（7 区）及左肺内淋巴结（11L 和 12L）。右肺上叶转移瘤 CT 图像中的 * 为右肺上叶转移性肿瘤，箭头所示为增厚的肺内间隔。7 区淋巴结转移 CT 图像中可发现隆嵴下淋巴结转移。

胸部连续横断层 47 （FH.12570）

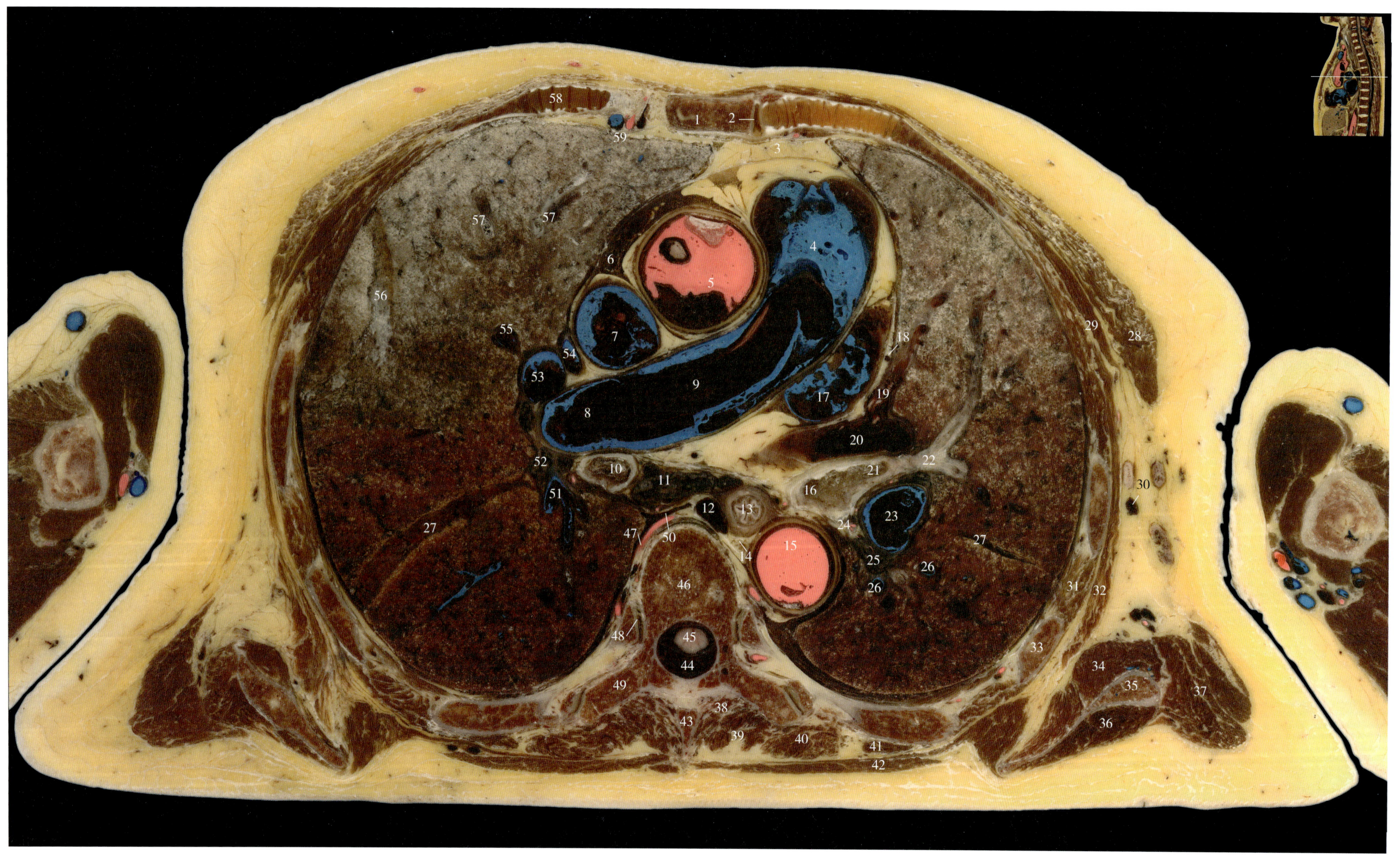

A. 断层标本图像

1. 胸骨体 body of sternum
2. 第3胸肋关节 3rd sternocostal joint
3. 胸腺 thymus
4. 肺动脉干 pulmonary trunk
5. 升主动脉 ascending aorta
6. 右心耳 right auricle
7. 上腔静脉 superior vena cava
8. 右肺叶间动脉 right interlobar artery
9. 右肺动脉 right pulmonary artery
10. 中间支气管 intermediate bronchus
11. 隆嵴下淋巴结（7区）subcarinal lymph nodes
12. 奇静脉 azygos vein
13. 食管 esophagus
14. 胸导管 thoracic duct
15. 胸主动脉 thoracic aorta
16. 左肺下叶支气管 left inferior lobar bronchus
17. 左心耳 left auricle
18. 膈神经和心包膈血管 phrenic nerve and pericardiacophrenic vessels
19. 左肺前段静脉（V3）left anterior segmental vein
20. 左上肺静脉 left superior pulmonary vein
21. 左肺上叶支气管 superior lobar bronchus of left lung
22. 上舌段支气管（B4）superior lingular segmental bronchus
23. 左肺下叶动脉 left inferior lobar artery
24. 左肺上段支气管（B6）left superior segmental bronchus
25. 左肺叶间淋巴结（11L）left interlobar lymph nodes
26. 左肺上段动脉（A6）left superior segmental artery
27. 斜裂 oblique fissure
28. 胸大肌 pectoralis major
29. 胸小肌 pectoralis minor
30. 胸外侧静脉 lateral thoracic vein
31. 肋间内、外肌 intercostales interni and externi
32. 前锯肌 serratus anterior
33. 第5肋骨 5th costal bone
34. 肩胛下肌 subscapularis
35. 肩胛骨 scapula
36. 冈下肌 infraspinatus
37. 大圆肌 teres major
38. 横突棘肌 transversospinales
39. 棘肌 spinales
40. 最长肌 longissimus
41. 髂肋肌 iliocostalis
42. 斜方肌 trapezius
43. 棘突 spinous process
44. 硬膜外隙 epidural space
45. 脊髓 spinal cord
46. 第6胸椎椎体 body of 6th thoracic vertebra
47. 肋间后动脉 posterior intercostal artery
48. 肋头关节 joint of costal head
49. 横突 transverse process
50. 奇静脉食管隐窝 azygoesophageal recess
51. 右肺上段动脉（A6）right superior segmental artery
52. 右肺叶间淋巴结（11R）right interlobar lymph nodes
53. 右肺后段静脉（V2）right posterior segmental vein
54. 右肺尖前段静脉（V1+3）right apicoanterior segmental vein
55. 右肺前段静脉（V3）right anterior segmental vein
56. 水平裂 horizontal fissure
57. 右肺前段支气管（B3）和动脉（A3）right anterior segmental bronchus and artery
58. 第3肋软骨 3rd costal cartilage
59. 胸廓内动、静脉 internal thoracic artery and vein

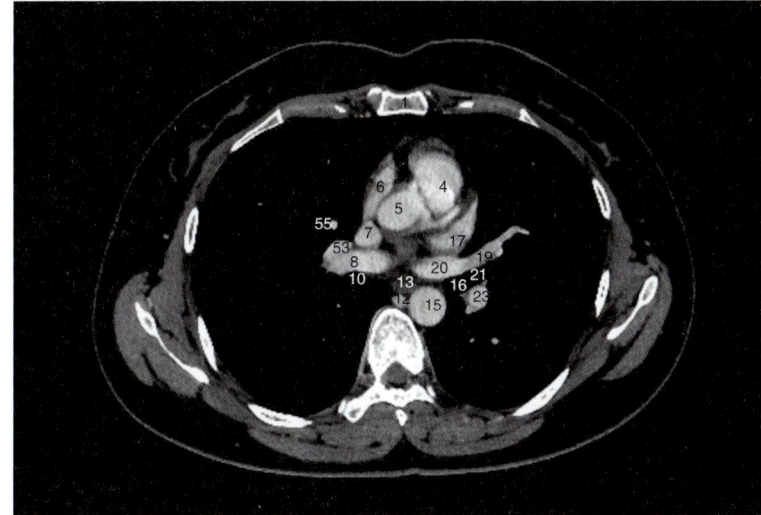

B. CT 纵隔窗增强图像

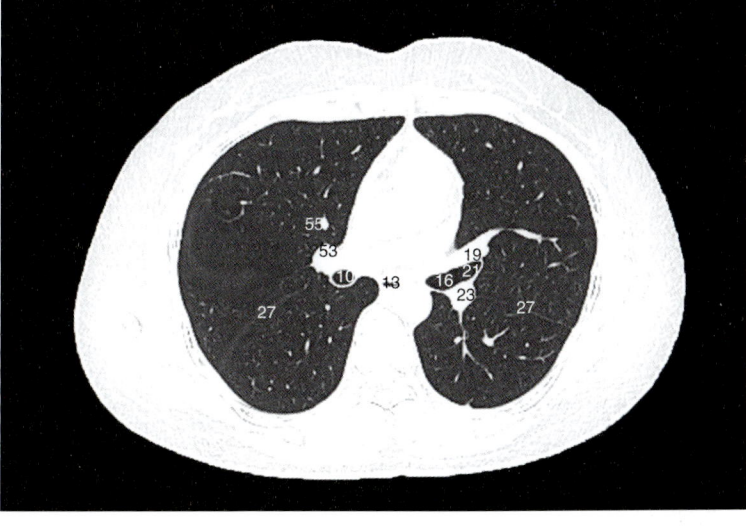

C. CT 肺窗图像

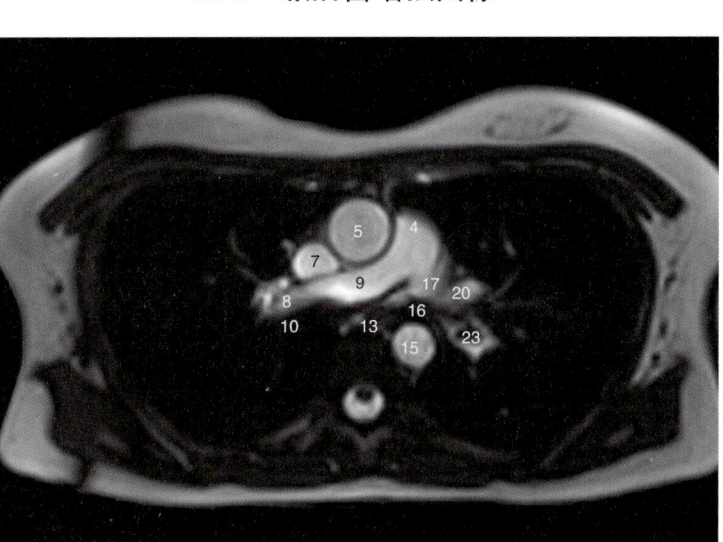

D. MR T2WI 平扫图像

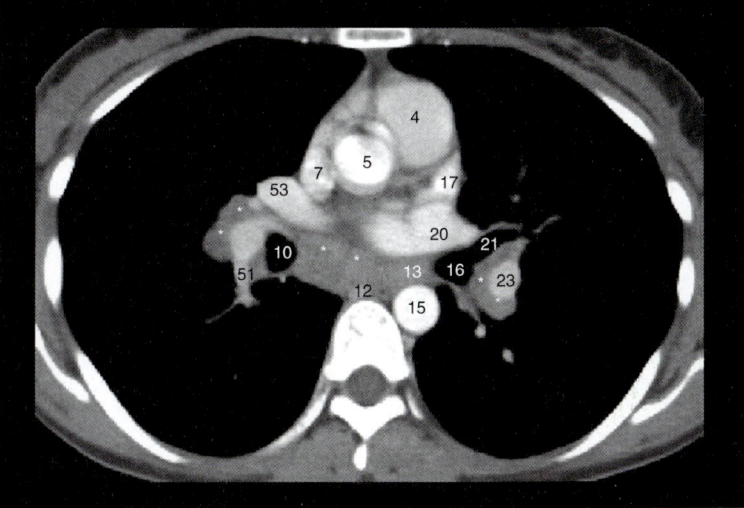

E. 7区、11区淋巴结转移 CT 图像

关键结构：左肺上叶支气管下干，上、下舌段支气管，左肺下叶支气管。

此断面经第6胸椎椎体上份。

左肺门处，因左上肺静脉从肺门前部穿出进入纵隔，故左肺门结构从"支气管+动脉"变为"静脉+支气管+动脉"从前至后排列。上叶支气管向上发出上干后，其下壁向外下发出下干，分布于左肺上叶的前下部（左肺小舌），相当于右肺中叶的范围，也称舌干。下干长度为 1.0 cm ± 0.3 cm，多重叠于左肺上叶支气管的远端，在横断面上常难以辨认，90% ± 3.0% 的下干分支为上、下舌段支气管[36]。发出上叶支气管后，左主支气管继续下行变为下叶支气管。下叶支气管较短，发出上段支气管后很快移行为基底干支气管。此断面仍可见隆嵴下淋巴结（7区）及左、右肺门内的叶间淋巴结（11L 和 11R）。在7区、11区淋巴结转移 CT 图像可见该区肿大的淋巴结。

胸部连续横断层 48（FH.12550）

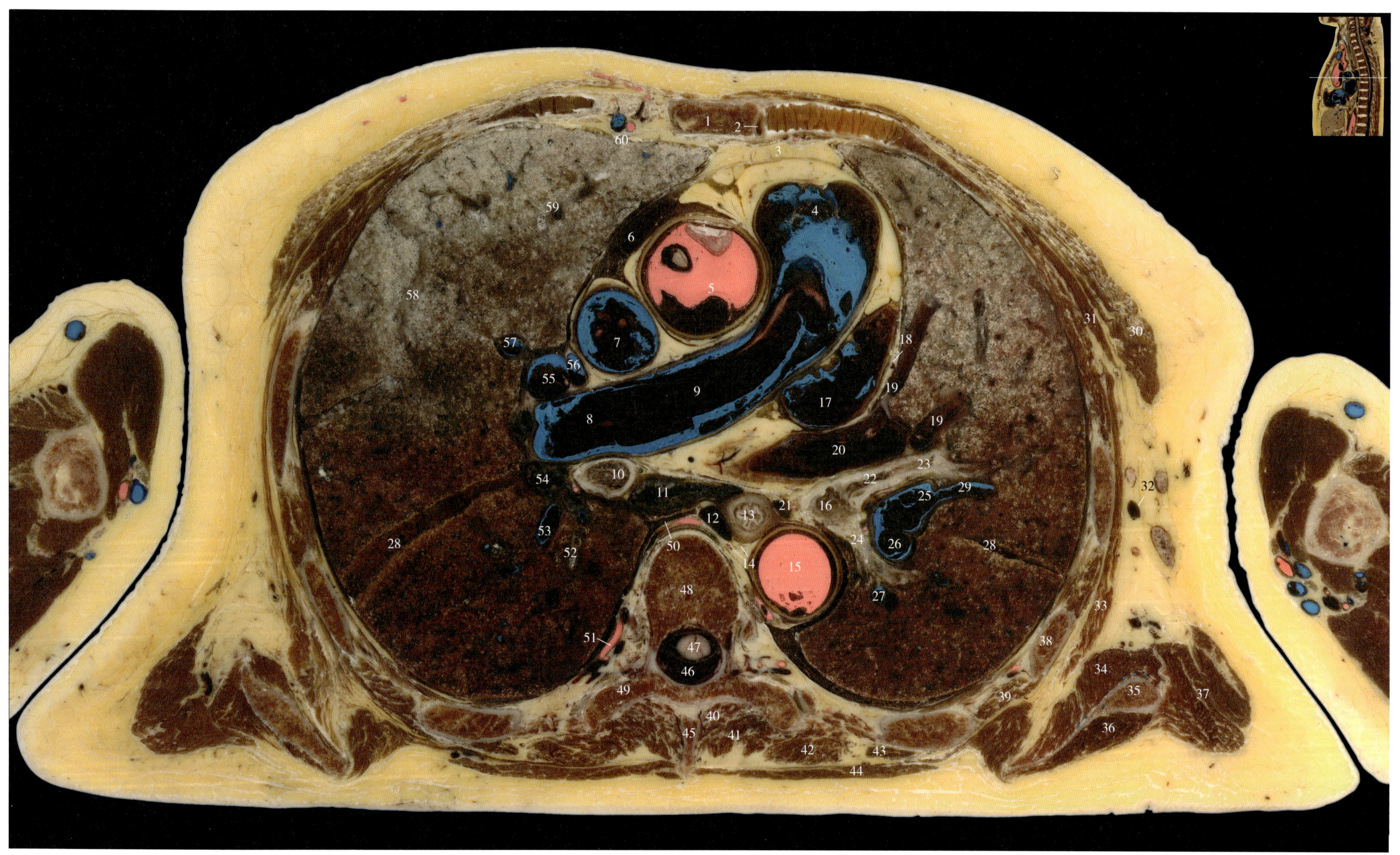

A. 断层标本图像

1. 胸骨体 body of sternum
2. 第 3 胸肋关节 3rd sternocostal joint
3. 胸腺 thymus
4. 肺动脉干 pulmonary trunk
5. 升主动脉 ascending aorta
6. 右心耳 right auricle
7. 上腔静脉 superior vena cava
8. 右肺叶间动脉 right interlobar artery
9. 右肺动脉 right pulmonary artery
10. 中间支气管 intermediate bronchus
11. 隆嵴下淋巴结（7 区）subcarinal lymph nodes
12. 奇静脉 azygos vein
13. 食管 esophagus
14. 胸导管 thoracic duct
15. 胸主动脉 thoracic aorta
16. 左肺下叶支气管 left inferior lobar bronchus
17. 左心耳 left auricle
18. 膈神经和心包膈血管 phrenic nerve and pericardiacophrenic vessels
19. 左肺前段静脉（V3）left anterior segmental vein
20. 左上肺静脉 left superior pulmonary vein
21. 左食管旁淋巴结（8L）left paraesophageal lymph nodes
22. 上叶支气管下干 inferior trunk of superior lobar bronchus
23. 上舌段支气管（B4）superior lingular segmental bronchus
24. 左肺上段支气管（B6）left superior segmental bronchus
25. 舌动脉干（A4+5）lingular arterial trunk
26. 左肺外后底段动脉（A9+10）left lateroposterior basal segmental artery
27. 左肺上段静脉（V6）left superior segmental vein
28. 斜裂 oblique fissure
29. 上舌段动脉（A4）superior lingular artery
30. 胸大肌 pectoralis major
31. 胸小肌 pectoralis minor
32. 胸外侧静脉 lateral thoracic vein
33. 前锯肌 serratus anterior
34. 肩胛下肌 subscapularis
35. 肩胛骨 scapula
36. 冈下肌 infraspinatus
37. 大圆肌 teres major
38. 第 5 肋骨 5th costal bone
39. 肋间内、外肌 intercostales interni and externi
40. 横突棘肌 transversospinales
41. 棘肌 spinales
42. 最长肌 longissimus
43. 髂肋肌 iliocostalis
44. 斜方肌 trapezius
45. 棘突 spinous process
46. 硬膜外隙 epidural space
47. 脊髓 spinal cord
48. 第 6 胸椎椎体 body of 6th thoracic vertebra
49. 横突 transverse process
50. 奇静脉食管隐窝 azygoesophageal recess
51. 肋间后动脉 posterior intercostal artery
52. 右肺上段支气管（B6）right superior segmental bronchus
53. 右肺上段动脉（A6）right superior segmental artery
54. 右肺叶间淋巴结（11R）right interlobar lymph nodes
55. 右肺后段静脉（V2）right posterior segmental vein
56. 右肺尖前段静脉（V1+3）right apicoanterior segmental vein
57. 右肺前段静脉（V3）right anterior segmental vein
58. 水平裂 horizontal fissure
59. 右肺前段支气管（B3）和动脉（A3）right anterior segmental bronchus and artery
60. 胸廓内动、静脉 internal thoracic artery and vein
61. 左肺下叶动脉 left inferior lobar artery

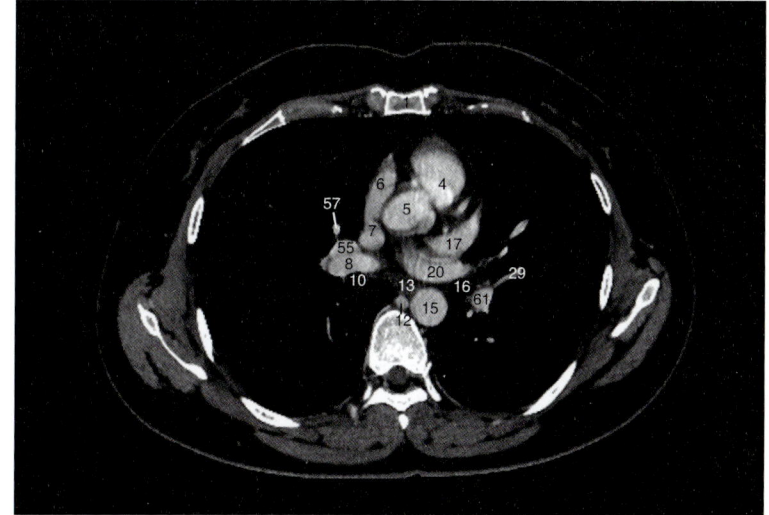

B. CT 纵隔窗增强图像

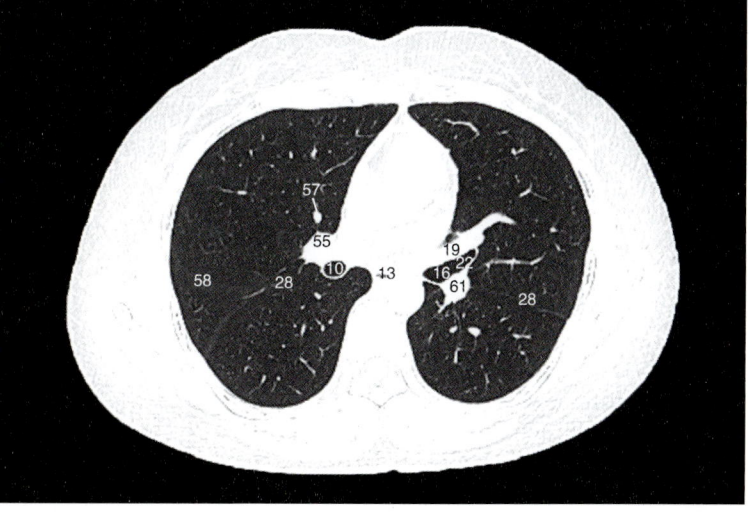

C. CT 肺窗图像

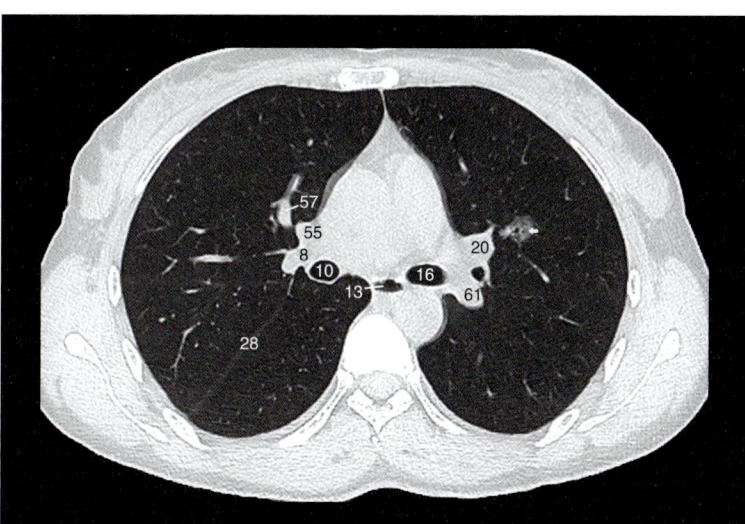

D. 左肺上叶磨玻璃病变 CT 图像

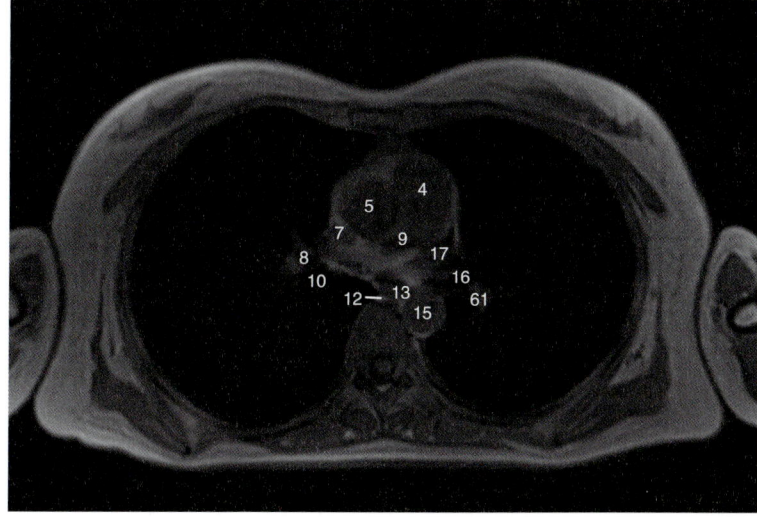

E. MR T1WI 平扫图像

关键结构：右肺上叶静脉，左上肺静脉。

此断面经第 6 胸椎椎体上份。

右肺上叶的管道中，肺静脉的主干位置偏下，故在此断面及相邻层面中，右肺门前部主要结构为右肺上叶静脉及其属支，常为尖段静脉和前段静脉逐渐后行，与后段静脉汇合。尖段静脉、后段静脉和前段静脉各自独立，共同汇合成上叶静脉，占 18%；尖段静脉先与前段静脉汇合成尖前段静脉（V1+3），再与后段面合成上叶静脉，占 30%；尖段静脉与后段静脉先汇合成尖后段静脉（V1+2），再与前段静脉合成上叶静脉，占 30%；3 支静脉互相有属支汇合，形成尖前段静脉（V1+3），尖后段静脉（V1+2）和前后段静脉（V2+3），再逐渐合成上叶静脉，占 22%。3 组段静脉常围成固定的"倒三角"形，随着断面下移，"倒三角"逐渐变小。后段静脉位置较为恒定，较为粗大，可作为前、后段分界的解剖标志。左肺门处，左上肺静脉进入纵隔，提示左心房即将出现。左上肺静脉的属支以 3 支最多见，占 70%，分别为尖后段静脉、前段静脉和舌段静脉干。前段静脉见 2 条属支，前方的为上支，后方的为下支，分隔前段与上舌段[38]。当肺内病变导致肺密度呈模糊的云雾样增高称为磨玻璃病变，如新冠肺炎或早期肺癌病变，常表现为片状、地图样分布或边缘不清的小叶中心性结节，不掩盖其中的血管或支气管。在左肺上叶磨玻璃病变 CT 图像可发现，左肺上叶呈结节样磨玻璃病灶，内有血管和支气管穿过，术后病理结果为浸润性腺癌。

胸部连续横断层 49（FH.12530）

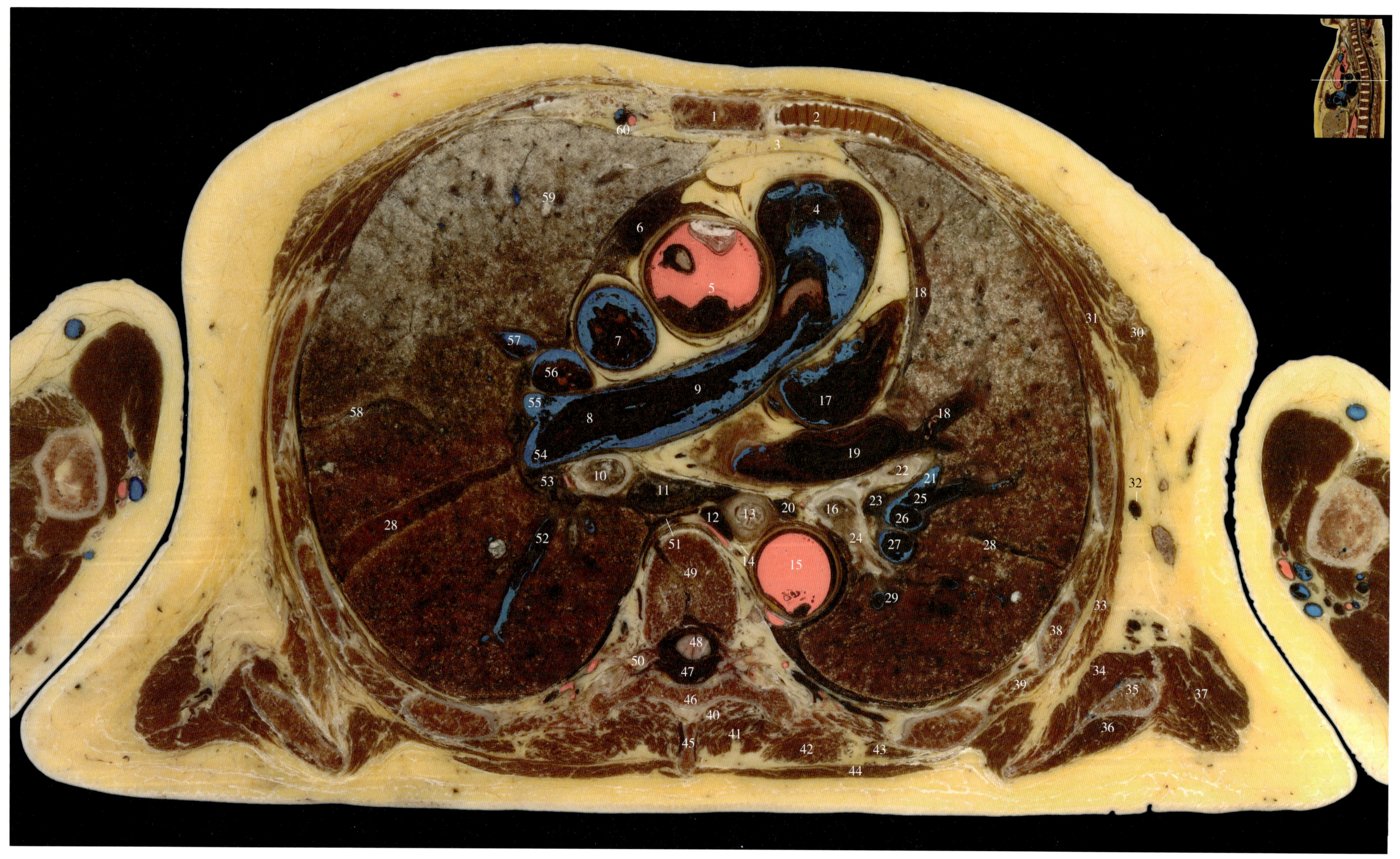

A. 断层标本图像

1. 胸骨体 body of sternum
2. 第 3 肋软骨 3rd costal cartilage
3. 胸腺 thymus
4. 肺动脉干 pulmonary trunk
5. 升主动脉 ascending aorta
6. 右心耳 right auricle
7. 上腔静脉 superior vena cava
8. 右肺叶间动脉 right interlobar artery
9. 右肺动脉 right pulmonary artery
10. 中间支气管 intermediate bronchus
11. 隆嵴下淋巴结（7 区）subcarinal lymph nodes
12. 奇静脉 azygos vein
13. 食管 esophagus
14. 胸导管 thoracic duct
15. 胸主动脉 thoracic aorta
16. 左肺下叶支气管 left inferior lobar bronchus
17. 左心耳 left auricle
18. 左肺前段静脉（V3）left anterior segmental vein
19. 左上肺静脉 left superior pulmonary vein
20. 左食管旁淋巴结（8L）left paraesophageal lymph nodes
21. 上舌段动脉（A4）superior lingular segmental artery
22. 左肺上叶支气管下干 inferior trunk of left superior lobar bronchus
23. 左肺叶淋巴结（12L）left lobar lymph nodes
24. 左肺上段支气管（B6）left superior segmental bronchus
25. 舌动脉干（A4+5）lingular arterial trunk
26. 内前底段动脉（A7+8）medioanterior basal segmental artery
27. 左肺外后底段动脉（A9+10）left lateroposterior basal segmental artery
28. 斜裂 oblique fissure
29. 左肺上段动脉（A6）left superior segmental artery
30. 胸大肌 pectoralis major
31. 胸小肌 pectoralis minor
32. 胸外侧静脉 lateral thoracic vein
33. 前锯肌 serratus anterior
34. 肩胛下肌 subscapularis
35. 肩胛骨 scapula
36. 冈下肌 infraspinatus
37. 大圆肌 teres major
38. 第 5 肋骨 5th costal bone
39. 肋间内、外肌 intercostales interni and externi
40. 横突棘肌 transversospinales
41. 棘肌 spinales
42. 最长肌 longissimus
43. 髂肋肌 iliocostalis
44. 斜方肌 trapezius
45. 棘突 spinous process
46. 椎弓板 lamina of vertebral arch
47. 硬膜外隙 epidural space
48. 脊髓 spinal cord
49. 第 6 胸椎椎体 body of 6th thoracic vertebra
50. 第 6 胸神经 6th thoracic nerve
51. 奇静脉食管隐窝 azygoesophageal recess
52. 右肺上段动脉（A6）right superior segmental artery
53. 右肺叶间淋巴结（11R）right interlobar lymph nodes
54. 右肺下叶动脉 right inferior lobar artery
55. 右肺中叶动脉 right middle lobar artery
56. 右肺上叶静脉 right superior lobar vein
57. 右肺前段静脉（V3）right anterior segmental vein
58. 水平裂 horizontal fissure
59. 右肺前段支气管（B3）和动脉（A3）right anterior segmental bronchus and artery
60. 胸廓内动、静脉 internal thoracic artery and vein
61. 左肺下叶动脉 left inferior lobar artery

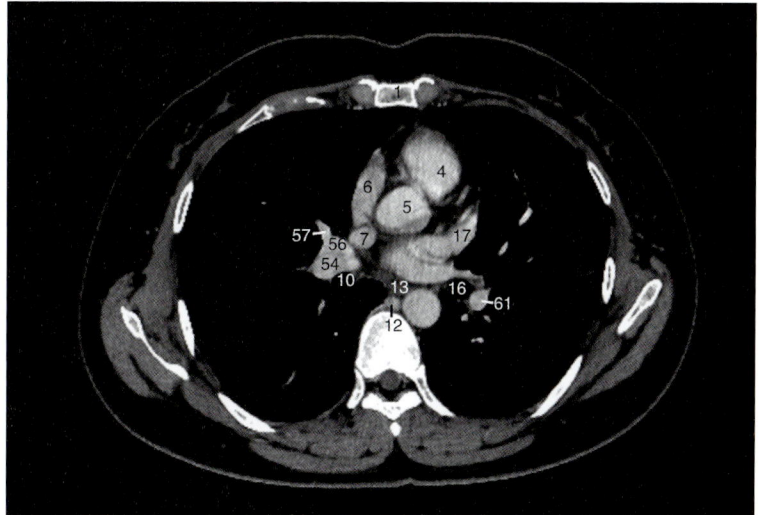

B. CT 纵隔窗增强图像

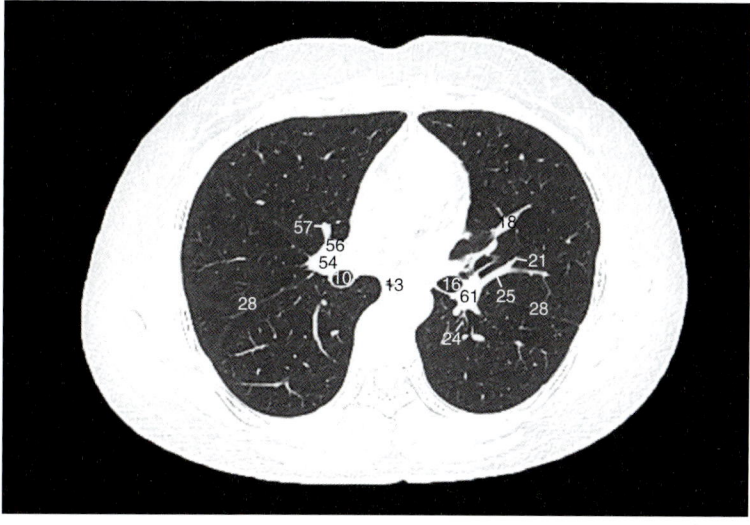

C. CT 肺窗图像

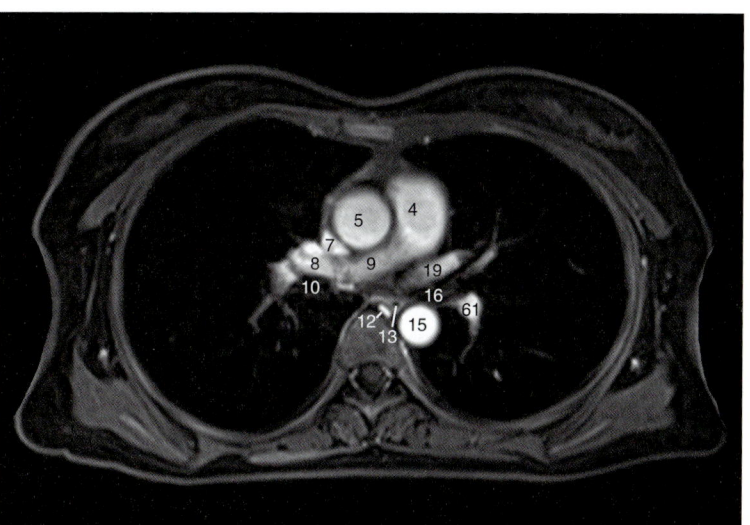

D. MR T1WI 增强图像

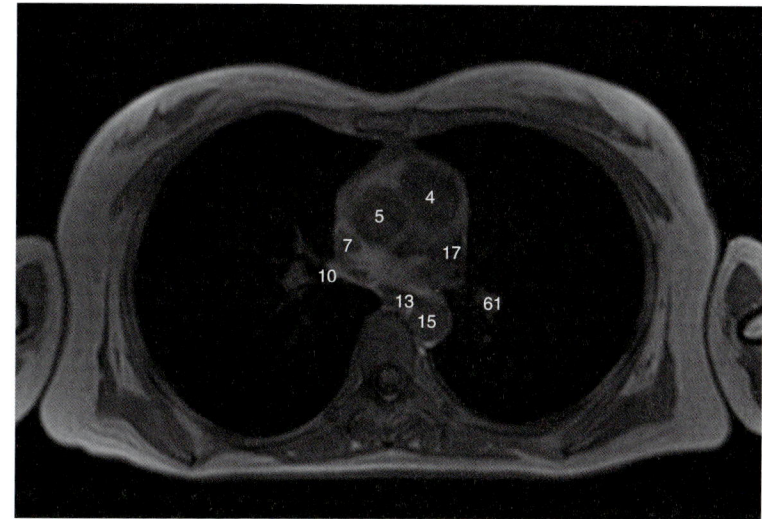

E. MR T1WI 平扫图像

关键结构：右肺中叶动脉，右肺下叶动脉，左肺上段支气管。

此断面经第 6 胸椎椎体中份。

右肺门中部可见右肺叶间动脉已两分为中叶动脉和下叶动脉。前方较细的为中叶动脉，行向前外侧下方，中叶动脉多数情况为 1 支，占 56.4% ± 3.0%；也可为 2 支，占 41.3% ± 3.1%[36]；后方粗且连于斜裂的为下叶动脉，在斜裂内进一步下行，发出上段动脉后移行为基底干动脉，分出底段动脉分支辐射状至各底段。CT 测量显示，收缩期中叶动脉直径为 0.6 cm ± 0.2 cm，长度为 1.6 cm ± 1.4 cm，下叶动脉直径为 1.2 cm ± 0.4 cm，长度为 0.9 cm ± 1.2 cm[43]。左肺门处，约距下叶支气管发出部 0.5~1 cm 处，下叶支气管后壁发出上段支气管，84.1% 的标本可见这种情况，起始部水平，较为粗大，行向后上方，是右肺吸入异物容易停留的部位。上段支气管多数分为 2 支或 3 支，上段动脉和静脉位于上段支气管的后外侧[47]。肺段支气管的走行可分为纵行、横行和斜行 3 种，上段支气管是横行支气管的典型代表。其他横行的支气管还包括：①右肺，有上叶支气管、后段支气管、前段支气管、外侧段支气管、内侧段支气管和上段支气管；②左肺，有左肺上叶支气管和上段支气管。横行支气管在断面上表现为横向的长条形。

99

胸部连续横断层 50（FH.12510）

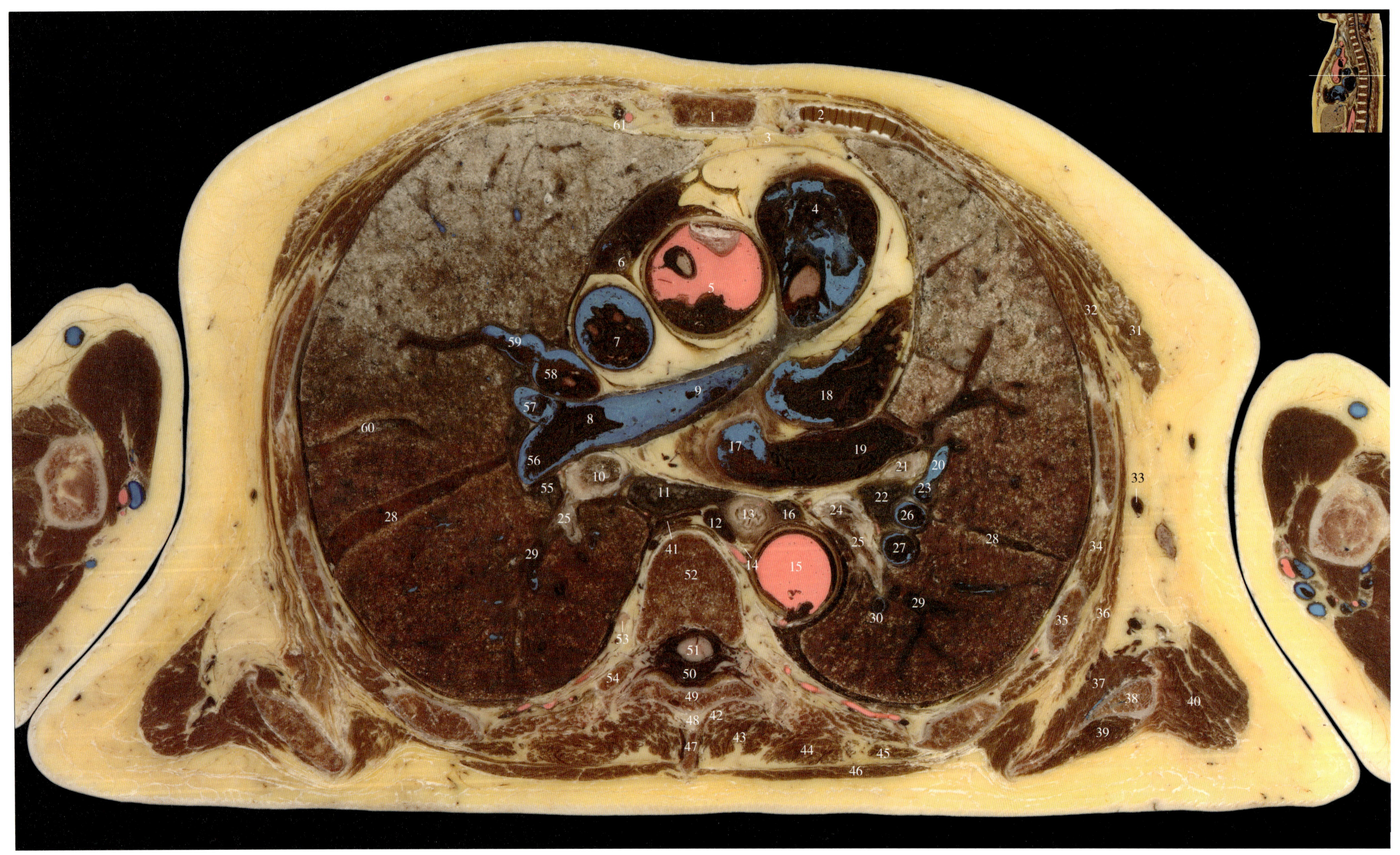

A. 断层标本图像

1. 胸骨体 body of sternum
2. 第 3 肋软骨 3rd costal cartilage
3. 胸腺 thymus
4. 肺动脉干 pulmonary trunk
5. 升主动脉 ascending aorta
6. 右心耳 right auricle
7. 上腔静脉 superior vena cava
8. 右肺叶间动脉 right interlobar artery
9. 右肺动脉 right pulmonary artery
10. 中间支气管 intermediate bronchus
11. 隆嵴下淋巴结（7区）subcarinal lymph nodes
12. 奇静脉 azygos vein
13. 食管 esophagus
14. 胸导管 thoracic duct
15. 胸主动脉 thoracic aorta
16. 左食管旁淋巴结（8L）left paraesophageal lymph nodes
17. 左心房 left atrium
18. 左心耳 left auricle
19. 左上肺静脉 left superior pulmonary vein
20. 上舌段动脉（A4）superior lingular segmental artery
21. 左肺上叶支气管下干 inferior trunk of left superior lobar bronchus
22. 左肺叶淋巴结（12L）left lobar lymph nodes
23. 舌动脉干（A4+5）lingular arterial trunk
24. 左肺下叶支气管 left inferior lobar bronchus
25. 上段支气管（B6）superior segmental bronchus
26. 内前底段动脉（A7+8）medioanterior basal segmental artery
27. 左肺外后底段动脉（A9+10）left lateroposterior basal segmental artery
28. 斜裂 oblique fissure
29. 上段静脉（V6）superior segmental vein
30. 左肺上段动脉（A6）left superior segmental artery
31. 胸大肌 pectoralis major
32. 胸小肌 pectoralis minor
33. 胸外侧静脉 lateral thoracic vein
34. 肋间内、外肌 intercostales interni and externi
35. 第 5 肋骨 5th costal bone
36. 前锯肌 serratus anterior
37. 肩胛下肌 subscapularis
38. 肩胛骨 scapula
39. 冈下肌 infraspinatus
40. 大圆肌 teres major
41. 奇静脉食管隐窝 azygoesophageal recess
42. 横突棘肌 transversospinales
43. 棘肌 spinales
44. 最长肌 longissimus
45. 髂肋肌 iliocostalis
46. 斜方肌 trapezius
47. 棘突 spinous process
48. 棘间韧带 interspinous ligament
49. 椎弓板 lamina of vertebral arch
50. 硬膜外隙 epidural space
51. 脊髓 spinal cord
52. 第 6 胸椎椎体 body of 6th thoracic vertebra
53. 胸交感神经节 thoracic sympathetic ganglion
54. 第 7 肋骨 7th costal bone
55. 右叶间淋巴结（11R）right interlobar lymph nodes
56. 右肺下叶动脉 right inferior lobar artery
57. 右肺中叶动脉 right middle lobar artery
58. 右肺上叶静脉 right superior lobar vein
59. 右肺前段静脉（V3）right anterior segmental vein
60. 水平裂 horizontal fissure
61. 胸廓内动、静脉 internal thoracic artery and vein
62. 上舌段支气管（B4）superior lingular segmental bronchus
63. 上舌段动脉（A4）superior lingular artery
64. 下舌段支气管（B5）inferior lingular segmental bronchus
65. 左肺下叶动脉 left inferior lobar artery

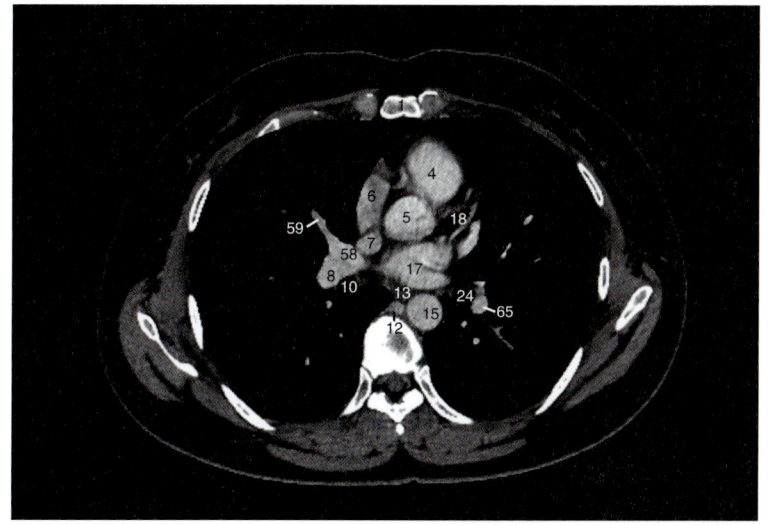

B. CT 纵隔窗增强图像

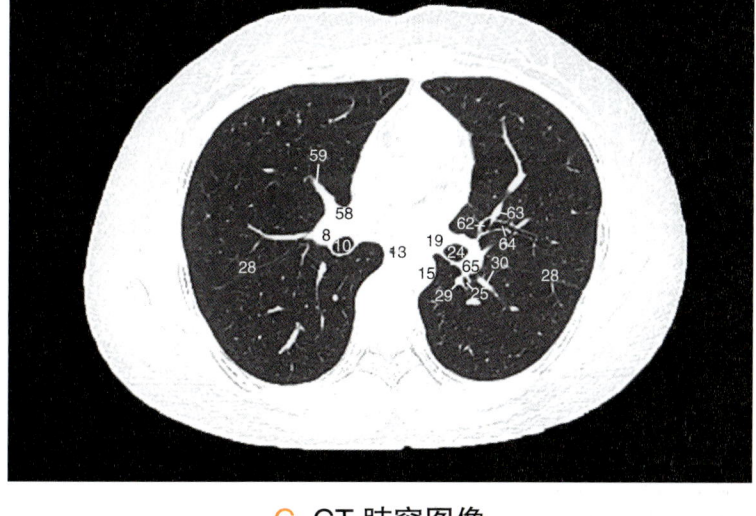

C. CT 肺窗图像

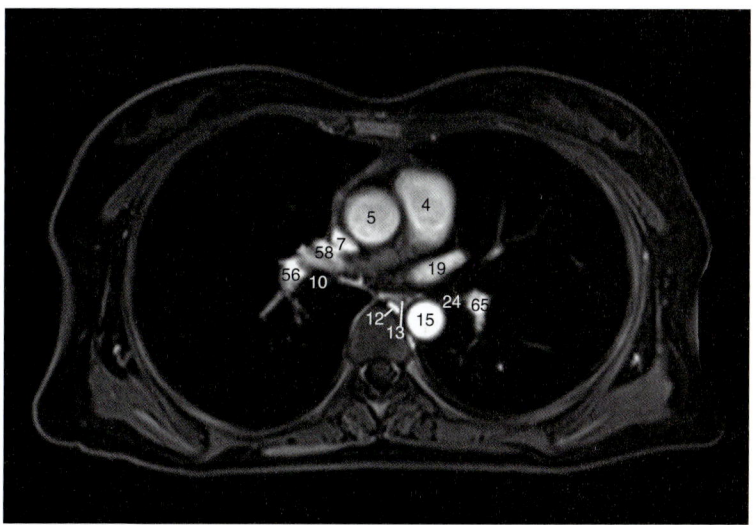

D. MR T1WI 增强图像

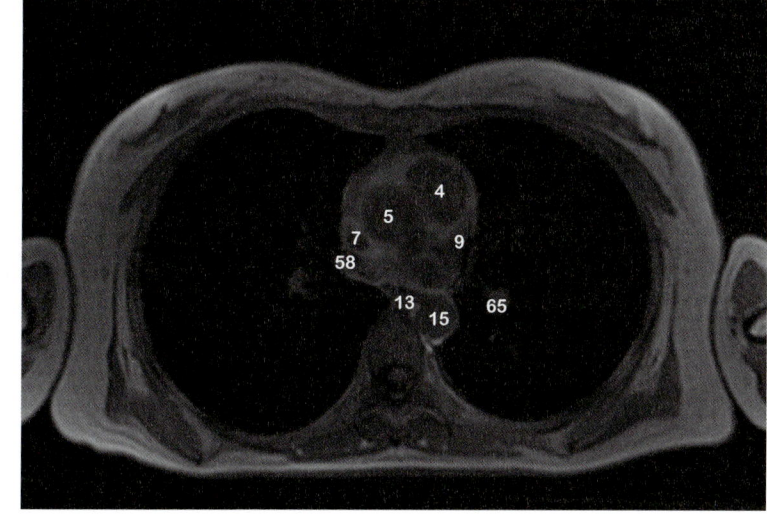

E. MR T1WI 平扫图像

关键结构：水平裂，斜裂。

此断面经第 6 胸椎椎体中份。

叶间裂位于相邻肺叶之间，是 CT 定位肺叶和肺段的重要依据，叶间裂包括斜裂和水平裂，右侧斜裂深部常见右肺叶间动脉，进一步向中叶和下叶门发出中叶动脉和下叶动脉，左肺斜裂深部见左肺下叶动脉或其分支。叶间裂的 CT 表现与层厚关系密切，层厚越薄，分辨率越高，扫描角度与叶间裂越垂直，叶间裂线影越常见，高密度带影及乏血管带影越少见。除水平裂和斜裂，还常见肺裂不全和副肺裂等异常[48]。叶间裂发育不全最常见的区域位于肺门和纵隔旁区，可观察到血管、支气管穿行于两叶之间，最常见的穿过肺叶间的结构是肺静脉，其次是肺动脉和支气管。水平裂是最常见的不完整叶间裂，其变异的出现率可达 56.1%，主要表现为水平裂阙如或发育不全[49]。肺裂不全可使肺感染在肺间互相蔓延，融合处有血管、淋巴管及神经通过，导致手术时难于剥离或出血。副肺裂多见于左肺上叶和右肺下叶，出现位置多与肺段一致，如左肺舌段与其他肺段之间出现肺裂，使舌段与上叶分离，左肺出现中叶。右肺下叶的上段（背段）与基底段之间出现肺裂，从而出现背叶等[50]。CT 横断面图像中，水平裂和斜裂多出现于肺门中部平面和右肺下叶动脉平面，均表现为低密度直带影[51]。

胸部连续横断层 51（FH.12490）

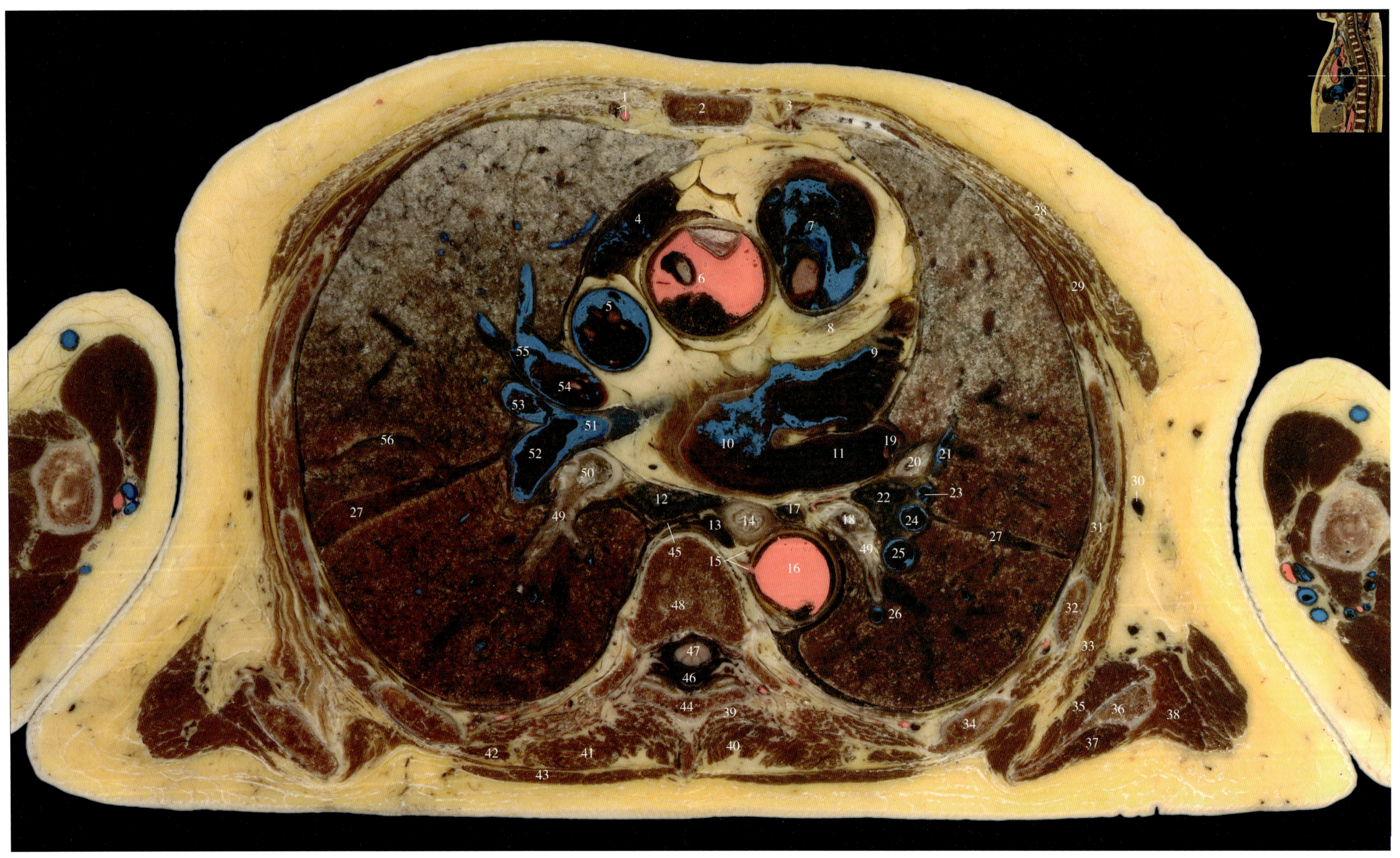

A. 断层标本图像

1. 胸廓内动、静脉 internal thoracic artery and vein
2. 胸骨体 body of sternum
3. 第3肋软骨 3rd costal cartilage
4. 右心耳 right auricle
5. 上腔静脉 superior vena cava
6. 升主动脉 ascending aorta
7. 肺动脉干 pulmonary trunk
8. 前室间支 anterior interventricular branch
9. 左心耳 left auricle
10. 左心房 left atrium
11. 左上肺静脉 left superior pulmonary vein
12. 隆嵴下淋巴结（7区）subcarinal lymph nodes
13. 奇静脉 azygos vein
14. 食管 esophagus
15. 胸导管和肋间后动脉 thoracic duct and posterior intercostal artery
16. 胸主动脉 thoracic aorta
17. 左食管旁淋巴结（8L）left paraesophageal lymph nodes
18. 左肺下叶支气管 left inferior lobar bronchus
19. 舌静脉干（V4+5）lingular venous trunk
20. 左肺上叶支气管下干 inferior trunk of left superior lobar bronchus
21. 上舌段动脉（A4）superior lingular segmental artery
22. 左肺叶淋巴结（12R）left lobar lymph nodes
23. 下舌段动脉（A5）inferior lingular segmental artery
24. 内前底段动脉（A7+8）medioanterior basal segmental artery
25. 左肺外后底段动脉（A9+10）left lateroposterior basal segmental artery
26. 左肺上段动脉（A6）left superior segmental artery
27. 斜裂 oblique fissure
28. 胸大肌 pectoralis major
29. 胸小肌 pectoralis minor
30. 胸外侧静脉 lateral thoracic vein
31. 肋间内、外肌 intercostales interni and externi
32. 第5肋骨 5th costal bone
33. 前锯肌 serratus anterior
34. 第6肋骨 6th costal bone
35. 肩胛下肌 subscapularis
36. 肩胛骨 scapula
37. 冈下肌 infraspinatus
38. 大圆肌 teres major
39. 横突棘肌 transversospinales
40. 棘肌 spinales
41. 最长肌 longissimus
42. 髂肋肌 iliocostalis
43. 斜方肌 trapezius
44. 椎弓板 lamina of vertebral arch
45. 奇静脉食管隐窝 azygoesophageal recess
46. 硬膜外隙 epidural space
47. 脊髓 spinal cord
48. 第6胸椎椎体 body of 6th thoracic vertebra
49. 上段支气管（B6）superior segmental bronchus
50. 右肺下叶支气管 right inferior lobar bronchus
51. 右肺叶间动脉 right interlobar artery
52. 右肺下动脉 right inferior lobar artery
53. 右肺中叶动脉 right middle lobar artery
54. 右上肺静脉 right superior pulmonary vein
55. 右肺前段静脉（V3）right anterior segmental vein
56. 水平裂 horizontal fissure
57. 上舌段支气管（B4）superior lingular segmental bronchus
58. 右肺下叶支气管 right inferior lobar bronchus
59. 左肺下叶动脉 left inferior lobar artery

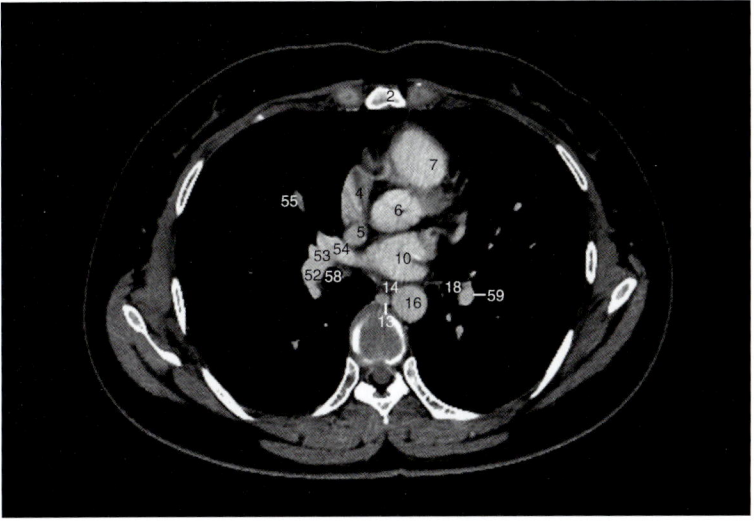

B. CT 纵隔窗增强图像

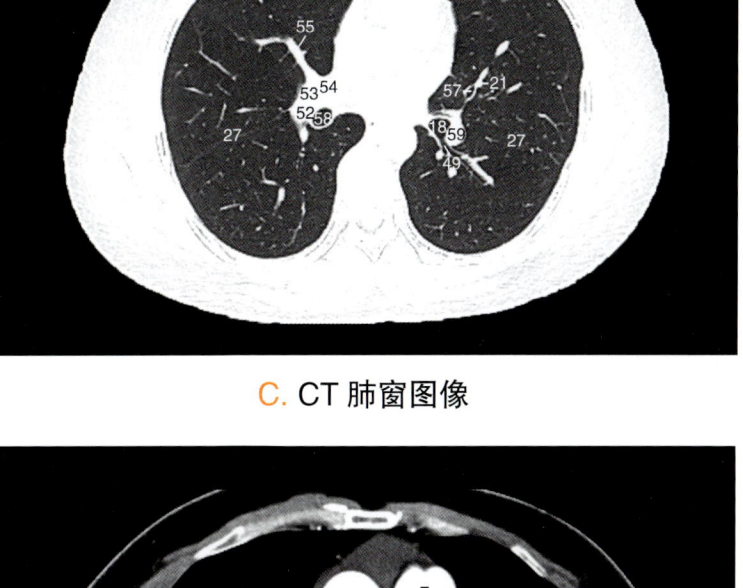

C. CT 肺窗图像

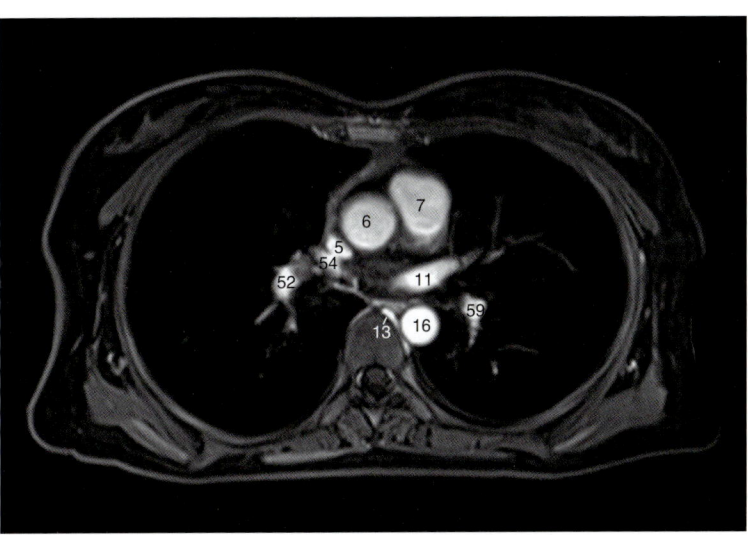

D. MR T1WI 增强图像

E. 心包横窦积液图像

关键结构：心包横窦，基底干支气管。

此断面经第6胸椎椎体下份。

心包横窦一般在左冠状动脉平面开始出现，位于升主动脉、左冠状动脉、肺动脉窦和右心耳、上腔静脉、左心房、左心耳之间。横窦窦体出现在升主动脉根部的后方、主动脉窦口稍上方。右侧出口在右心耳、右心室壁之间。左侧出口在左冠状动脉、右心室壁和左心耳之间。成年人横窦长度平均为 50.4 mm，CT 显示率为 100%，MRI 检查发现 71.4% 的病例可显示横窦[52]。CT 图像中，横窦在心包无积液时表现为线形或三角形；积液时，为新月形或三角形，如图 E 所示。右肺门处，上叶结构仅剩居前的上叶静脉，即将汇入左心房；中叶见中叶动脉进入中叶门，下叶有两组管道进入下叶门，位于内侧的为右肺下叶支气管，右肺下叶动脉从支气管外侧进入下叶内。下叶支气管后壁水平发出上段支气管，发出位置略低于中叶支气管发出的位置[53]。右肺基底干支气管的常见分支类型包括：外侧底段与前底段共干型，占 50.4%；各底段单独分支型，占 38.4%；内侧底段与前底段共干型，占 9.1%；内侧底段支气管、前底段支气管、外侧底段支气管和后底段支气管呈逆时针排列。左肺基底干支气管的分支类型包括：分为内前底段支气管、外后底段支气管，占 75%；分为内前底段支气管、外侧底段支气管、后底段支气管，占 18%。内前底段支气管、外侧底段支气管和后底段支气管呈顺时针排列。

胸部连续横断层 52（FH.12470）

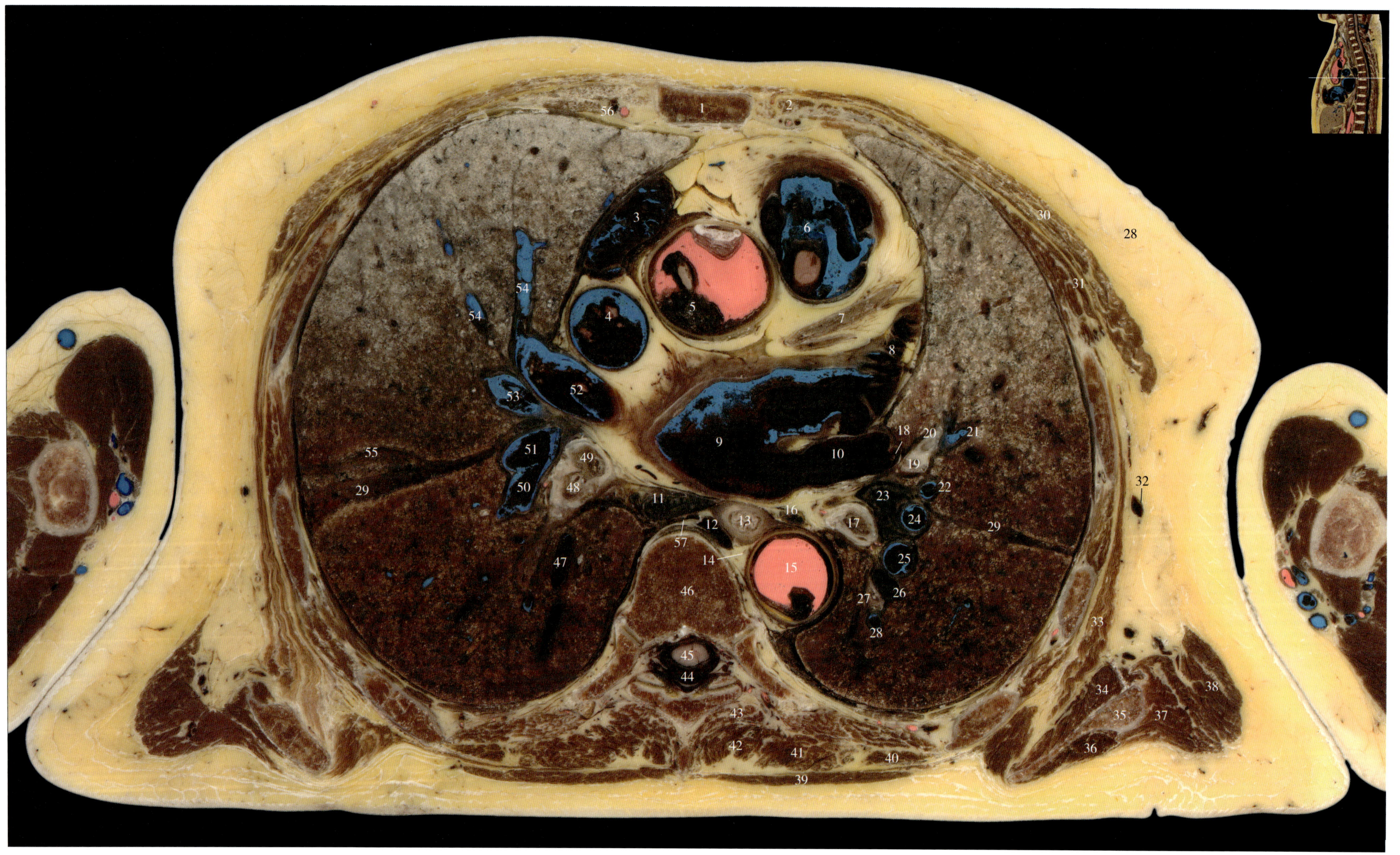

A. 断层标本图像

1. 胸骨体 body of sternum
2. 第 3 肋软骨 3rd costal cartilage
3. 右心耳 right auricle
4. 上腔静脉 superior vena cava
5. 升主动脉 ascending aorta
6. 右心室 right ventricle
7. 前室间支 anterior interventricular branch
8. 左心耳 left auricle
9. 左心房 left atrium
10. 左上肺静脉 left superior pulmonary vein
11. 隆嵴下淋巴结（7 区）subcarinal lymph nodes
12. 奇静脉 azygos vein
13. 食管 esophagus
14. 胸导管 thoracic duct
15. 胸主动脉 thoracic aorta
16. 左食管旁淋巴结（8L）left paraesophageal lymph nodes
17. 左肺基底干支气管 left common basal bronchus
18. 舌静脉干（V4+5）lingular venous trunk
19. 下舌段支气管（B5）inferior lingular segmental bronchus
20. 上舌段支气管（B4）superior lingular segmental bronchus
21. 上舌段动脉（A4）superior lingular segmental artery
22. 下舌段动脉（A5）inferior lingular segmental artery
23. 左肺叶淋巴结（12L）left lobar lymph nodes
24. 内前底段动脉（A7+8）medioanterior basal segmental artery
25. 左肺外后底段动脉（A9+10）left posterolateral basal segmental artery
26. 左肺上段静脉（V6）left superior segmental vein
27. 左肺上段支气管（B6）和动脉（A6）left superior segmental bronchus and artery
28. 乳腺 mammary gland
29. 斜裂 oblique fissure
30. 胸大肌 pectoralis major
31. 胸小肌 pectoralis minor
32. 胸外侧静脉 lateral thoracic vein
33. 前锯肌 serratus anterior
34. 肩胛下肌 subscapularis
35. 肩胛骨 scapula
36. 冈下肌 infraspinatus
37. 大圆肌 teres major
38. 背阔肌 latissimus dorsi
39. 斜方肌 trapezius
40. 髂肋肌 iliocostalis
41. 最长肌 longissimus
42. 棘肌 spinales
43. 横突棘肌 transversospinales
44. 硬膜外隙 epidural space
45. 脊髓 spinal cord
46. 第 6 胸椎体 body of 6th thoracic vertebra
47. 右肺上段静脉（V6）right superior segmental vein
48. 右肺基底干支气管 right common basal bronchus
49. 右肺中叶支气管 right middle lobar bronchus
50. 右肺后底段动脉（A10）right posterior basal segmental artery
51. 右肺内前外底段动脉（A7+8+9）right common trunk of medial, anterior and lateral basal segmental arteries
52. 右肺上叶静脉 right superior lobar vein
53. 右肺中叶动脉 right middle lobar artery
54. 右肺前段静脉（V3）right anterior segmental vein
55. 水平裂 horizontal fissure
56. 胸廓内动、静脉 internal thoracic artery and vein
57. 奇静脉食管隐窝 azygoesophageal recess
58. 左肺下叶动脉 left inferior lobar artery
59. 右肺下叶动脉 right inferior lobar artery
60. 右肺上段动脉（A6）right superior segmental artery
61. 右肺下叶支气管 right inferior lobar bronchus

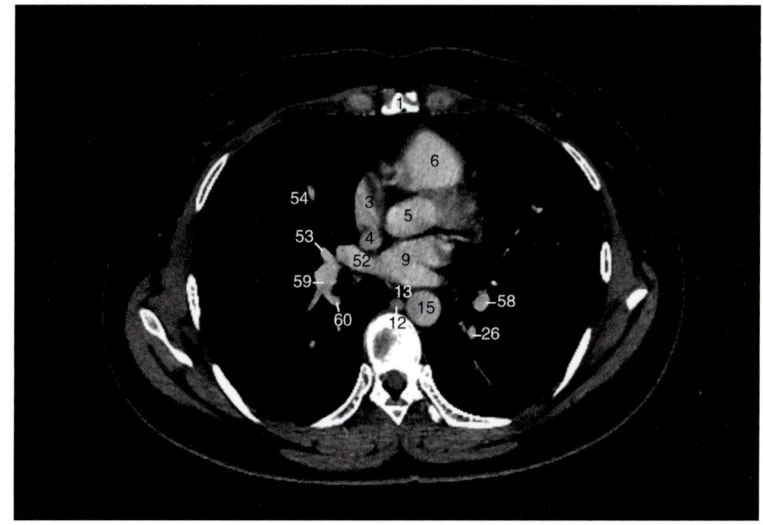

B. CT 纵隔窗增强图像

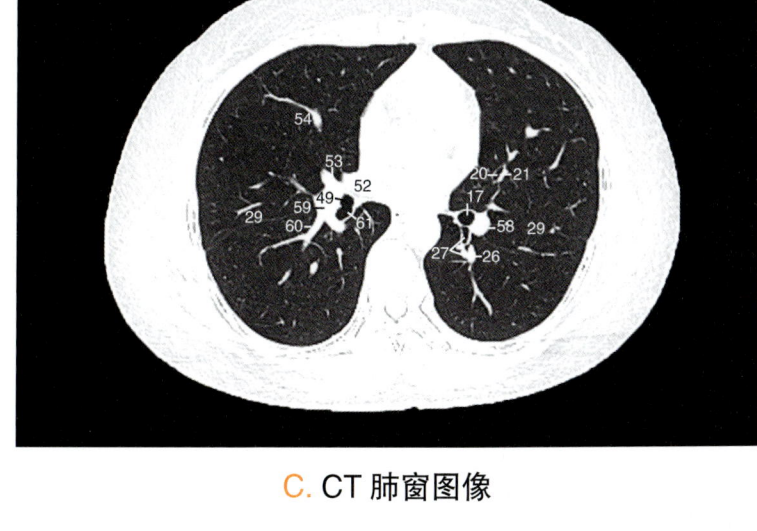

C. CT 肺窗图像

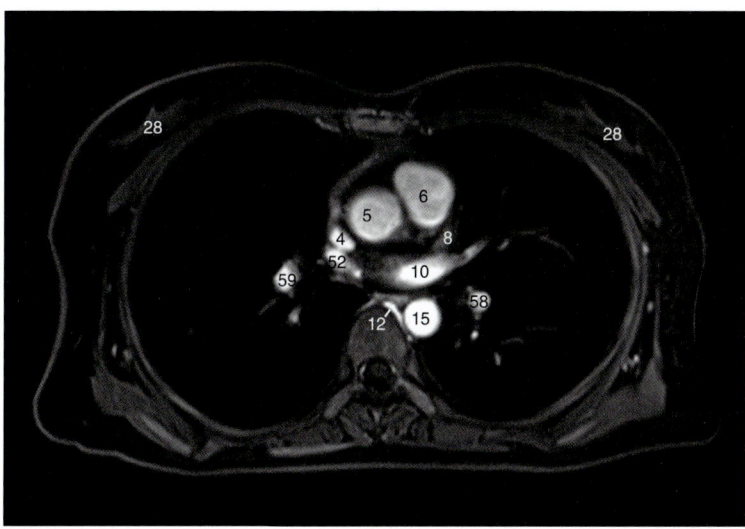

D. MR T1WI 增强图像

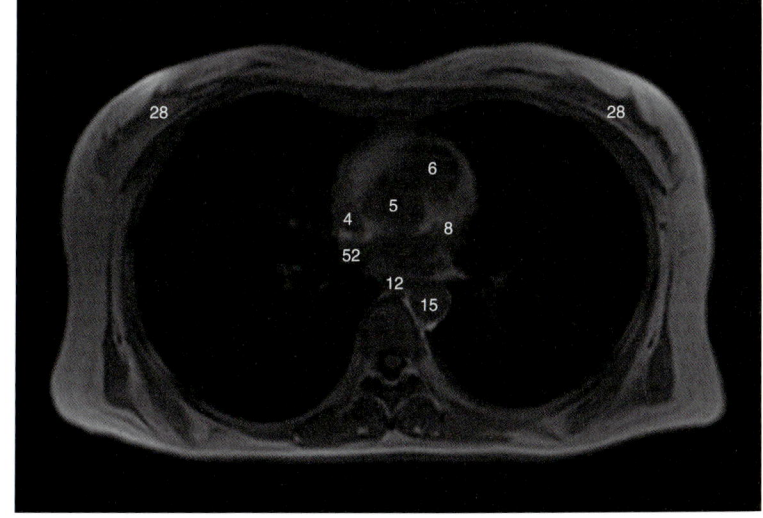

E. MR T1WI 平扫图像

关键结构：右肺中叶支气管，舌静脉干。

此断面经过第 6 胸椎体下份。

右肺斜裂前方，随着上叶静脉汇入左心房，上叶管道几乎消失；中间支气管和叶间动脉均前后两分，二者前方为中叶动脉和中叶支气管，伴行进入中叶门，二者后方为下叶动脉和基底干支气管，伴行进入下叶门。中叶支气管长度为 1.4 cm ± 0.3 cm，外横径为 0.8 cm ± 0.1 cm，94.9% ± 1.3% 的中叶支气管进一步两分为外侧段和内侧段支气管[36]。左肺门处，斜裂前方的舌叶内，上、下舌段的管道逐渐分离；左肺上叶支气管以下层面，前段和尖后段结构逐渐消失，上叶内主要出现的为舌叶的结构，断面结构分布规律与右肺中叶管道有相似处：段动脉与段支气管伴行，动脉通常位于支气管的前外侧或外侧。舌静脉干和下舌段静脉为段间静脉，分隔上、下舌段的结构。舌静脉干出现在左上肺静脉下方的平面，逐渐离开左心房，初始位于左肺纵隔面中部，下舌段管道的前内侧，逐渐行至下舌段管道的前方（或上、下舌段管道之间），再演变为下舌段静脉。左肺上叶上、下舌段静脉（V4、V5）多共干形成舌静脉干，约占 61.3%，也可单独汇入左上肺静脉，占 38.8%[54]。下叶内，紧靠斜裂的下叶动脉已两分为内前底段动脉和外后底段动脉，动脉内侧为基底干支气管。

105

胸部连续横断层 53 (FH.12450)

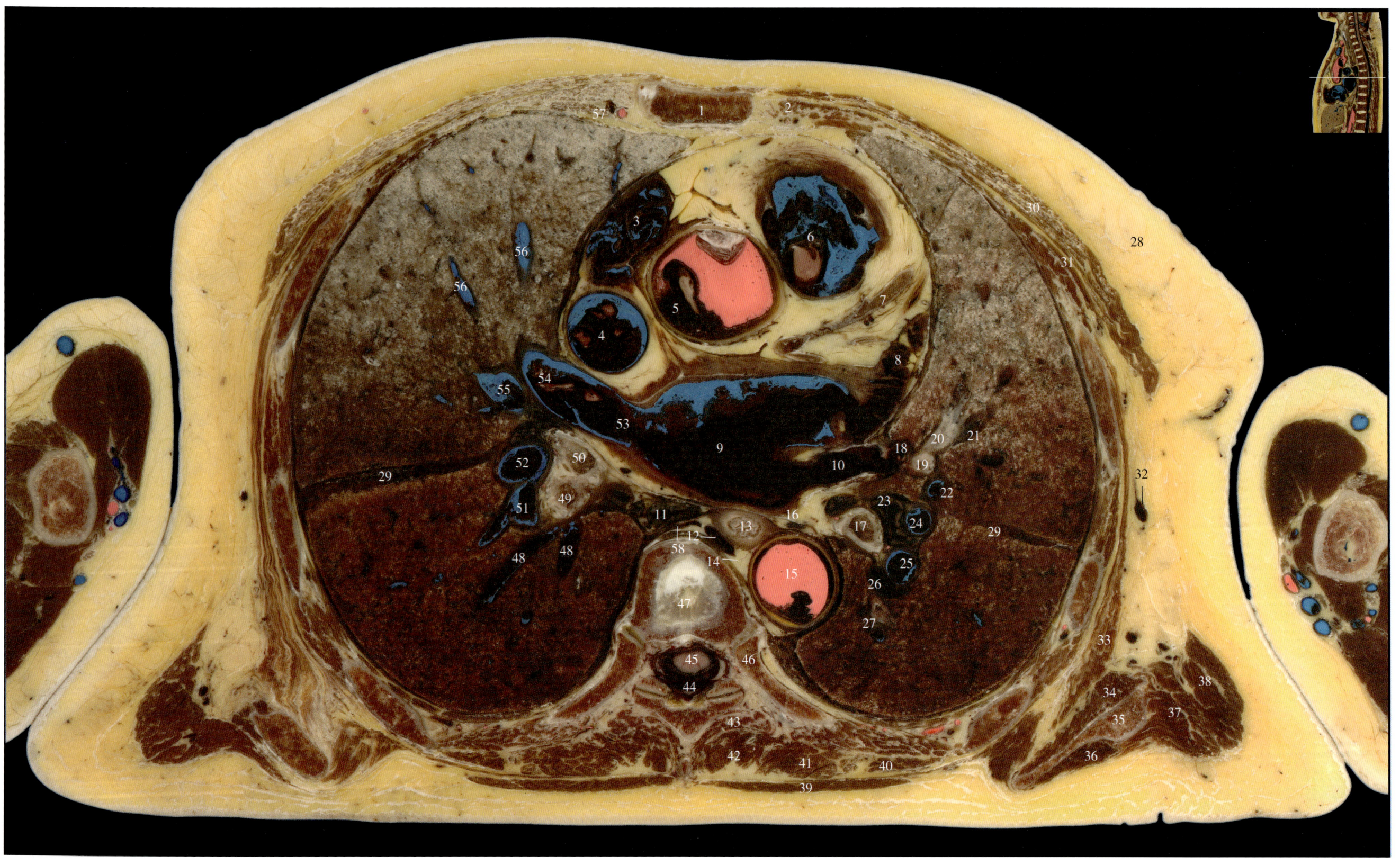

A. 断层标本图像

1. 胸骨体 body of sternum
2. 第 3 肋软骨 3rd costal cartilage
3. 右心耳 right auricle
4. 上腔静脉 superior vena cava
5. 升主动脉 ascending aorta
6. 右心室 right ventricle
7. 前室间支 anterior interventricular branch
8. 左心耳 left auricle
9. 左心房 left atrium
10. 左上肺静脉 left superior pulmonary vein
11. 隆嵴下淋巴结（7 区）subcarinal lymph nodes
12. 奇静脉 azygos vein
13. 食管 esophagus
14. 胸导管 thoracic duct
15. 胸主动脉 thoracic aorta
16. 左食管旁淋巴结（8L）left paraesophageal lymph nodes
17. 左肺基底干支气管 left common basal bronchus
18. 舌静脉干（V4+5）lingular venous trunk
19. 下舌段支气管（B5）inferior lingular segmental bronchus
20. 上舌段支气管（B4）superior lingular segmental bronchus
21. 上舌段动脉（A4）superior lingular segmental artery
22. 下舌段动脉（A5）inferior lingular segmental artery
23. 左肺叶淋巴结（12L）left lobar lymph nodes
24. 内前底段动脉（A7+8）medioanterior basal segmental artery
25. 左肺外后底段动脉（A9+10）left posterolateral basal segmental artery
26. 左肺上段静脉（V6）left superior segmental vein
27. 左肺上段支气管（B6）和动脉（A6）left superior segmental bronchus and artery
28. 乳腺 mammary gland
29. 斜裂 oblique fissure
30. 胸大肌 pectoralis major
31. 胸小肌 pectoralis minor
32. 胸外侧静脉 lateral thoracic vein
33. 前锯肌 serratus anterior
34. 肩胛下肌 subscapularis
35. 肩胛骨 scapula
36. 冈下肌 infraspinatus
37. 大圆肌 teres major
38. 背阔肌 latissimus dorsi
39. 斜方肌 trapezius
40. 髂肋肌 iliocostalis
41. 最长肌 longissimus
42. 棘肌 spinales
43. 横突棘肌 transversospinales
44. 硬膜外隙 epidural space
45. 脊髓 spinal cord
46. 第 7 肋骨 7th costal bone
47. T6-7 椎间盘 T6-7 intervertebral disc
48. 右肺上段静脉（V6）right superior segmental vein
49. 右肺基底干支气管 right common basal bronchus
50. 右肺中叶支气管 right middle lobar bronchus
51. 右肺后底段动脉（A10）right posterior basal segmental artery
52. 右肺内前外侧底段动脉（A7+8+9）right common trunk of medial, anterior and lateral basal segmental arteries
53. 右上肺静脉 right superior pulmonary vein
54. 右肺上叶静脉 right superior lobar vein
55. 右肺中叶动脉 right middle lobar artery
56. 右肺前段静脉（V3）right anterior segmental vein
57. 胸廓内动、静脉 internal thoracic artery and vein
58. 奇静脉食管隐窝 azygoesophageal recess
59. 右肺下叶支气管 right inferior lobar bronchus
60. 右肺上段支气管（B6）right superior segmental bronchus
61. 右肺下叶动脉 right inferior lobar artery
62. 外侧段动脉（A4）lateral segmental artery
63. 左下肺静脉 left inferior pulmonary vein
64. 左肺下叶动脉 left inferior lobar artery

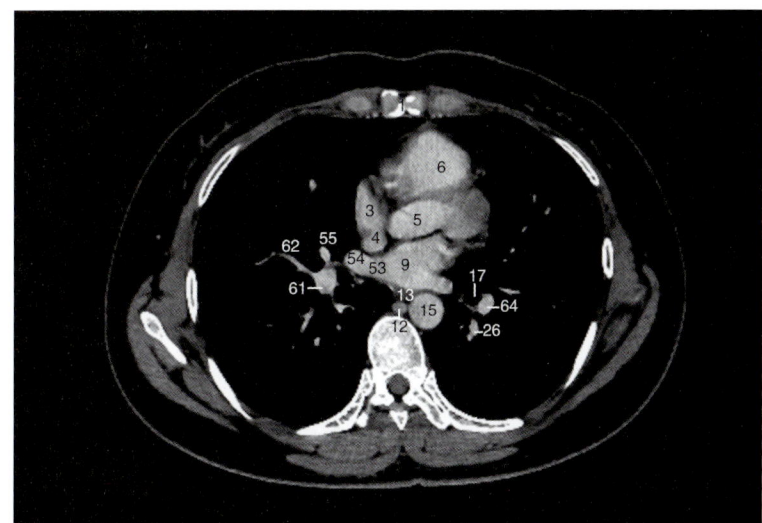

B. CT 纵隔窗增强图像

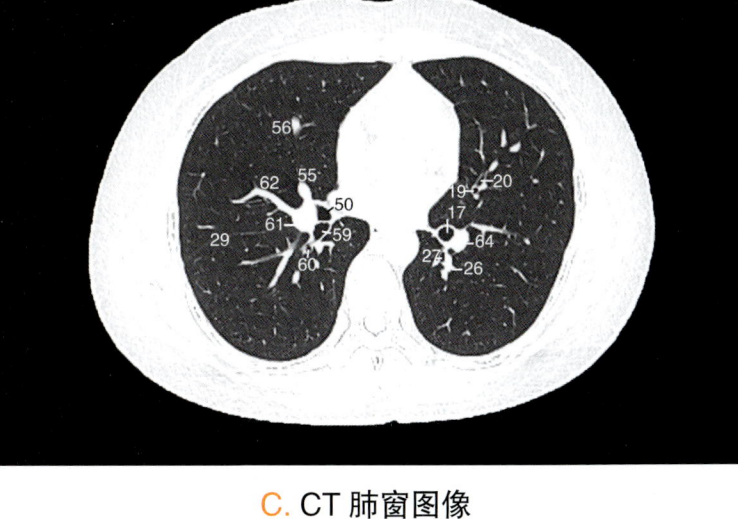

C. CT 肺窗图像

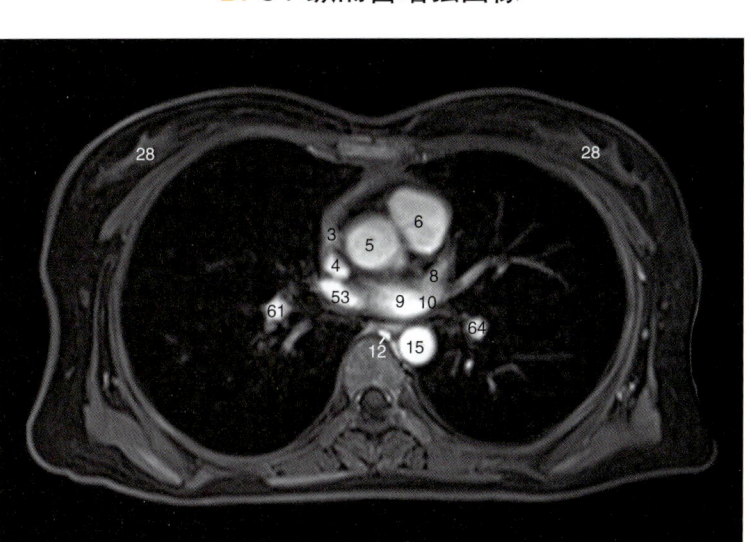

D. MR T1WI 增强图像

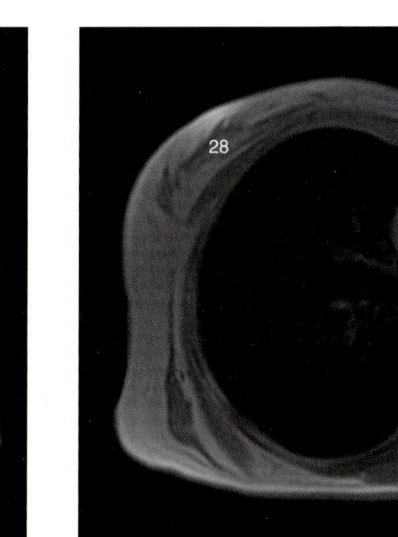

E. MR T1WI 平扫图像

关键结构：左心耳，右心耳。

此断面经过 T6-7 椎间盘上份。

纵隔内左、右心耳均出现，因左、右心耳在心腔中的位置较高，所以均较其他心腔结构先出现。右心耳是右心房上部向前突出的囊袋状结构，是电生理和起搏器电极植入的重要部位[55]。断面上右心耳位于上腔静脉口水平面以上的层面，表现为紧靠在升主动脉的右侧、从前向后连于上腔静脉的长条状空腔，前部尖，横径随着层面的下移逐渐增大，前部也逐渐钝圆，内壁因有梳状肌而表现得较为粗糙。右心耳向下与上腔静脉汇合，汇合处见上腔静脉口。右心耳的形态主要受左侧的动脉圆锥、升主动脉及上腔静脉和下方的右心室及后方的右心房的影响，同时也受到心包的限制。CT 测量显示，右心耳容积为 12.4 mL ± 3.9 mL，高度为 31.2 mm ± 3.2 mm，基底部长径为 33.8 mm ± 4.0 mm，基底部短径 27.8 mm ± 4.3 mm。左冠状动脉的前室间支位于右心室与左心耳之间，横行向外侧，在下方断面进入前室间沟并进一步向前下行向心尖处。此断面于纵隔内见后部左心房随断面下移变得更加明显，有多个结构从其侧壁汇入。右前壁汇入的结构为右上肺静脉，左前壁有左心耳汇入，其后方紧邻左上肺静脉汇入。右上肺静脉有 2 个属支，分别是右肺上叶静脉和右肺中叶静脉，此断面见右肺上叶静脉粗大，为右上肺静脉向上叶内的延续，中叶静脉未见，位置相对较低，将在下方断面单独汇入左心房。

107

胸部连续横断层 54 (FH.12430)

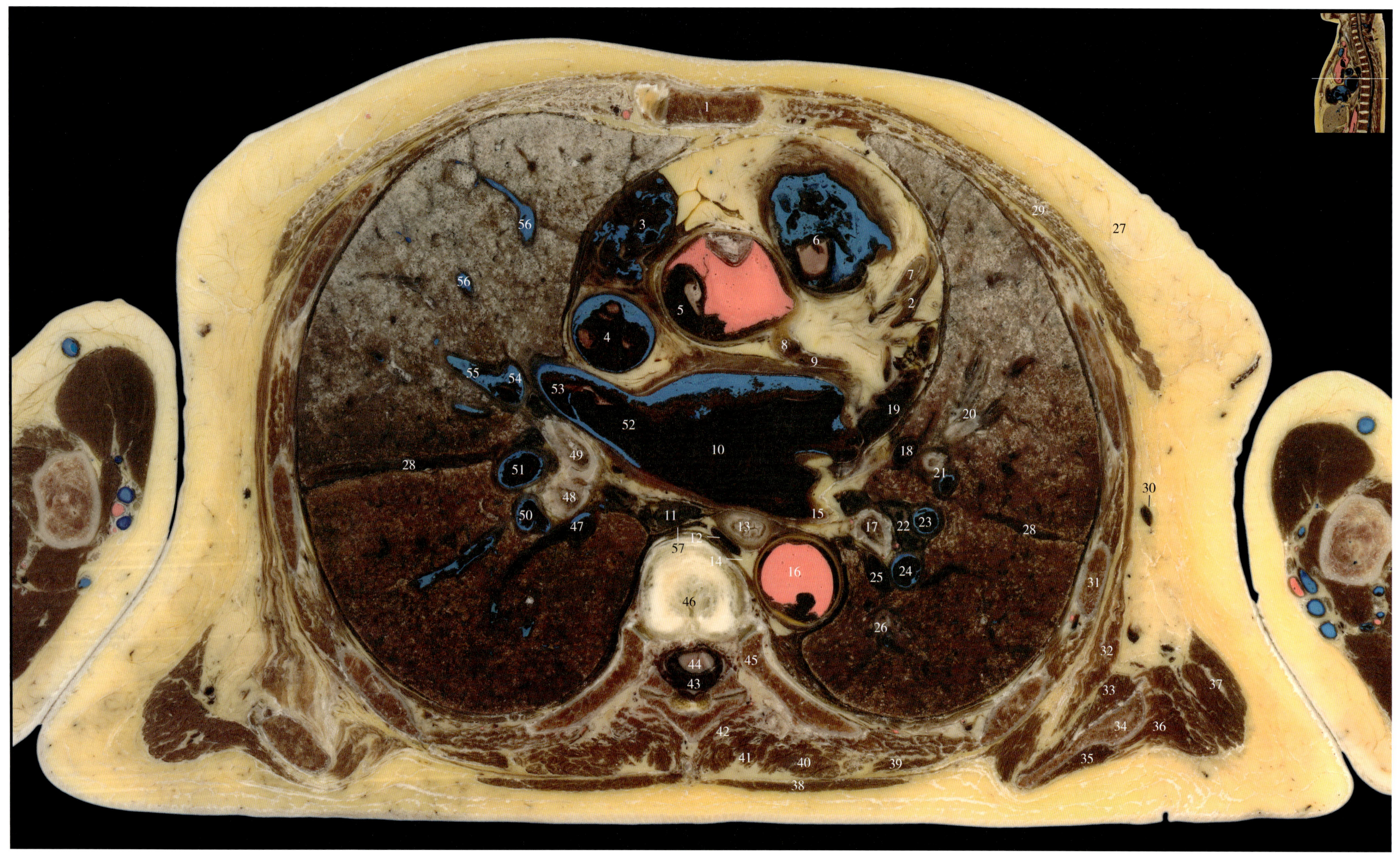

A. 断层标本图像

1. 胸骨体 body of sternum
2. 心大静脉 great cardiac vein
3. 右心耳 right auricle
4. 上腔静脉 superior vena cava
5. 升主动脉 ascending aorta
6. 右心室 right ventricle
7. 前室间支 anterior interventricular branch
8. 左冠状动脉 left coronary artery
9. 旋支 circumflex branch
10. 左心房 left atrium
11. 右食管旁淋巴结（8R）right paraesophageal lymph nodes
12. 奇静脉 azygos vein
13. 食管 esophagus
14. 胸导管 thoracic duct
15. 左下肺静脉 left inferior pulmonary vein
16. 胸主动脉 thoracic aorta
17. 左肺基底干支气管 left common basal bronchus
18. 舌静脉干（V4+5）lingular venous trunk
19. 左心耳 left auricle
20. 上舌段支气管（B4）和动脉（A4）superior lingular segmental bronchus and artery
21. 下舌段支气管（B5）和动脉（A5）inferior lingular segmental bronchus and artery
22. 左肺叶淋巴结（12L）left lobar lymph nodes
23. 内前底段动脉（A7+8）medioanterior basal segmental artery
24. 左肺外后底段动脉（A9+10）left posterolateral basal segmental artery
25. 左肺上段静脉（V6）left superior segmental vein
26. 左肺上段支气管（B6）和动脉（A6）left superior segmental bronchus and artery
27. 乳腺 mammary gland
28. 斜裂 oblique fissure
29. 胸大肌 pectoralis major
30. 胸外侧静脉 lateral thoracic vein
31. 第 5 肋骨 5th costal bone
32. 前锯肌 serratus anterior
33. 肩胛下肌 subscapularis
34. 肩胛骨 scapula
35. 冈下肌 infraspinatus
36. 大圆肌 teres major
37. 背阔肌 latissimus dorsi
38. 斜方肌 trapezius
39. 髂肋肌 iliocostalis
40. 最长肌 longissimus
41. 棘肌 spinales
42. 横突棘肌 transversospinales
43. 硬膜外隙 epidural space
44. 脊髓 spinal cord
45. 第 7 肋骨 7th costal bone
46. T6-7 椎间盘 T6-7 intervertebral disc
47. 右肺上段静脉（V6）right superior segmental vein
48. 右肺基底干支气管 right common basal bronchus
49. 右肺中叶支气管 right middle lobar bronchus
50. 右肺后底段动脉（A10）right posterior basal segmental artery
51. 右肺内前外侧底段动脉（A7+8+9）right common trunk of medial, anterior and lateral basal segmental arteries
52. 右上肺静脉 right superior pulmonary vein
53. 右肺上叶静脉 right superior lobar vein
54. 内侧段动脉（A5）medial segmental artery
55. 外侧段动脉（A4）lateral segmental artery
56. 右肺前段静脉（V3）right anterior segmental vein
57. 奇静脉食管隐窝 azygoesophageal recess
58. 右肺下叶支气管 right inferior lobar bronchus
59. 右肺上段支气管（B6）right superior segmental bronchus
60. 右肺下叶动脉 right inferior lobar artery
61. 右肺中叶动脉 right middle lobar artery
62. 左肺下叶动脉 left inferior lobar artery
63. 右冠状动脉 right coronary artery
64. 斜角支 diagonal branch

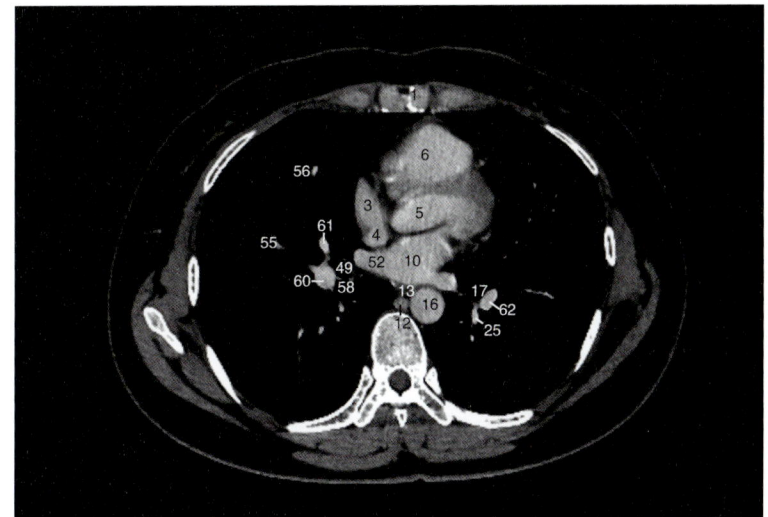

B. CT 纵隔窗增强图像

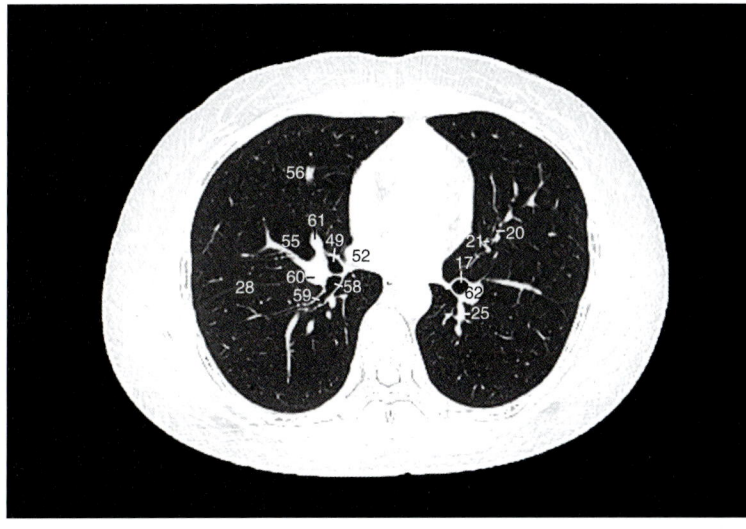

C. CT 肺窗图像

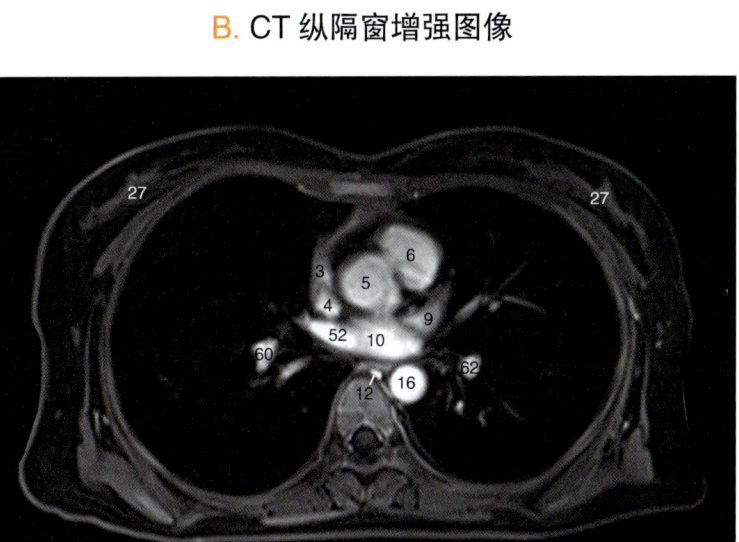

D. MR T1WI 增强图像

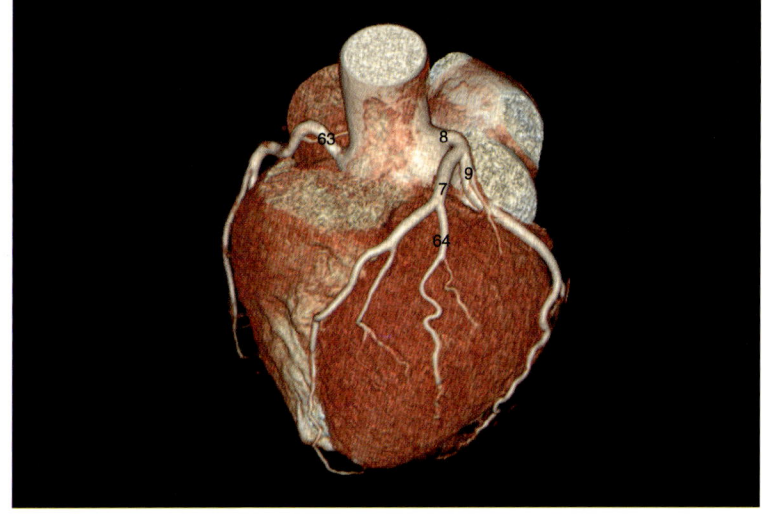

E. 冠状动脉 CT 三维重建图像（前面观）

关键结构：左冠状动脉，奇静脉食管隐窝。

此断面经第 3 肋软骨和 T6~7 椎间盘中部层面。

纵隔内见左冠状动脉发自主动脉左窦，左冠状动脉口距窦底 14~18 mm，占 68.5%，左冠状动脉口一般比右冠状动脉口高 2~4 mm。左冠状动脉与升主动脉的夹角为 $110.1° ± 15.0°$ [56]。左冠状动脉主干较短，发出后即进入冠状沟左侧部，肺动脉干后部，经左心耳与肺动脉干之间左行，长度多介于 5~10 mm 间，外径为 $5.3\ mm ± 0.2\ mm$，左冠状动脉大于右冠状动脉占 $67.7\% ± 2.8\%$。

心脏的血供以左冠状动脉为主（左优势型）的情况较少，仅占 6.8%~18.57% [57]。约 9.4% 冠状动脉存在变异，主要包括冠状动脉走行异常和冠状动脉起源开口异常。左冠状动脉的分支较多，最大的分支为前室间支和旋支，两分支夹角介于 20°~120° 之间，以 50°~80° 多见，占 62.3% [36]。在冠脉 VR 图像中可见左冠状动脉分支为前室间支和旋支，二者分叉处下方，有斜角支发出，斜向左下分布于左心室前壁一部分。

胸部连续横断层 55（FH.12410）

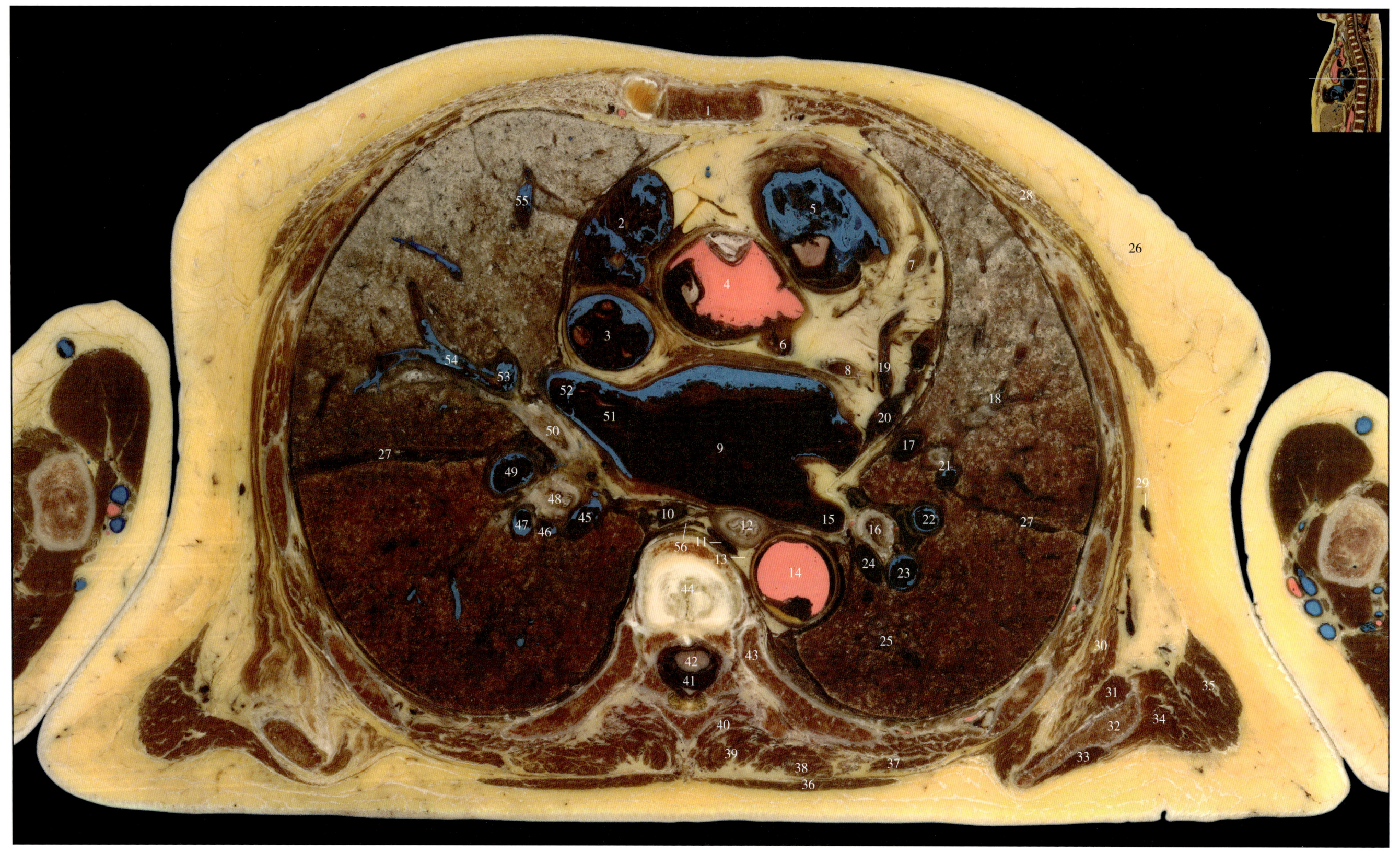

A. 断层标本图像

1. 胸骨体 body of sternum
2. 右心耳 right auricle
3. 上腔静脉 superior vena cava
4. 升主动脉 ascending aorta
5. 右心室 right ventricle
6. 左冠状动脉 left coronary artery
7. 前室间支 anterior interventricular branch
8. 旋支 circumflex branch
9. 左心房 left atrium
10. 右食管旁淋巴结（8R）right paraesophageal lymph nodes
11. 奇静脉 azygos vein
12. 食管 esophagus
13. 胸导管 thoracic duct
14. 胸主动脉 thoracic aorta
15. 左下肺静脉 left inferior pulmonary vein
16. 左肺基底干支气管 left common basal bronchus
17. 舌静脉干（V4+5）lingular venous trunk
18. 上舌段支气管（B4）和动脉（A4）superior lingular segmental bronchus and artery
19. 心大静脉 great cardiac vein
20. 左心耳 left auricle
21. 下舌段支气管（B5）和动脉（A5）inferior lingular segmental bronchus and artery
22. 内前底段动脉（A7+8）medioanterior basal segmental artery
23. 左肺外后底段动脉（A9+10）left posterolateral basal segmental artery
24. 左肺上段静脉（V6）left superior segmental vein
25. 左肺上段支气管（B6）和动脉（A6）left superior segmental bronchus and artery
26. 乳腺 mammary gland
27. 斜裂 oblique fissure
28. 胸大肌 pectoralis major
29. 胸外侧静脉 lateral thoracic vein
30. 前锯肌 serratus anterior
31. 肩胛下肌 subscapularis
32. 肩胛骨 scapula
33. 冈下肌 infraspinatus
34. 大圆肌 teres major
35. 背阔肌 latissimus dorsi
36. 斜方肌 trapezius
37. 髂肋肌 iliocostalis
38. 最长肌 longissimus
39. 棘肌 spinales
40. 横突棘肌 transversospinales
41. 硬膜外隙 epidural space
42. 脊髓 spinal cord
43. 第7肋骨 7th costal bone
44. T6-7椎间盘 T6-7 intervertebral disc
45. 右肺上段静脉（V6）right superior segmental vein
46. 内侧底段动脉（A7）medial basal segmental artery
47. 右肺后底段动脉（A10）right posterior basal segmental artery
48. 右肺基底干支气管 right common basal bronchus
49. 右肺内前外侧底段动脉（A7+8+9）right common trunk of medial, anterior and lateral basal segmental arteries
50. 右肺中叶支气管 right middle lobar bronchus
51. 右上肺静脉 right superior pulmonary vein
52. 右肺上叶静脉 right superior lobar vein
53. 内侧段动脉（A5）medial segmental artery
54. 外侧段动脉（A4）lateral segmental artery
55. 右肺前段静脉（V3）right anterior segmental vein
56. 奇静脉食管隐窝 azygoesophageal recess
57. 左肺内前外侧底段动脉（A7+8+9）left common trunk of medial, anterior and lateral basal segmental arteries
58. 左肺后底段动脉（A10）left posterior basal segmental artery
59. 内侧段支气管（B5）medial segmental bronchus
60. 外侧段支气管（B4）lateral segmental bronchus
61. 右肺中叶动脉 right middle lobar artery
62. 右肺下叶动脉 right inferior lobar artery
63. 右肺上段支气管（B6）right superior segmental bronchus

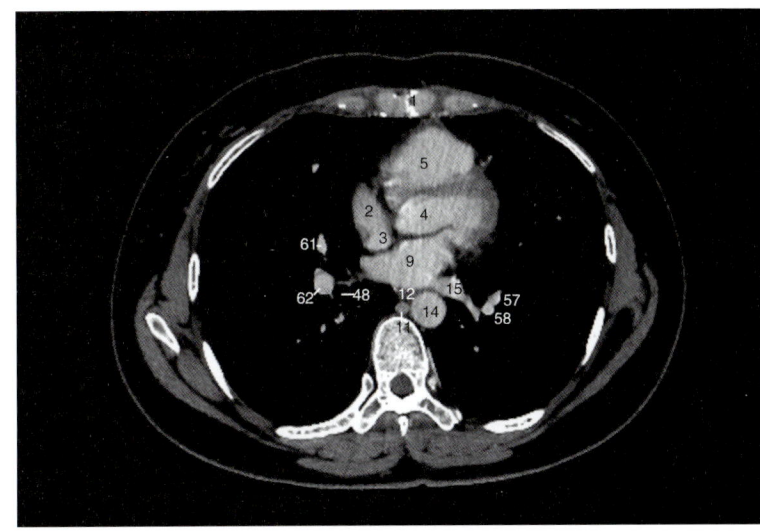

B. CT 纵隔窗增强图像

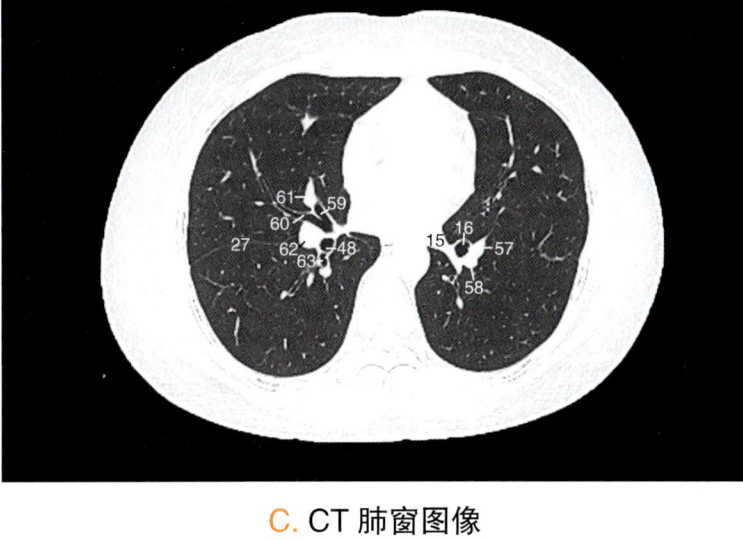

C. CT 肺窗图像

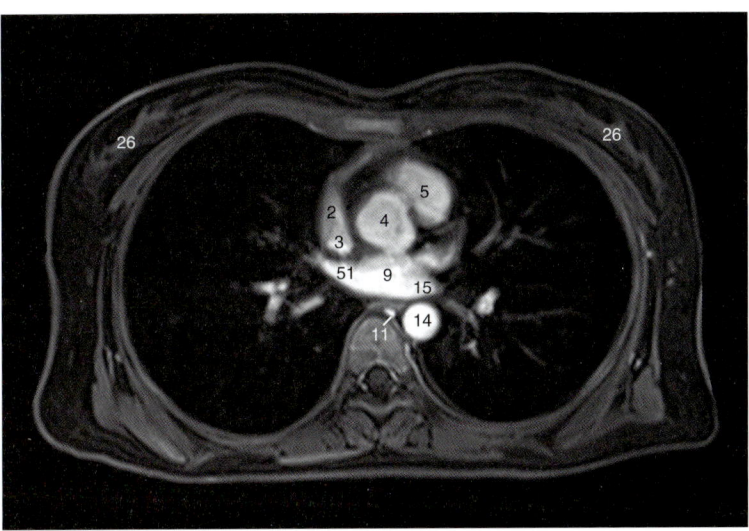

D. MR T1WI 增强图像

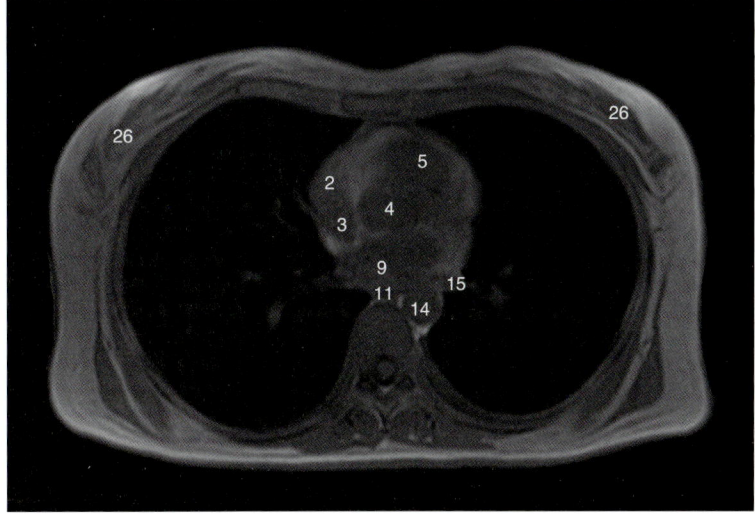

E. MR T1WI 平扫图像

关键结构：左肺上、下舌段支气管和动脉。

此断面经过 T6-7 椎间盘下份。

左肺舌叶的主要管道包括支气管下（舌）干、舌动脉干和舌静脉干。这 3 组管道中，动脉与支气管伴行，先进入舌叶门，静脉随后进入舌叶门。故在伴行位置关系中，段动脉分支位于最外侧，段支气管位于段动脉内侧，段静脉位于最内侧，这种关系与右肺中叶类似，而与上叶其他位置不同。90%±3.0% 的支气管下干两分为上、下舌段支气管，发出后行向左肺舌叶的前外侧上方和下方，其中，上舌段支气管通常不分支，占 83.1%±1.5%。上、下舌段动脉与支气管伴行，位于支气管的前外侧或后外侧。上、下舌段动脉可来自舌动脉干，占 59%±3.5%，也可单独发自下叶动脉，占 39.5%±3.5%。且舌段动脉发出的高度多数情况下低于上舌段动脉发出高度，占 78.5%±4.7%[36]。随着断面下移，上、下舌段支气管及动脉距离逐渐拉开，两组管道之间逐渐见舌静脉干插入，可作为区分上、下舌段的解剖标志[40]。

胸部连续横断层 56（FH.12390）

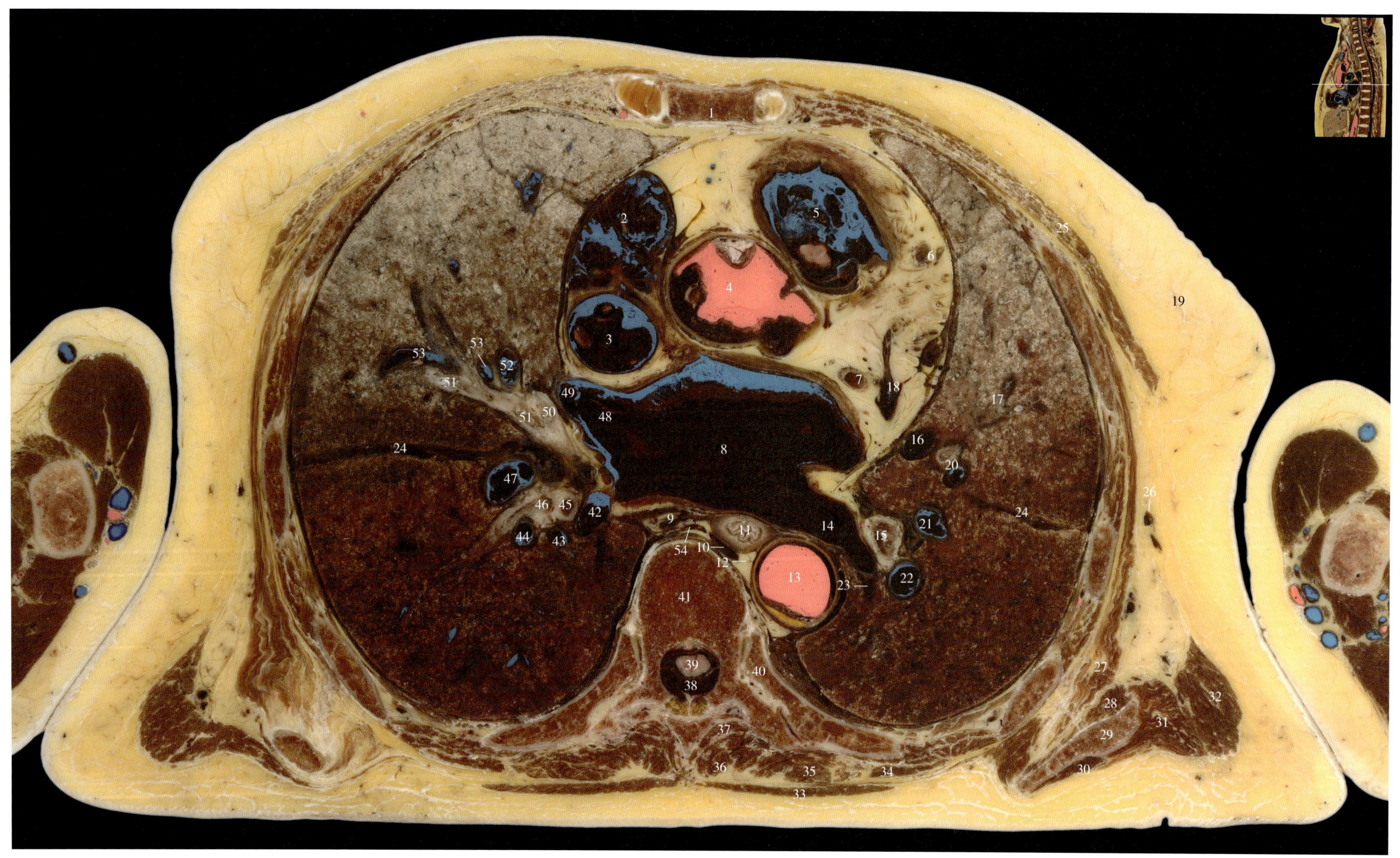

A. 断层标本图像

1. 胸骨体 body of sternum
2. 右心耳 right auricle
3. 上腔静脉 superior vena cava
4. 升主动脉 ascending aorta
5. 右心室 right ventricle
6. 前室间支 anterior interventricular branch
7. 旋支 circumflex branch
8. 左心房 left atrium
9. 右食管旁淋巴结（8R）right paraesophageal lymph nodes
10. 奇静脉 azygos vein
11. 食管 esophagus
12. 胸导管 thoracic duct
13. 胸主动脉 thoracic aorta
14. 左下肺静脉 left inferior pulmonary vein
15. 左肺基底干支气管 left common basal bronchus
16. 舌静脉干（V4+5）lingular venous trunk
17. 上舌段支气管（B4）和动脉（A4）superior lingular segmental bronchus and artery
18. 心大静脉 great cardiac vein
19. 乳腺 mammary gland
20. 下舌段支气管（B5）和动脉（A5）inferior lingular segmental bronchus and artery
21. 内前底段动脉（A7+8）medioanterior basal segmental artery
22. 左肺外后底段动脉（A9+10）left posterolateral basal segmental artery
23. 左肺上段静脉（V6）left superior segmental vein
24. 斜裂 oblique fissure
25. 胸大肌 pectoralis major
26. 胸外侧静脉 lateral thoracic vein
27. 前锯肌 serratus anterior
28. 肩胛下肌 subscapularis
29. 肩胛骨 scapula
30. 冈下肌 infraspinatus
31. 大圆肌 teres major
32. 背阔肌 latissimus dorsi
33. 斜方肌 trapezius
34. 髂肋肌 iliocostalis
35. 最长肌 longissimus
36. 棘肌 spinales
37. 横突棘肌 transversospinales
38. 硬膜外隙 epidural space
39. 脊髓 spinal cord
40. 第 7 肋骨 7th costal bone
41. 第 7 胸椎椎体 body of 7th thoracic vertebra
42. 右肺上段静脉（V6）right superior segmental vein
43. 右肺内侧底段动脉（A7）right medial basal segmental artery
44. 右肺后底段动脉（A10）right posterior basal segmental artery
45. 内侧底段支气管（B7）medial basal segmental bronchus
46. 右肺前外后底段支气管（B8+9+10）right common trunk of anterior, lateral, posterior basal segmental bronchi
47. 右肺内前外侧底段动脉（A7+8+9）right common trunk of medial, anterior and lateral basal segmental arteries
48. 右上肺静脉 right superior pulmonary vein
49. 右肺上叶静脉 right superior lobar vein
50. 内侧段支气管（B5）medial segmental bronchus
51. 外侧段支气管（B4）lateral segmental bronchus
52. 内侧段动脉（A5）medial segmental artery
53. 外侧段动脉（A4）lateral segmental artery
54. 奇静脉食管隐窝 azygoesophageal recess
55. 左肺内前外侧底段动脉（A7+8+9）left common trunk of medial, anterior and lateral basal segmental arteries
56. 左肺后底段动脉（A10）left posterior basal segmental artery
57. 右肺基底干支气管 right common basal bronchus
58. 右肺上段支气管（B6）right superior segmental bronchus
59. 右肺下叶动脉 right inferior lobar artery
60. 右肺上段动脉（A6）right superior segmental artery
61. 右下肺静脉 right inferior pulmonary vein

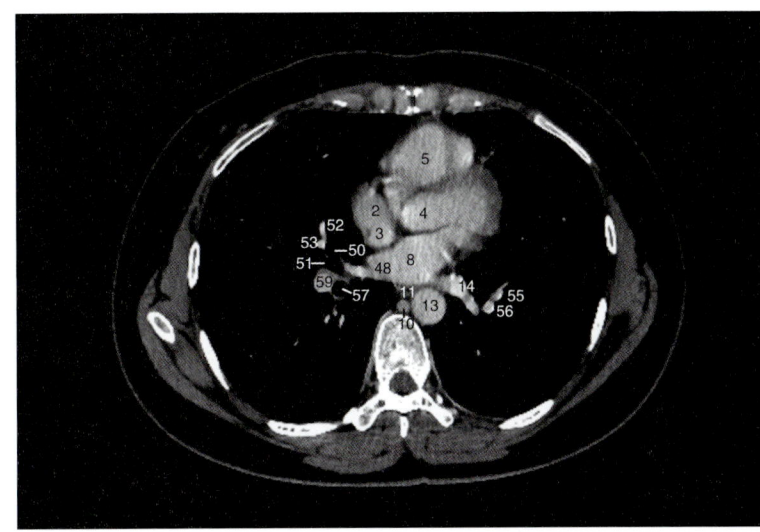

B. CT 纵隔窗增强图像

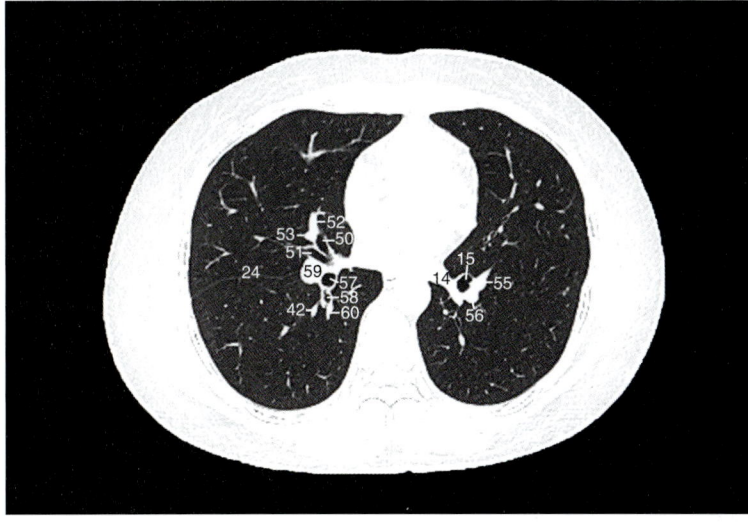

C. CT 肺窗图像

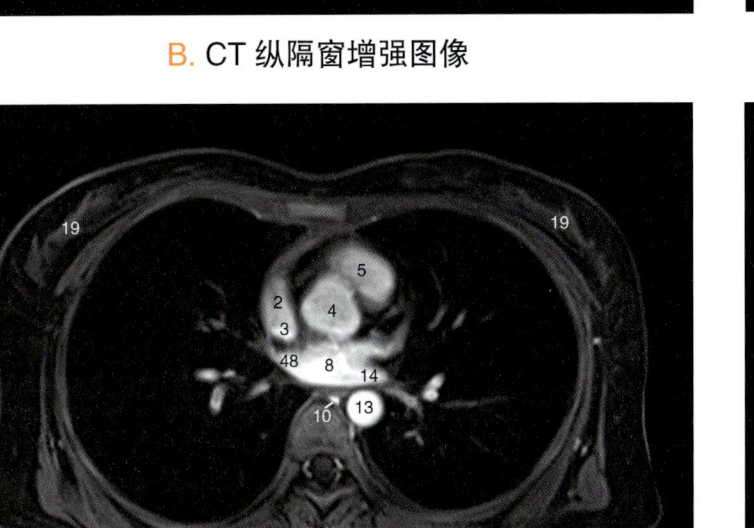

D. MR T1WI 增强图像

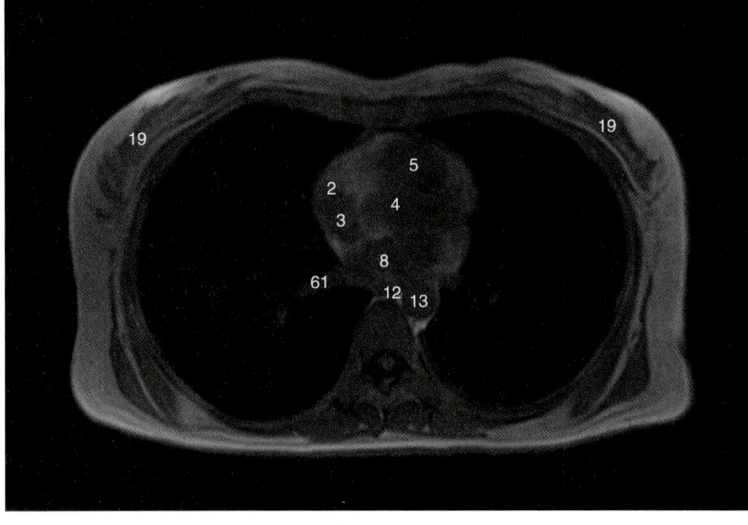

E. MR T1WI 平扫图像

关键结构：右上肺静脉，奇静脉食管隐窝。

此断面经第 4 肋软骨和第 7 胸椎椎体上份。

升主动脉到其根部，左冠状动脉已发出，右冠状动脉窦即将发出右冠状动脉。左心房在 4 个心腔中位置最高，最早出现，位于中纵隔最后部，两侧壁接受肺静脉的汇入。在此断面左心房左侧后壁见左下肺静脉已出现，右侧壁前部有右上肺静脉的汇入。右上肺静脉收集右肺上叶和中叶的静脉，正常情况下右肺上叶静脉和中叶静脉汇合，形成右上肺静脉，占 82.8%；有时上叶静脉和中叶静脉各自汇入左心房，占 7.3%[58]。在奇静脉弓以下断面，右胸膜腔深入食管后方、脊柱的前方，称奇静脉食管隐窝，此隐窝凸面向左，向下达膈肌。奇静脉食管隐窝的深度因胸廓的发育程度而异，年老肺气肿患者该隐窝深；青年胸腔前后径小，该隐窝较浅[59]。奇静脉食管隐窝可越过中线至脊柱左侧，左侧入路行食管和胸导管手术时，可误伤奇静脉食管隐窝而导致右侧气胸。当隐窝内占位性病变如隆突下淋巴结肿大可导致该隐窝消失[60]。

胸部连续横断层 57（FH.12370）

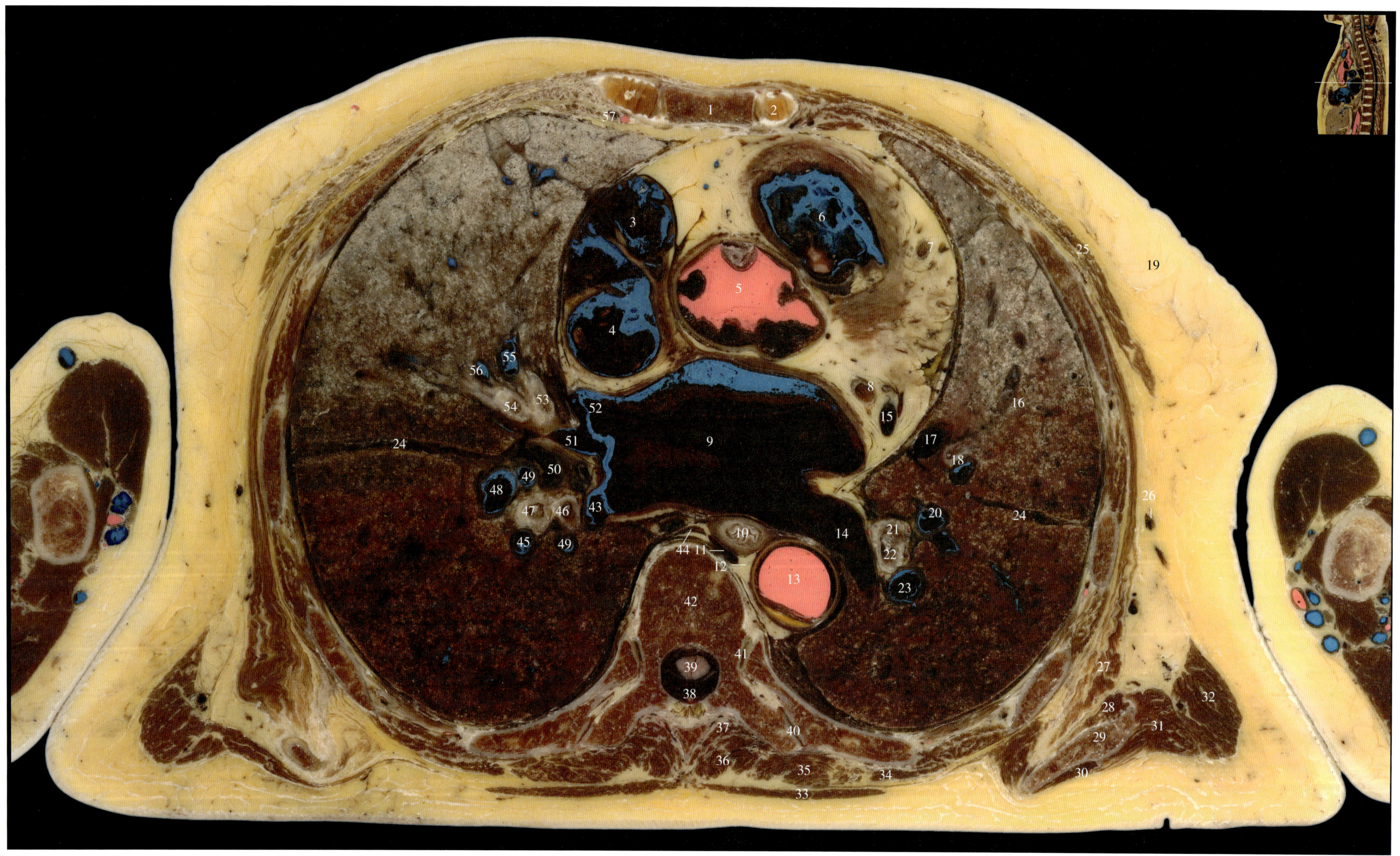

A. 断层标本图像

1. 胸骨体 body of sternum
2. 第 4 肋软骨 4th costal cartilage
3. 右心耳 right auricle
4. 上腔静脉口 orifice of superior vena cava
5. 升主动脉 ascending aorta
6. 右心室 right ventricle
7. 前室间支 anterior interventricular branch
8. 旋支 circumflex branch
9. 左心房 left atrium
10. 食管 esophagus
11. 奇静脉 azygos vein
12. 胸导管 thoracic duct
13. 胸主动脉 thoracic aorta
14. 左下肺静脉 left inferior pulmonary vein
15. 心大静脉 great cardiac vein
16. 上舌段支气管（B4）和动脉（A4）superior lingular segmental bronchus and artery
17. 舌静脉干（V4+5）lingular venous trunk
18. 下舌段支气管（B5）和动脉（A5）inferior lingular segmental bronchus and artery
19. 乳腺 mammary gland
20. 内前底段动脉（A7+8）medioanterior basal segmental artery
21. 内前底段支气管（B7+8）medioanterior basal segmental bronchus
22. 左肺外后底段支气管（B9+10）left posterolateral basal segmental bronchus
23. 左肺外后底段动脉（A9+10）left posterolateral basal segmental artery
24. 斜裂 oblique fissure
25. 胸大肌 pectoralis major
26. 胸外侧静脉 lateral thoracic vein
27. 前锯肌 serratus anterior
28. 肩胛下肌 subscapularis
29. 肩胛骨 scapula
30. 冈下肌 infraspinatus
31. 大圆肌 teres major
32. 背阔肌 latissimus dorsi
33. 斜方肌 trapezius
34. 髂肋肌 iliocostalis
35. 最长肌 longissimus
36. 棘肌 spinales
37. 横突棘肌 transversospinales
38. 硬膜外隙 epidural space
39. 脊髓 spinal cord
40. 肋横突关节 costotransverse joint
41. 肋头关节 joints of costal head
42. 第 7 胸椎椎体 body of 7th thoracic vertebra
43. 右下肺静脉 right inferior pulmonary vein
44. 奇静脉食管隐窝 azygoesophageal recess
45. 右肺后底段动脉（A10）right posterior basal segmental artery
46. 右肺内侧底段支气管（B7）right medial basal segmental bronchus
47. 右肺前外后底段支气管（B8+9+10）right common trunk of anterior, lateral, posterior basal segmental bronchi
48. 右肺前外侧底段动脉（A8+9）right anterolateral basal segmental artery
49. 右肺内侧底段动脉（A7）right medial basal segmental artery
50. 右肺段淋巴结（13R）right segmental lymph nodes
51. 右肺中叶静脉 right middle lobar vein
52. 右肺上叶静脉 right superior lobar vein
53. 内侧段支气管（B5）medial segmental bronchus
54. 外侧段支气管（B4）lateral segmental bronchus
55. 内侧段动脉（A5）medial segmental artery
56. 外侧段动脉（A4）lateral segmental artery
57. 胸廓内动、静脉 internal thoracic artery and vein
58. 左肺内前外侧底段动脉（A7+8+9）left common trunk of medial, anterior and lateral basal segmental arteries
59. 左肺后底段动脉（A10）left posterior basal segmental artery
60. 右肺下叶动脉 right inferior lobar artery
61. 右肺基底干支气管 right common basal bronchus
62. 右肺上段静脉（V6）right superior segmental vein

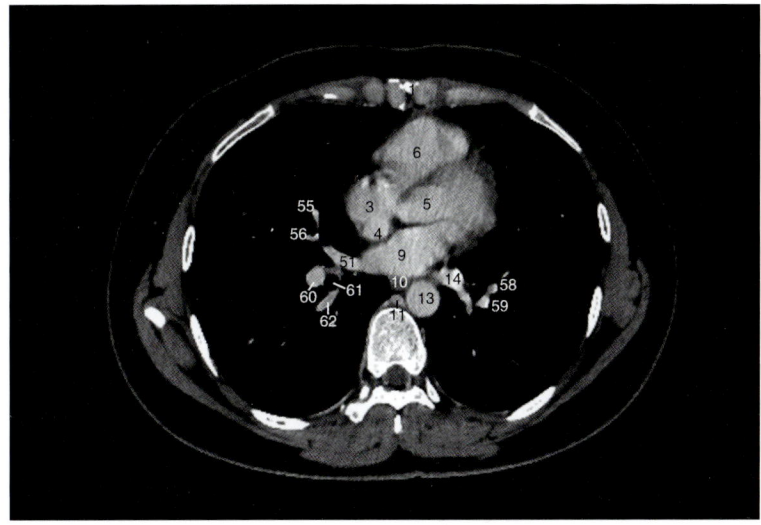

B. CT 纵隔窗增强图像

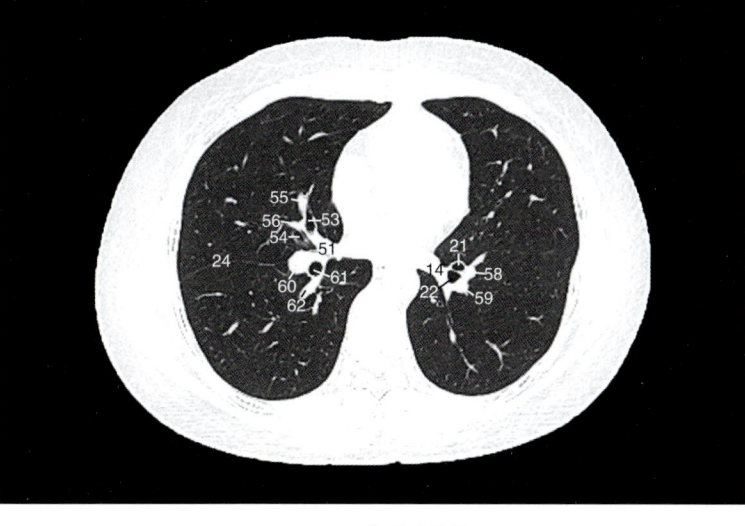

C. CT 肺窗图像

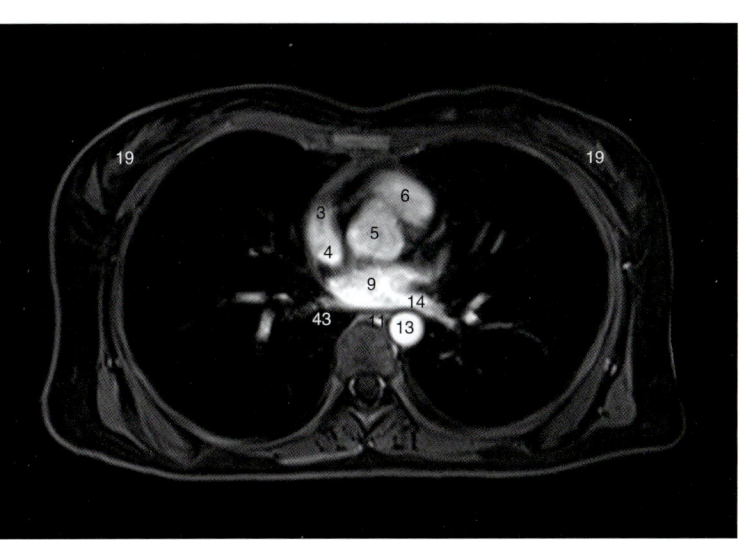

D. MR T1WI 增强图像

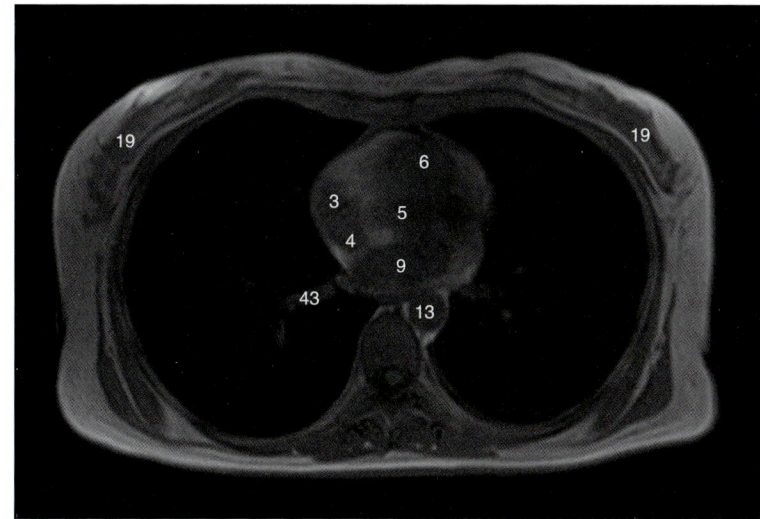

E. MR T1WI 平扫图像

关键结构：内、外侧段支气管和动脉。

此断面经第 7 胸椎椎体上份。

纵隔右侧见右心耳与上腔静脉融合成右心房，标志性结构是上腔静脉口壁开始变得不完整。右心室位置逐渐移向前方中部，左心室腔未见，仅见少量左心室顶壁肌，左心房居后，侧壁接受肺静脉的汇入。随着层面的下移，右肺上叶结构逐渐消失，右肺中叶门处，94.9% ± 1.3% 的中叶支气管两分为外侧段和内侧段支气管，且多数情况下内、外侧段支气管的直径相同，占 56.0% ± 5.0%；81.6% 的情况内、外侧段支气管高度一致，18.4% 的情况二者高度不一致[36]。由于中叶动脉先于支气管进入中叶并分支行向外下或内下，故支气管与伴行的动脉在断面上常表现为段动脉位于段支气管的前外侧。CT 测量显示，男性内侧段动脉的直径为 4.5 mm ± 0.1 mm，女性为 3.6 mm ± 0.1 mm；男性外侧段动脉的直径为 4.3 mm ± 0.1 mm，女性为 3.6 mm ± 0.1 mm[61]。中叶静脉及属支的位置相对较低，故静脉常伴行于相应段支气管的内侧，故在外侧段和内侧段内部，从外侧向内侧管道伴行的关系依次为段动脉、段支气管和段静脉。外侧段静脉有段间支，常出现于内侧段和外侧段支气管的夹角中。在下叶支气管分为各底段支气管后，其前方可出现肺段支气管。

胸部连续横断层 58（FH.12350）

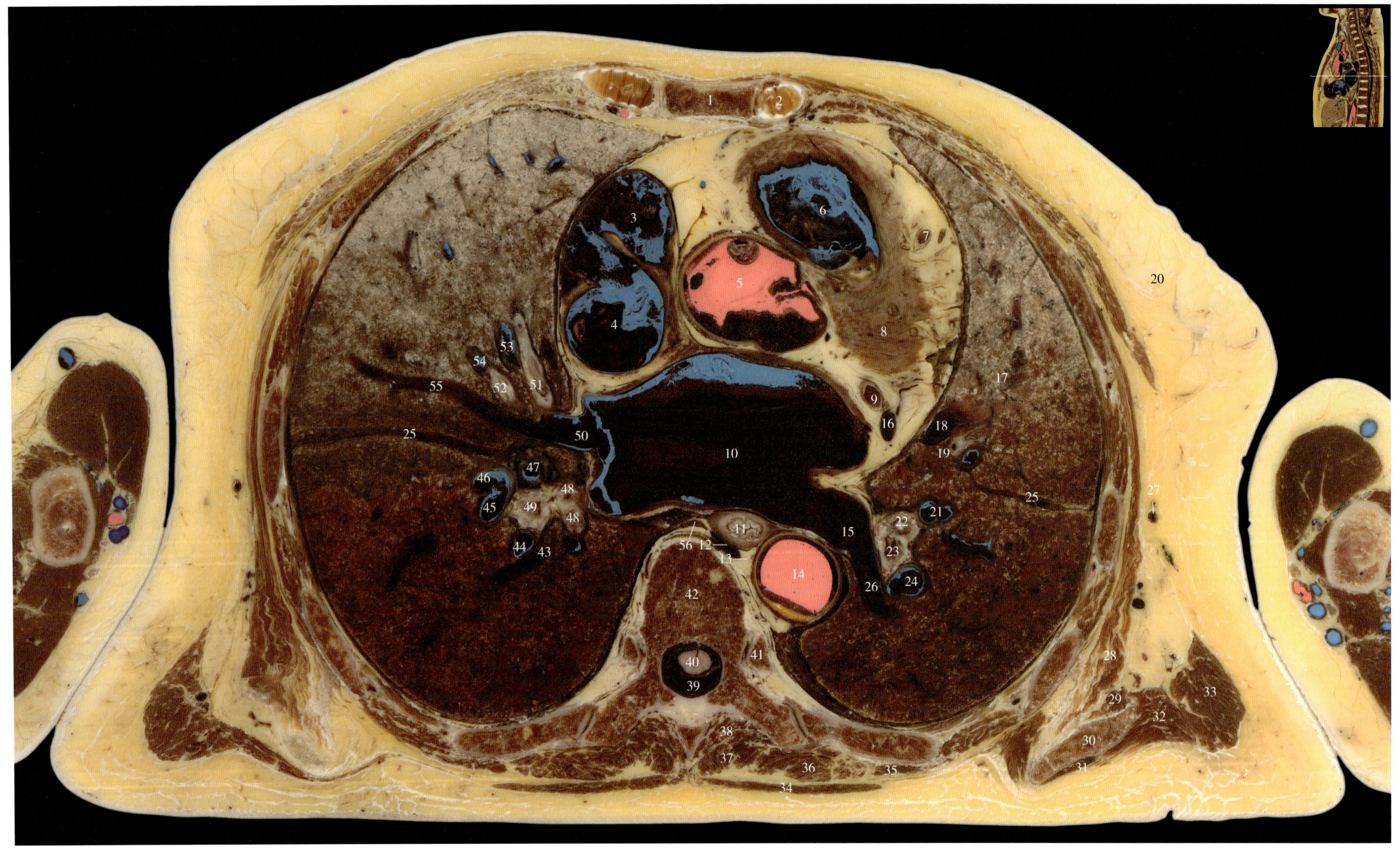

A. 断层标本图像

1. 胸骨体 body of sternum
2. 第 4 肋软骨 4th costal cartilage
3. 右心耳 right auricle
4. 上腔静脉口 orifice of superior vena cava
5. 升主动脉 ascending aorta
6. 右心室 right ventricle
7. 前室间支 anterior interventricular branch
8. 左心室顶壁 roof of left ventricle
9. 旋支 circumflex branch
10. 左心房 left atrium
11. 食管 esophagus
12. 奇静脉 azygos vein
13. 胸导管 thoracic duct
14. 胸主动脉 thoracic aorta
15. 左下肺静脉 left inferior pulmonary vein
16. 心大静脉 great cardiac vein
17. 上舌段支气管（B4）和动脉（A4） superior lingular segmental bronchus and artery
18. 舌静脉干（V4+5）lingular venous trunk
19. 下舌段支气管（B5）和动脉（A5）inferior lingular segmental bronchus and artery
20. 乳腺 mammary gland
21. 内前底段动脉（A7+8）medioanterior basal segmental artery
22. 内前底段支气管（B7+8）medioanterior basal segmental bronchus
23. 左肺外后底段支气管（B9+10） left posterolateral basal segmental bronchus
24. 左肺外后底段动脉（A9+10） left posterolateral basal segmental artery
25. 斜裂 oblique fissure
26. 左肺上段静脉（V6）left superior segmental vein
27. 胸外侧静脉 lateral thoracic vein
28. 前锯肌 serratus anterior
29. 肩胛下肌 subscapularis
30. 肩胛骨 scapula
31. 冈下肌 infraspinatus
32. 大圆肌 teres major
33. 背阔肌 latissimus dorsi
34. 斜方肌 trapezius
35. 髂肋肌 iliocostalis
36. 最长肌 longissimus
37. 棘肌 spinales
38. 横突棘肌 transversospinales
39. 硬膜外隙 epidural space
40. 脊髓 spinal cord
41. 第 7 肋骨 7th costal bone
42. 第 7 胸椎椎体 body of 7th thoracic vertebra
43. 右肺上段静脉（V6） right superior segmental vein
44. 右肺后底段动脉（A10） right posterior basal segmental artery
45. 右肺外侧底段动脉（A9） right lateral basal segmental artery
46. 右肺前底段动脉（A8） right anterior basal segmental artery
47. 右肺内侧底段动脉（A7） right medial basal segmental artery
48. 右肺内侧底段支气管（B7） right medial basal segmental bronchus
49. 右肺前外后底段支气管（B8+9+10） right common trunk of anterior, lateral, posterior basal segmental bronchi
50. 右肺中叶静脉 right middle lobar vein
51. 内侧段支气管（B5） medial segmental bronchus
52. 外侧段支气管（B4） lateral segmental bronchus
53. 内侧段动脉（A5） medial segmental artery
54. 外侧段动脉（A4） lateral segmental artery
55. 外侧段静脉（V4） lateral segmental vein
56. 奇静脉食管隐窝 azygoesophageal recess
57. 左肺内前外底段动脉（A7+8+9） left common trunk of medial, anterior and lateral basal segmental arteries
58. 左肺后底段动脉（A10） left posterior basal segmental artery
59. 右肺基底干支气管 right common basal bronchus
60. 右肺下叶动脉 right inferior lobar artery

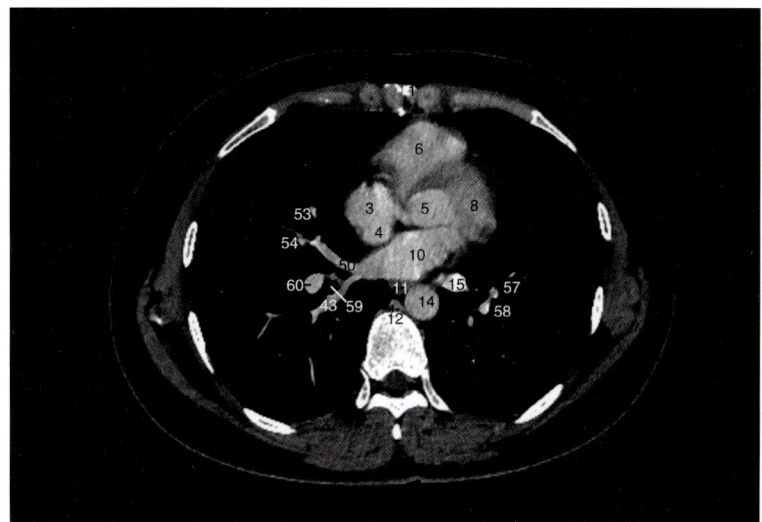

B. CT 纵隔窗增强图像

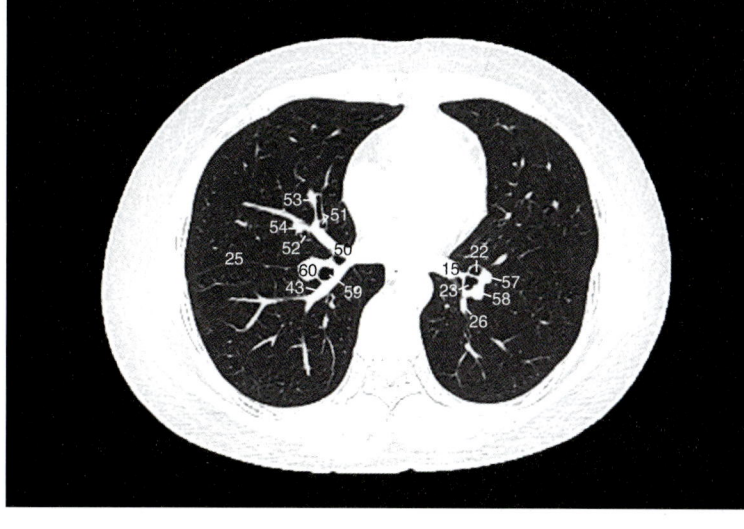

C. CT 肺窗图像

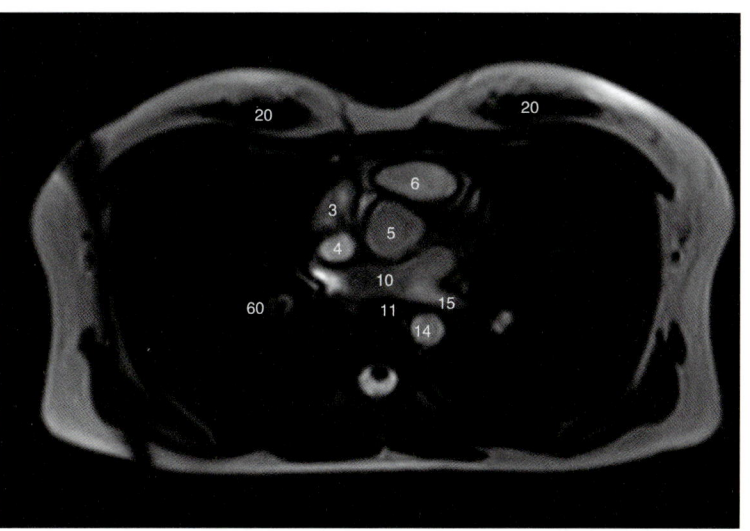

D. MR T2WI 平扫图像

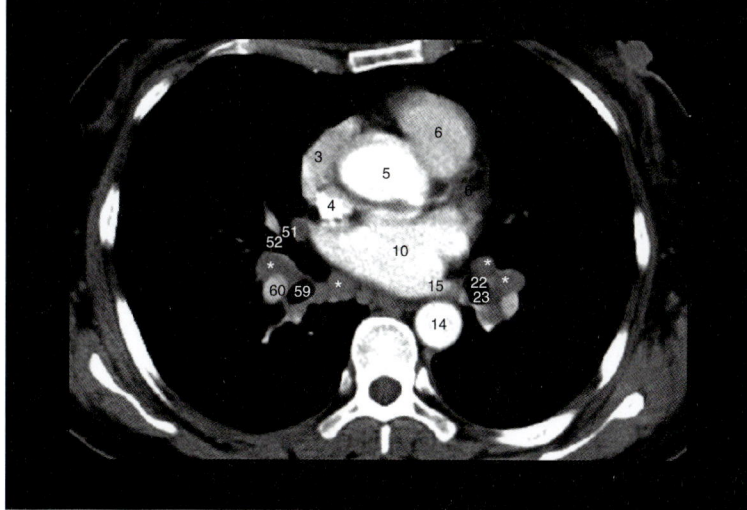

E. 淋巴结转移 CT 图像

关键结构：中叶静脉，外侧段静脉，内侧段静脉，左下肺静脉。

此断面经第 7 胸椎椎体上份平面。

纵隔后部的左心房大而明显，其右侧壁前部见中叶静脉汇入。中叶静脉多数情况汇入上叶静脉，占 83.6%，也可直接汇入左心房，占 9.1%，其他少见类型包括中叶静脉汇入下叶静脉，外侧段和内侧段静脉分别汇入左心房等[58]。中叶静脉多数情况只有 1 支，占 58.0%±4.0%；也可为 2 支，占 32.0%±3.8%。中叶静脉的属支包括外侧段静脉和内侧段静脉，通常外侧段静脉有分间支，占 54%，从外侧段和内侧段支气管分叉夹角处经过，始终位于两组管道之间的位置。左心房后部左侧有左下肺静脉汇入，右下肺静脉也即将出现。下肺静脉通常收集上段静脉和底段总静脉。正常型右肺下叶底段静脉的组合是：底段上静脉有前底段静脉和外侧底段静脉合成，底段下静脉由后底段静脉形成；抑或底段上静脉由前底段静脉形成，底段下静脉由外侧底段静脉和后底段静脉合成。左肺下叶的底段上静脉由内前底段形成，有上支和基底支 2 个属支，基底支是段间静脉，内前底段和外侧底段；外侧底段静脉是段间静脉，多汇入底段上静脉，后底段静脉为段内静脉，多汇入底段下静脉[62]。

胸部连续横断层 59（FH.12330）

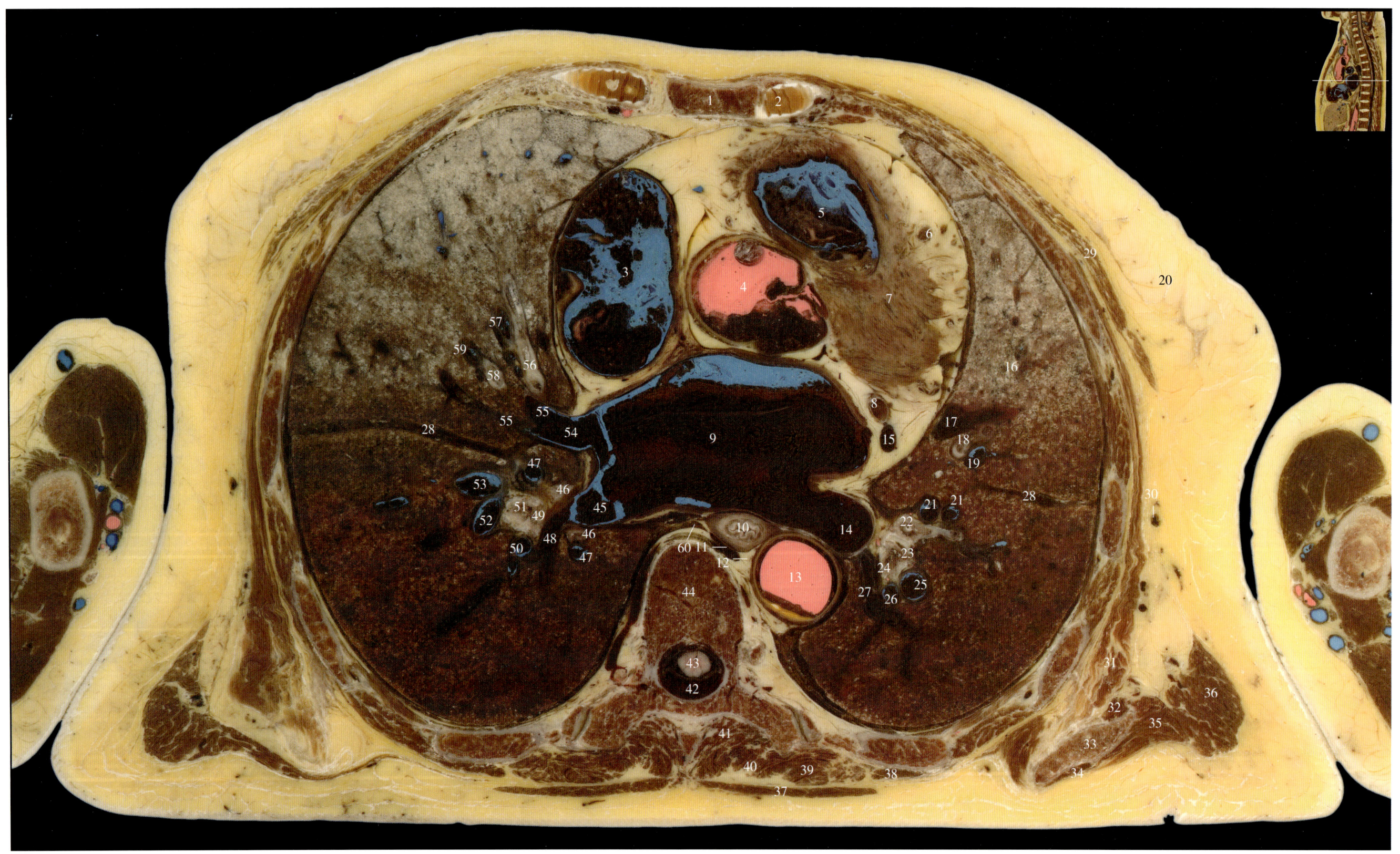

A. 断层标本图像

1. 胸骨体 body of sternum
2. 第 4 肋软骨 4th costal cartilage
3. 右心房 right atrium
4. 升主动脉 ascending aorta
5. 右心室 right ventricle
6. 前室间支 anterior interventricular branch
7. 左心室顶壁 roof of left ventricle
8. 旋支 circumflex branch
9. 左心房 left atrium
10. 食管 esophagus
11. 奇静脉 azygos vein
12. 胸导管 thoracic duct
13. 胸主动脉 thoracic aorta
14. 左下肺静脉 left inferior pulmonary vein
15. 心大静脉 great cardiac vein
16. 上舌段支气管（B4）和动脉（A4）superior lingular segmental bronchus and artery
17. 舌静脉干（V4+5）lingular venous trunk
18. 下舌段支气管（B5）inferior lingular segmental bronchus
19. 下舌段动脉（A5）inferior lingular segmental artery
20. 乳腺 mammary gland
21. 内前底段动脉（A7+8）medioanterior basal segmental artery
22. 内前底段支气管（B7+8）medioanterior basal segmental bronchus
23. 左肺外侧底段支气管（B9）left lateral basal segmental bronchus
24. 左肺后底段支气管（B10）left posterior basal segmental bronchus
25. 左肺外侧底段动脉（A9）left lateral basal segmental artery
26. 左肺后底段动脉（A10）left posterior basal segmental artery
27. 左肺上段静脉（V6）left superior segmental vein
28. 斜裂 oblique fissure
29. 胸大肌 pectoralis major
30. 胸外侧静脉 lateral thoracic vein
31. 前锯肌 serratus anterior
32. 肩胛下肌 subscapularis
33. 肩胛骨 scapula
34. 冈下肌 infraspinatus
35. 大圆肌 teres major
36. 背阔肌 latissimus dorsi
37. 斜方肌 trapezius
38. 髂肋肌 iliocostalis
39. 最长肌 longissimus
40. 棘肌 spinales
41. 横突棘肌 transversospinales
42. 硬膜外隙 epidural space
43. 脊髓 spinal cord
44. 第 7 胸椎椎体 body of 7th thoracic vertebra
45. 右下肺静脉 right inferior pulmonary vein
46. 右肺内侧底段支气管（B7）right medial basal segmental bronchus
47. 右肺内侧底段动脉（A7）right medial basal segmental artery
48. 右肺上段静脉（V6）right superior segmental vein
49. 右肺后底段支气管（B10）right posterior basal segmental bronchus
50. 右肺后底段动脉（A10）right posterior basal segmental artery
51. 右肺前外侧底段支气管（B8+9）right anterolateral basal segmental bronchus
52. 右肺外侧底段动脉（A9）right lateral basal segmental artery
53. 右肺前底段动脉（A8）right anterior basal segmental artery
54. 右肺中叶静脉 right middle lobar vein
55. 外侧段静脉（V4）lateral segmental vein
56. 内侧段支气管（B5）medial segmental bronchus
57. 内侧段动脉（A5）lateral segmental artery
58. 外侧段支气管（B4）lateral segmental bronchus
59. 外侧段动脉（A4）lateral segmental artery
60. 奇静脉食管隐窝 azygoesophageal recess
61. 左肺内前外侧底段支气管（A7+8+9）left common trunk of medial, anterior and lateral basal segmental arteries
62. 右肺前外后底段支气管（B8+9+10）right common trunk of anterior, lateral and posterior basal segmental bronchi
63. 右肺前外侧底段动脉（A8+9）right anterolateral basal segmental artery

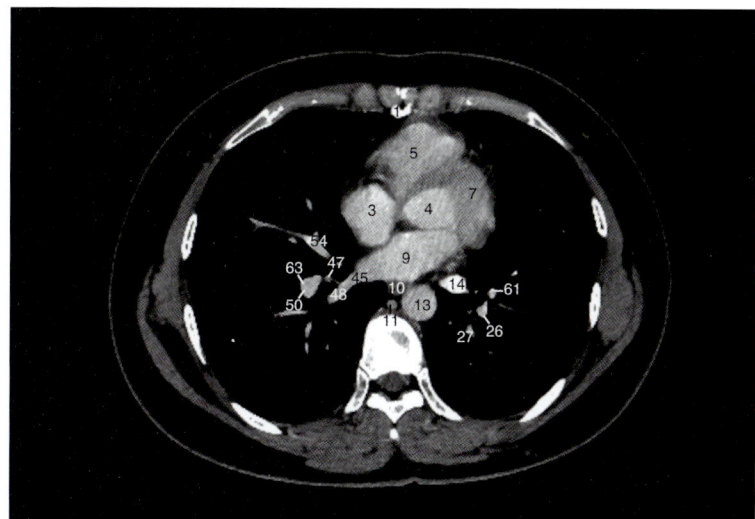

B. CT 纵隔窗增强图像

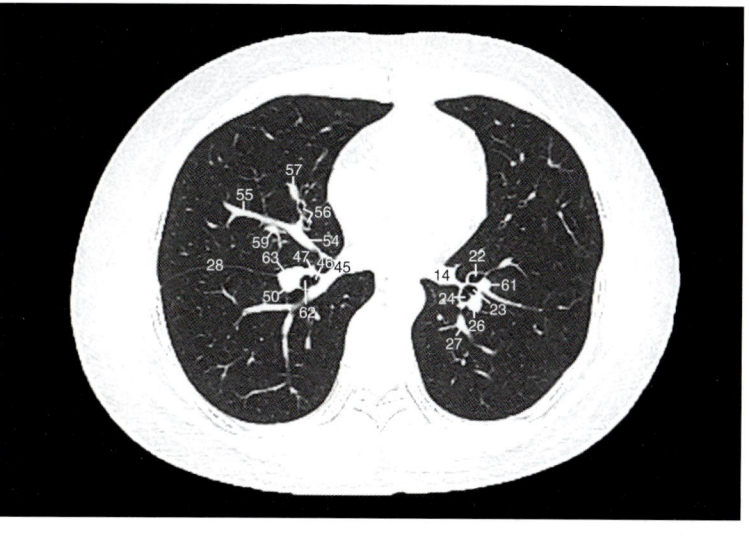

C. CT 肺窗图像

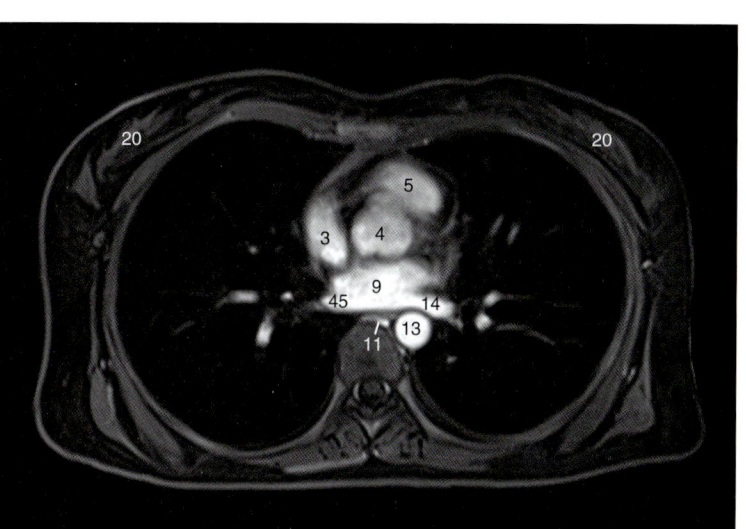

D. MR T1WI 增强图像

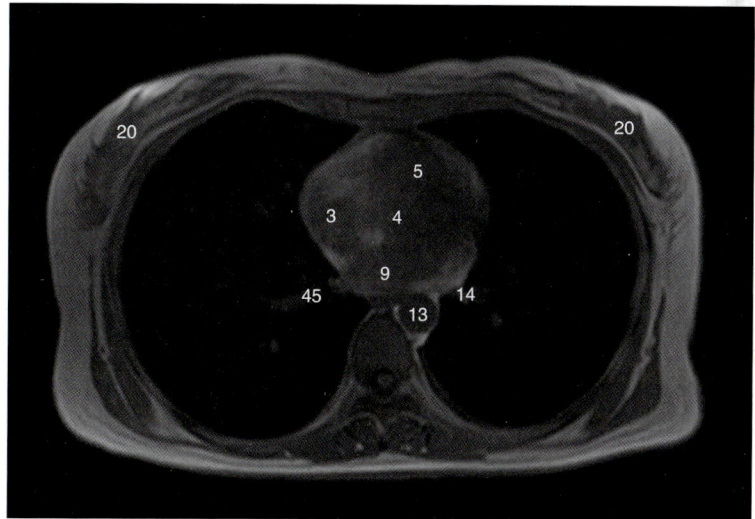

E. MR T1WI 平扫图像

关键结构：上段静脉，奇静脉食管隐窝。

此断面经第 7 胸椎椎体中份。

4 个心腔中左心室位置最低、本断面纵隔左侧仅见左心室顶壁，未见左心室腔。可依左、右心室交界确定前室间沟，内有前室间支和心大静脉；左心房、心室交界为冠状沟左侧部，内有旋支和心大静脉；右心房与右心室未紧贴，故冠状沟右侧部深且宽。左、右心房间的房间隔逐渐变为横位，在房间隔、主动脉右后窦和左心房之间为主动脉下隐窝。右肺门前部为中叶，后部为下叶，两叶均支气管和动脉已进入段内，静脉正穿过肺叶门。右肺中叶分内、外侧段，外侧段静脉为段间支，位于内、外侧段之间；左肺舌叶的舌静脉干为段间支，区分上、下舌段。两肺的上段居于下叶的最高处，在上段支气管、上段动脉和上段静脉这 3 组管道中，通常上段支气管和动脉伴行，在较高的位置进入上段门，上段静脉在稍低的位置出上段门。上段静脉可分为单干或双干型，其中单干型占 88%，双干型占 12%[36]，在单干型中，又通常由 3 支合成，包括内侧支、上支和外侧支。内、外侧支经段间，区分上段和其他底段。于右肺下叶内，内侧底段支气管、前外侧底段支气管和后底段支气管呈逆时针排列，各肺段动脉位于相应支气管的外周；左肺下叶内，内前底段支气管、外侧底段支气管和后底段支气管呈顺时针排列，其外周可见各底段动脉分布。

胸部连续横断层 60（FH.12310）

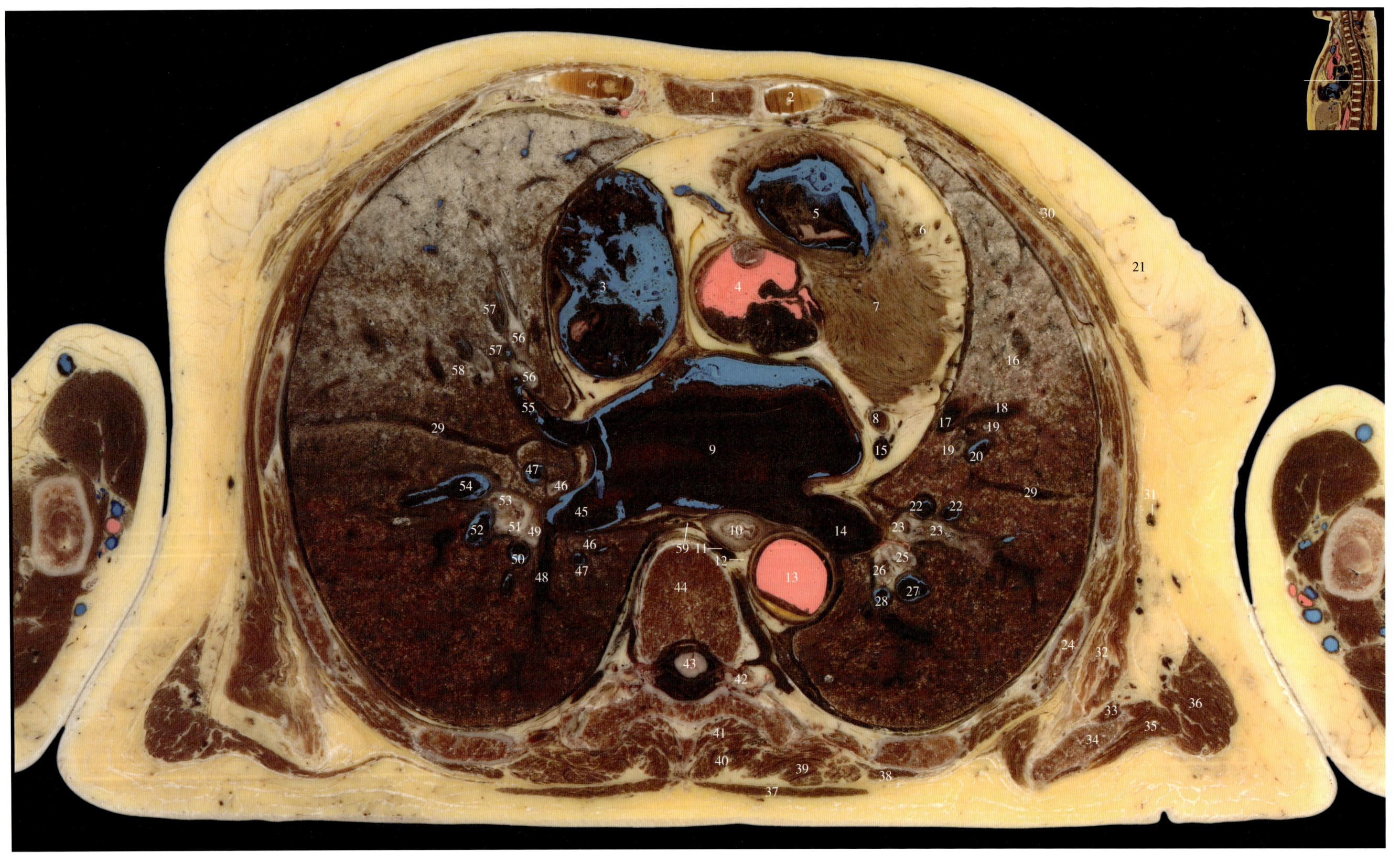

A. 断层标本图像

1. 胸骨体 body of sternum
2. 第 4 肋软骨 4th costal cartilage
3. 右心房 right atrium
4. 升主动脉 ascending aorta
5. 右心室 right ventricle
6. 前室间支 anterior interventricular branch
7. 左心室顶壁 roof of left ventricle
8. 旋支 circumflex branch
9. 左心房 left atrium
10. 食管 esophagus
11. 奇静脉 azygos vein
12. 胸导管 thoracic duct
13. 胸主动脉 thoracic aorta
14. 左下肺静脉 left inferior pulmonary vein
15. 心大静脉 great cardiac vein
16. 上舌段支气管（B4）和动脉（A4）superior lingular segmental bronchus and artery
17. 舌静脉干（V4+5）lingular venous trunk
18. 下舌段动脉（A5）inferior lingular segmental artery
19. 下舌段支气管（B5）inferior lingular segmental bronchus
20. 下舌段动脉（A5）inferior lingular segmental artery
21. 乳腺 mammary gland
22. 内前底段动脉（A7+8）medioanterior basal segmental artery
23. 内前底段支气管（B7+8）medioanterior basal segmental bronchus
24. 第 6 肋骨 6th costal bone
25. 左肺外侧底段支气管（B9）left lateral basal segmental bronchus
26. 左肺后底段支气管（B10）left posterior basal segmental bronchus
27. 左肺外侧底段动脉（A9）left lateral basal segmental artery
28. 左肺后底段动脉（A10）left posterior basal segmental artery
29. 斜裂 oblique fissure
30. 胸大肌 pectoralis major
31. 胸外侧静脉 lateral thoracic vein
32. 前锯肌 serratus anterior
33. 肩胛下肌 subscapularis
34. 肩胛骨 scapula
35. 大圆肌 teres major
36. 背阔肌 latissimus dorsi
37. 斜方肌 trapezius
38. 髂肋肌 iliocostalis
39. 最长肌 longissimus
40. 棘肌 spinales
41. 横突棘肌 transversospinales
42. 椎间孔 intervertebral foramen
43. 脊髓 spinal cord
44. 第 7 胸椎椎体 body of 7th thoracic vertebra
45. 右下肺静脉 right inferior pulmonary vein
46. 右肺内侧底段支气管（B7）right medial basal segmental bronchus
47. 右肺内侧底段动脉（A7）right medial basal segmental artery
48. 右肺上段静脉（V6）right superior segmental vein
49. 右肺后底段支气管（B10）right posterior basal segmental bronchus
50. 右肺后底段动脉（A10）right posterior basal segmental artery
51. 右肺外侧底段支气管（B9）right lateral basal segmental bronchus
52. 右肺外侧底段动脉（A9）right lateral basal segmental artery
53. 右肺前底段支气管（B8）right anterior basal segmental bronchus
54. 右肺前底段动脉（A8）right anterior basal segmental artery
55. 外侧段静脉（V4）lateral segmental vein
56. 内侧段支气管（B5）medial segmental bronchus
57. 内侧段动脉（A5）medial segmental artery
58. 外侧段支气管（B4）和动脉（A4）lateral segmental bronchus and artery
59. 奇静脉食管隐窝 azygoesophageal recess
60. 左肺内前外侧底段动脉（A7+8+9）left common trunk of medial, anterior and lateral basal segmental arteries
61. 右肺前外后底段支气管（B8+9+10）right common trunk of anterior, lateral and posterior basal segmental bronchi
62. 右肺前外侧底段动脉（A8+9）right anterolateral basal segmental artery

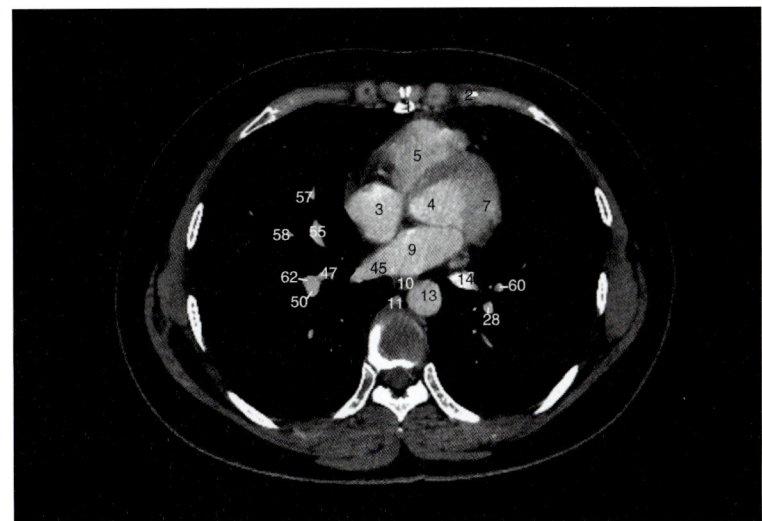

B. CT 纵隔窗增强图像

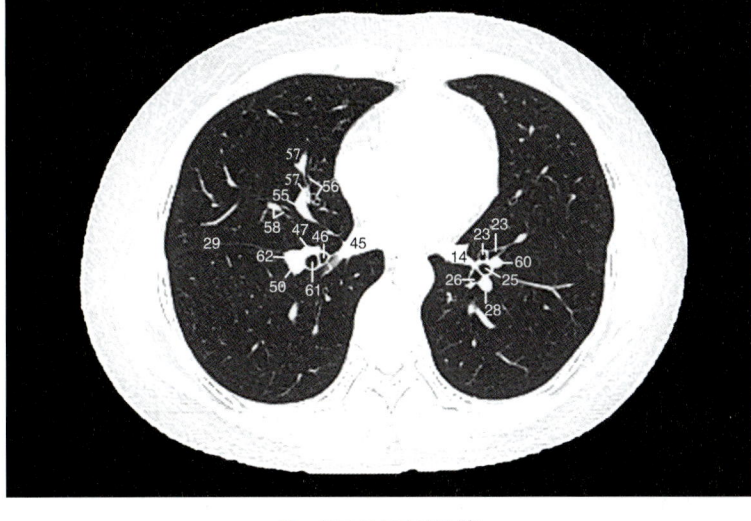

C. CT 肺窗图像

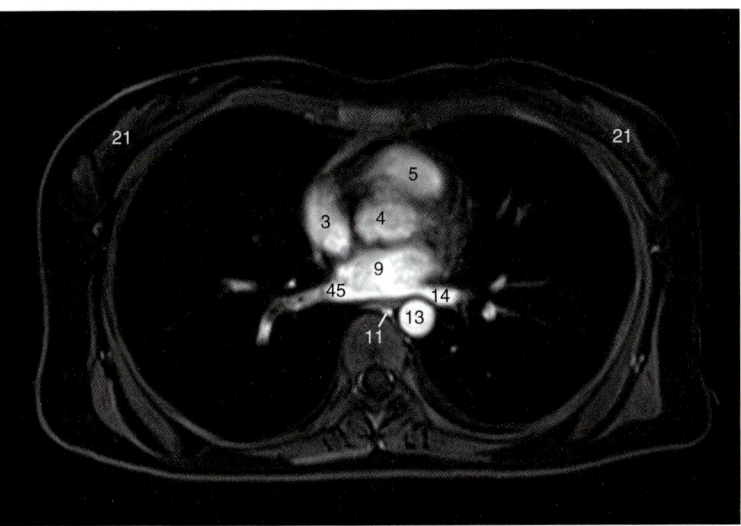

D. MR T1WI 增强图像

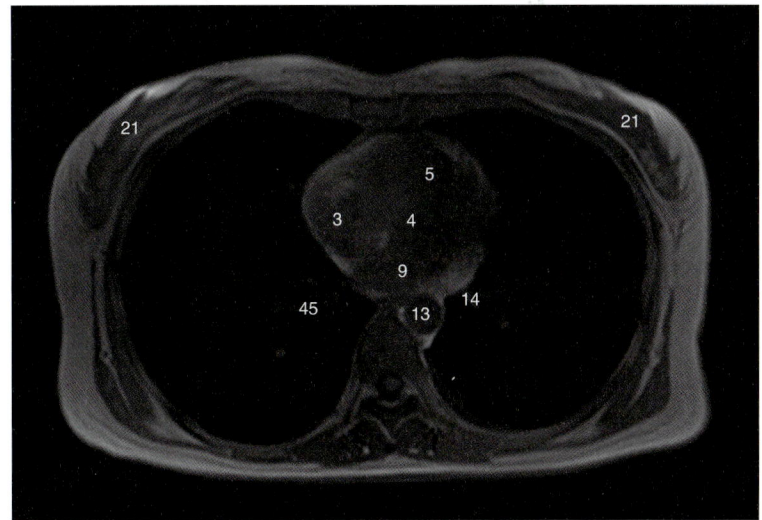

E. MR T1WI 平扫图像

关键结构：主动脉瓣，主动脉窦。

此断面前方经过第 4 肋软骨，后方经过第 7 胸椎体中份。

随着断面下移，左心室顶壁及左心室腔逐渐明显，可见升主动脉逐渐后移与左心室流出道融合的趋势。此时，升主动脉根部常位于纵隔中心位置，内壁有主动脉瓣附着，包括右冠状动脉瓣、左冠状动脉瓣和无冠状动脉瓣。标本测量显示主动脉瓣环周长为 62.3 mm ± 8.4 mm，瓣叶面积为 272.5 mm^2 ± 82.7 mm^2，游离缘距瓣底的距离为 15.2 mm ± 2.7 mm[63]。CT 和超声心动图测量主动脉瓣的面积可用于主动脉瓣狭窄患者的分级评估[64]。主动脉根部管壁与主动脉瓣围成的主动脉窦，左冠状动脉窦位于管腔前部，前 3/5 与左心室毗邻，后 2/5 与心包横窦相邻；右冠状动脉窦位于后外侧，前 3/5 与右心室相邻，后 2/5 与右心房相邻；无冠状动脉窦位于后内侧，与心包横窦及右心房同时相邻，临床主动脉窦瘤多发生于右冠状动脉窦，右冠状动脉窦瘤多破入右心室[65]。

胸部连续横断层 61（FH.12290）

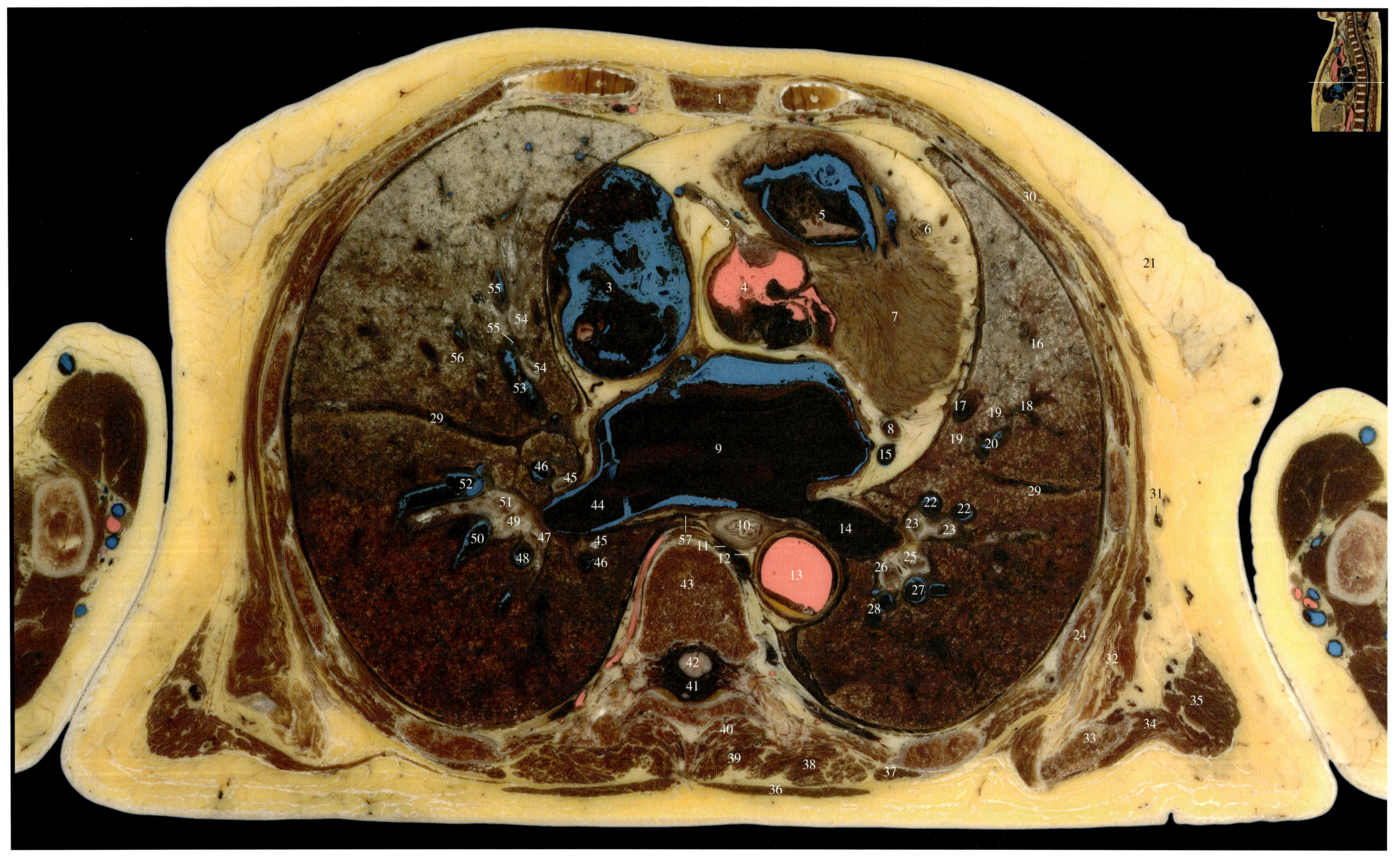

A. 断层标本图像

1. 胸骨体 body of sternum
2. 右冠状动脉 right coronary artery
3. 右心房 right atrium
4. 升主动脉 ascending aorta
5. 右心室 right ventricle
6. 前室间支 anterior interventricular branch
7. 左心室顶壁 roof of left ventricle
8. 旋支 circumflex branch
9. 左心房 left atrium
10. 食管 esophagus
11. 奇静脉 azygos vein
12. 胸导管 thoracic duct
13. 胸主动脉 thoracic aorta
14. 左下肺静脉 left inferior pulmonary vein
15. 心大静脉 great cardiac vein
16. 上舌段支气管（B4）和动脉（A4）superior lingular segmental bronchus and artery
17. 舌静脉干（V4+5）lingular venous trunk
18. 下舌段静脉（V5）inferior lingular segmental vein
19. 下舌段支气管（B5）inferior lingular segmental bronchus
20. 下舌段动脉（A5）inferior lingular segmental artery
21. 乳腺 mammary gland
22. 内前底段动脉（A7+8）medioanterior basal segmental artery
23. 内前底段支气管（B7+8）medioanterior basal segmental bronchus
24. 第 6 肋骨 6th costal bone
25. 左肺外侧底段支气管（B9）left lateral basal segmental bronchus
26. 左肺后底段支气管（B10）left posterior basal segmental bronchus
27. 左肺外侧底段动脉（A9）left lateral basal segmental artery
28. 左肺后底段动脉（A10）left posterior basal segmental artery
29. 斜裂 oblique fissure
30. 胸大肌 pectoralis major
31. 胸外侧静脉 lateral thoracic vein
32. 前锯肌 serratus anterior
33. 肩胛骨 scapula
34. 大圆肌 teres major
35. 背阔肌 latissimus dorsi
36. 斜方肌 trapezius
37. 髂肋肌 iliocostalis
38. 最长肌 longissimus
39. 棘肌 spinales
40. 横突棘肌 transversospinales
41. 硬膜外隙 epidural space
42. 脊髓 spinal cord
43. 第 7 胸椎椎体 body of 7th thoracic vertebra
44. 右下肺静脉 right inferior pulmonary vein
45. 内侧底段支气管（B7）medial basal segmental bronchus
46. 内侧底段动脉（A7）medial basal segmental artery
47. 右肺后底段支气管（B10）right posterior basal segmental bronchus
48. 右肺后底段动脉（A10）right posterior basal segmental artery
49. 右肺外侧底段支气管（B9）right lateral basal segmental bronchus
50. 右肺外侧底段动脉（A9）right lateral basal segmental artery
51. 右肺前底段支气管（B8）right anterior basal segmental bronchus
52. 右肺前底段动脉（A8）right anterior basal segmental artery
53. 外侧段静脉（V4）lateral segmental vein
54. 内侧段支气管（B5）medial segmental bronchus
55. 内侧段动脉（A5）medial segmental artery
56. 外侧段支气管（B4）和动脉（A4）lateral segmental bronchus and artery
57. 奇静脉食管隐窝 azygoesophageal recess
58. 左肺内前外侧底段动脉（A7+8+9）right common trunk of medial, anterior and lateral basal segmental arteries
59. 右肺前外后底段支气管（B8+9+10）right common trunk of anterior, lateral and posterior basal segmental bronchi
60. 右肺前外侧底段动脉（A8+9）right anterolateral basal segmental artery

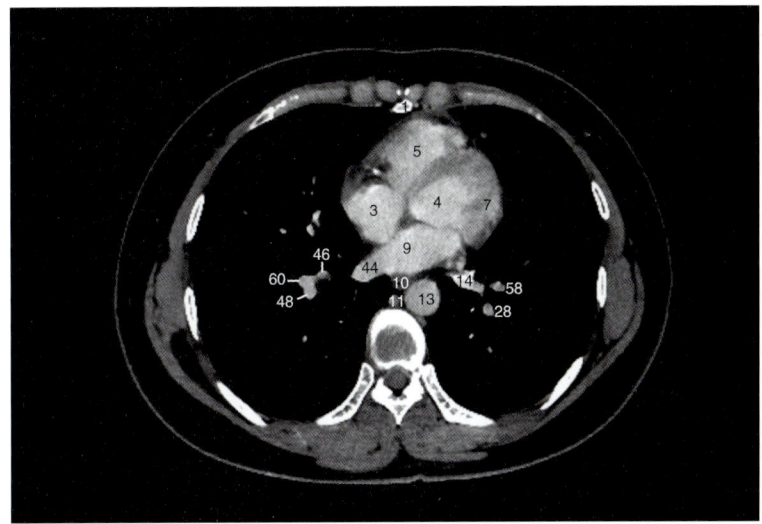

B. CT 纵隔窗增强图像

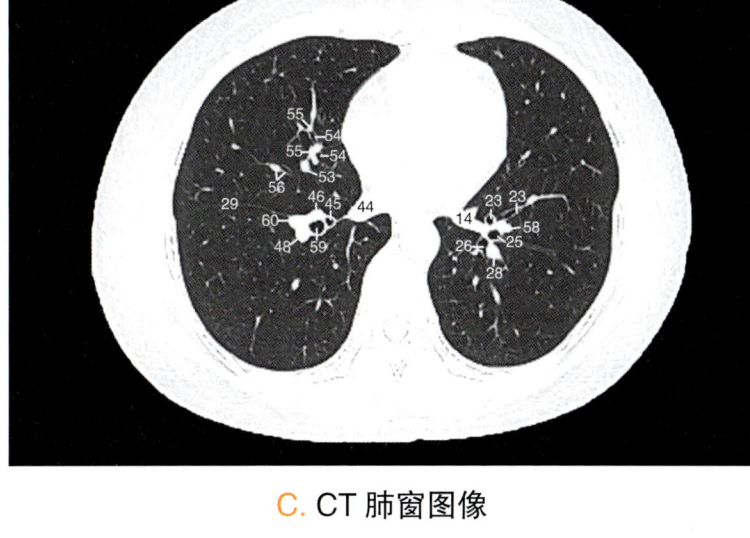

C. CT 肺窗图像

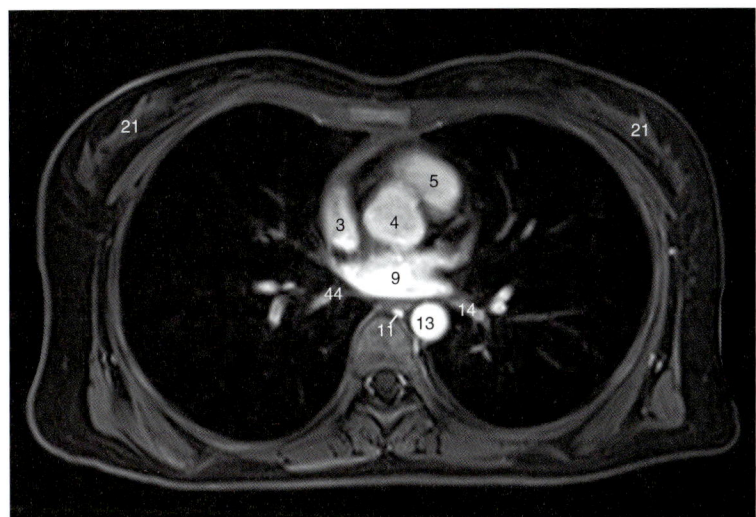

D. MR T1WI 增强图像

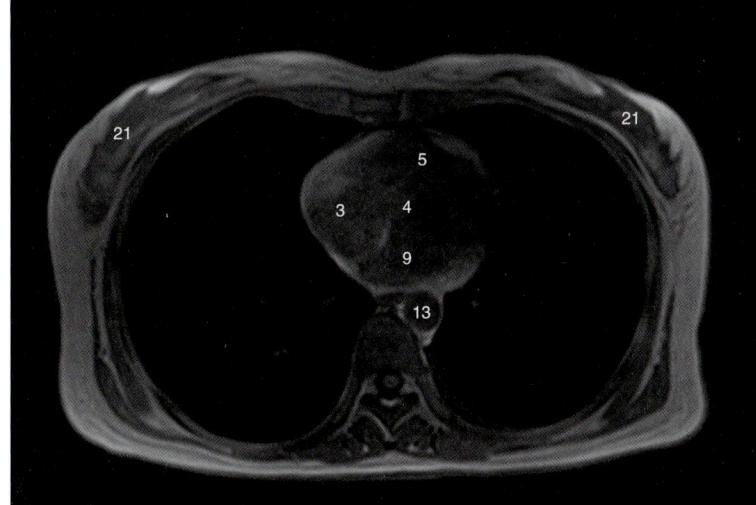

E. MR T1WI 平扫图像

关键结构：右下肺静脉，左下肺静脉。

此断面前方经过第 4 肋软骨，后方经过第 7 胸椎椎体中份。

纵隔后部的左心房腔大而明显，其后壁右侧见右下肺静脉汇入，左侧见左下肺静脉汇入，两下肺静脉均大而明显。正常肺静脉以典型四开口形式汇入左心房，CT 显示肺静脉的变异较多，主要为肺静脉数量和汇入点位置的变异[66]。在异位起搏患者中，36% 是由异常肺静脉引起的。国人以 4 支肺静脉为主，占 78.6%，极少部分有 3 支或 5 支。静脉共同开口的出现率为 22.5%，左侧较右侧出现的概率大。肺静脉口近似椭圆形，多不规则，其长轴多为上下走行，其短轴多为前后走行，上肺静脉口面积大于下肺静脉口[67]。心包内肺静脉的解剖参数分别为：左上肺静脉直径为 1.6 cm，长度为 1.0 cm；右上肺静脉直径为 1.7 cm，长度为 0.7 cm；左下肺静脉直径为 1.4 cm，长度为 0.7 cm；右下肺静脉直径为 1.5 cm，长度为 0.4 cm。下肺静脉主要收集 2 组属支，一组较小，为来自上方的上段静脉；另一组粗大，来自下方的各底段，为底段总静脉[36]。

胸部连续横断层 62（FH.12270）

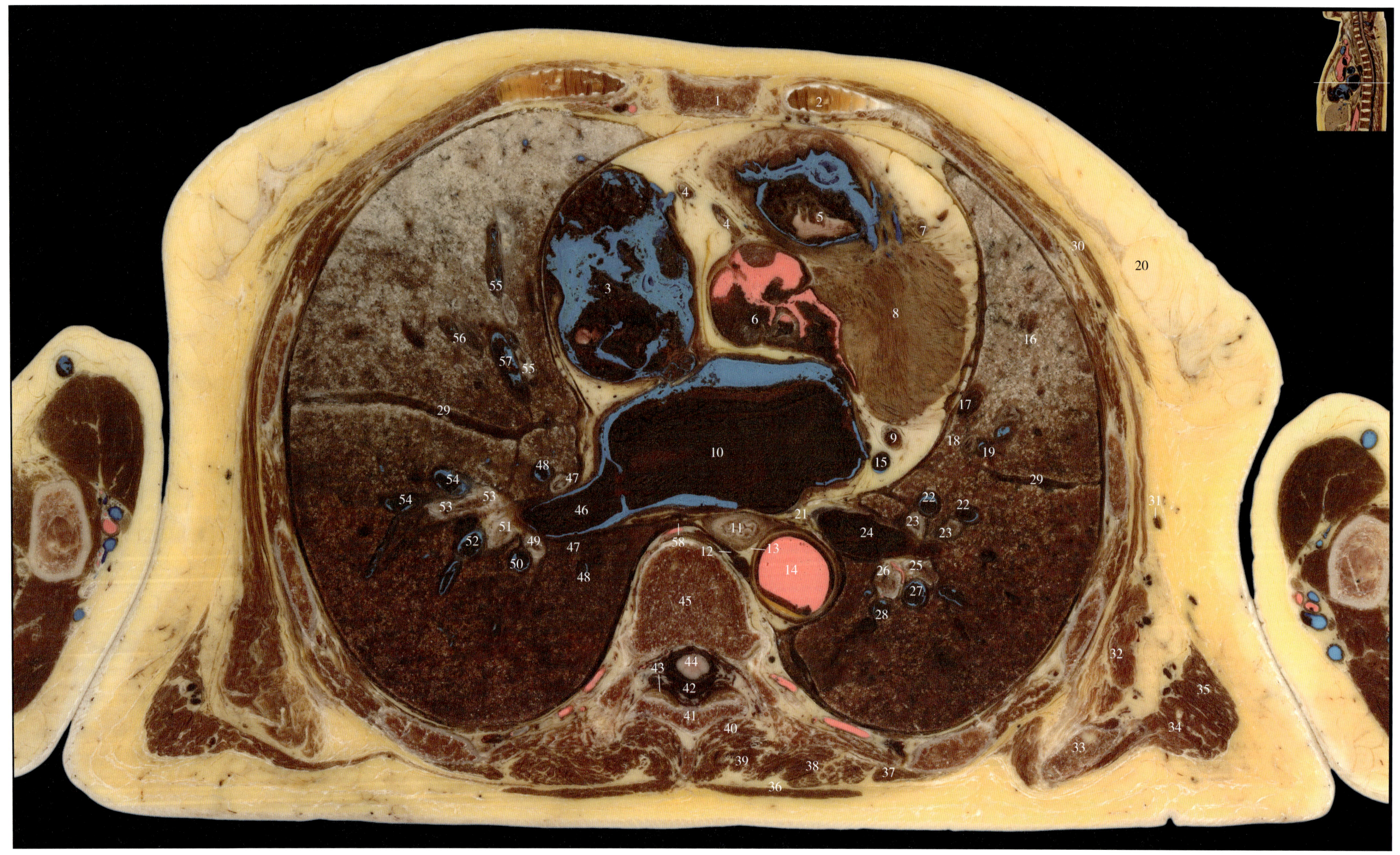

A. 断层标本图像

1. 胸骨体 body of sternum
2. 第 4 肋软骨 4th costal cartilage
3. 右心房 right atrium
4. 右冠状动脉 right coronary artery
5. 右心室 right ventricle
6. 升主动脉 ascending aorta
7. 前室间支 anterior interventricular branch
8. 左心室顶壁 roof of left ventricle
9. 旋支 circumflex branch
10. 左心房 left atrium
11. 食管 esophagus
12. 奇静脉 azygos vein
13. 胸导管 thoracic duct
14. 胸主动脉 thoracic aorta
15. 心大静脉 great cardiac vein
16. 上舌段支气管（B4）和动脉（A4） superior lingular segmental bronchus and artery
17. 舌静脉干（V4+5）lingular venous trunk
18. 下舌段支气管（B5）inferior lingular segmental bronchus
19. 下舌段动脉（A5）inferior lingular segmental artery
20. 乳腺 mammary gland
21. 肺韧带 pulmonary ligament
22. 内前底段动脉（A7+8）medioanterior basal segmental artery
23. 内前底段支气管（B7+8）medioanterior basal segmental bronchus
24. 左肺底段总静脉 left common basal vein
25. 左肺外侧底段支气管（B9）left lateral basal segmental bronchus
26. 左肺后底段支气管（B10）left posterior basal segmental bronchus
27. 左肺外侧底段动脉（A9）left lateral basal segmental artery
28. 左肺后底段动脉（A10）left posterior basal segmental artery
29. 斜裂 oblique fissure
30. 胸大肌 pectoralis major
31. 胸外侧静脉 lateral thoracic vein
32. 前锯肌 serratus anterior
33. 肩胛骨 scapula
34. 大圆肌 teres major
35. 背阔肌 latissimus dorsi
36. 斜方肌 trapezius
37. 髂肋肌 iliocostalis
38. 最长肌 longissimus
39. 棘肌 spinales
40. 横突棘肌 transversospinales
41. 椎弓板 lamina of vertebral arch
42. 硬膜外隙 epidural space
43. 黄韧带 ligamenta flava
44. 脊髓 spinal cord
45. 第 7 胸椎椎体 body of 7th thoracic vertebra
46. 右下肺静脉 right inferior pulmonary vein
47. 内侧底段支气管（B7）medial basal segmental bronchus
48. 内侧底段动脉（A7）medial basal segmental artery
49. 右肺后底段支气管（B10）right posterior basal segmental bronchus
50. 右肺后底段动脉（A10）right posterior basal segmental artery
51. 右肺外侧底段支气管（B9）right lateral basal segmental bronchus
52. 右肺外侧底段动脉（A9）right lateral basal segmental artery
53. 右肺前底段支气管（B8）right anterior basal segmental bronchus
54. 右肺前底段动脉（A8）right anterior basal segmental artery
55. 内侧段支气管（B5）和动脉（A5）medial segmental bronchus and artery
56. 外侧段支气管（B4）和动脉（A4）lateral segmental bronchus and artery
57. 外侧段静脉（V4）lateral segmental vein
58. 奇静脉食管隐窝 azygoesophageal recess
59. 右肺前外侧底段动脉（A8+9）right anterolateral basal segmental artery
60. 右肺前外侧底段支气管（B8+9）right anterolateral basal segmental bronchus
61. 左冠状动脉 left coronary artery

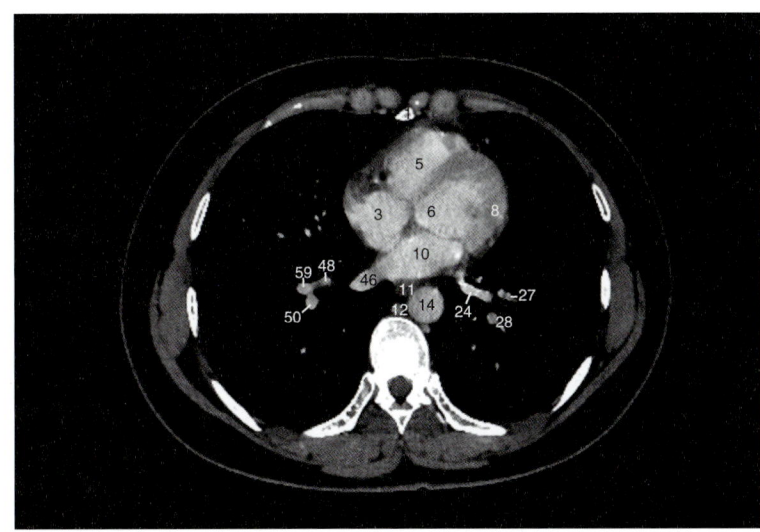

B. CT 纵隔窗增强图像

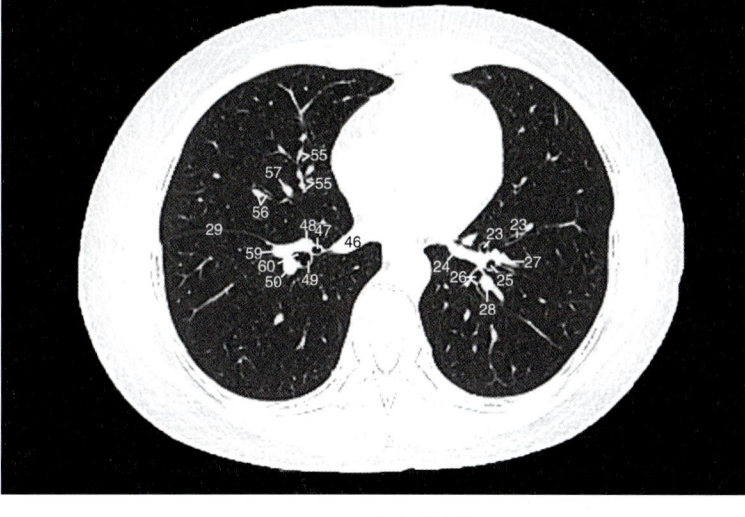

C. CT 肺窗图像

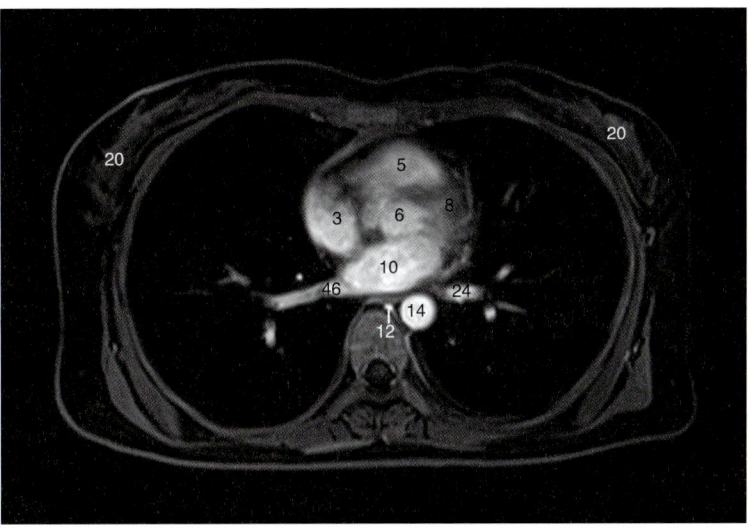

D. MR T1WI 增强图像

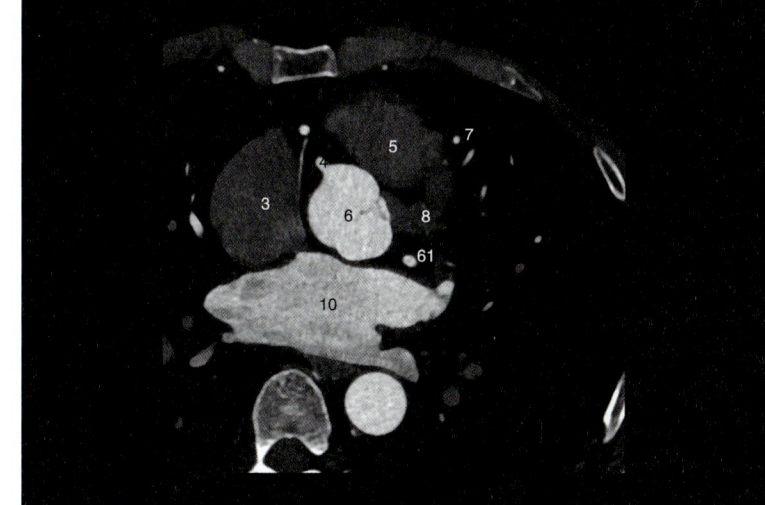

E. 冠状动脉 CT 增强图像

关键结构：底段总静脉。

此断面经第 4 肋软骨和第 7 胸椎椎体下份。

纵隔左侧见左心室顶壁内侧逐渐凹陷，与升主动脉根部逐渐融合，表明左心室流出道逐渐出现，至此 4 个心腔全都出现。心在发育过程中出现沿纵轴的轻度右旋转，故左半心位于右半心的左后方。右心房是最靠右侧的心腔，右心室是最前方的心腔，左心室是最靠左侧的心腔，左心房是最后方的心腔，同时位置较高[68]。可据心腔位置判断冠状沟、室间沟和房间沟的位置：两心房和心室之间为冠状沟，可分为右侧部和左侧部，中间隔以主动脉根部；两心室间前方为前室间沟；两心房间为房间沟。冠状沟右侧部内可定位右冠状动脉，冠状沟左侧部内可定位左冠状动脉旋支及伴行的心大静脉，前室间沟内可定位左冠状动脉前室间支。左心房侧壁后部接受下肺静脉的汇入，断面中当下肺静脉离开左心房进入下叶门后，即形成底段总静脉。底段总静脉由底段上静脉和底段下静脉合成[69]。

胸部连续横断层 63（FH.12250）

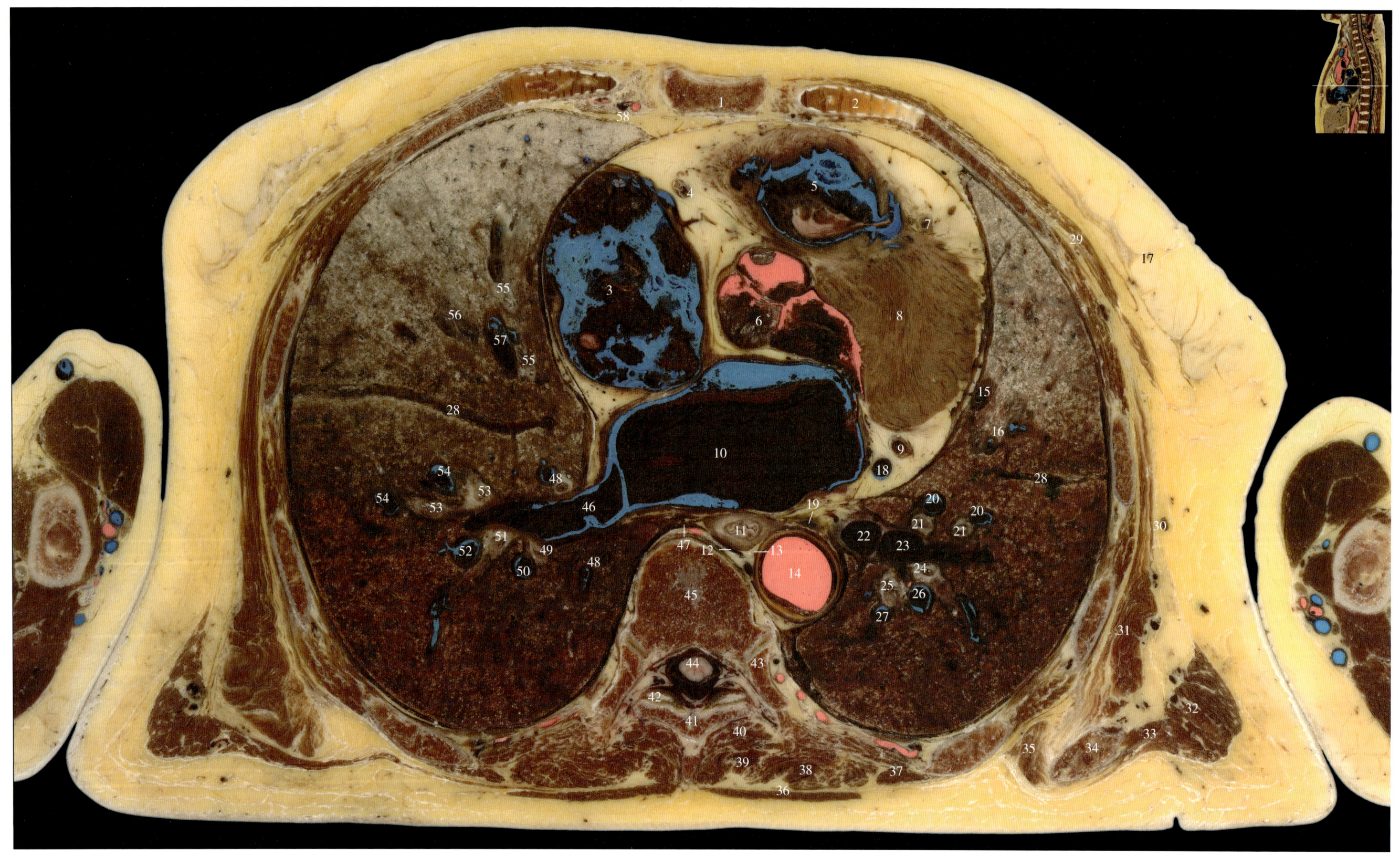

A. 断层标本图像

1. 胸骨体 body of sternum
2. 第 4 肋软骨 4th costal cartilage
3. 右心房 right atrium
4. 右冠状动脉 right coronary artery
5. 右心室 right ventricle
6. 升主动脉 ascending aorta
7. 前室间支 anterior interventricular branch
8. 左心室顶壁 roof of left ventricle
9. 旋支 circumflex branch
10. 左心房 left atrium
11. 食管 esophagus
12. 奇静脉 azygos vein
13. 胸导管 thoracic duct
14. 胸主动脉 thoracic aorta
15. 舌静脉干（V4+5）lingular venous trunk
16. 下舌段支气管（B4）和动脉（A4）inferior lingular segmental bronchus and artery
17. 乳腺 mammary gland
18. 心大静脉 great cardiac vein
19. 肺韧带淋巴结（9 区）pulmonary ligament lymph nodes
20. 内前底段动脉（A7+8）medioanterior basal segmental artery
21. 内前底段支气管（B7+8）medioanterior basal segmental bronchus
22. 左肺底段下静脉 left inferior basal vein
23. 左肺底段上静脉 left superior basal vein
24. 左肺外侧底段支气管（B9）left lateral basal segmental bronchus
25. 左肺后底段支气管（B10）left posterior basal segmental bronchus
26. 左肺外侧底段动脉（A9）left lateral basal segmental artery
27. 左肺后底段动脉（A10）left posterior basal segmental artery
28. 斜裂 oblique fissure
29. 胸大肌 pectoralis major
30. 胸外侧静脉 lateral thoracic vein
31. 前锯肌 serratus anterior
32. 背阔肌 latissimus dorsi
33. 大圆肌 teres major
34. 肩胛骨 scapula
35. 菱形肌 rhomboideus
36. 斜方肌 trapezius
37. 髂肋肌 iliocostalis
38. 最长肌 longissimus
39. 棘肌 spinales
40. 横突棘肌 transversospinales
41. 椎弓板 lamina of vertebral arch
42. 关节突关节 zygapophysial joint
43. 第 8 肋骨 8th costal bone
44. 脊髓 spinal cord
45. 第 7 胸椎椎体 body of 7th thoracic vertebra
46. 右下肺静脉 right inferior pulmonary vein
47. 奇静脉食管隐窝 azygoesophageal recess
48. 内侧底段支气管（B7）和动脉（A7）medial basal segmental bronchus and artery
49. 右肺后底段支气管（B10）right posterior basal segmental bronchus
50. 右肺后底段动脉（A10）right posterior basal segmental artery
51. 右肺外侧底段支气管（B9）right lateral basal segmental bronchus
52. 右肺外侧底段动脉（A9）right lateral basal segmental artery
53. 右肺前底段支气管（B8）right anterior basal segmental bronchus
54. 右肺前底段动脉（A8）right anterior basal segmental artery
55. 内侧段支气管（B5）和动脉（A5）medial segmental bronchus and artery
56. 外侧段支气管（B4）和动脉（A4）lateral segmental bronchus and artery
57. 外侧段静脉（V4）lateral segmental vein
58. 胸廓内动、静脉 internal thoracic artery and vein
59. 右肺前外侧底段支气管（B8+9）right anterolateral basal segmental bronchus
60. 右肺前外侧底段动脉（A8+9）right anterolateral basal segmental artery

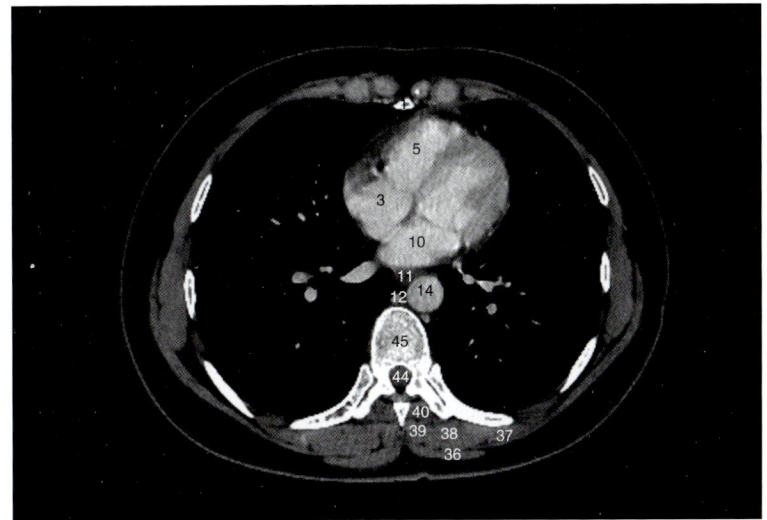

B. CT 纵隔窗增强图像

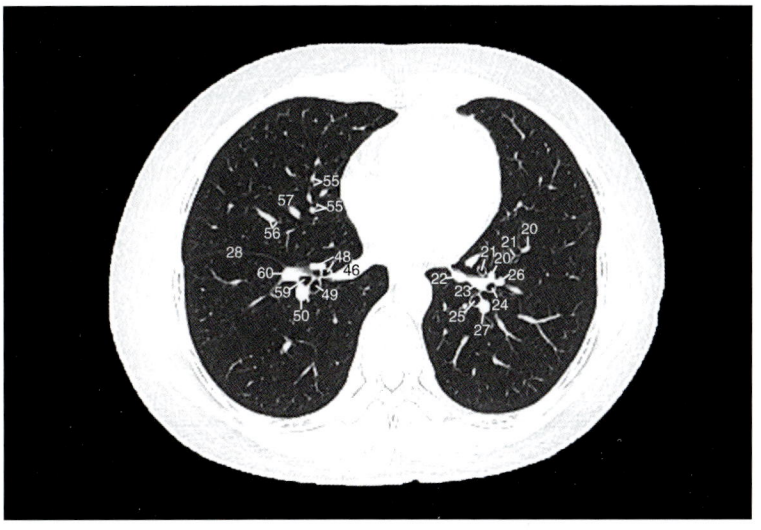

C. CT 肺窗图像

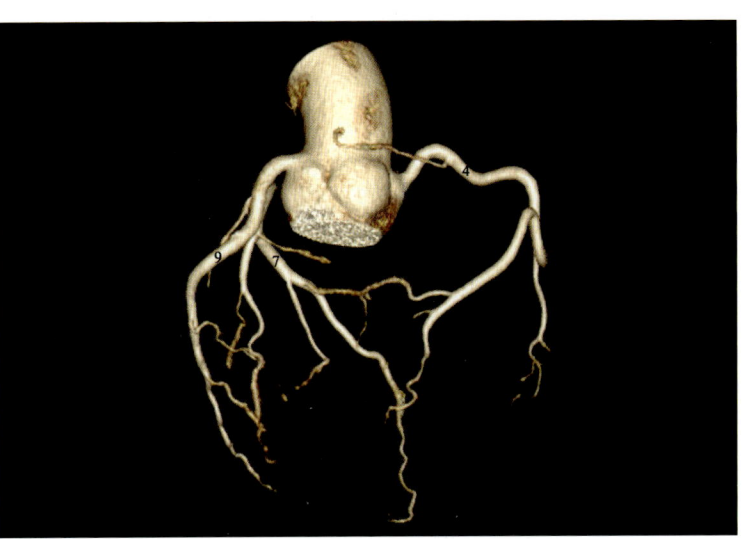

D. 冠状动脉 VR 重建图像

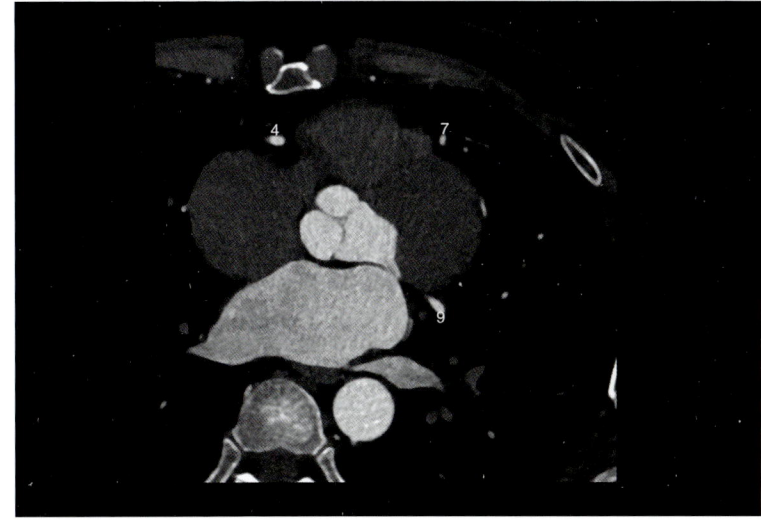

E. 冠状动脉 CT 增强图像

关键结构：肺韧带，肺韧带淋巴结。

此断面经第 7 胸椎椎体中份。

随着左下肺静脉消失，其下方出现肺韧带，内部有肺韧带淋巴结。根据 IASLC 肺癌淋巴结分区，肺韧带淋巴结为 9 区，其范围上界为下肺静脉，下界为膈。肺韧带为下肺静脉下方的叶状双层胸膜结构，附着于肺下叶内侧缘，游离在肺上者，称为不完全型肺韧带（多见）或称"三角韧带"；继续向下伸延，并同时附着于膈肌者，称为完全型肺韧带或称"肺膈韧带"。左、右侧肺韧带的上部附着点各不相同，右肺韧带位于下腔静脉与奇静脉之间附着于食管，左侧则附着于食管或降主动脉。肺韧带的形态因人而存在明显差异，而同一人的左、右侧肺韧带的长度也多不相等，左侧较右侧长者多见[70]。CT 图像中，肺韧带在下肺静脉下方连续层面上显示，为后纵隔两旁向肺内延伸的线样影，该线样影无分支。CT 上肺韧带的出现率可达 77.6%，其中右侧占 37.2%，左侧为 67.4%，左侧肺韧带较右侧显示率高，两侧同时显示者占 27.1%。肺韧带固定肺下叶，影响下胸部疾病的影像学表现：肺底积液时，肺韧带将胸腔积液分隔成前、后两部分，导致所产生"膈顶外移"和类似椎旁阴影增宽的假象；肺下叶肿瘤或炎症，以及食管的肿瘤转移常累及肺韧带，呈不规则增厚和鸟嘴状增厚，或肺韧带淋巴结肿大[71]。

胸部连续横断层 64（FH.12230）

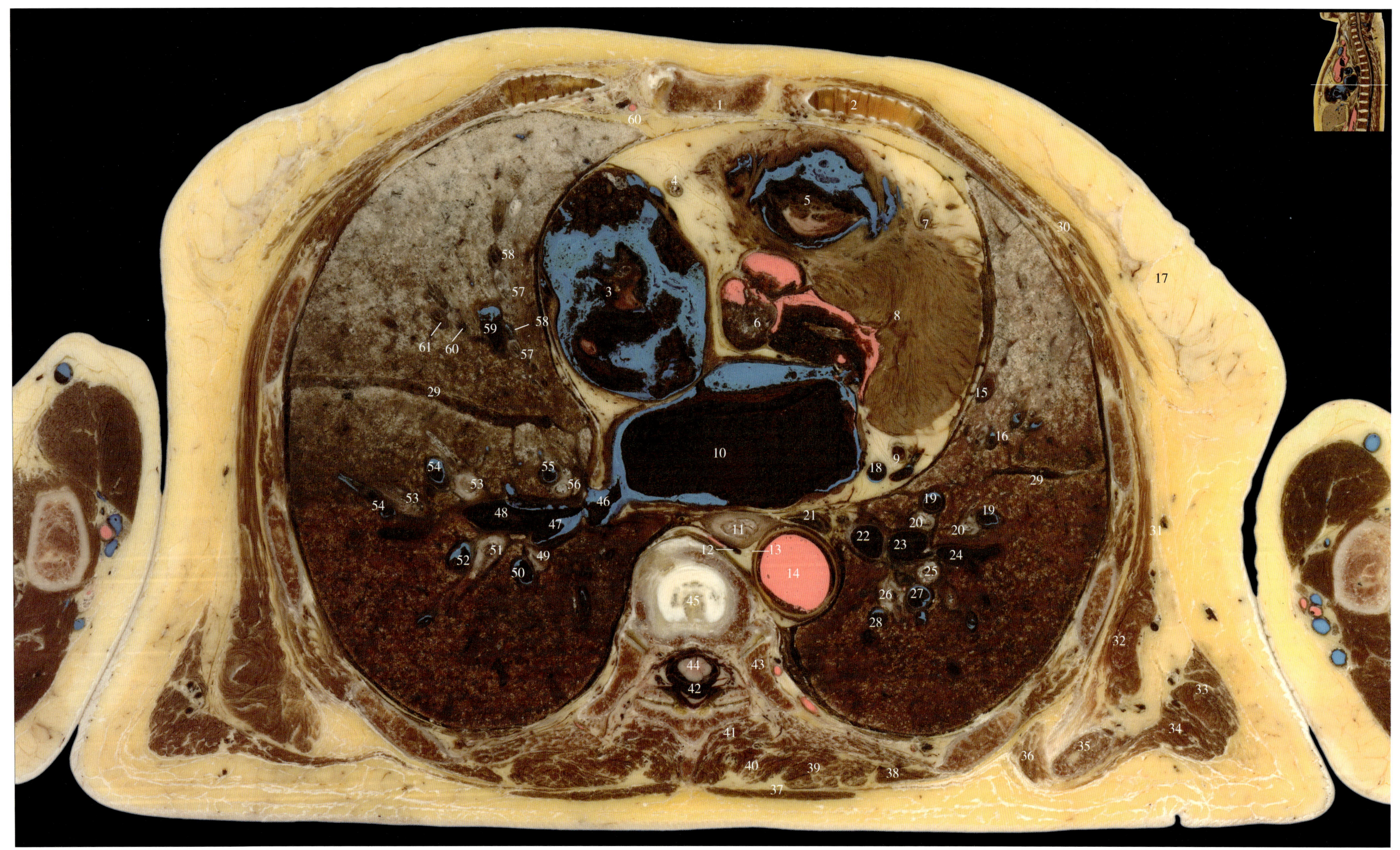

A. 断层标本图像

1. 胸骨体 body of sternum
2. 第 4 肋软骨 4th costal cartilage
3. 右心房 right atrium
4. 右冠状动脉 right coronary artery
5. 右心室 right ventricle
6. 主动脉窦 aortic sinus
7. 前室间支 anterior interventricular branch
8. 左心室顶壁 roof of left ventricle
9. 旋支 circumflex coronary artery
10. 左心房 left atrium
11. 食管 esophagus
12. 奇静脉 azygos vein
13. 胸导管 thoracic duct
14. 胸主动脉 thoracic aorta
15. 舌静脉干（V4+5）lingular venous trunk
16. 下舌段支气管（B4）和动脉（A4） inferior lingular segmental bronchus and artery
17. 乳腺 mammary gland
18. 心大静脉 great cardiac vein
19. 内前底段动脉（A7+8）medioanterior basal segmental artery
20. 内前底段支气管（B7+8）medioanterior basal segmental bronchus
21. 肺韧带淋巴结（9 区）pulmonary ligament lymph nodes
22. 左肺底段下静脉 left inferior basal vein
23. 左肺底段上静脉 left superior basal vein
24. 左肺前底段静脉（V8）left anterior basal segmental vein
25. 左肺外侧底段支气管（B9）left lateral basal segmental bronchus
26. 左肺后底段支气管（B10）left posterior basal segmental bronchus
27. 左肺外侧底段动脉（A9）left lateral basal segmental artery
28. 左肺后底段动脉（A10）left posterior basal segmental artery
29. 斜裂 oblique fissure
30. 胸大肌 pectoralis major
31. 胸外侧静脉 lateral thoracic vein
32. 前锯肌 serratus anterior
33. 背阔肌 latissimus dorsi
34. 大圆肌 teres major

35. 肩胛骨 scapula
36. 菱形肌 rhomboideus
37. 斜方肌 trapezius
38. 髂肋肌 iliocostalis
39. 最长肌 longissimus
40. 棘肌 spinales
41. 横突棘肌 transversospinales
42. 硬膜外隙 epidural space
43. 第 8 肋骨 8th costal bone
44. 脊髓 spinal cord
45. T7-8 椎间盘 T7-8 intervertebral disc
46. 右下肺静脉 right inferior pulmonary vein
47. 右肺底段下静脉 right inferior basal vein
48. 右肺底段上静脉 right superior basal vein
49. 右肺后底段支气管（B10）right posterior basal segmental bronchus
50. 右肺后底段动脉（A10）right posterior basal segmental artery
51. 右肺外侧底段支气管（B9）right lateral basal segmental bronchus
52. 右肺外侧底段动脉（A9）right lateral basal segmental artery
53. 右肺前底段支气管（B8）right anterior basal segmental bronchus
54. 右肺前底段动脉（A8）right anterior basal segmental artery
55. 右肺内侧底段动脉（A7）right medial basal segmental artery
56. 右肺内侧底段支气管（B7）right medial basal segmental bronchus
57. 内侧段支气管（B5）和动脉（A5）medial segmental bronchus and artery
58. 外侧段支气管（B4）和动脉（A4）lateral segmental bronchus and artery
59. 外侧段静脉（V4）lateral segmental vein
60. 胸廓内动、静脉 internal thoracic artery and vein
61. 右肺前外侧底段动脉（A8+9）right anterolateral basal segmental artery
62. 右肺前外侧底段支气管（B8+9）right anterolateral basal segmental bronchus

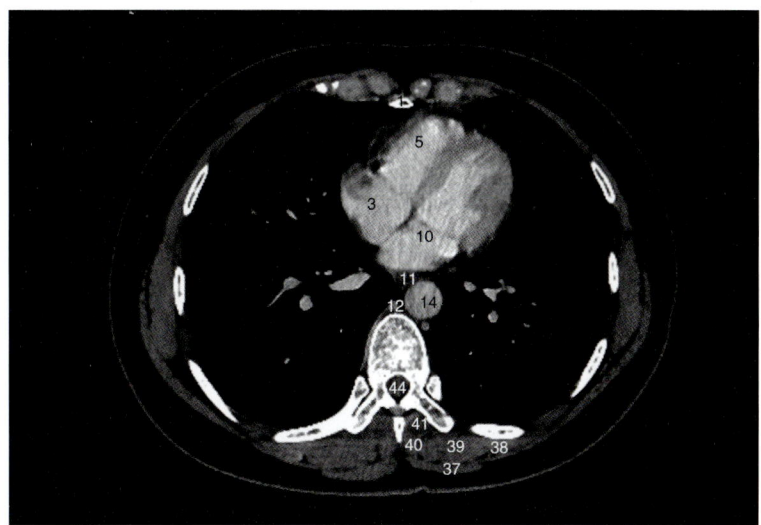

B. CT 纵隔窗增强图像

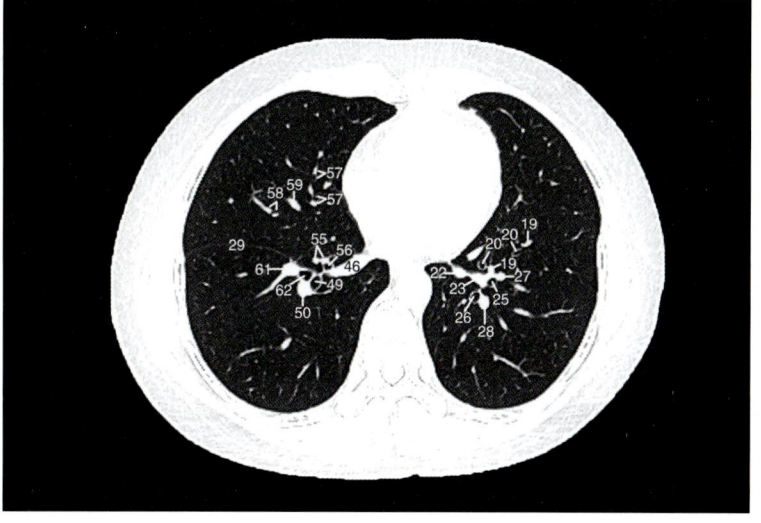

C. CT 肺窗图像

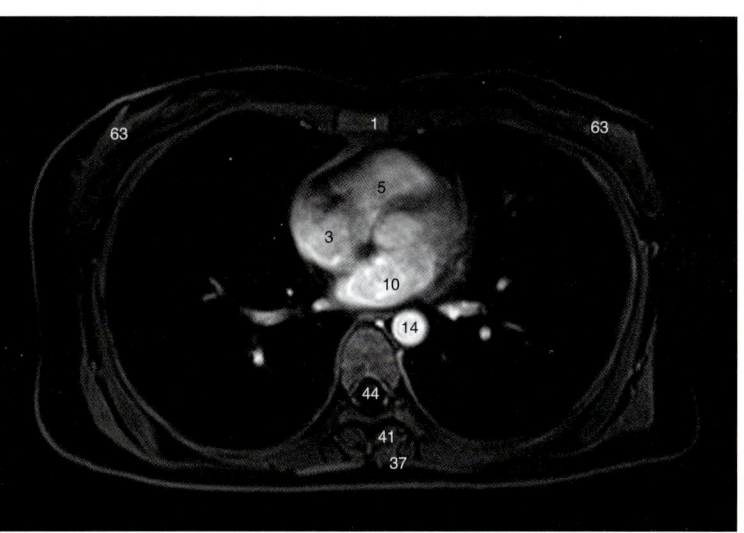

D. MR T1WI 增强图像

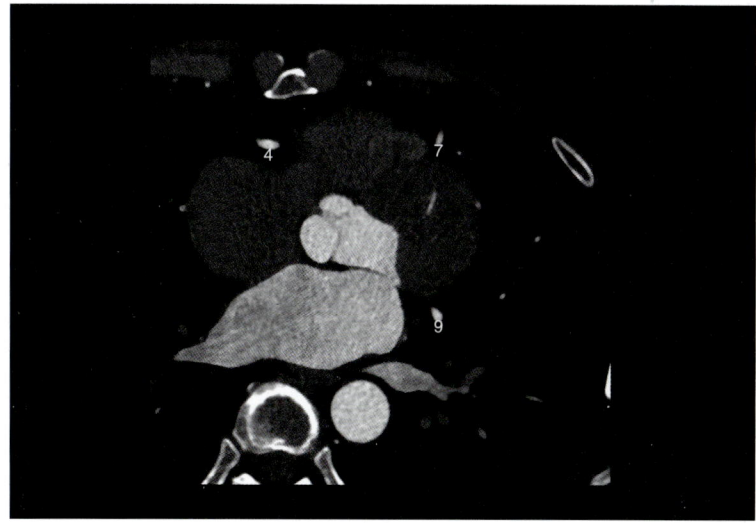

E. 冠状动脉 CT 增强图像

关键结构：乳腺，底段支气管和动脉。

此断面经过 T7-8 椎间盘上份。

右肺中叶及左肺舌叶均接近下部，两肺下叶进入各底段层面，各肺段内部的管道排列有较为明显的规律。首先，段间静脉位于段与段之间，管径略粗于段内支气管和伴行动脉。右肺中叶内、内外侧段支气管和动脉在各自段内伴行，两段管道之间见管径明显较大的外侧段静脉，可作为区分内、外侧段的标志；左肺舌叶内，下舌段动脉与段支气管伴行，区分上、下舌段的舌静脉干管径明显较粗，位于舌叶内侧面中部紧贴纵隔面处或下舌段支气管前内侧或前方；两肺下叶均见明显的底段上、下静脉，管径较周围其他底段管道粗大，位置在 4 个底段中心，相较于其他底段管道更靠近左心房。其次，各个段内的段支气管和段动脉均伴行[72]。乳腺位于胸壁浅层，为复管泡状腺体，包括乳管和腺泡两部分。乳腺癌是一种危害性大、死亡率高的恶性肿瘤，早期诊断、早期治疗是改善预后的关键[73]，目前临床应用的影像学方法有彩色多普勒超声、钼靶 X 线和 MRI，尤其是彩色多普勒超声已成为乳腺癌普查和诊疗的重要手段。乳腺癌的超声表现因病理分型繁杂而呈现复杂多样性，特别是早期乳腺癌，声像表现多不典型，给超声诊断带来一定困难，可通过联合钼靶 X 线、MRI 提高癌灶的检出率[74]，并指导治疗方案的制订。

胸部连续横断层 65（FH.12210）

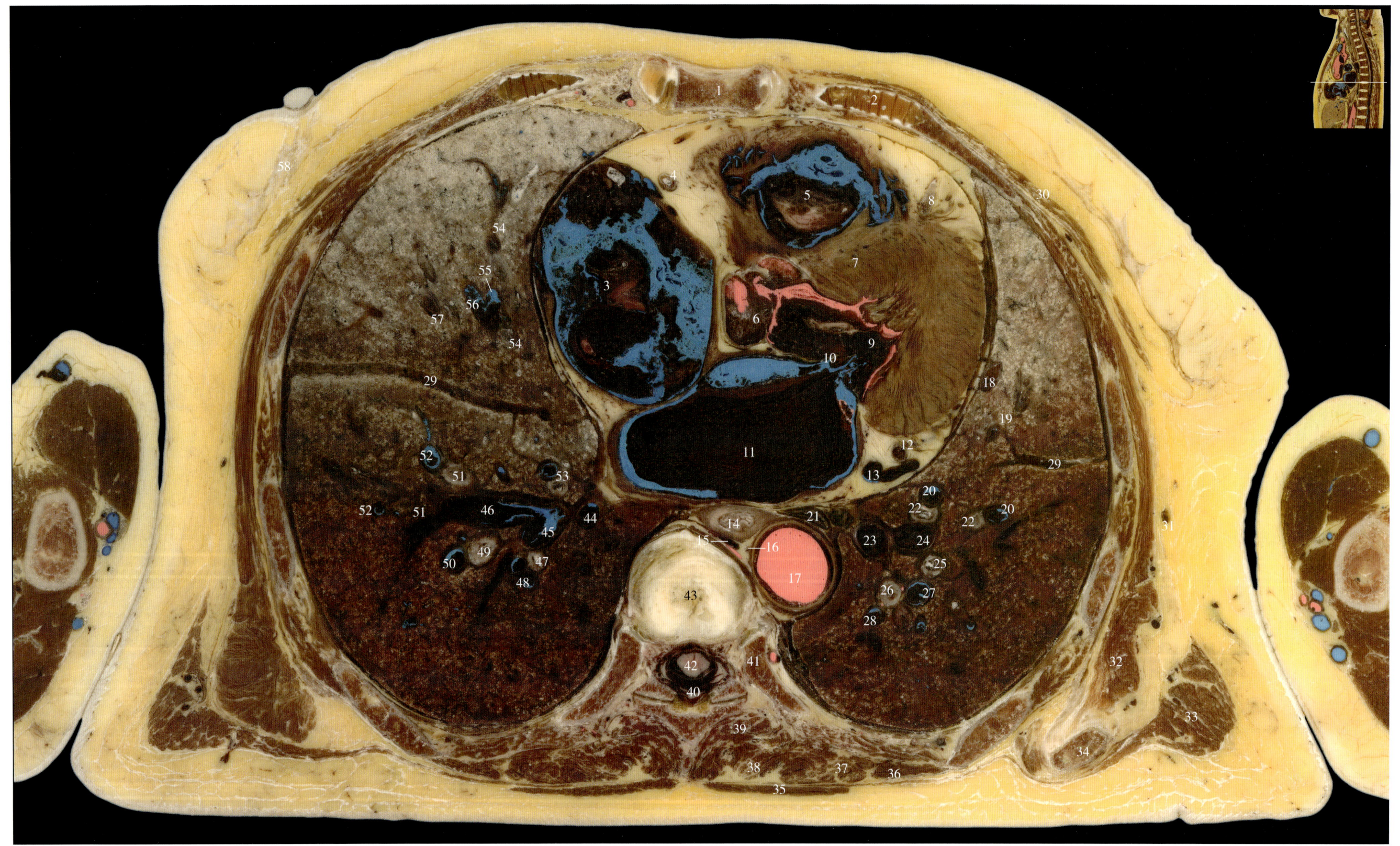

A. 断层标本图像

1. 胸骨体 body of sternum
2. 第 4 肋软骨 4th costal cartilage
3. 右心房 right atrium
4. 右冠状动脉 right coronary artery
5. 右心室 right ventricle
6. 主动脉窦 aortic sinus
7. 室间隔 interventricular septum
8. 前室间支 anterior interventricular branch
9. 左心室 left ventricle
10. 二尖瓣 mitral valve
11. 左心房 left atrium
12. 旋支 circumflex branch
13. 心大静脉 great cardiac vein
14. 食管 esophagus
15. 奇静脉 azygos vein
16. 胸导管 thoracic duct
17. 胸主动脉 thoracic aorta
18. 舌静脉干（V4+5）lingular venous trunk
19. 下舌段支气管（B5）和动脉（A5）inferior lingular segmental bronchus and artery
20. 内前底段动脉（A7+8）medioanterior basal segmental artery
21. 肺韧带淋巴结（9 区）pulmonary ligament lymph nodes
22. 内前底段支气管（B7+8）medioanterior basal segmental bronchus
23. 外后底段静脉（V9+10）posterolateral basal segmental vein
24. 内前底段静脉（V7+8）medioanterior basal segmental vein
25. 左肺外侧底段支气管（B9）left lateral basal segmental bronchus
26. 左肺后底段支气管（B10）left posterior basal segmental bronchus
27. 左肺外侧底段动脉（A9）left lateral basal segmental artery
28. 左肺后底段动脉（A10）left posterior basal segmental artery
29. 斜裂 oblique fissure
30. 胸大肌 pectoralis major
31. 胸外侧静脉 lateral thoracic vein
32. 前锯肌 serratus anterior
33. 背阔肌 latissimus dorsi
34. 肩胛骨 scapula
35. 斜方肌 trapezius
36. 髂肋肌 iliocostalis
37. 最长肌 longissimus
38. 棘肌 spinales
39. 横突棘肌 transversospinales
40. 硬膜外隙 epidural space
41. 第 8 肋骨 8th costal bone
42. 脊髓 spinal cord
43. T7-8 椎间盘 T7-8 intervertebral disc
44. 内侧底段静脉（V7）medial basal segmental vein
45. 右肺底段下静脉 right inferior basal vein
46. 右肺底段上静脉 right superior basal vein
47. 右肺后底段支气管（B10）right posterior basal segmental bronchus
48. 右肺后底段动脉（A10）right posterior basal segmental artery
49. 右肺外侧底段支气管（B9）right lateral basal segmental bronchus
50. 右肺外侧底段动脉（A9）right lateral basal segmental artery
51. 前底段支气管（B8）anterior basal segmental bronchus
52. 前底段动脉（A8）anterior basal segmental artery
53. 内侧底段支气管（B7）和动脉（A7）medial basal segmental bronchus and artery
54. 内侧段支气管（B5）和动脉（A5）medial segmental bronchus and artery
55. 内侧段静脉（V5）medial segmental vein
56. 外侧段静脉（V4）lateral segmental vein
57. 外侧段支气管（B4）和动脉（A4）lateral segmental bronchus and artery
58. 乳腺 mammary gland
59. 右肺底段总静脉 right common basal vein
60. 右肺前外侧底段支气管（B8+9）和动脉（A8+9）right anterolateral basal segmental bronchus and artery
61. 左肺外侧底段静脉（V9）left lateral basal segmental vein
62. 左肺后底段静脉（V10）left posterior basal segmental vein

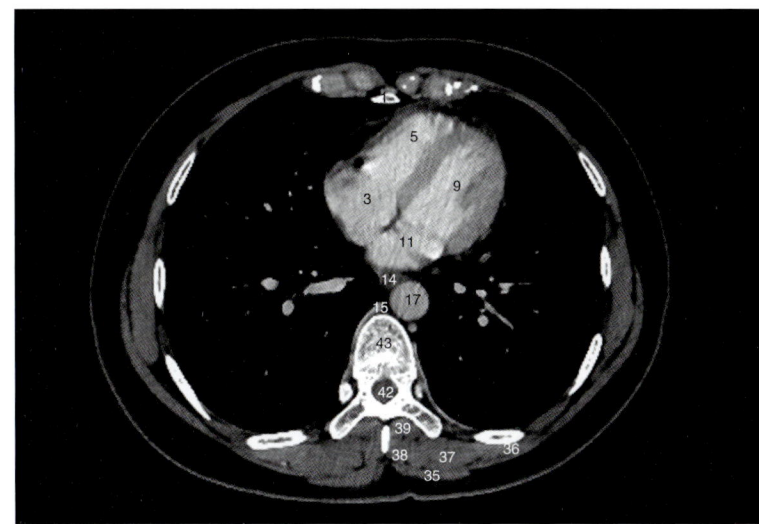

B. CT 纵隔窗增强图像

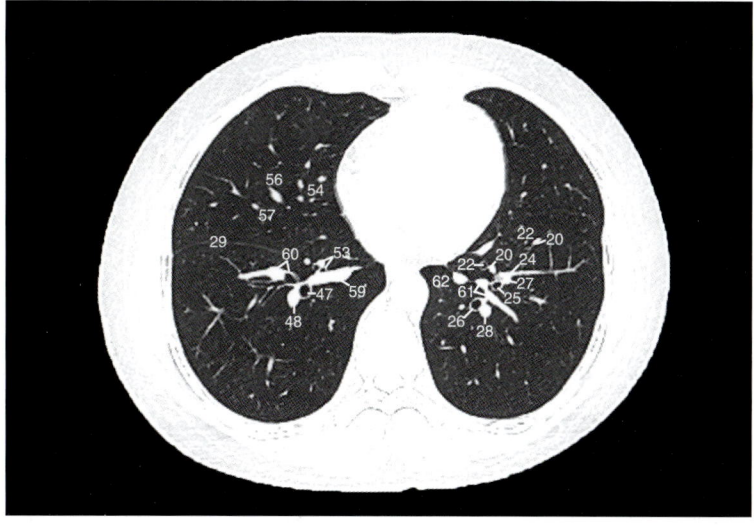

C. CT 肺窗图像

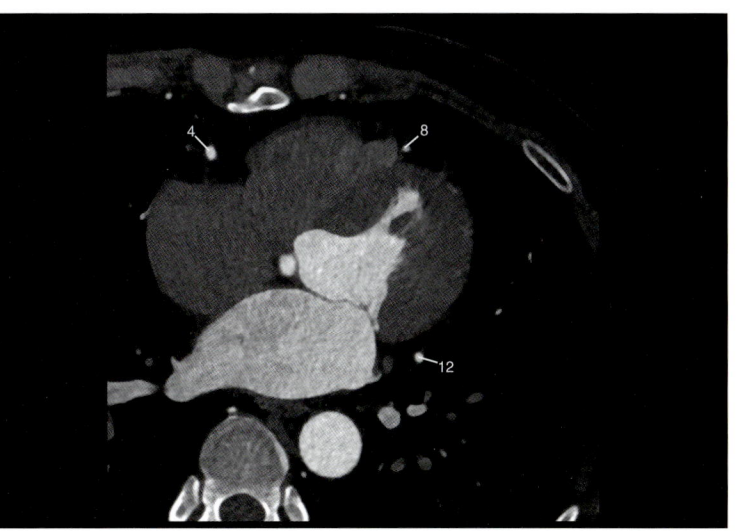
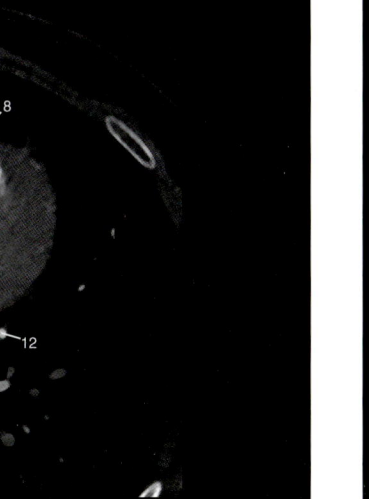

D. 冠状动脉 CT 增强图像

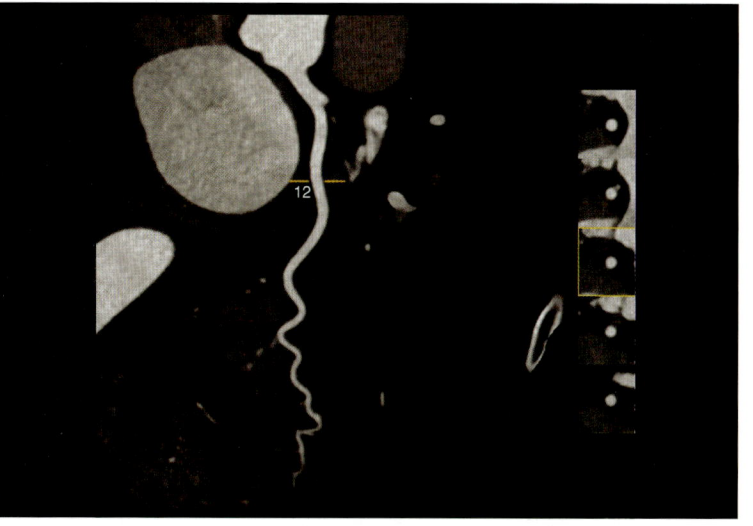

E. 左冠状动脉旋支 CT 重建图像

关键结构：左心房，旋支，心大静脉。

此断面经 T7-8 椎间盘中份。

左心房构成心底的大部分，居 4 个心腔中的最后方，其左前方突出的部分称左心耳，后方紧邻食管，当左心房扩大时可压迫食管，导致食管 X 线钡餐检查时心房压迹明显增大甚至食管后曲。左心房有 4 条肺静脉汇入，开口于左心房的后壁。左心房的出口为左房室口，位于左心房的前下部。左心房腔前部（即左心耳部分）梳状肌发达，而后部腔壁光滑。心表面的冠状沟右侧见右冠状动脉，左侧见左冠状动脉的旋支和心大静脉即将注入冠状窦。旋支是左冠状动脉的主要分支之一，直径为 2.8 mm ± 0.8 mm，在冠状沟左侧部行向外下，绕心左缘至膈面，其供血范围是左心房、左心室前壁的小部分、左室侧壁和后壁的大部分，甚至可达左室后乳头肌、窦房结和房室结。旋支长短不定，分布范围与右冠状动脉在膈面的分布互相配合。有 48% 终止于左室后面，40% 终止于左心缘，9% 的旋支至房室交点处，甚至延续为后室间支，2%~3% 到右心室膈面形成右室后支，极少数的心脏，旋支阙如[20]。心大静脉起于心尖或前室间沟的下 1/3，伴随前室间支上行，多位于动脉的浅面，于室间沟上 1/3 处斜向左上方，进入冠状沟，绕过心左缘至心后面的冠状沟，于左房斜静脉注入处移行为冠状窦。心大静脉沿途收纳左、右心室前壁，左房前壁和外侧壁，室间隔前部，左心耳及大动脉根部等的静脉血。

胸部连续横断层 66（FH.12190）

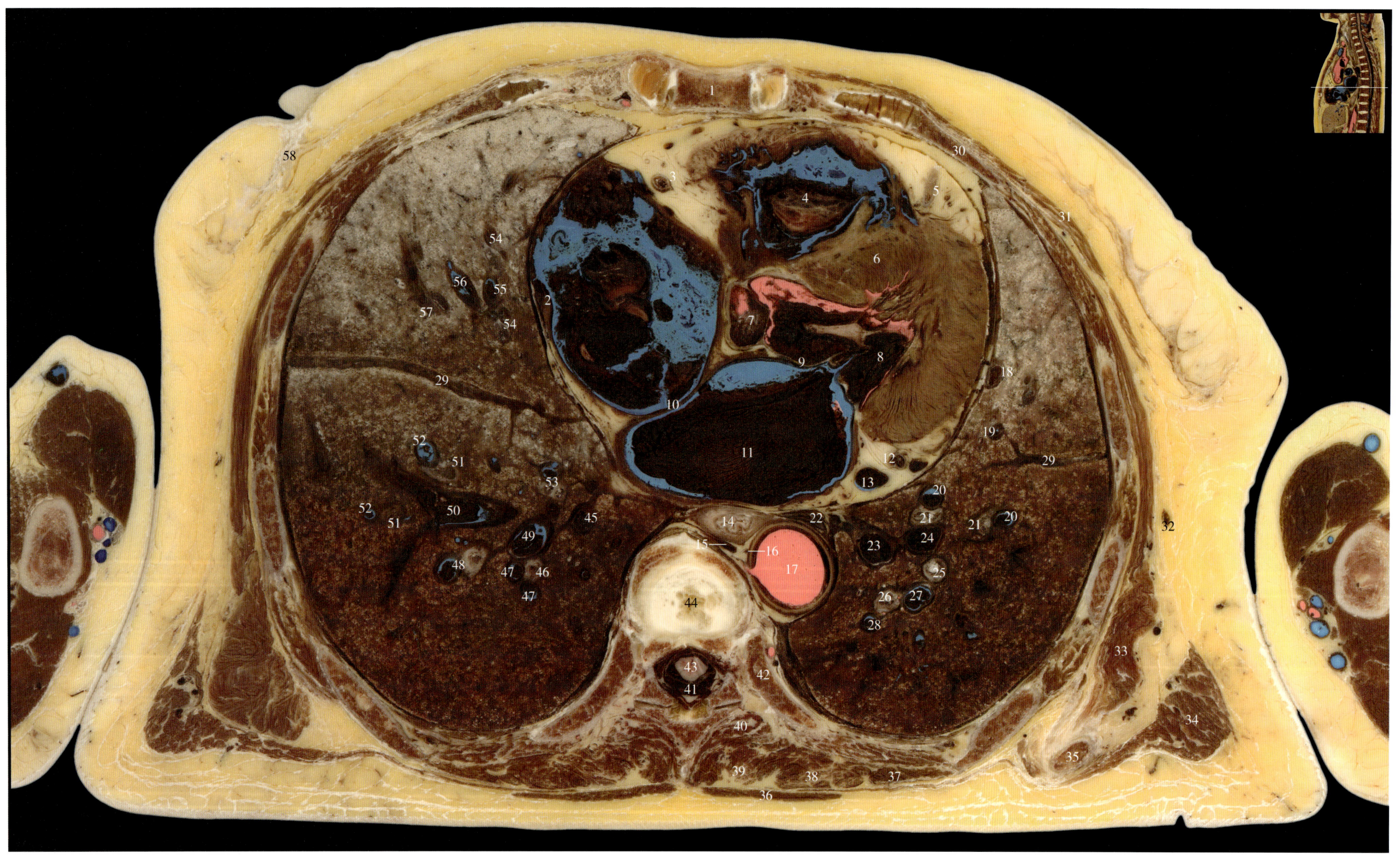

A. 断层标本图像

1. 胸骨体 body of sternum
2. 界嵴 crista terminalis
3. 右冠状动脉 right coronary artery
4. 右心室 right ventricle
5. 前室间支 anterior interventricular branch
6. 室间隔 interventricular septum
7. 主动脉窦 aortic sinus
8. 左心室 left ventricle
9. 二尖瓣 mitral valve
10. 房间隔 interatrial septum
11. 左心房 left atrium
12. 旋支 circumflex branch
13. 冠状窦 coronary sinus
14. 食管 esophagus
15. 奇静脉 azygos vein
16. 胸导管 thoracic duct
17. 胸主动脉 thoracic aorta
18. 舌静脉干（V4+5）lingular venous trunk
19. 下舌段支气管（B5）和动脉（A5）inferior lingular segmental bronchus and artery
20. 内前底段动脉（A7+8）medioanterior basal segmental artery
21. 内前底段支气管（B7+8）medioanterior basal segmental bronchus
22. 肺韧带淋巴结（9区）pulmonary ligament lymph nodes
23. 左肺外后底段静脉（V9+10）left posterolateral basal segmental vein
24. 内前底段静脉（V7+8）medioanterior basal segmental vein
25. 左肺外侧底段支气管（B9）left lateral basal segmental bronchus
26. 左肺后底段支气管（B10）left posterior basal segmental bronchus
27. 左肺外侧底段动脉（A9）left lateral basal segmental artery
28. 左肺后底段动脉（A10）left posterior basal segmental artery
29. 斜裂 oblique fissure
30. 第 4 肋骨 4th costal bone
31. 胸大肌 pectoralis major
32. 胸外侧静脉 lateral thoracic vein
33. 前锯肌 serratus anterior
34. 背阔肌 latissimus dorsi
35. 肩胛骨 scapula
36. 斜方肌 trapezius
37. 髂肋肌 iliocostalis
38. 最长肌 longissimus
39. 棘肌 spinales
40. 横突棘肌 transversospinales
41. 硬膜外隙 epidural space
42. 第 8 肋骨 8th costal bone
43. 脊髓 spinal cord
44. T7-8 椎间盘 T7-8 intervertebral disc
45. 内侧底段静脉（V7）medial basal segmental vein
46. 右肺后底段支气管（B10）right posterior basal segmental bronchus
47. 右肺后底段动脉（A10）right posterior basal segmental artery
48. 右肺外侧底段支气管（B9）和动脉（A9）right lateral basal segmental bronchus and artery
49. 右肺底段下静脉 right inferior basal vein
50. 右肺底段上静脉 right superior basal vein
51. 前底段支气管（B8）anterior basal segmental bronchus
52. 前底段动脉（A8）anterior basal segmental artery
53. 内侧底段支气管（B7）和动脉（A7）medial basal segmental bronchus and artery
54. 内侧段支气管（B5）和动脉（A5）medial segmental bronchus and artery
55. 内侧段静脉（V5）medial segmental vein
56. 外侧段静脉（V4）lateral segmental vein
57. 外侧段支气管（B4）和动脉（A4）lateral segmental bronchus and artery
58. 乳腺 mammary gland
59. 左肺外侧段静脉（V9）left lateral basal segmental vein
60. 左肺后底段静脉（V10）left posterior basal segmental vein
61. 右肺前外侧底段支气管（B8+9）和动脉（A8+9）right anterolateral basal segmental bronchus and artery

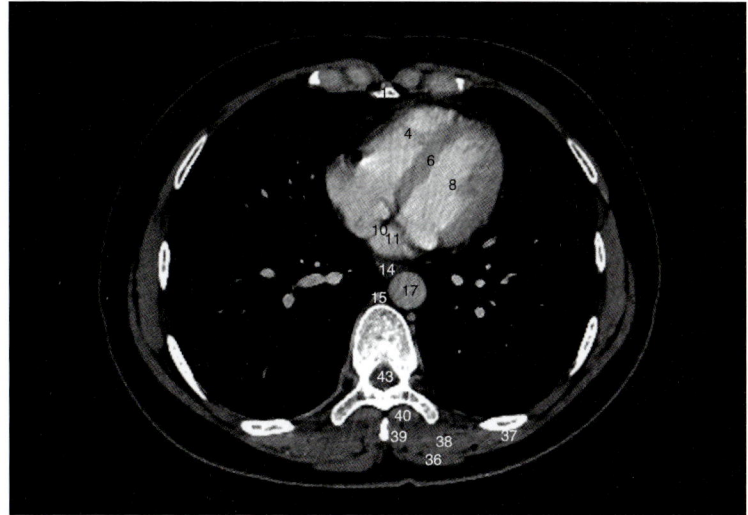

B. CT 纵隔窗增强图像

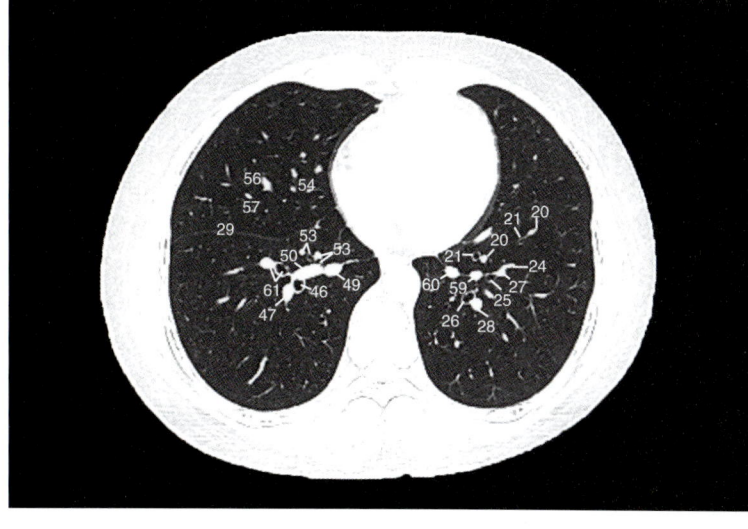

C. CT 肺窗图像

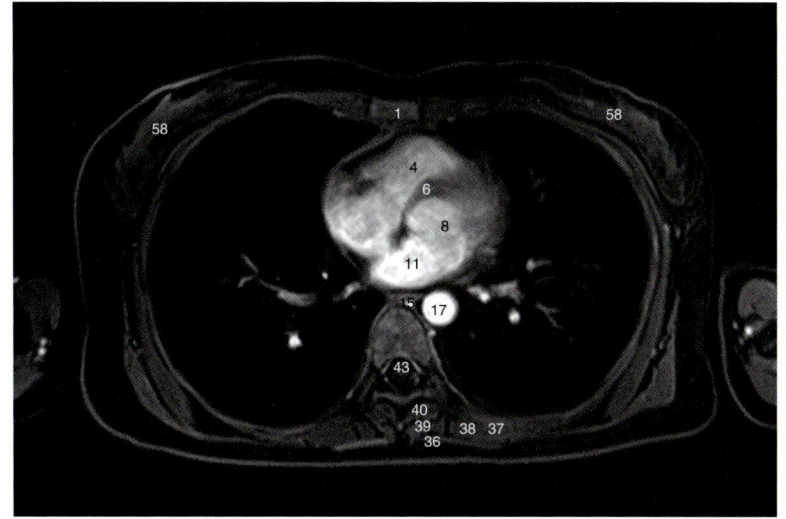

D. MR T1WI 增强图像

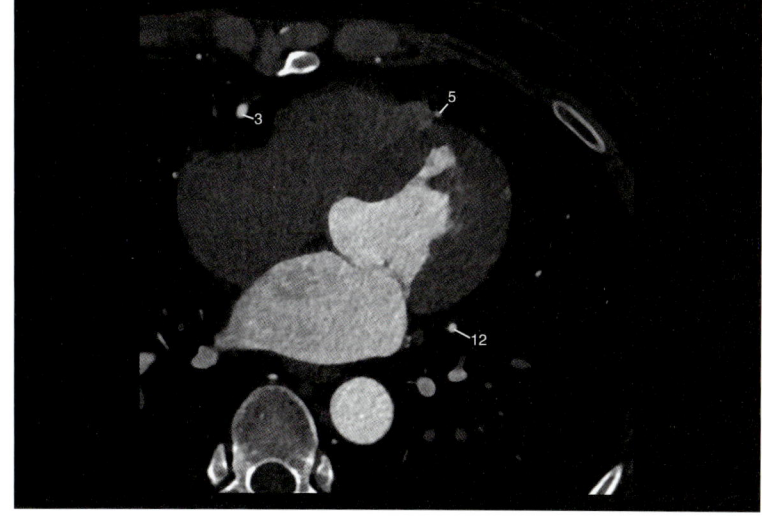

E. 冠状动脉 CT 增强图像

关键结构：左心房，冠状窦。

此断面经 T7-8 椎间盘下份。

左心房和左心室后方的冠状沟左侧部，见冠状窦及左冠状动脉旋支走行。冠状窦及其属支是心脏最主要的静脉系，主要功能是汇集来自心肌的静脉血，并将其引流回右心房。冠状窦也是许多心脏疾病诊断治疗的通道和重要标志，尤其是在心律失常的射频消融、多心腔起搏器的置入及心脏逆向灌注治疗中发挥着极为重要的作用。正常情况下，冠状窦位于心脏后部、心包斜窦下缘的冠状沟内，向右越过房间隔，于下腔静脉口和右房室口之间注入右心房。其主要属支有心大静脉、心中静脉、心小静脉、左心室后静脉和左心房斜静脉。CT 图像中，71.4% 的冠状窦呈管状，喇叭状占 28.6%。解剖学多以左心房斜静脉汇入处作为冠状窦与心大静脉分界点，但左心房斜静脉细小，造影及多层螺旋 CT 常不能清晰显示，故也可选用冠状窦突然变细处作为起始点。冠状窦长度为 36.2 mm ± 8.8 mm，起始处外径为 6.9 mm ± 2.0 mm，中段的外径为 8.5 mm ± 2.9 mm，末端外径为 10.4 mm ± 3.2 mm。冠状窦口有不完整的冠状窦瓣（Thebesian 瓣），出现率约为 79.2%，可为半月形、网状或条索状，其中半月形最多见，而当瓣膜呈条索状横架于冠状窦口时，可能会阻挡导管的进入，增加插管的难度[75]。

胸部连续横断层 67（FH.12170）

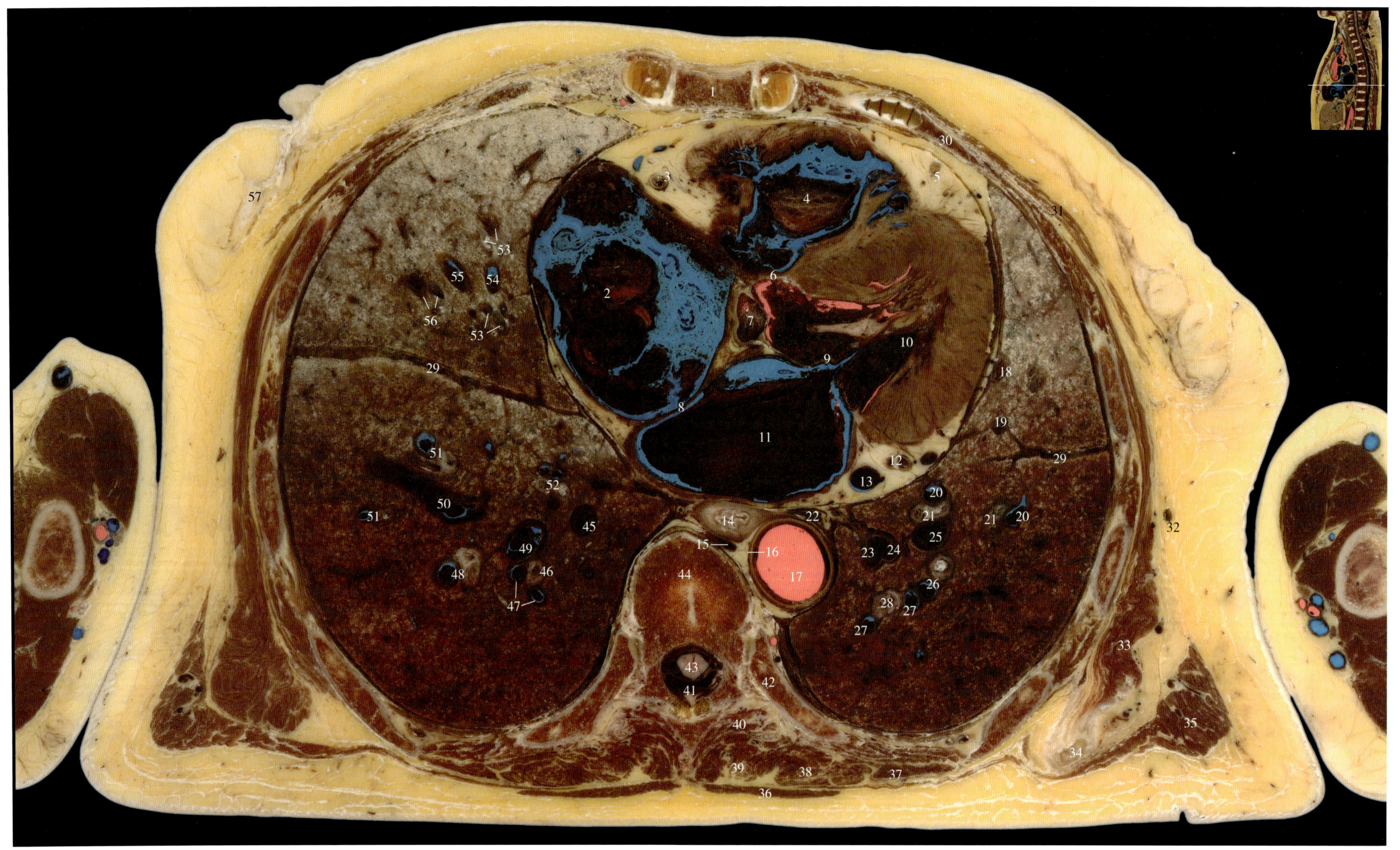

A. 断层标本图像

1. 胸骨体 body of sternum
2. 右心房 right atrium
3. 右冠状动脉 right coronary artery
4. 右心室 right ventricle
5. 前室间支 anterior interventricular branch
6. 室间隔膜部 membranous part of interventricular septum
7. 主动脉窦 aortic sinus
8. 房间隔 interatrial septum
9. 二尖瓣 mitral valve
10. 左心室 left ventricle
11. 左心房 left atrium
12. 旋支 circumflex branch
13. 冠状窦 coronary sinus
14. 食管 esophagus
15. 奇静脉 azygos vein
16. 胸导管 thoracic duct
17. 胸主动脉 thoracic aorta
18. 舌静脉干（V4+5）lingular venous trunk
19. 下舌段支气管（B5）和动脉（A5）inferior lingular segmental bronchus and artery
20. 内前底段动脉（A7+8）medioanterior basal segmental artery
21. 内前底段支气管（B7+8）medioanterior basal segmental bronchus
22. 肺韧带 pulmonary ligament
23. 左肺后底段静脉（V10）left posterior basal segmental vein
24. 左肺外侧底段静脉（V9）left lateral basal segmental vein
25. 内前底段静脉（V7+8）medioanterior basal segmental vein
26. 左肺外侧底段支气管（B9）和动脉（A9）left lateral basal segmental bronchus and artery
27. 左肺后底段动脉（A10）left posterior basal segmental artery
28. 左肺后底段支气管（B10）left posterior basal segmental bronchus
29. 斜裂 oblique fissure
30. 第 4 肋骨 4th costal bone
31. 胸大肌 pectoralis major
32. 胸外侧静脉 lateral thoracic vein
33. 前锯肌 serratus anterior
34. 肩胛骨下角 inferior angle of scapula
35. 背阔肌 latissimus dorsi
36. 斜方肌 trapezius
37. 髂肋肌 iliocostalis
38. 最长肌 longissimus
39. 棘肌 spinales
40. 横突棘肌 transversospinales
41. 硬膜外隙 epidural space
42. 第 8 肋骨 8th costal bone
43. 脊髓 spinal cord
44. 第 8 胸椎椎体 body of 8th thoracic vertebra
45. 内侧底段静脉（V7）medial basal segmental vein
46. 右肺后底段支气管（B10）right posterior basal segmental bronchus
47. 右肺后底段动脉（A10）right posterior basal segmental artery
48. 右肺外侧底段支气管（B9）和动脉（A9）right lateral basal segmental bronchus and artery
49. 右肺外后底段静脉（V9+10）right posterolateral basal segmental vein
50. 前底段静脉（V8）anterior basal segmental vein
51. 前底段支气管（B8）和动脉（A8）right anterior basal segmental bronchus and artery
52. 内侧底段支气管（B7）和动脉（A7）medial basal segmental bronchus and artery
53. 内侧段支气管（B5）和动脉（A5）medial segmental bronchus and artery
54. 内侧段静脉（V5）medial segmental vein
55. 外侧段静脉（V4）lateral segmental vein
56. 外侧段支气管（B4）和动脉（A4）lateral segmental bronchus and artery
57. 乳腺 mammary gland
58. 右肺底段上静脉 right superior basal vein
59. 右肺底段下静脉 right inferior basal vein
60. 右肺前外侧底段支气管（B8+9）和动脉（A8+9）right anterolateral basal segmental bronchus and artery

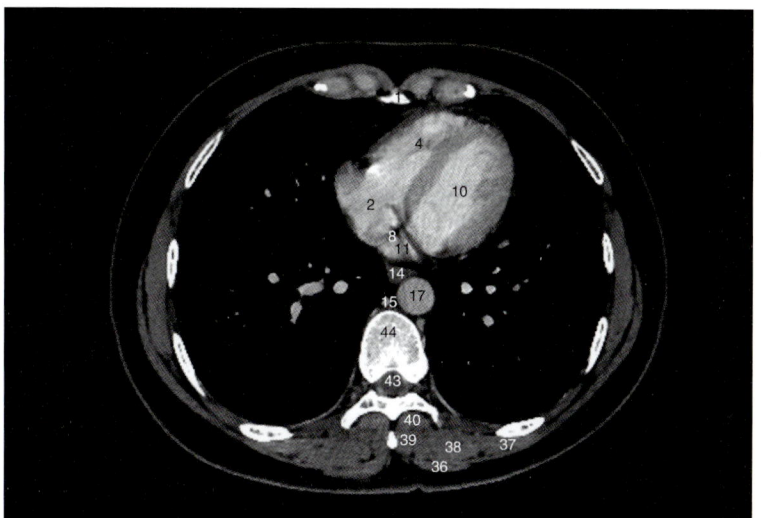

B. CT 纵隔窗增强图像

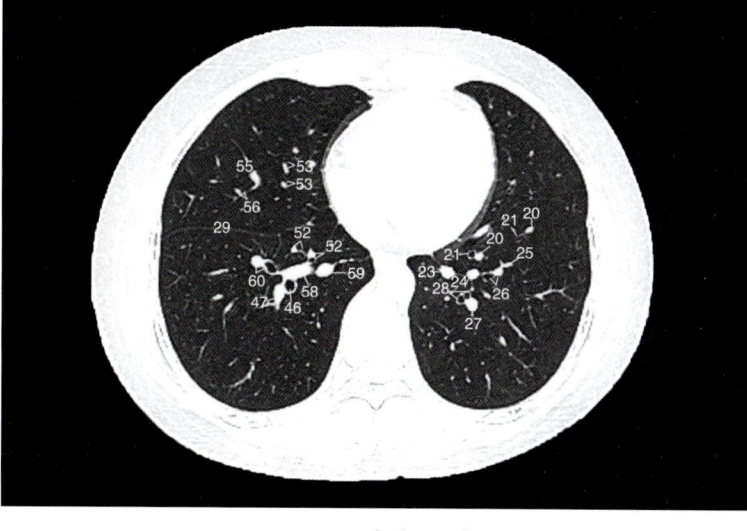

C. CT 肺窗图像

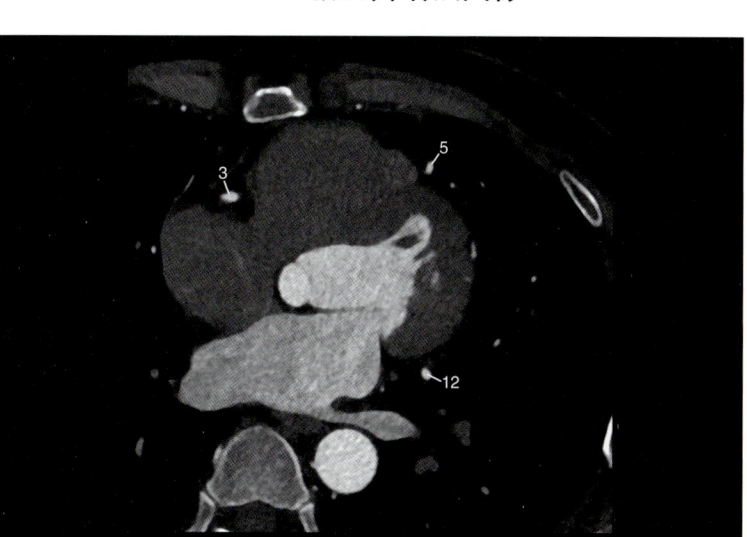

D. 冠状动脉 CT 增强图像

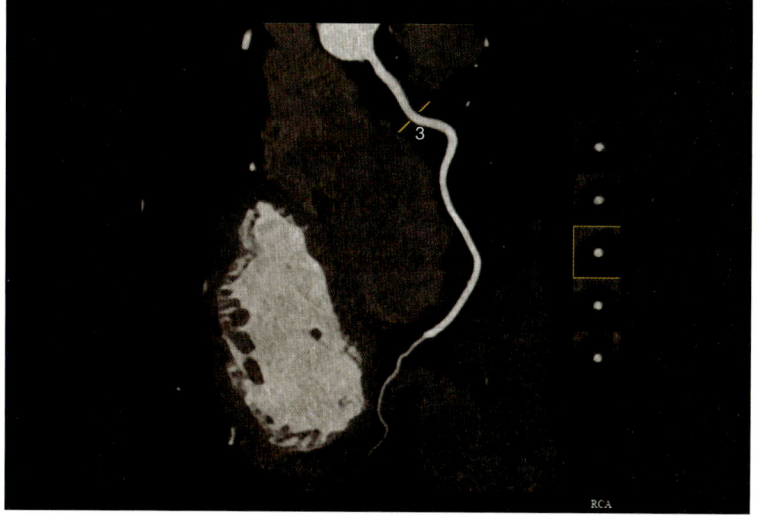

E. 右冠状动脉 CT 重建图像

关键结构：冠状沟，前室间沟。

此断面经第 8 胸椎上份。

近心底处呈额状位的环状沟即为冠状沟，是心表面分隔后方心室与前方心室的标志。在横断面中，冠状沟右侧前部位于右心房与右心室之间，沟内有右冠状动脉；冠状沟左侧后部位于左心房和左心室间，沟内见冠状窦。前室间沟是心的胸肋面自冠状沟向心尖延伸的浅沟，与室间隔的前缘一致，是左、右心室在心前表面的分界，沟内有左冠状动脉的前室间支（临床上常称为左前降支）和心大静脉。心脏表面有 4 条沟，可作为 4 个心腔的表面分界。

冠状沟分隔心房和心室，前方被肺动脉干所中断；前、后室间沟分隔左、右心室，在心尖右侧的交汇处稍凹陷，称心尖切迹；房间沟分隔左、右心房。冠状沟和前、后室间沟内被心的血管和脂肪组织等填充，使心脏表面沟的轮廓不清晰。本断面纵隔内 4 个心腔的结构均清晰显示，4 个心腔的位置亦较为典型：右心室位于纵隔前方，右心房位于纵隔右侧，左心室位于纵隔左侧，左心房位于后部。4 个心腔中，通常左心房的位置较高，在横断面从上至下的连续断面中，左心房较早出现，亦较早消失。

胸部连续横断层 68（FH.12150）

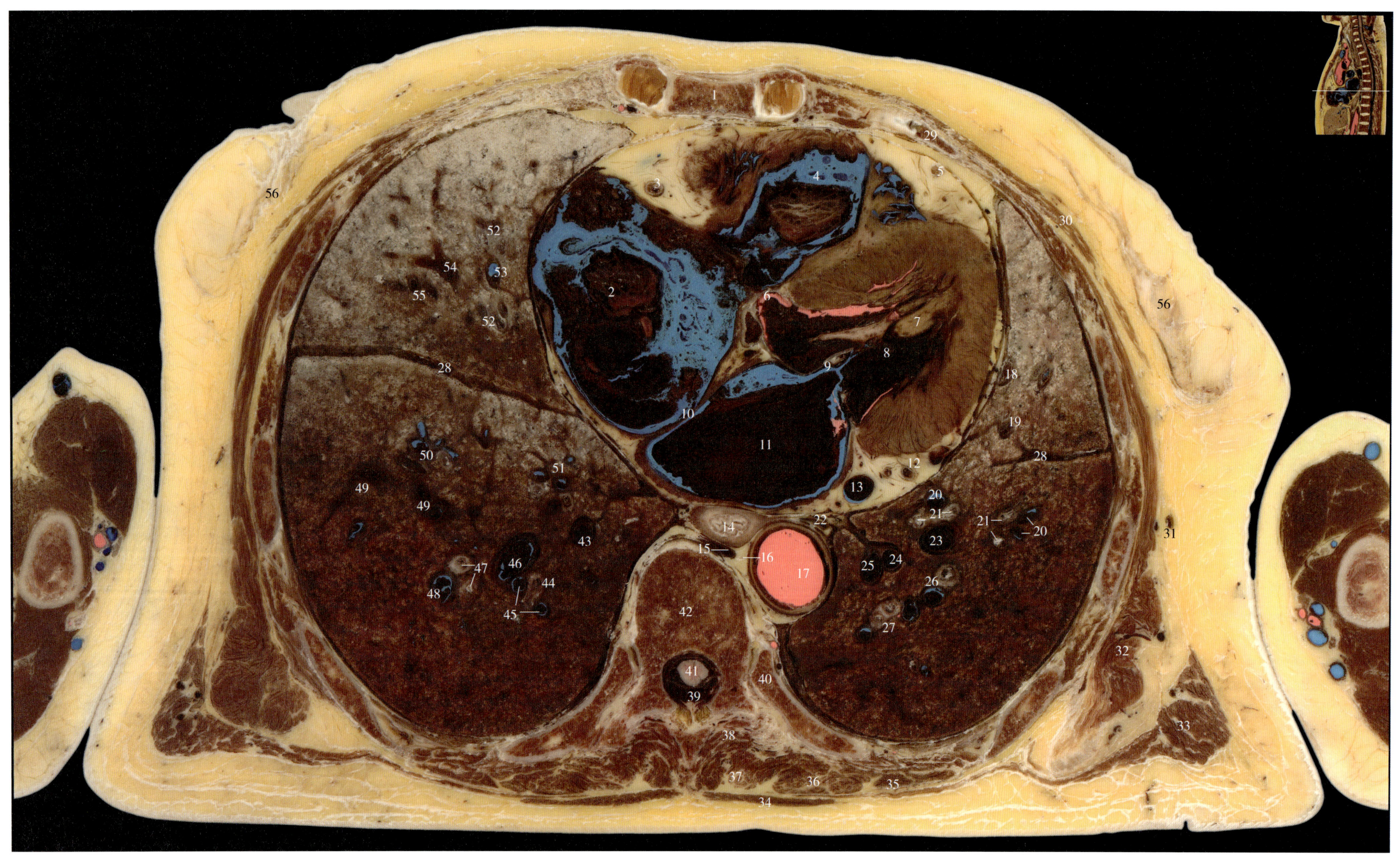

A. 断层标本图像

1. 胸骨体 body of sternum
2. 右心房 right atrium
3. 右冠状动脉 right coronary artery
4. 右心室 right ventricle
5. 前室间支 anterior interventricular branch
6. 室间隔膜部 membranous part of interventricular septum
7. 乳头肌 papillary muscle
8. 左心室 left ventricle
9. 二尖瓣 mitral valve
10. 房间隔 interatrial septum
11. 左心房 left atrium
12. 旋支 circumflex branch
13. 冠状窦 coronary sinus
14. 食管 esophagus
15. 奇静脉 azygos vein
16. 胸导管 thoracic duct
17. 胸主动脉 thoracic aorta
18. 舌静脉干（V4+5）lingular venous trunk
19. 下舌段支气管（B5）和动脉（A5）inferior lingular segmental bronchus and artery
20. 内前底段动脉（A7+8）medioanterior basal segmental artery
21. 内前底段支气管（B7+8）medioanterior basal segmental bronchus
22. 肺韧带 pulmonary ligament
23. 内前底段静脉（V7+8）medioanterior basal segmental vein
24. 左肺外侧底段静脉（V9）left lateral basal segmental vein
25. 左肺后底段静脉（V10）left posterior basal segmental vein
26. 左肺外侧底段支气管（B9）和动脉（A9）left lateral basal segmental bronchus and artery
27. 左肺后底段支气管（B10）和动脉（A10）left posterior basal segmental bronchus and artery
28. 斜裂 oblique fissure
29. 第 4 肋骨 4th costal bone
30. 胸大肌 pectoralis major
31. 胸外侧静脉 lateral thoracic vein
32. 前锯肌 serratus anterior
33. 背阔肌 latissimus dorsi

34. 斜方肌 trapezius
35. 髂肋肌 iliocostalis
36. 最长肌 longissimus
37. 棘肌 spinales
38. 横突棘肌 transversospinales
39. 硬膜外隙 epidural space
40. 第 8 肋骨 8th costal bone
41. 脊髓 spinal cord
42. 第 8 胸椎椎体 body of 8th thoracic vertebra
43. 内侧底段静脉（V7）medial basal segmental vein
44. 右肺后底段支气管（B10）right posterior basal segmental bronchus
45. 右肺后底段动脉（A10）right posterior basal segmental artery
46. 右肺外后底段静脉（V9+10）right posterolateral basal segmental vein
47. 右肺外侧底段支气管（B9）right lateral basal segmental bronchus
48. 右肺外侧底段动脉（A9）right lateral basal segmental artery
49. 前底段静脉（V8）anterior basal segmental vein
50. 前底段支气管（B8）和动脉（A8）anterior basal segmental bronchus and artery
51. 内侧底段支气管（B7）和动脉（A7）medial basal segmental bronchus and artery
52. 内侧底段支气管（B5）和动脉（A5）medial segmental bronchus and artery
53. 内侧段静脉（V5）medial segmental vein
54. 外侧段静脉（V4）lateral segmental vein
55. 外侧段支气管（B4）和动脉（A4）lateral segmental bronchus and artery
56. 乳腺 mammary gland
57. 右肺底段上静脉 right superior basal vein
58. 右肺底段下静脉 right inferior basal vein
59. 前底段支气管（B8）anterior basal segmental bronchus
60. 右肺前外侧底段动脉（A8+9）right anterolateral basal segmental artery

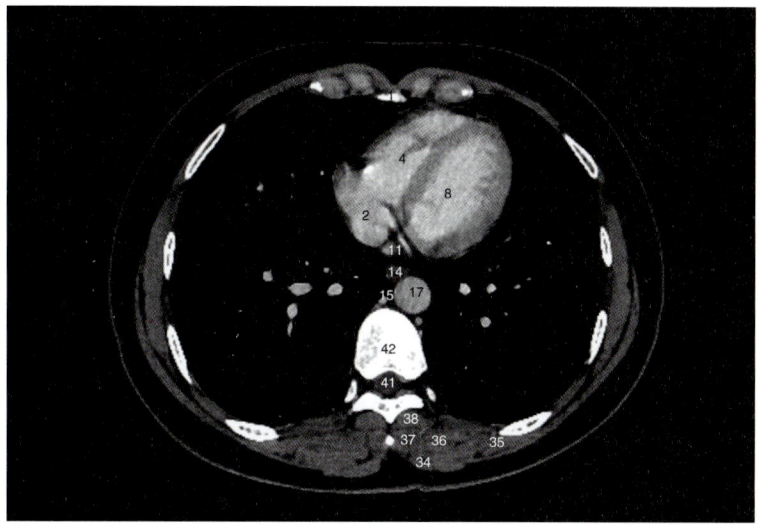

B. CT 纵隔窗增强图像

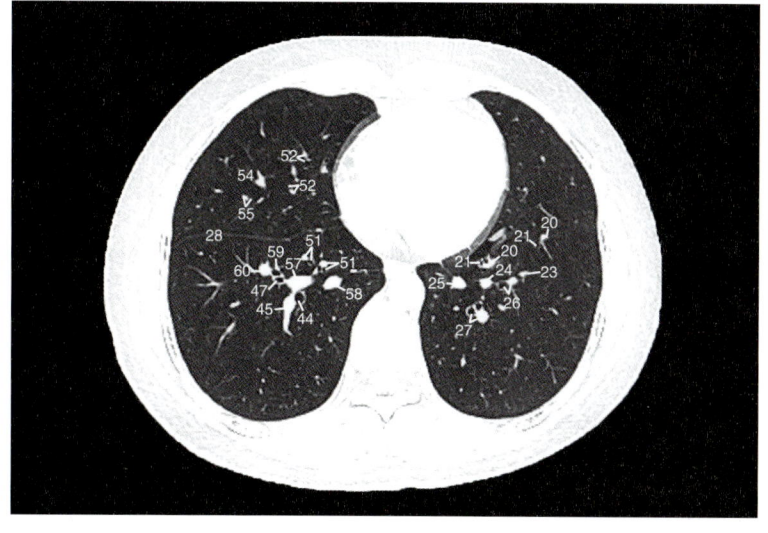

C. CT 肺窗图像

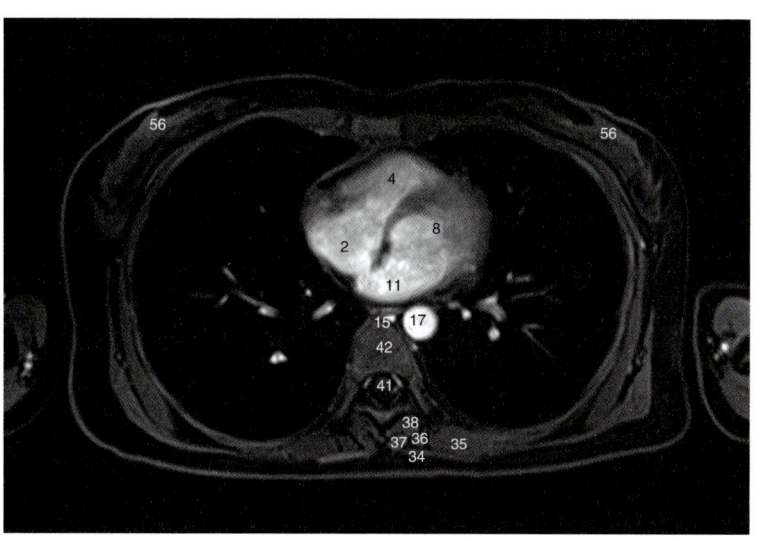

D. MR T1WI 增强图像

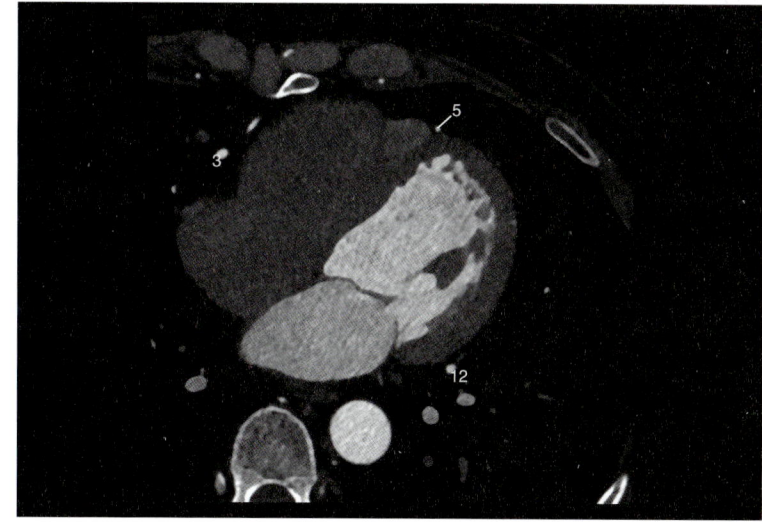

E. 冠状动脉 CT 增强图像

关键结构：房间隔，卵圆窝，乳头肌。

此断面经第 8 胸椎椎体上份。

房间隔由原发隔和继发隔发育而来，位于左、右心房之间，呈矢状位，前缘向左前方倾斜。房间隔右侧面中下部有卵圆窝，为胚胎时期卵圆孔闭合后的遗迹，是房间隔缺损的好发部位，也是右心房进入左心房导管穿刺的理想部位。卵圆窝的面积与房间隔的总面积相比，成人为 24%，儿童为 28%。约有 50% 的标本，卵圆窝上缘存在着斜位的裂缝，探针可由右心房通入左心房，但由于左心房压力高于右心房，故不存在血液的分流。房间隔前上部的右心房内侧壁，由主动脉窦向右心房凸起形成主动脉隆凸，为心导管术的重要标志[76]。房间隔的左侧面较平整，只在前缘上部附近可见一肌性弓状边缘，此为原发房间隔边缘缺损。当房间隔未完全闭合时，此处可呈一小的半月形裂隙使左右房相通，心导管可通过这一裂隙由右心房通至左心房。左心室流入道内见前乳头肌连于心室前壁。左心室乳头肌较右心室粗大，分为前、后两组，发自左心室壁的前上和后下，不发自室间隔。前乳头肌 1~5 个，位于左心室前外侧壁的中部，常为单个粗大的锥状肌束；后乳头肌 1~5 个，位于左心室后壁的内侧部。前乳头肌主要接受左冠状动脉的前室间支、对角支和旋支的血液供应，后乳头肌主要接受右冠状动脉的分支。

胸部连续横断层 69（FH.12130）

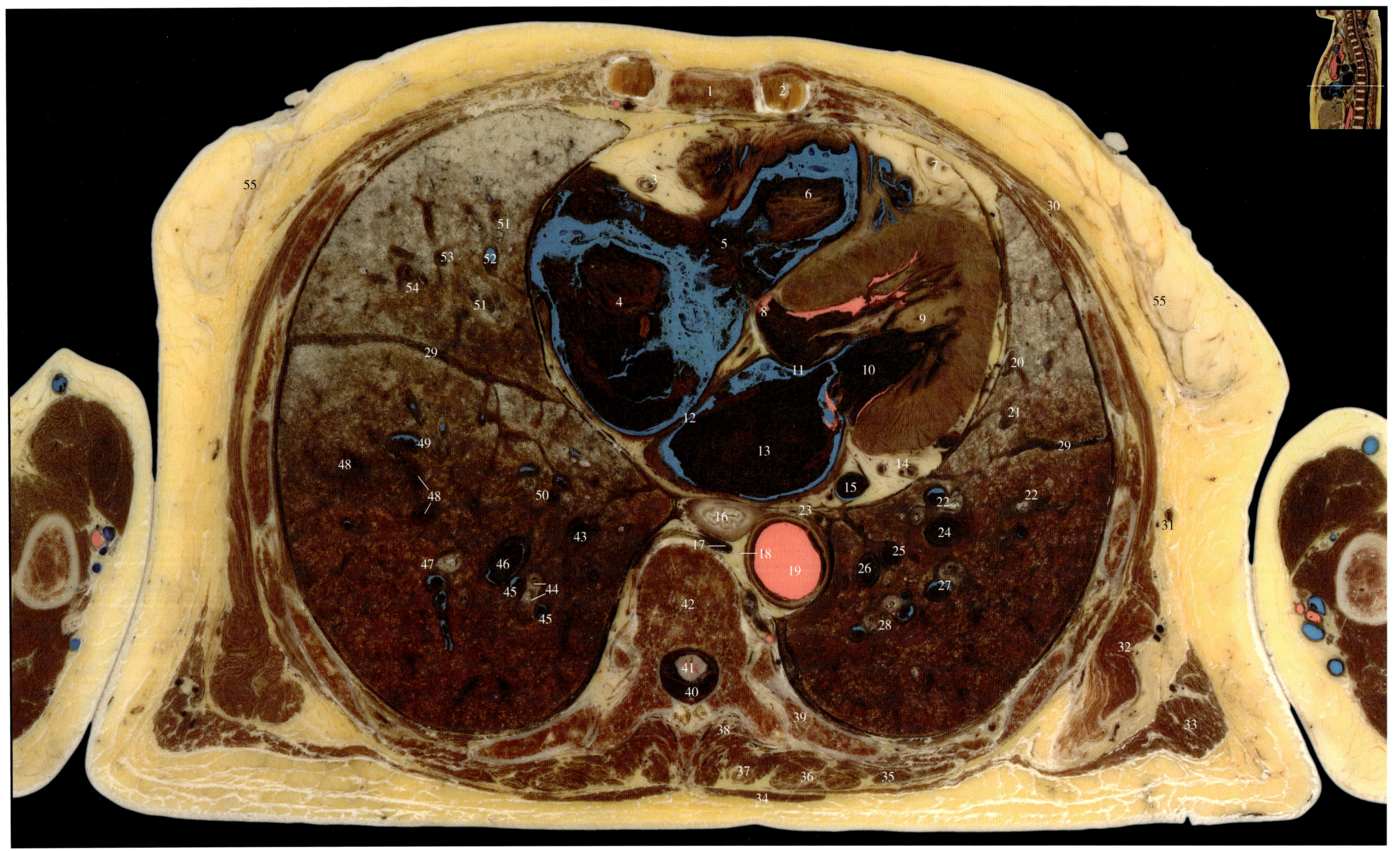

A. 断层标本图像

1. 胸骨体 body of sternum
2. 第 5 肋软骨 5th costal cartilage
3. 右冠状动脉 right coronary artery
4. 右心房 right atrium
5. 三尖瓣 tricuspid valve
6. 右心室 right ventricle
7. 前室间支 anterior interventricular branch
8. 室间隔膜部 membranous part of interventricular septum
9. 乳头肌 papillary muscle
10. 左心室 left ventricle
11. 二尖瓣 mitral valve
12. 房间隔 interatrial septum
13. 左心房 left atrium
14. 旋支 circumflex branch
15. 冠状窦 coronary sinus
16. 食管 esophagus
17. 奇静脉 azygos vein
18. 胸导管 thoracic duct
19. 胸主动脉 thoracic aorta
20. 舌静脉干（V4+5）lingular venous trunk
21. 下舌段支气管（B5）和动脉（A5）inferior lingular segmental bronchus and artery
22. 内前底段支气管（B7+8）和动脉（A7+8）medioanterior basal segmental artery
23. 肺韧带 pulmonary ligament
24. 内前底段静脉（V7+8）medioanterior basal segmental vein
25. 左肺外侧底段静脉（V9）left lateral basal segmental vein
26. 左肺后底段静脉（V10）left posterior basal segmental vein
27. 左肺外侧底段支气管（B9）和动脉（A9）left lateral basal segmental bronchus and artery
28. 左肺后底段支气管（B10）和动脉（A10）left posterior basal segmental bronchus and artery
29. 斜裂 oblique fissure
30. 胸大肌 pectoralis major
31. 胸外侧静脉 lateral thoracic vein
32. 前锯肌 serratus anterior
33. 背阔肌 latissimus dorsi
34. 斜方肌 trapezius
35. 髂肋肌 iliocostalis
36. 最长肌 longissimus
37. 棘肌 spinales
38. 横突棘肌 transversospinales
39. 第 8 肋骨 8th costal bone
40. 硬膜外隙 epidural space
41. 脊髓 spinal cord
42. 第 8 胸椎椎体 body of 8th thoracic vertebra
43. 内侧底段静脉（V7）medial basal segmental vein
44. 右肺后底段支气管（B10）right posterior basal segmental bronchus
45. 右肺后底段动脉（A10）right posterior basal segmental bronchus
46. 右肺外后底段静脉（V9+10）right posterolateral basal segmental vein
47. 右肺外侧底段支气管（B9）和动脉（A9）right lateral basal segmental bronchus and artery
48. 前底段静脉（V8）anterior basal segmental vein
49. 前底段支气管（B8）和动脉（A8）anterior basal segmental bronchus and artery
50. 内侧底段支气管（B7）和动脉（A7）medial basal segmental bronchus and artery
51. 内侧段支气管（B5）和动脉（A5）medial segmental bronchus and artery
52. 内侧段静脉（V5）medial segmental vein
53. 外侧段静脉（V4）lateral segmental vein
54. 外侧段支气管（B4）和动脉（A4）lateral segmental bronchus and artery
55. 乳腺 mammary gland
56. 右肺外侧底段静脉（V9）right lateral basal segmental vein
57. 右肺后底段静脉（V10）right posterior basal segmental vein

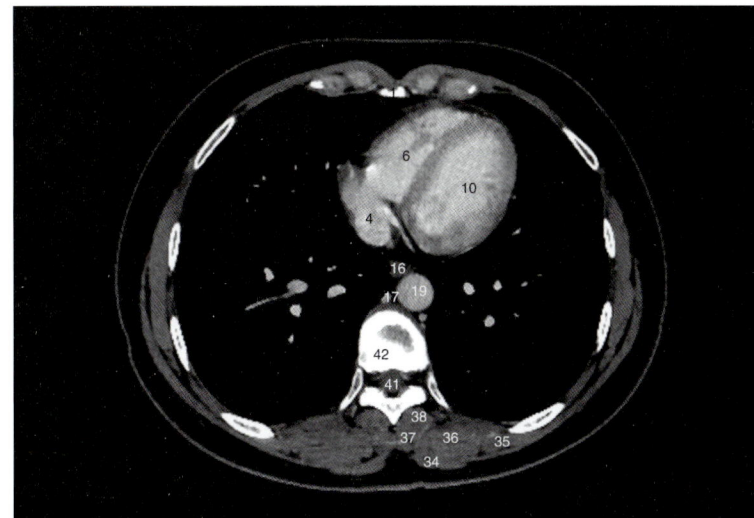

B. CT 纵隔窗增强图像

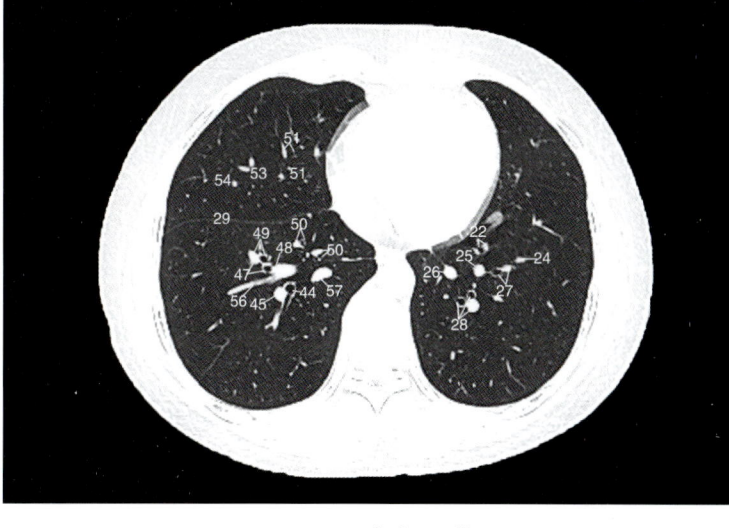

C. CT 肺窗图像

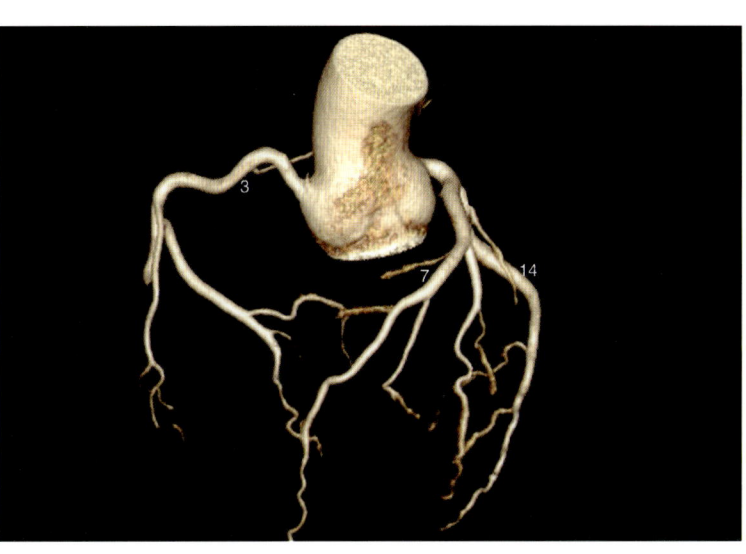

D. 冠状动脉 VR 重建图像前面观

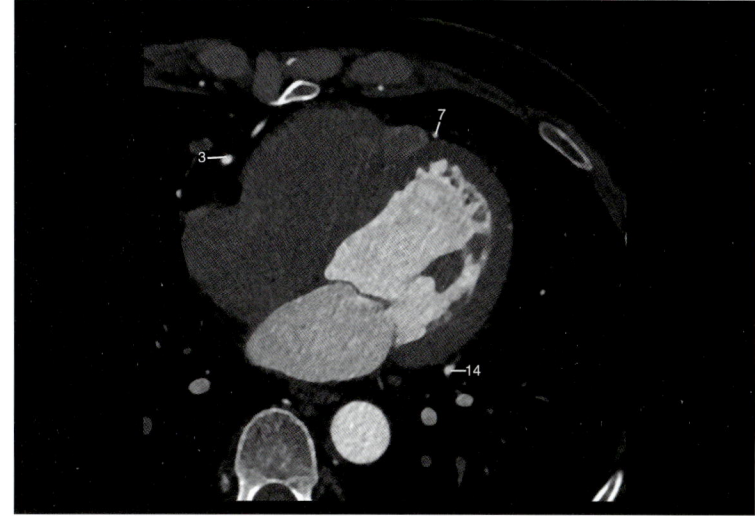

E. 冠状动脉 CT 增强图像

关键结构：室间隔膜部，室间隔。

此层面经第 8 胸椎椎体中份。

室间隔位于左、右心室之间，分为肌部和膜部，肌部占室间隔的大部分，主要由心肌纤维及两侧的心内膜构成，厚 1~2 cm。膜部是室间隔上缘较小的区域，由致密结缔组织和两侧的心内膜构成。从左心室腔面观察，室间隔膜部位于主动脉前瓣环与后瓣环相对缘的下方和室间隔肌部上缘之间。随其形态和大小不同，其边缘位置和毗邻也有相应的变化：室间隔膜部与主动脉前瓣和后瓣相对缘的瓣环直接相连，占 37.5%；室间隔膜部只与主动脉后瓣环直接相连，占 29.7%；与主动脉前瓣环直接相接，占 6.3%；低于两瓣环，占 26.6%[77]。室间隔膜部右侧面被三尖瓣的隔侧尖附着，故其上方介于右心房和左心室之间，称为房室间部；下方位于左、右心室之间，称室间部。膜部的后下缘有房室束通过，下缘与肌部之间为房室束的分叉部。膜部是室间隔缺损的好发部位，手术时注意这些结构关系。室间隔的供血常来自左冠状动脉前室间支的分支－室间隔支，可多达 12~17 支，供应其前 2/3。右冠状动脉的后室间支（亦称后降支，94% 来自右冠状动脉，其余来自旋支）发出分支供应室间隔的后 1/3。室间隔供血障碍可导致束支阻滞和室间隔肌纤维功能失调。

胸部连续横断层 70（FH.12110）

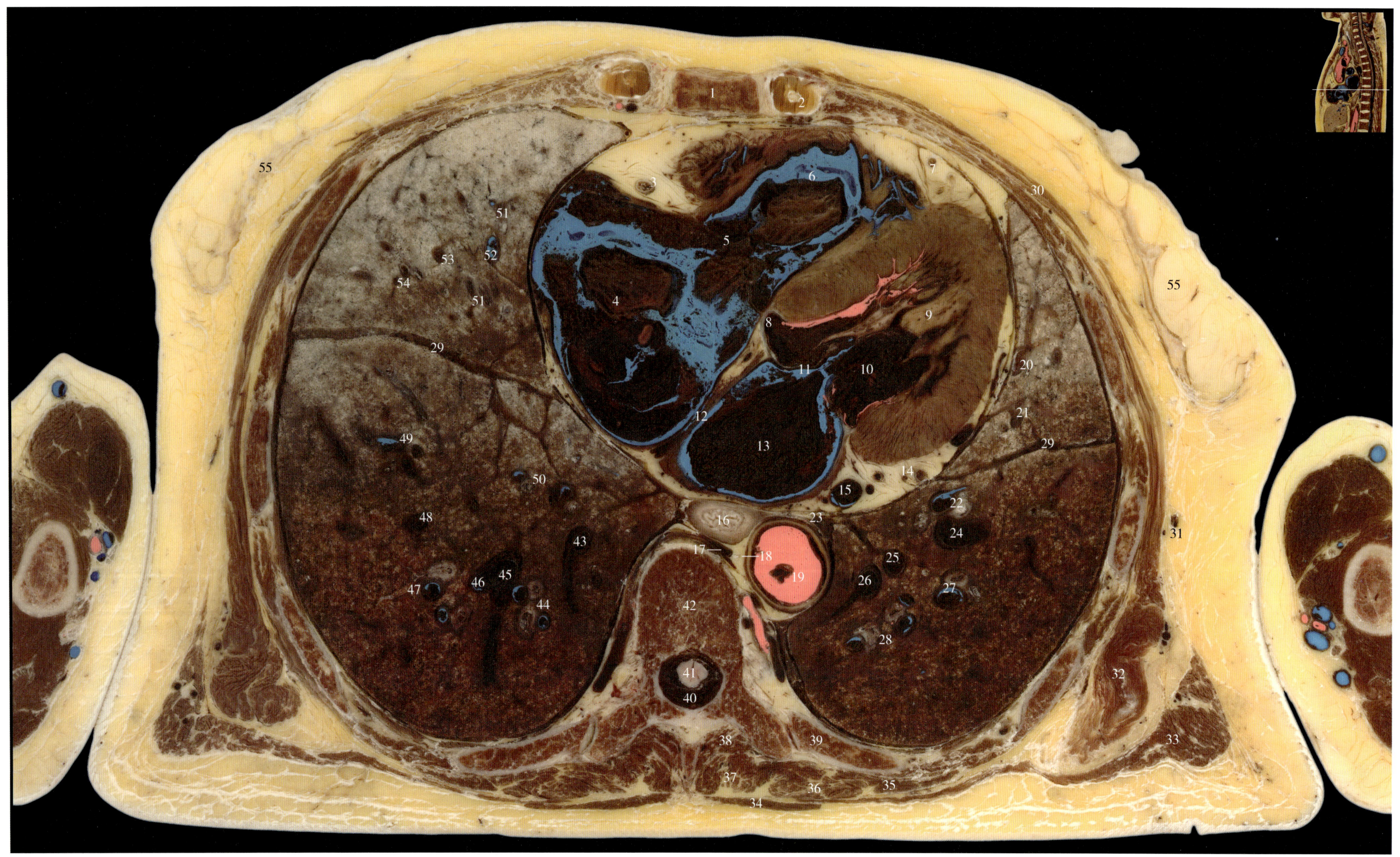

A. 断层标本图像

1. 胸骨体 body of sternum
2. 第 5 肋软骨 5th costal cartilage
3. 右冠状动脉 right coronary artery
4. 右心房 right atrium
5. 三尖瓣 tricuspid valve
6. 右心室 right ventricle
7. 前室间支 anterior interventricular branch
8. 室间隔膜部 membranous part of interventricular septum
9. 乳头肌 papillary muscle
10. 左心室 left ventricle
11. 二尖瓣 mitral valve
12. 房间隔 interatrial septum
13. 左心房 left atrium
14. 旋支 circumflex branch
15. 冠状窦 coronary sinus
16. 食管 esophagus
17. 奇静脉 azygos vein
18. 胸导管 thoracic duct
19. 胸主动脉 thoracic aorta
20. 舌静脉干（V4+5）lingular venous trunk
21. 下舌段支气管（B5）和动脉（A5）inferior lingular segmental bronchus and artery
22. 内前底段支气管（B7+8）和动脉（A7+8）medioanterior basal segmental bronchus and artery
23. 肺韧带 pulmonary ligament
24. 内前底段静脉（V7+8）medioanterior basal segmental vein
25. 左肺外侧底段静脉（V9）left lateral basal segmental vein
26. 左肺后底段静脉（V10）left posterior basal segmental vein
27. 左肺外侧底段支气管（B9）和动脉（A9）left lateral basal segmental bronchus and artery
28. 左肺后底段支气管（B10）和动脉（A10）left posterior basal segmental bronchus and artery
29. 斜裂 oblique fissure
30. 胸大肌 pectoralis major
31. 胸外侧静脉 lateral thoracic vein
32. 前锯肌 serratus anterior
33. 背阔肌 latissimus dorsi
34. 斜方肌 trapezius
35. 髂肋肌 iliocostalis
36. 最长肌 longissimus
37. 棘肌 spinales
38. 横突棘肌 transversospinales
39. 第 8 肋骨 8th costal bone
40. 硬膜外隙 epidural space
41. 脊髓 spinal cord
42. 第 8 胸椎椎体 body of 8th thoracic vertebra
43. 内侧底段静脉（V7）medial basal segmental vein
44. 右肺后底段支气管（B10）和动脉（A10）right posterior basal segmental bronchus and artery
45. 右肺后底段静脉（V10）right posterior basal segmental vein
46. 右肺外侧底段静脉（V9）right lateral basal segmental vein
47. 右肺外侧底段支气管（B9）和动脉（A9）right lateral basal segmental bronchus and artery
48. 前底段静脉（V8）anterior basal segmental vein
49. 前底段支气管（B8）和动脉（A8）anterior basal segmental bronchus and artery
50. 内侧底段支气管（B7）和动脉（A7）medial basal segmental bronchus and artery
51. 内侧段支气管（B5）和动脉（A5）medial segmental bronchus and artery
52. 内侧段静脉（V5）medial segmental vein
53. 外侧段静脉（V4）lateral segmental vein
54. 外侧段支气管（B4）和动脉（A4）lateral segmental bronchus and artery
55. 乳腺 mammary gland

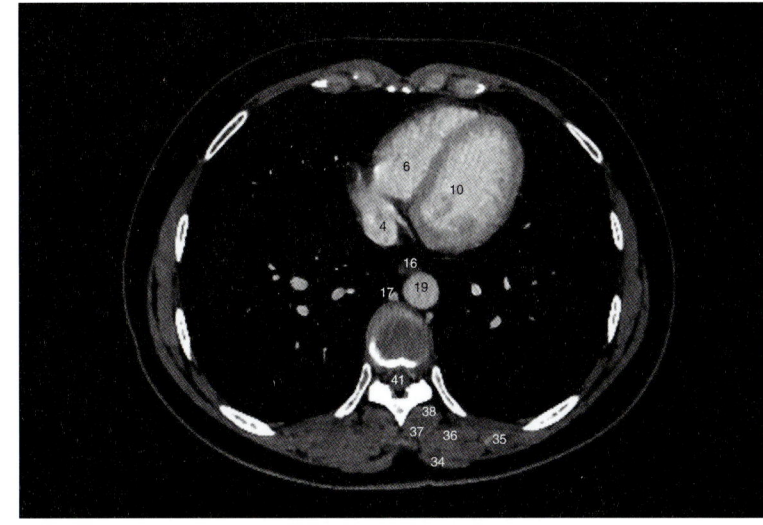

B. CT 纵隔窗增强图像

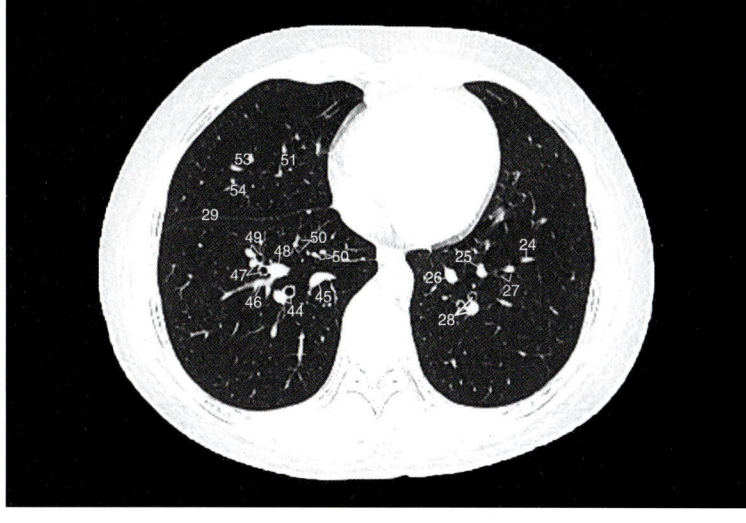

C. CT 肺窗图像

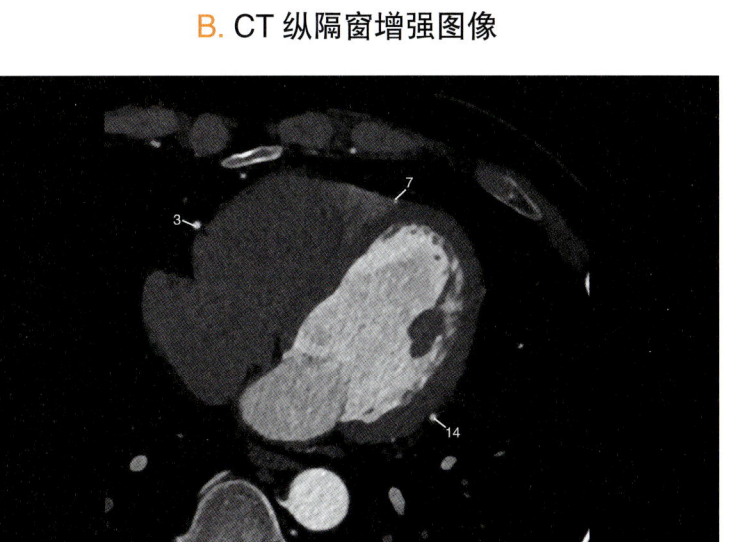

D. 冠状动脉 CT 增强图像

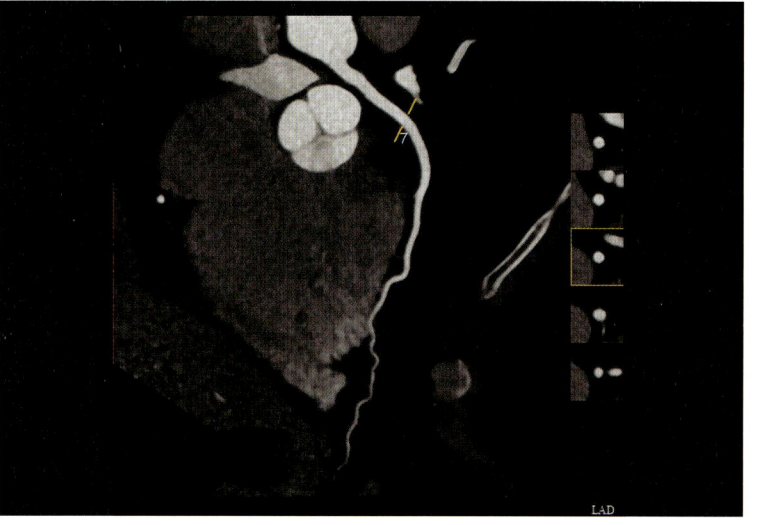

E. 左冠状动脉前室间支 CT 重建图像

关键结构：二尖瓣，三尖瓣。

此断面经第 8 胸椎椎体中份。

左、右心室内可见乳头肌及腱索，分别与左、右房室口的二尖瓣和三尖瓣以及瓣环形成二尖瓣复合体和三尖瓣复合体，它们在功能上是一个整体，保证血液只能从心房流入心室，而不能逆流。二尖瓣分为前尖和后尖；前尖较大，略呈三角形或新月形，是区分左心室流入道和流出道的解剖标志，介于左房室口与主动脉口之间；后尖略小，位于后外侧，呈波浪状。三尖瓣分为前尖、后尖和隔侧尖，面积大小几乎一致[78]。三尖瓣隔侧尖的前上 2/3 不附着于三尖瓣环上，而下移附着在室间隔的膜部和肌部，下移最大的距离在成人为 6.1 mm ± 0.9 mm。CT 测量显示，二尖瓣前尖长度为 25.9 mm ± 4.7 mm，尖长度为 13.2 mm ± 2.5 mm。二尖瓣环的前 1/3 为前瓣的附着缘，最为坚韧牢固，其后 2/3 为后瓣附着缘，纤维组织比较薄弱。在心动周期的不同阶段，二尖瓣环的形态和周径有所改变，瓣环在心动周期中主要保持椭圆形，国人二尖瓣环口接近于圆形，积为 413.4 mm^2 ± 69.9 mm^2。二尖瓣环在心室收缩期进一步缩小，使瓣口面积减少 20%~40%。心脏舒张期，环的长轴方向从右后斜行至左前，与瓣叶的前后交界一致，其长径平均为 2.6 cm，其周径为 8.5~11.5 cm[79]。

胸部连续横断层 71（FH.12090）

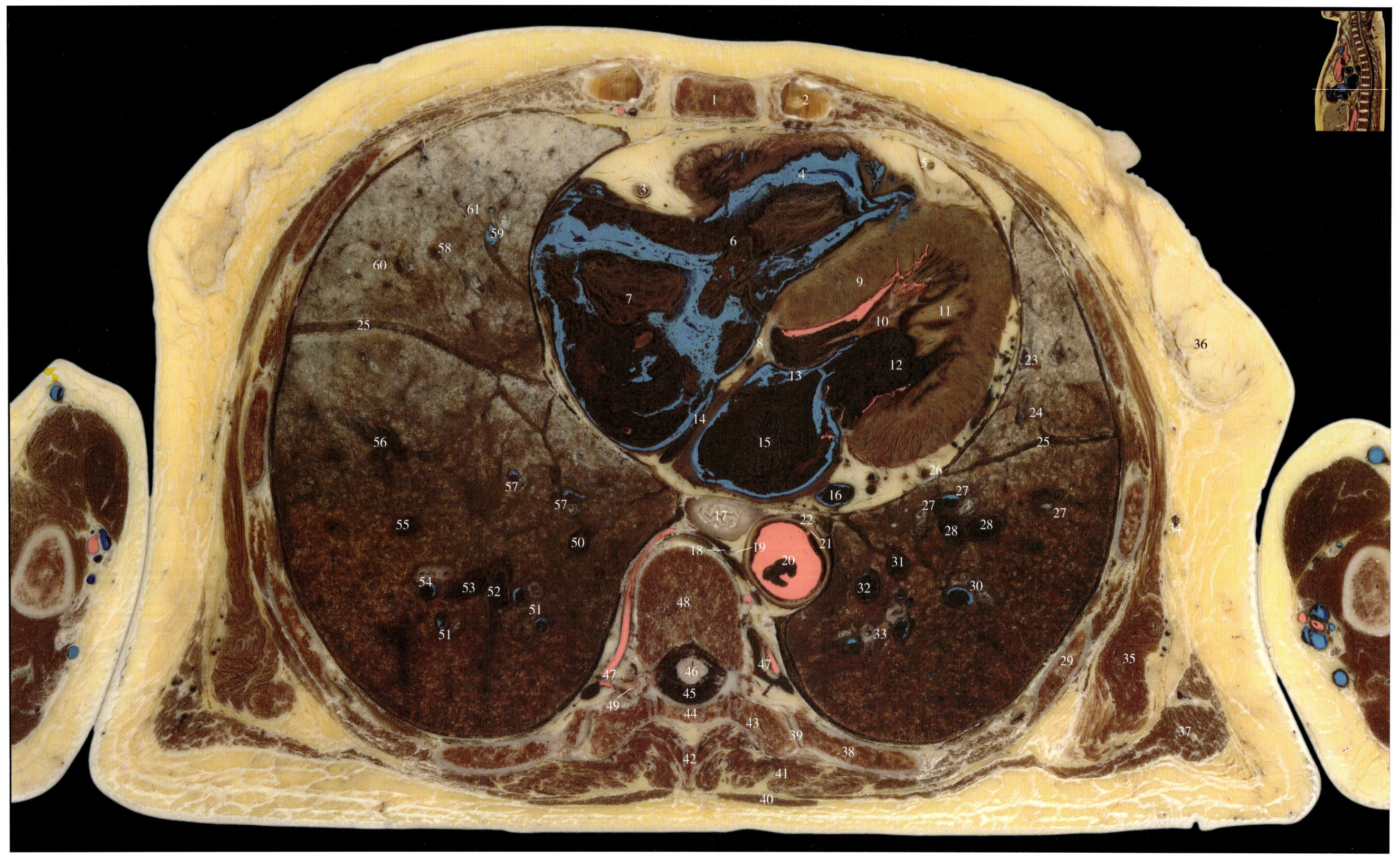

A. 断层标本图像

1. 胸骨体 body of sternum
2. 第 5 肋软骨 5th costal cartilage
3. 右冠状动脉 right coronary artery
4. 右心室 right ventricle
5. 前室间支 anterior interventricular branch
6. 三尖瓣 tricuspid valve
7. 右心房 right atrium
8. 室间隔膜部 membranous part of interventricular septum
9. 室间隔肌部 muscular part of interventricular septum
10. 腱索 tendinous cord
11. 乳头肌 papillary muscle
12. 左心室 left ventricle
13. 二尖瓣 mitral valve
14. 房间隔 interatrial septum
15. 左心房 left atrium
16. 冠状窦 coronary sinus
17. 食管 esophagus
18. 奇静脉 azygos vein
19. 胸导管 thoracic duct
20. 胸主动脉 thoracic aorta
21. 胸主动脉食管支 esophageal branch of thoracic aorta
22. 肺韧带 pulmonary ligament
23. 舌静脉干（V4+5）lingular venous trunk
24. 下舌段支气管（B5）和动脉（A5）inferior lingular segmental bronchus and artery
25. 斜裂 oblique fissure
26. 旋支 circumflex branch
27. 内前底段支气管（B7+8）和动脉（A7+8）medioanterior basal segmental bronchus and artery
28. 内前底段静脉（V7+8）medioanterior basal segmental vein
29. 第 7 肋骨 7th costal bone
30. 左肺外侧底段支气管（B9）和动脉（A9）left lateral basal segmental bronchus and artery
31. 左肺外侧底段静脉（V9）left lateral basal segmental vein
32. 左肺后底段静脉（V10）left posterior basal segmental vein
33. 左肺后底段支气管（B10）和动脉（A10）left posterior basal segmental bronchus and artery
34. 胸外侧静脉 lateral thoracic vein
35. 前锯肌 serratus anterior
36. 乳腺 mammary gland
37. 背阔肌 latissimus dorsi
38. 第 8 肋骨 8th costal bone
39. 肋横突关节 costotransverse joint
40. 斜方肌 trapezius
41. 竖脊肌 erector spinae
42. 棘突 spinous process
43. 横突 transverse process
44. 椎弓板 lamina of vertebral arch
45. 硬膜外腔 epidural space
46. 脊髓 spinal cord
47. 肋间后动、静脉 posterior intercostal artery and vein
48. 第 8 胸椎椎体 body of 8th thoracic vertebra
49. 脊神经节 spinal ganglion
50. 内侧底段静脉（V7）medial basal segmental vein
51. 右肺后底段支气管（B10）和动脉（A10）right posterior basal segmental bronchus and artery
52. 右肺后底段静脉（V10）right posterior basal segmental vein
53. 右肺外侧底段静脉（V9）right lateral basal segmental vein
54. 右肺外侧底段支气管（B9）和动脉（A9）right lateral basal segmental bronchus and artery
55. 前底段静脉（V8）anterior basal segmental vein
56. 前底段支气管（B8）和动脉（A8）anterior basal segmental bronchus and artery
57. 内侧段支气管（B7）和动脉（A7）medial basal segmental bronchus and artery
58. 外侧段静脉（V4）lateral segmental vein
59. 内侧段静脉（V5）medial segmental vein
60. 外侧段支气管（B4）和动脉（A4）lateral segmental bronchus and artery
61. 内侧段支气管（B5）和动脉（A5）medial segmental bronchus and artery

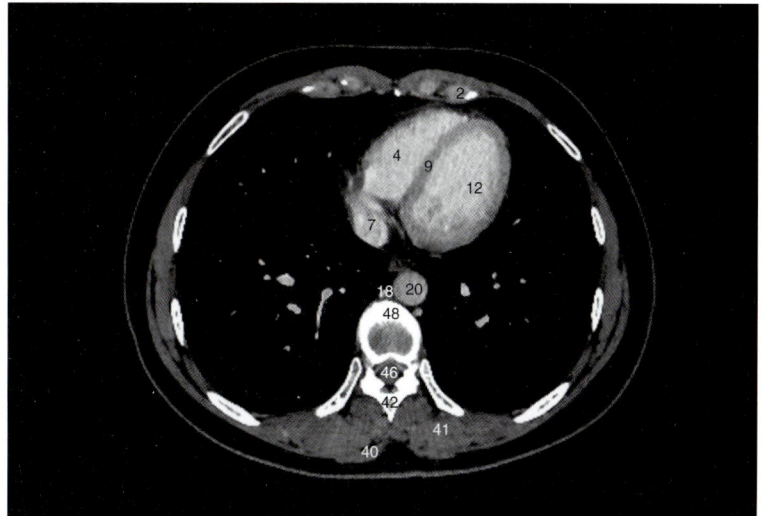

B. CT 纵隔窗增强图像

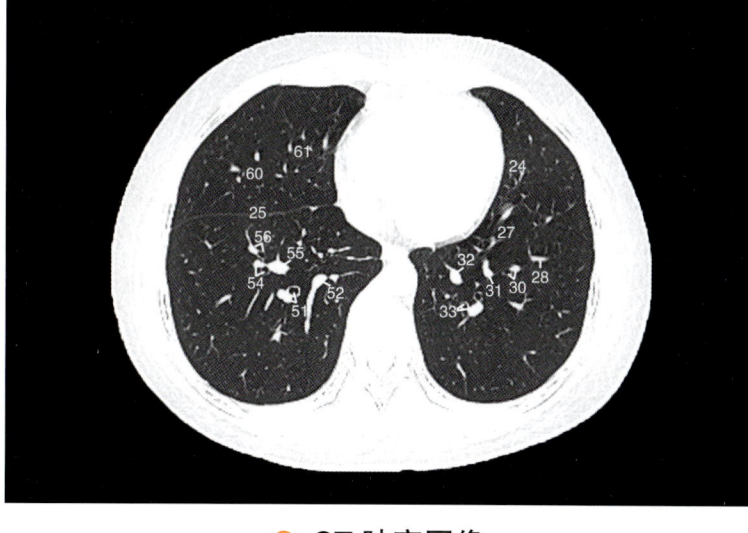

C. CT 肺窗图像

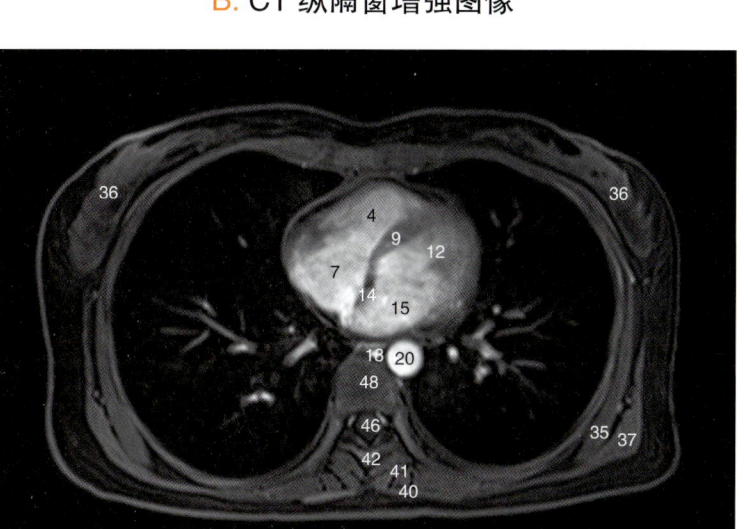

D. MR T1WI 增强图像

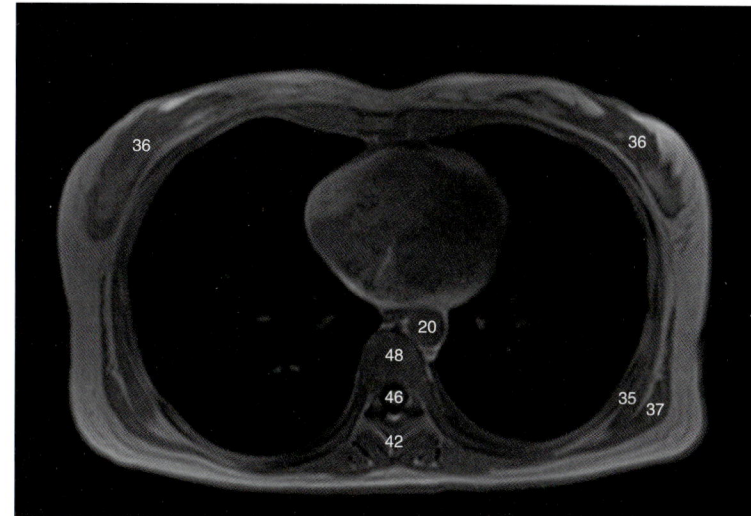

E. MR T1WI 平扫图像

关键结构：心房，心室，椎管。

此断面第 8 胸椎椎体下份。

纵隔内，4 个心腔仍清晰可见，左心室壁厚，腔内可见乳头肌。心脏中隔呈"一"字形自右后斜向左前，与矢状面约成 45°角，仍可见室间隔膜部。心脏 CT 和 MRI 能从三维结构角度，提供心脏结构的详细信息，能够无创地从多个角度对心血管系统进行评估[80]。右肺中叶内，外侧段静脉作为段间支，分隔内侧和外侧段。右肺下叶内，前底段静脉和后底段静脉是段间支，分别位于前底段和外侧底段，以及外侧底段和后底段之间。底段的支气管和伴行动脉都较为细小，出现在各底段中央，各段动脉位于相应支气管的外侧。左肺上叶内，主要为下舌段支气管、动脉和静脉。左肺下叶内，内侧底段静脉和前底段静脉分隔了内前底段和外侧底段，外侧底段静脉分隔外侧底段和后底段[81]。脊柱区椎管由各椎骨椎孔连结而成，上至枕骨大孔，下经骶管终于骶管裂孔。椎管前壁由椎体、椎间盘和后纵韧带构成，后壁是椎弓板及韧带，后外侧壁为关节突关节，两侧壁为椎弓根和椎间孔。椎管内有脊髓及其被膜、脊神经根、血管和脂肪组织等结构。椎弓横突伸向后外上方，其末端前面与同序数肋骨构成肋横突关节，但第 11、12 胸椎的横突不与同序数肋构成肋横突关节。

胸部连续横断层 72 (FH.12070)

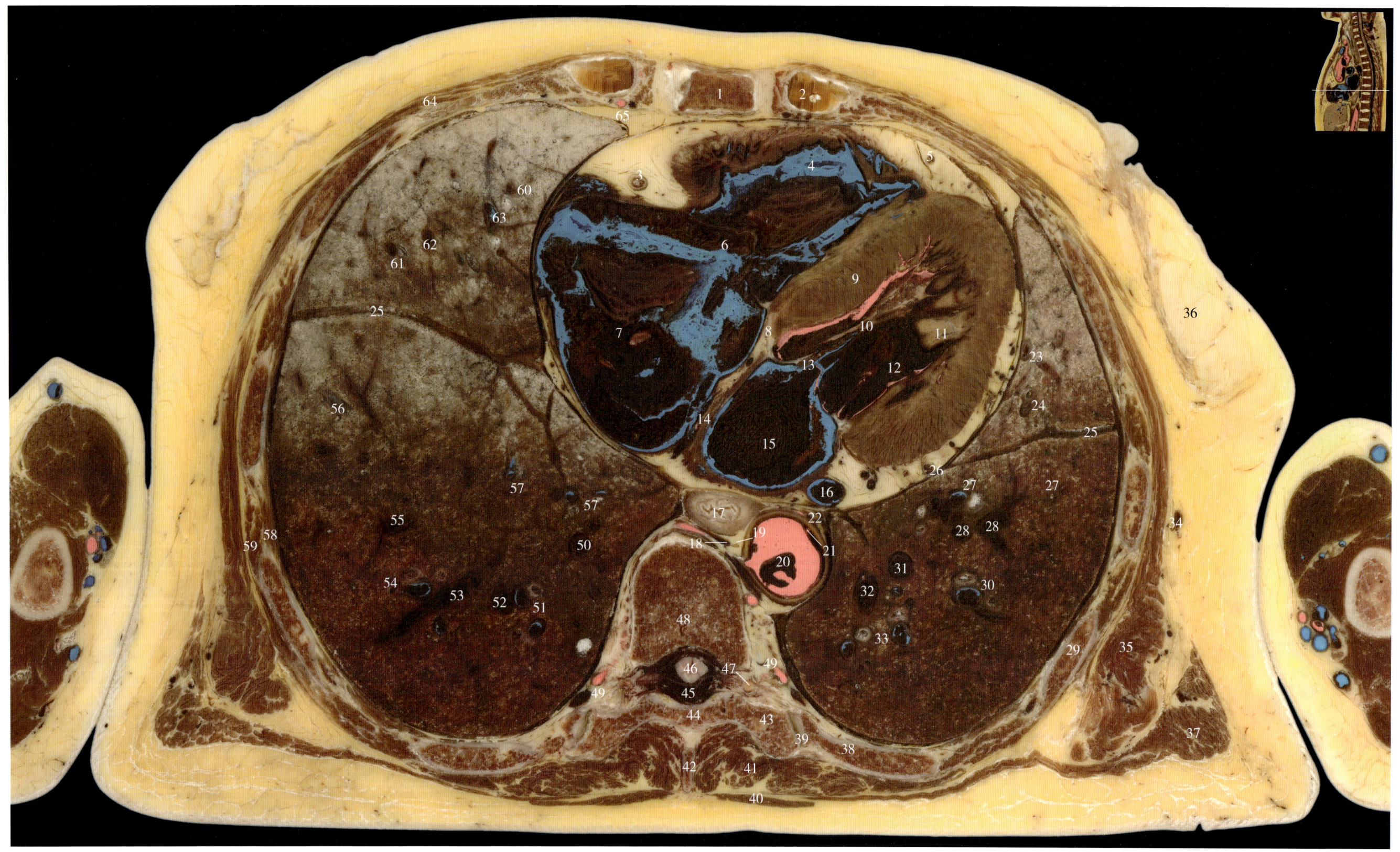

A. 断层标本图像

1. 胸骨体 body of sternum
2. 第 5 肋软骨 5th costal cartilage
3. 右冠状动脉 right coronary artery
4. 右心室 right ventricle
5. 前室间支 anterior interventricular branch
6. 三尖瓣 tricuspid valve
7. 右心房 right atrium
8. 室间隔膜部 membranous part of interventricular septum
9. 室间隔肌部 muscular part of interventricular septum
10. 腱索 tendinous cord
11. 乳头肌 papillary muscle
12. 左心室 left ventricle
13. 二尖瓣 mitral valve
14. 房间隔 interatrial septum
15. 左心房 left atrium
16. 冠状窦 coronary sinus
17. 食管 esophagus
18. 奇静脉 azygos vein
19. 胸导管 thoracic duct
20. 胸主动脉 thoracic aorta
21. 胸主动脉食管支 esophageal branch of thoracic aorta
22. 肺韧带 pulmonary ligament
23. 舌静脉干（V4+5）lingular venous trunk
24. 下舌段支气管（B5）和动脉（A5）inferior lingular segmental bronchus and artery
25. 斜裂 oblique fissure
26. 旋支 circumflex branch
27. 内前底段支气管（B7+8）和动脉（A7+8）medioanterior basal segmental bronchus and artery
28. 内前底段静脉（V7+8）medioanterior basal segmental vein
29. 第 7 肋骨 7th costal bone
30. 左肺外侧底段支气管（B9）和动脉（A9）left lateral basal segmental bronchus and artery
31. 左肺外侧底段静脉（V9）left lateral basal segmental vein
32. 左肺后底段静脉（V10）left posterior basal segmental vein
33. 左肺后底段支气管（B10）和动脉（A10）left posterior basal segmental bronchus and artery

34. 胸外侧静脉 lateral thoracic vein
35. 前锯肌 serratus anterior
36. 乳腺 mammary gland
37. 背阔肌 latissimus dorsi
38. 第 8 肋骨 8th costal bone
39. 肋横突关节 costotransverse joint
40. 斜方肌 trapezius
41. 竖脊肌 erector spinae
42. 棘突 spinous process
43. 横突 transverse process
44. 椎弓板 lamina of vertebral arch
45. 硬膜外隙 epidural space
46. 脊髓 spinal cord
47. 脊神经节 spinal ganglion
48. 第 8 胸椎椎体 body of 8th thoracic vertebra
49. 肋间后动、静脉 posterior intercostal artery and vein
50. 内侧底段静脉（V7）medial basal segmental vein
51. 右肺后底段支气管（B10）和动脉（A10）right posterior basal segmental bronchus and artery
52. 右肺后底段静脉（V10）right posterior basal segmental vein
53. 右肺外侧底段静脉（V9）right lateral basal segmental vein
54. 右肺外侧底段支气管（B9）和动脉（A9）right lateral basal segmental bronchus and artery
55. 前底段静脉（V8）anterior basal segmental vein
56. 前底段支气管（B8）和动脉（A8）anterior basal segmental bronchus and artery
57. 内侧底段支气管（B7）和动脉（A7）medial basal segmental bronchus and artery
58. 肋间内肌 intercostales interni
59. 肋间外肌 intercostales externi
60. 内侧段支气管（B5）和动脉（A5）medial segmental bronchus and artery
61. 外侧段支气管（B4）和动脉（A4）lateral segmental bronchus and artery
62. 外侧段静脉（V4）lateral segmental vein
63. 内侧段静脉（V5）medial segmental vein
64. 胸大肌 pectoralis major
65. 胸廓内动、静脉 internal thoracic artery and vein

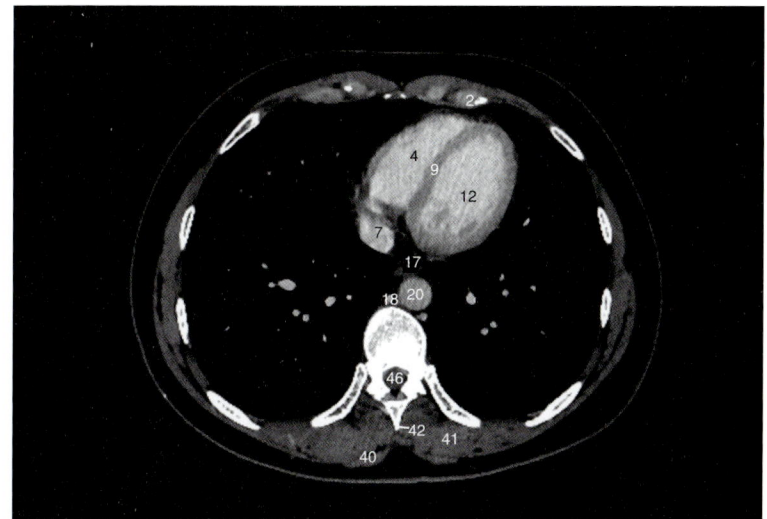

B. CT 纵隔窗增强图像

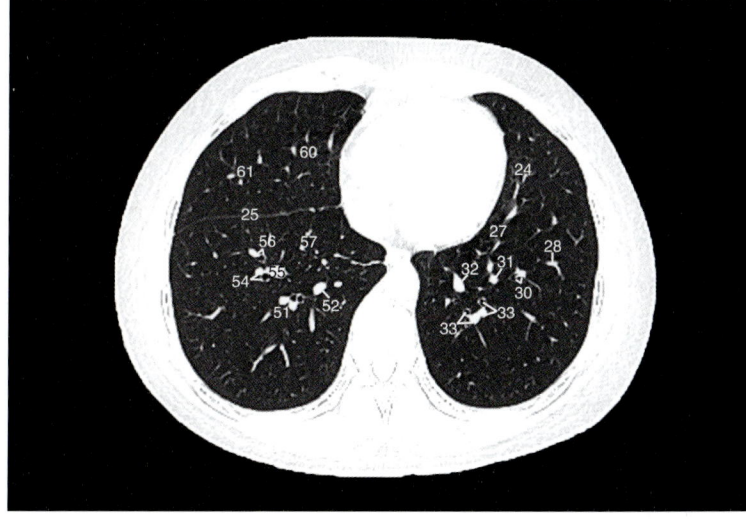

C. CT 肺窗图像

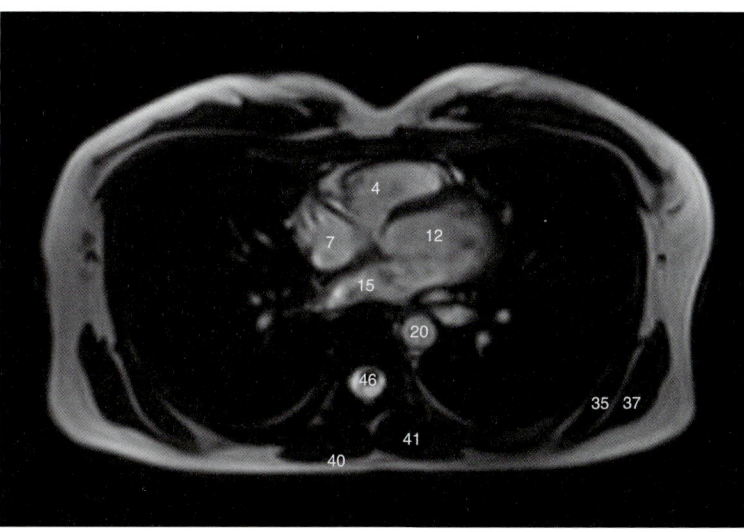

D. MR T2WI 平扫图像

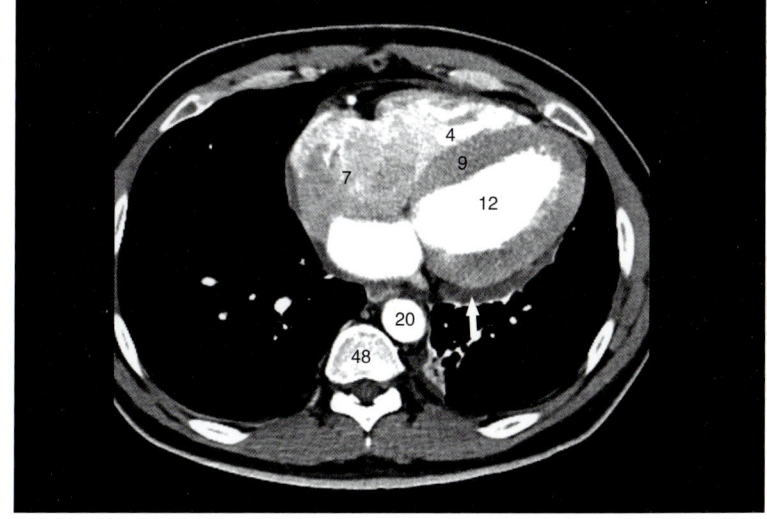

E. 心包斜窦积液 CT 增强图像

关键结构：心包腔，心包斜窦。

此断面前方经胸骨体下端，后方经第 8 胸椎椎体下份。

纵隔内，4 个心腔及心脏中隔不变，左心室壁最厚，室腔内可见乳头肌与腱索相连。心脏表面包被心包，分为纤维心包和浆膜心包，浆膜心包的脏、壁两层在进出心的大血管根部互相反折移行，形成密闭的心包腔，内有少量浆液[82]。当心包腔积液时，可见其内增宽的低密度影，如 E 图所见，左心房和左心室后方的心包斜窦内有明显增厚的积液区。心包斜窦为心包腔在左心房后壁、两侧肺静脉、下腔静脉与心包后壁（食管前方）之间的部分，是平卧位心包腔的最低点[83]。斜窦的形态与肺静脉间隐窝的发育密切相关，多见肺静脉间隐窝与斜窦皆发育，斜窦底及左、右肺静脉间隐窝底均可达肺动脉下缘或其后壁水平，故此型左、右肺静脉间隐窝与斜窦相互靠近，此型占 72.5%；其次为肺静脉间隐窝不发育、斜窦发育型，此型通常是上、下肺静脉合干，斜窦较大，几乎占据了整个左心房后壁，此型占 19.6%[52]。当上、下肺静脉合干，而左、右肺静脉注入左心房的位置相距较近时，则心包斜窦不伸入到左、右肺静脉间，故而较浅，与其他窦或隐窝亦不相毗邻。心包斜窦少量积液时，CT 图像呈线状或窄带状。

胸部连续横断层 73（FH.12050）

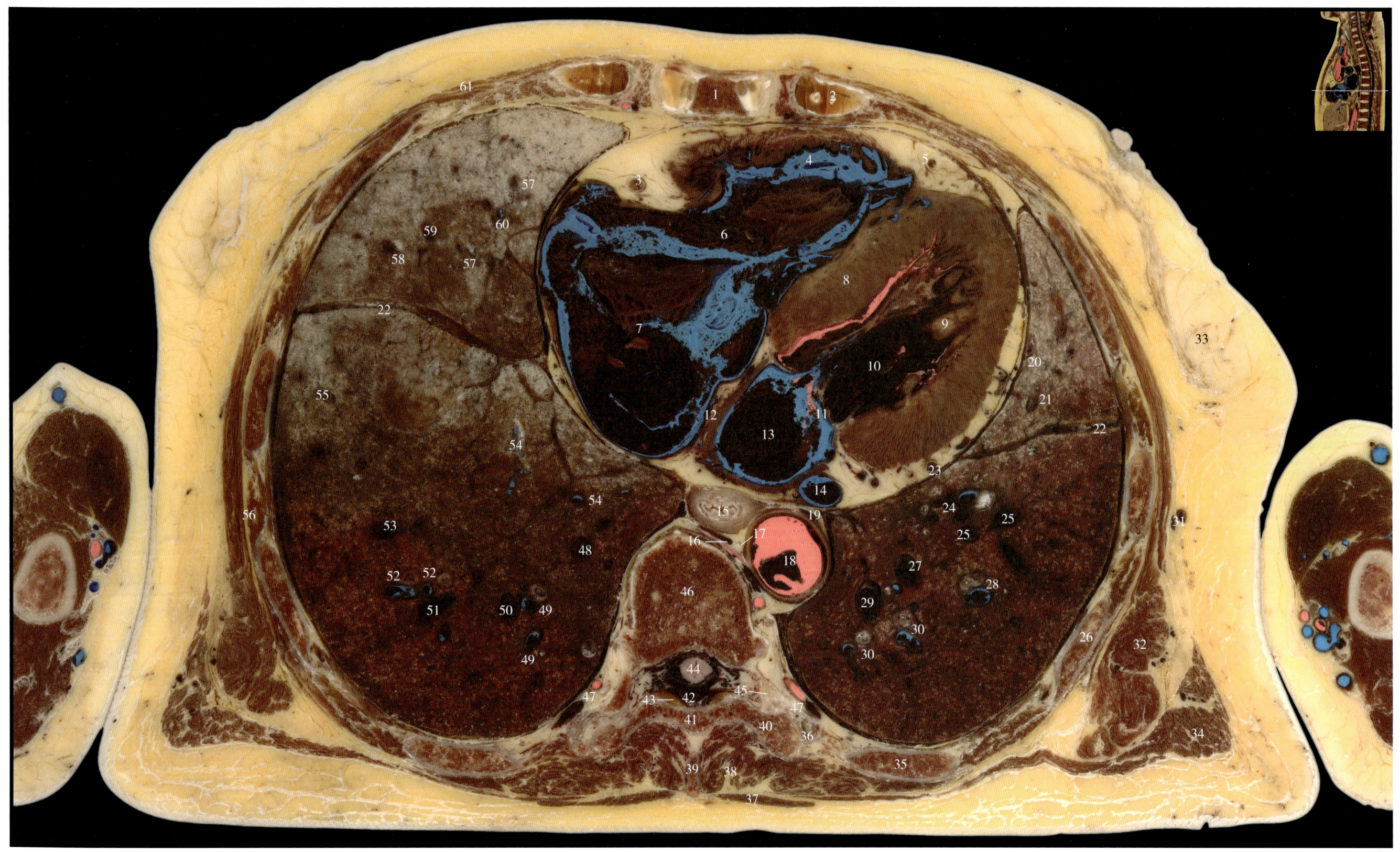

A. 断层标本图像

1. 胸骨体 body of sternum
2. 第 5 肋软骨 5th costal cartilage
3. 右冠状动脉 right coronary artery
4. 右心室 right ventricle
5. 前室间支 anterior interventricular branch
6. 三尖瓣 tricuspid valve
7. 右心房 right atrium
8. 室间隔 interventricular septum
9. 乳头肌 papillary muscle
10. 左心室 left ventricle
11. 二尖瓣 mitral valve
12. 房间隔 interatrial septum
13. 左心房 left atrium
14. 冠状窦 coronary sinus
15. 食管 esophagus
16. 奇静脉 azygos vein
17. 胸导管 thoracic duct
18. 胸主动脉 thoracic aorta
19. 肺韧带 pulmonary ligament
20. 下舌段静脉（V5）inferior lingular segmental vein
21. 下舌段支气管（B5）和动脉（A5）inferior lingular segmental bronchus and artery
22. 斜裂 oblique fissure
23. 旋支 circumflex branch
24. 内前底段支气管（B7+8）和动脉（A7+8）medioanterior basal segmental bronchus and artery
25. 内前底段静脉（V7+8）medioanterior basal segmental vein
26. 第 7 肋骨 7th costal bone
27. 左肺外侧底段静脉（V9）left lateral basal segmental vein
28. 左肺外侧底段支气管（B9）和动脉（A9）left lateral basal segmental bronchus and artery
29. 左肺后底段静脉（V10）left posterior basal segmental vein
30. 左肺后底段支气管（B10）和动脉（A10）left posterior basal segmental bronchus and artery
31. 胸外侧静脉 lateral thoracic vein
32. 前锯肌 serratus anterior
33. 乳腺 mammary gland
34. 背阔肌 latissimus dorsi
35. 第 8 肋骨 8th costal bone
36. 肋横突关节 costotransverse joint
37. 斜方肌 trapezius
38. 竖脊肌 erector spinae
39. 棘突 spinous process
40. 横突 transverse process
41. 椎弓板 lamina of vertebral arch
42. 硬膜外隙 epidural space
43. 黄韧带 ligamenta flava
44. 脊髓 spinal cord
45. 脊神经节 spinal ganglion
46. 第 8 胸椎椎体 body of 8th thoracic vertebra
47. 肋间后动、静脉 posterior intercostal artery and vein
48. 内侧底段静脉（V7）medial basal segmental vein
49. 右肺后底段支气管（B10）和动脉（A10）right posterior basal segmental bronchus and artery
50. 右肺后底段静脉（V10）right posterior basal segmental vein
51. 右肺外侧底段静脉（V9）right lateral basal segmental vein
52. 右肺外侧底段支气管（B9）和动脉（A9）right lateral basal segmental bronchus and artery
53. 前底段静脉（V8）anterior basal segmental vein
54. 内侧底段支气管（B7）和动脉（A7）medial basal segmental bronchus and artery
55. 前底段支气管（B8）和动脉（A8）anterior basal segmental bronchus and artery
56. 肋间外肌 intercostales externi
57. 内侧段支气管（B5）和动脉（A5）medial segmental bronchus and artery
58. 外侧段支气管（B4）和动脉（A4）lateral segmental bronchus and artery
59. 外侧段静脉（V4）lateral segmental vein
60. 内侧段静脉（V5）medial segmental vein
61. 胸大肌 pectoralis major
62. 蛛网膜下隙 subarachnoid space

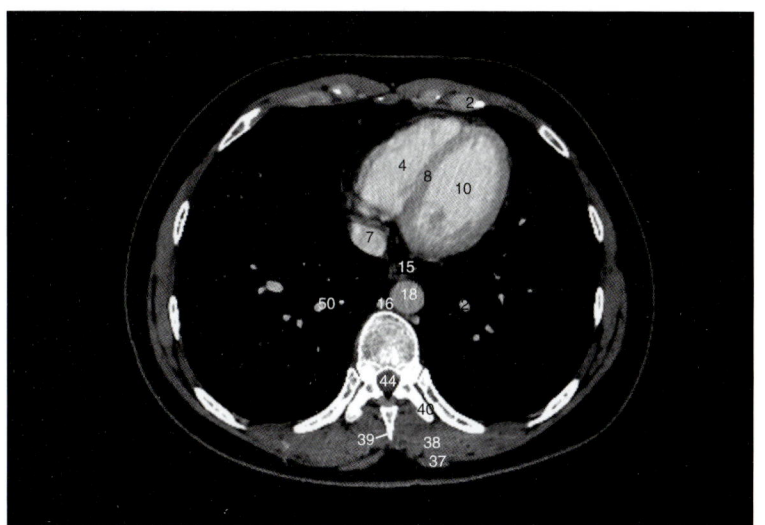

B. CT 纵隔窗增强图像

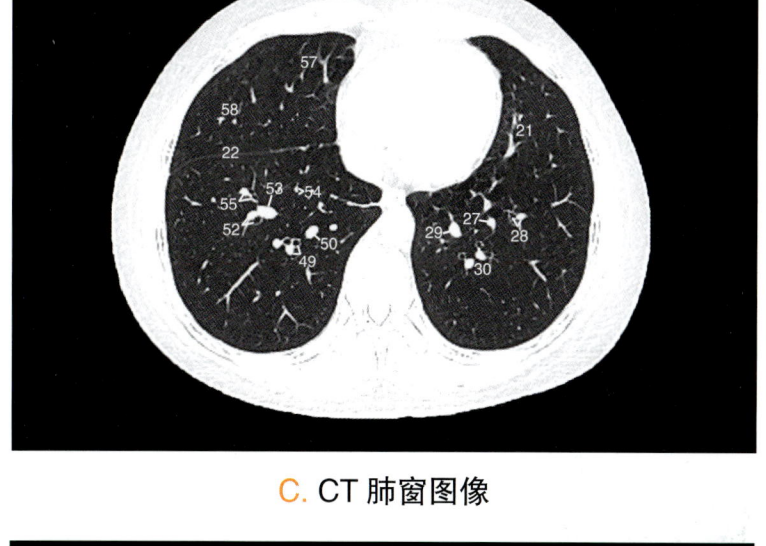

C. CT 肺窗图像

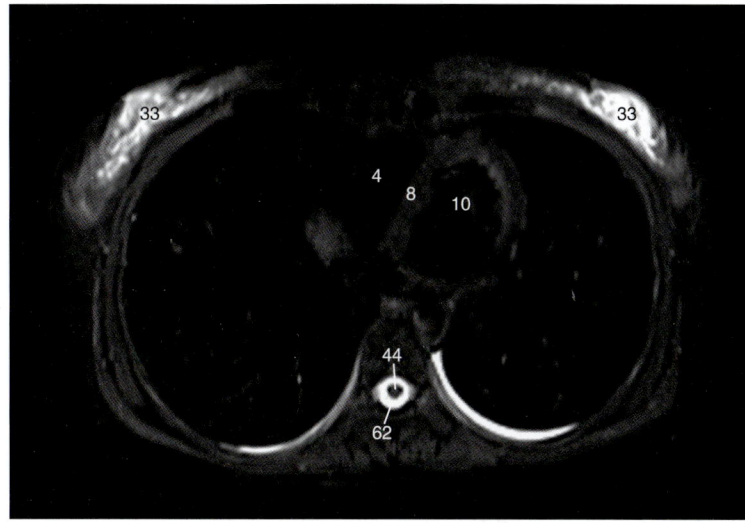

D. MR T2WI 抑脂图像

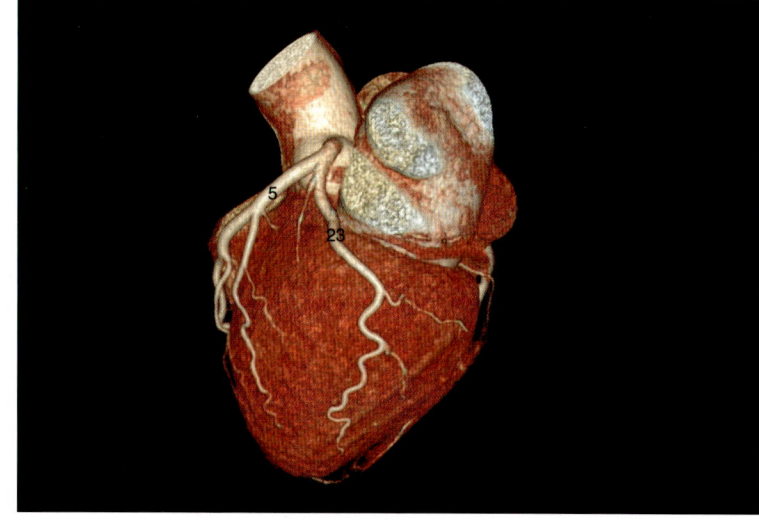

E. 左冠状动脉 CT 三维重建图像

关键结构：椎弓板，食管（下胸段），肺下叶。

此断面前方经胸骨体下端，后方经第 8 胸椎椎体下份。

胸椎椎体后方为椎管和椎间孔，椎间孔为相邻椎弓根之间的孔隙，由脊神经根穿出。椎弓根向后的板状突起是椎弓板，相邻椎弓板由黄韧带连接，构成椎管的后壁。纵隔内，左心房进一步缩小，通过左房室口通向左心室，开口处可见二尖瓣，左心室内可见前、后组乳头肌。右心房居于右侧，腔大而明显，通过右房室口通向右心室，开口处见三尖瓣。冠状窦逐渐变大，随着左心房的变小而逐渐靠近右心房。随着断面下移，两肺均接近肺底，肺底形态前高后底，故两肺下叶底段中，前底段最先消失。本断面见右肺内前底段内支气管和动脉已近消失，其他各底段管道仍清晰可见，排列同上一断面。左肺内，各底段支气管和动脉均分出亚段分支。食管下胸段具有稳定的供血动脉来源，即直接发自主动脉胸部的食管支，因为这种食管支较为恒定，故又被称为食管固有动脉。食管固有动脉在选择性食管动脉造影及食管癌的介入治疗有特别意义[84]。CT 图像因活体肺部较充盈，两肺底段的各管道还较清晰，纵隔层面低于标本层面，仍可见右心房和左、右心室，后纵隔为食管、胸主动脉、奇静脉和半奇静脉。

胸部连续横断层 74（FH.12030）

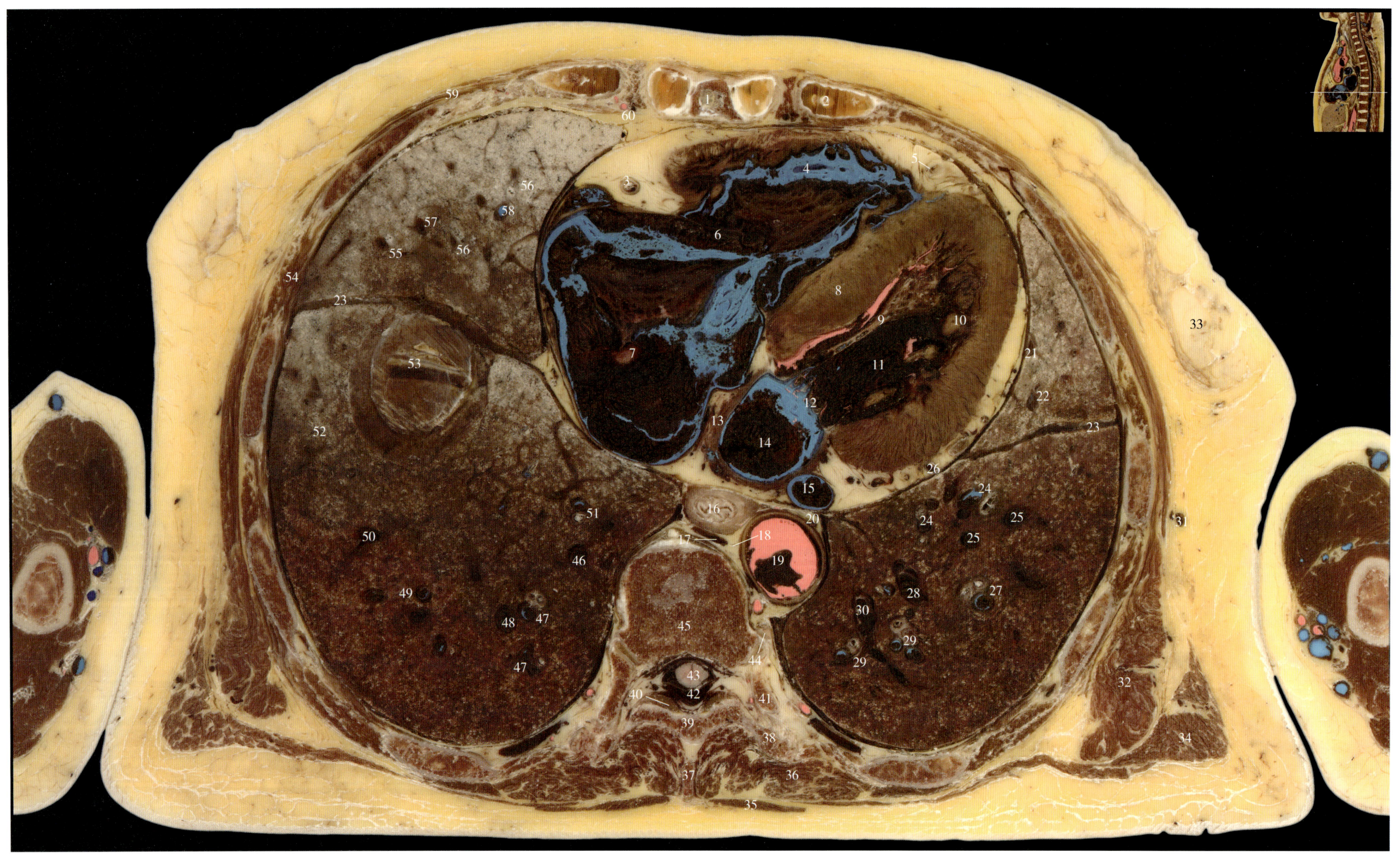

A. 断层标本图像

1. 胸骨体 body of sternum
2. 第 5 肋软骨 5th costal cartilage
3. 右冠状动脉 right coronary artery
4. 右心室 right ventricle
5. 前室间支 anterior interventricular branch
6. 三尖瓣 tricuspid valve
7. 右心房 right atrium
8. 室间隔 interventricular septum
9. 腱索 tendinous cord
10. 乳头肌 papillary muscle
11. 左心室 left ventricle
12. 二尖瓣 mitral valve
13. 房间隔 interatrial septum
14. 左心房 left atrium
15. 冠状窦 coronary sinus
16. 食管 esophagus
17. 奇静脉 azygos vein
18. 胸导管 thoracic duct
19. 胸主动脉 thoracic aorta
20. 肺韧带 pulmonary ligament
21. 下舌段静脉（V5）inferior lingular segmental vein
22. 下舌段支气管（B5）和动脉（A5）inferior lingular segmental bronchus and artery
23. 斜裂 oblique fissure
24. 内前底段支气管（B7+8）和动脉（A7+8）medioanterior basal segmental bronchus and artery
25. 内前底段静脉（V7+8）medioanterior basal segmental vein
26. 旋支 circumflex branch
27. 左肺外侧底段支气管（B9）和动脉（A9）left lateral basal segmental bronchus and artery
28. 左肺外侧底段静脉（V9）left lateral basal segmental vein
29. 左肺后底段支气管（B10）和动脉（A10）left posterior basal segmental bronchus and artery
30. 左肺后底段静脉（V10）left posterior basal segmental vein
31. 胸外侧静脉 lateral thoracic vein
32. 前锯肌 serratus anterior
33. 乳腺 mammary gland
34. 背阔肌 latissimus dorsi
35. 斜方肌 trapezius
36. 竖脊肌 erector spinae
37. 棘突 spinous process
38. 横突 transverse process
39. 椎弓板 lamina of vertebral arch
40. 黄韧带 ligamenta flava
41. 第 9 肋骨 9th costal bone
42. 硬膜外隙 epidural space
43. 脊髓 spinal cord
44. 交感干神经节 ganglia of sympathetic trunk
45. 第 8 胸椎椎体 body of 8th thoracic vertebra
46. 内侧底段静脉（V7）medial basal segmental vein
47. 右肺后底段支气管（B10）和动脉（A10）right posterior basal segmental bronchus and artery
48. 右肺后底段静脉（V10）right posterior basal segmental vein
49. 右肺外侧底段支气管（B9）和动脉（A9）right lateral basal segmental bronchus and artery
50. 前底段静脉（V8）anterior basal segmental vein
51. 内侧底段支气管（B7）和动脉（A7）medial basal segmental bronchus and artery
52. 前底段支气管（B8）和动脉（A8）anterior basal segmental bronchus and artery
53. 膈右穹窿 right fornix of diaphragm
54. 肋间内肌 intercostales interni
55. 外侧段支气管（B4）和动脉（A4）lateral segmental bronchus and artery
56. 内侧段支气管（B5）和动脉（A5）medial segmental bronchus and artery
57. 外侧段静脉（V4）lateral segmental vein
58. 内侧段静脉（V5）medial segmental vein
59. 胸大肌 pectoralis major
60. 胸廓内动、静脉 internal thoracic artery and vein

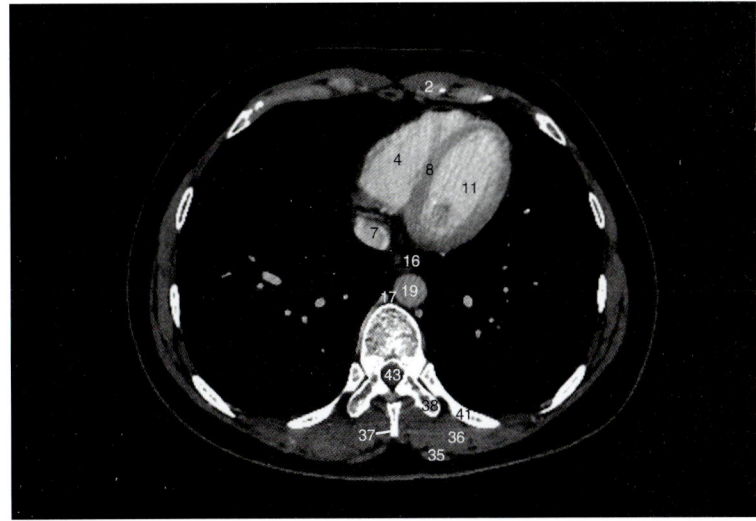

B. CT 纵隔窗增强图像

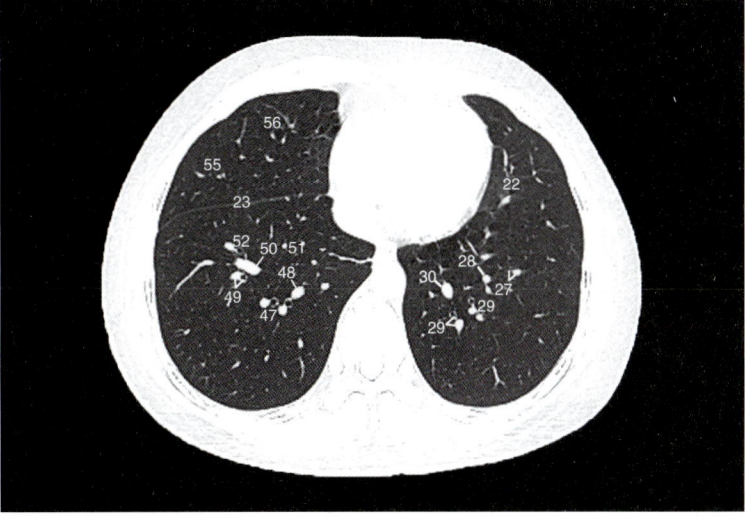

C. CT 肺窗图像

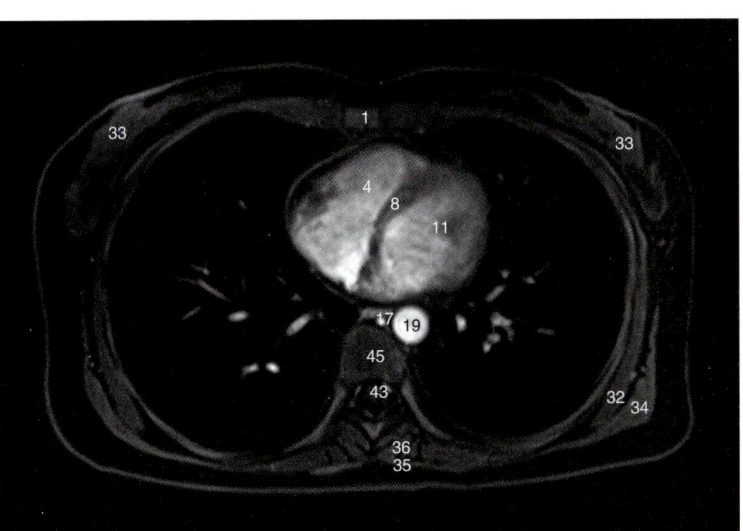

D. MR T1WI 增强图像

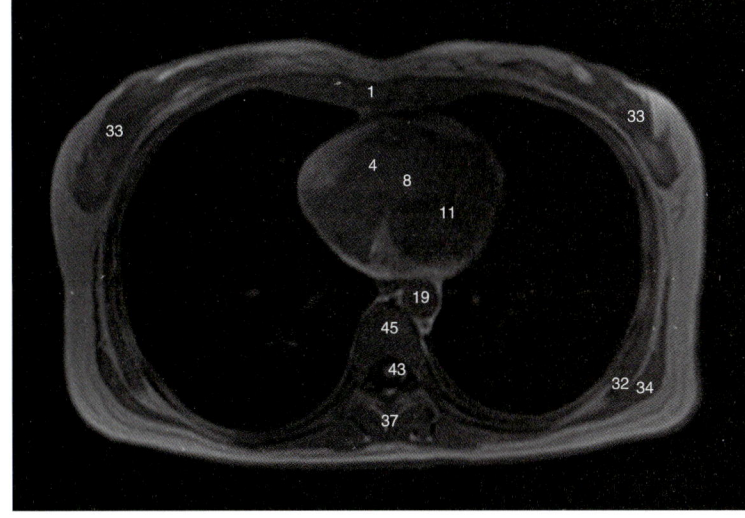

E. MR T1WI 平扫图像

关键结构：冠状窦，斜裂，左心房，左心室。

此断面前方经第 6 胸肋关节，后方经第 8 胸椎椎体下份。

纵隔内，左心房已明显变小，房间隔显示其中下部。其他 3 个心腔仍较为明显，右心室居前，右心房居右，左心室居于左侧。冠状窦直径较大，位于冠状沟后部，因左心房变小，冠状窦逐渐靠近右心房，并最终汇入之。右肺下叶内，前底段消失，相应部位出现膈穹窿。其他底段内管道变细，仍清晰可见，前底段静脉、后底段静脉和内侧底段静脉为段间支，分隔 3 个底段。左肺下叶内，内前底段、外侧底段和后底段的管道依然较易识别，且均为亚段分支。两肺斜裂均位于肺前部，其走行方向呈现一定规律：上胸部层面，斜裂由后外至前内；中胸部层面，由外向内，几呈冠状位；下胸部层面，由前外走向后内。明确斜裂的位置，有助于肺内疾病的定位诊断和观察病变对邻叶的侵犯情况。CT 图像中肺内管道变化不大，中纵隔内主要为右心房和左、右心室。后纵隔见右肋间后静脉注入奇静脉。

胸部连续横断层 75（FH.12010）

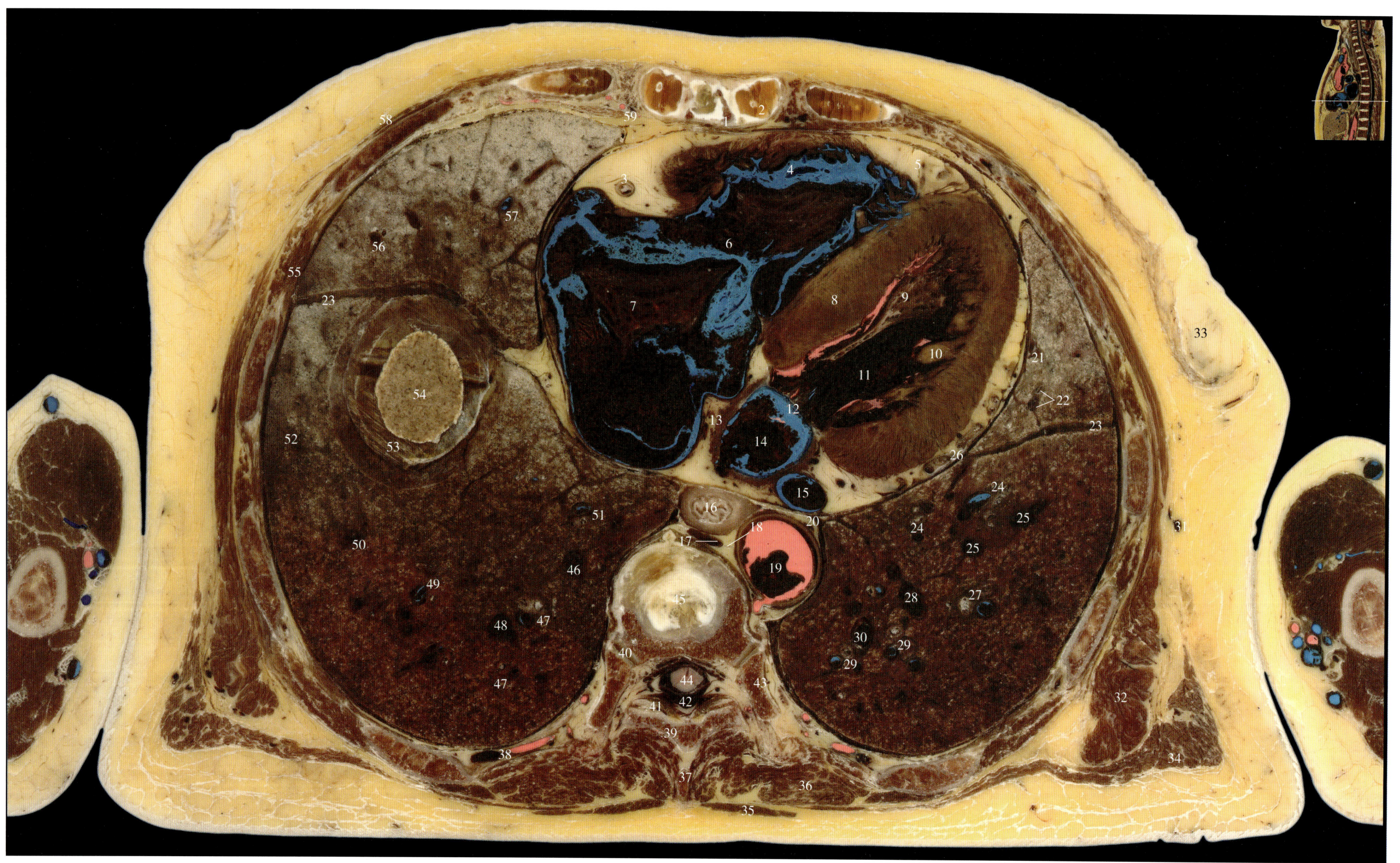

A. 断层标本图像

1. 胸骨体 body of sternum
2. 第 6 肋软骨 6th costal cartilage
3. 右冠状动脉 right coronary artery
4. 右心室 right ventricle
5. 前室间支 anterior interventricular branch
6. 三尖瓣 tricuspid valve
7. 右心房 right atrium
8. 室间隔 interventricular septum
9. 腱索 tendinous cord
10. 乳头肌 papillary muscle
11. 左心室 left ventricle
12. 二尖瓣 mitral valve
13. 房间隔 interatrial septum
14. 左心房 left atrium
15. 冠状窦 coronary sinus
16. 食管 esophagus
17. 奇静脉 azygos vein
18. 胸导管 thoracic duct
19. 胸主动脉 thoracic aorta
20. 肺韧带 pulmonary ligament
21. 下舌段静脉（V5）inferior lingular segmental vein
22. 下舌段支气管（B5）和动脉（A5）inferior lingular segmental bronchus and artery
23. 斜裂 oblique fissure
24. 内前底段支气管（B7+8）和动脉（A7+8）medioanterior basal segmental bronchus and artery
25. 内前底段静脉（V7+8）medioanterior basal segmental vein
26. 旋支 circumflex branch
27. 左肺外侧底段支气管（B9）和动脉（A9）left lateral basal segmental bronchus and artery
28. 左肺外侧底段静脉（V9）left lateral basal segmental vein
29. 左肺后底段支气管（B10）和动脉（A10）left posterior basal segmental bronchus and artery
30. 左肺后底段静脉（V10）left posterior basal segmental vein
31. 胸外侧静脉 lateral thoracic vein
32. 前锯肌 serratus anterior

33. 乳腺 mammary gland
34. 背阔肌 latissimus dorsi
35. 斜方肌 trapezius
36. 竖脊肌 erector spinae
37. 棘突 spinous process
38. 肋间后动、静脉 posterior intercostal artery and vein
39. 椎弓板 lamina of vertebral arch
40. 肋头关节 joints of costal head
41. 黄韧带 ligamenta flava
42. 硬膜外隙 epidural space
43. 第 9 肋骨 9th costal bone
44. 脊髓 spinal cord
45. T8-9 椎间盘 T8-9 intervertebral disc
46. 内侧底段静脉（V7）medial basal segmental vein
47. 右肺后底段支气管（B10）和动脉（A10）right posterior basal segmental bronchus and artery
48. 右肺后底段静脉（V10）right posterior basal segmental vein
49. 右肺外侧底段支气管（B9）和动脉（A9）right lateral basal segmental bronchus and artery
50. 前底段静脉（V8）anterior basal segmental vein
51. 内侧底段支气管（B7）和动脉（A7）medial basal segmental bronchus and artery
52. 前底段支气管（B8）和动脉（A8）anterior basal segmental bronchus and artery
53. 膈 diaphragm
54. 肝 liver
55. 肋间内肌 intercostales interni
56. 外侧段（S4）lateral segment
57. 内侧段（S5）medial segment
58. 胸大肌 pectoralis major
59. 胸廓内动、静脉 internal thoracic artery and vein
60. 后室间支 posterior interventricular branch
61. 左室后支 posterior branch of left ventricle
62. 右缘支 right marginal branch

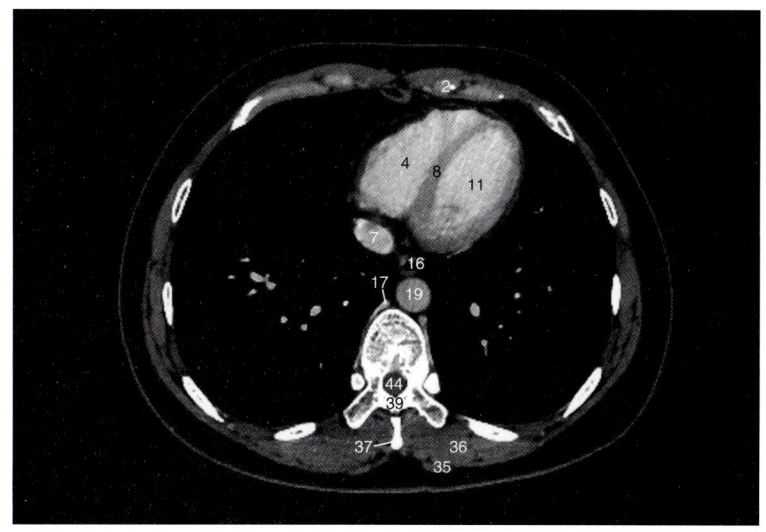

B. CT 纵隔窗增强图像

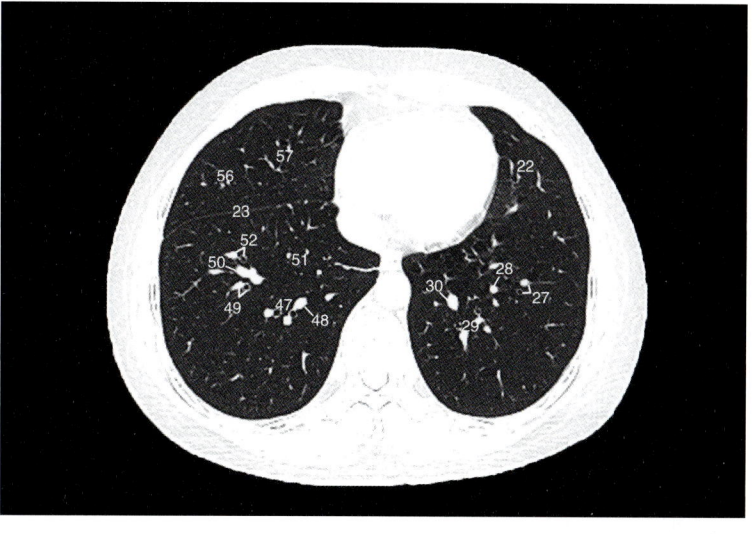

C. CT 肺窗图像

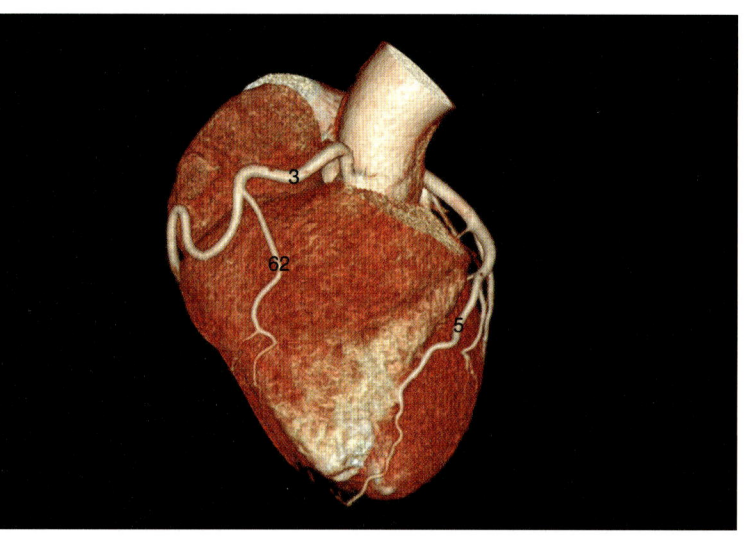

D. 冠状动脉 CT 三维重建图像（前面观）

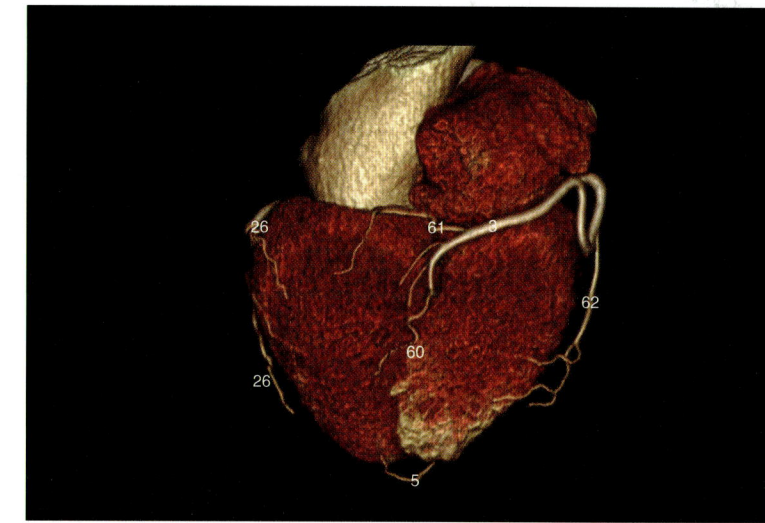

E. 冠状动脉 CT 三维重建图像（后面观）

关键结构：右冠状动脉，后室间支，左室后支。

此断面经 T8-9 椎间盘上份。

纵隔右侧的右心房和前部的右心室之间隔以冠状沟的右侧部，右冠状动脉主干从主动脉右窦发出后，随即进入冠状沟右侧部，绕心右缘至膈面的冠状沟内，行至房室交点附近或右侧，分为 2 个终末支：后室间支（后降支）和左室后支（右旋支）[85]。右冠状动脉的其他分支还包括右缘支、窦房结支、房室结支、右室支、右房支等，一般分布于右心房、右心室前壁大部、右心室侧壁和后壁、左心室后壁一部分和室间隔后 1/3，包括左束支的后半以及房室结和窦房结，如右冠状动脉阻塞，可发生左室后壁及右心室肌的梗死，如果病变累及窦房结或房室结，可发生各种缓慢型心律失常[86]。右冠状动脉外径为 4.5 mm ± 0.2 mm，左冠状动脉外径常大于右冠状动脉。心脏供血常见以右冠状动脉为主（右优势型），右冠状动脉在房室交点附近呈倒"U"形弯曲，一旦出现即为冠状动脉造影的一个有用的辨认标志，并分为后室间支和左室后支[87]。其中后室间支粗大，为终末支，沿室间沟下行，终止于后室间沟中 1/3 的占 40.3% ± 3.1%，终止于后室间沟下 1/3 的占 30.3% ± 3.0%。64.9% ± 2.4% 的右冠状动脉分布终点到达左室后部[36]。在冠状动脉 CT 三维重建图像的前面和后面观中显示了右冠状动脉的主要分支及其走行。

胸部连续横断层 76（FH.11990）

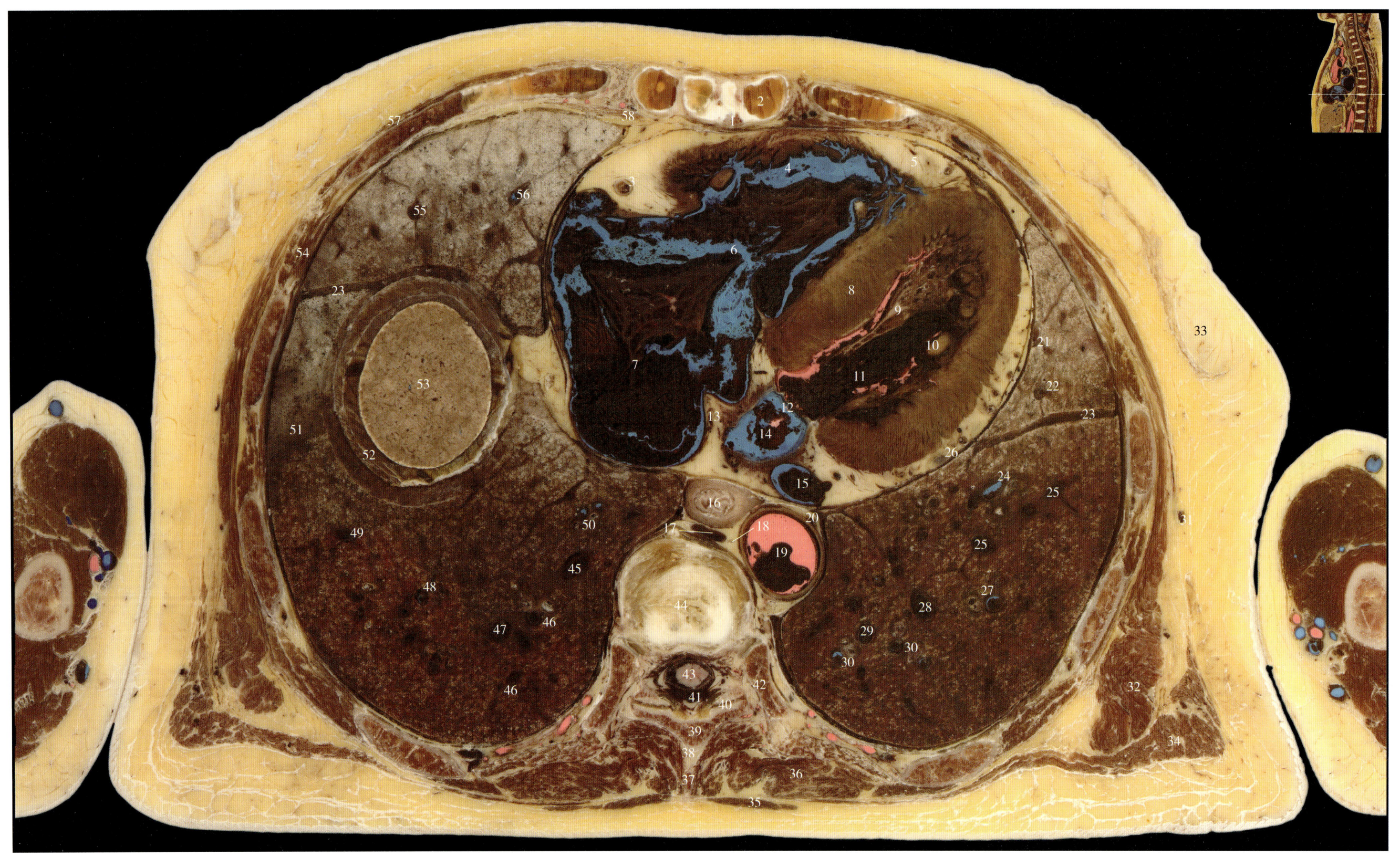

A. 断层标本图像

1. 胸骨体 body of sternum
2. 第 6 肋软骨 6th costal cartilage
3. 右冠状动脉 right coronary artery
4. 右心室 right ventricle
5. 前室间支 anterior interventricular branch
6. 三尖瓣 tricuspid valve
7. 右心房 right atrium
8. 室间隔 interventricular septum
9. 腱索 tendinous cord
10. 乳头肌 papillary muscle
11. 左心室 left ventricle
12. 二尖瓣 mitral valve
13. 房间隔 interatrial septum
14. 左心房 left atrium
15. 冠状窦 coronary sinus
16. 食管 esophagus
17. 奇静脉 azygos vein
18. 胸导管 thoracic duct
19. 胸主动脉 thoracic aorta
20. 肺韧带 pulmonary ligament
21. 下舌段静脉（V5）inferior lingular segmental vein
22. 下舌段支气管（B5）和动脉（A5）inferior lingular segmental bronchus and artery
23. 斜裂 oblique fissure
24. 内前底段支气管（B7+8）和动脉（A7+8）medioanterior basal segmental bronchus and artery
25. 内前底段静脉（V7+8）medioanterior basal segmental vein
26. 旋支 circumflex branch
27. 左肺外侧底段支气管（B9）和动脉（A9）left lateral basal segmental bronchus and artery
28. 左肺外侧底段静脉（V9）left lateral basal segmental vein
29. 左肺后底段静脉（V10）left posterior basal segmental vein
30. 左肺后底段支气管（B10）和动脉（A10）left posterior basal segmental bronchus and artery
31. 胸外侧静脉 lateral thoracic vein
32. 前锯肌 serratus anterior
33. 乳腺 mammary gland
34. 背阔肌 latissimus dorsi
35. 斜方肌 trapezius
36. 竖脊肌 erector spinae
37. 棘突 spinous process
38. 棘间韧带 interspinous ligament
39. 椎弓板 lamina of vertebral arch
40. 关节突关节 zygapophysial joint
41. 硬膜外隙 epidural space
42. 第 9 肋骨 9th costal bone
43. 脊髓 spinal cord
44. T8-9 椎间盘 T8-9 intervertebral disc
45. 内侧底段静脉（V7）medial basal segmental vein
46. 右肺后底段支气管（B10）和动脉（A10）right posterior basal segmental bronchus and artery
47. 右肺后底段静脉（V10）right posterior basal segmental vein
48. 右肺外侧底段支气管（B9）和动脉（A9）right lateral basal segmental bronchus and artery
49. 前底段静脉（V8）anterior basal segmental vein
50. 内侧底段支气管（B7）和动脉（A7）medial basal segmental bronchus and artery
51. 前底段（S8）anterior basal segment
52. 膈 diaphragm
53. 肝 liver
54. 肋间肌 intercostal muscle
55. 外侧段（S4）lateral segment
56. 内侧段（S5）medial segment
57. 胸大肌 pectoralis major
58. 胸廓内动、静脉 internal thoracic artery and vein
59. 后室间支 posterior interventricular branch
60. 前底段支气管（B8）和动脉（A8）anterior basal segmental bronchus and artery

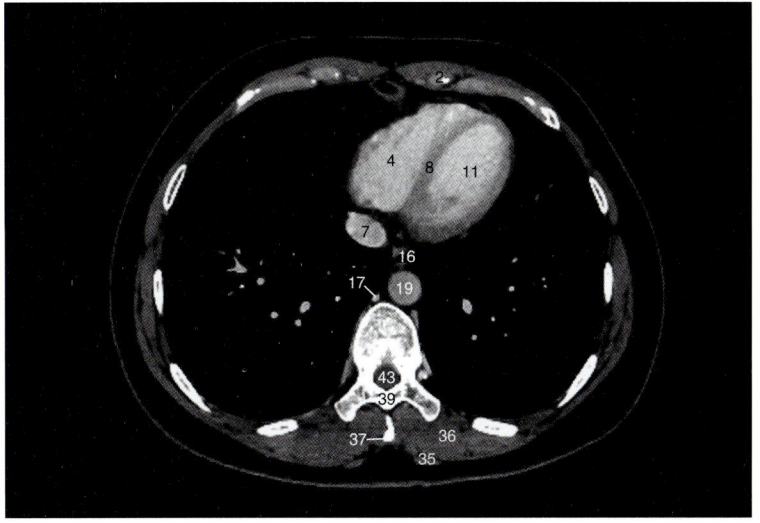

B. CT 纵隔窗增强图像

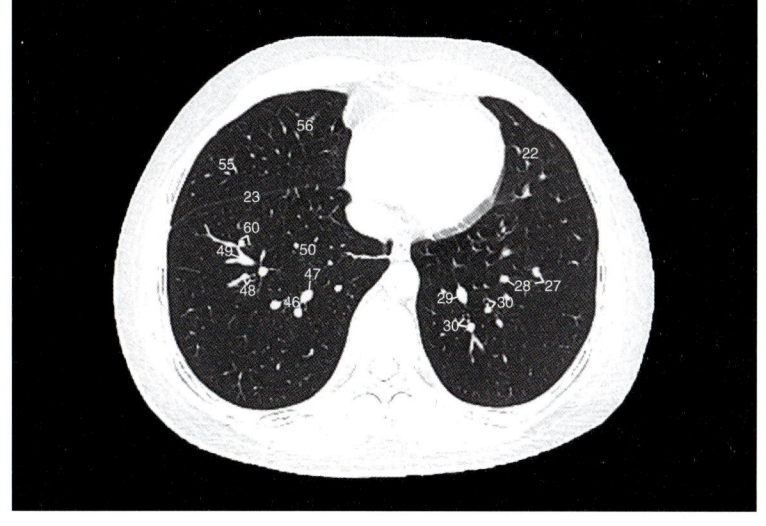

C. CT 肺窗图像

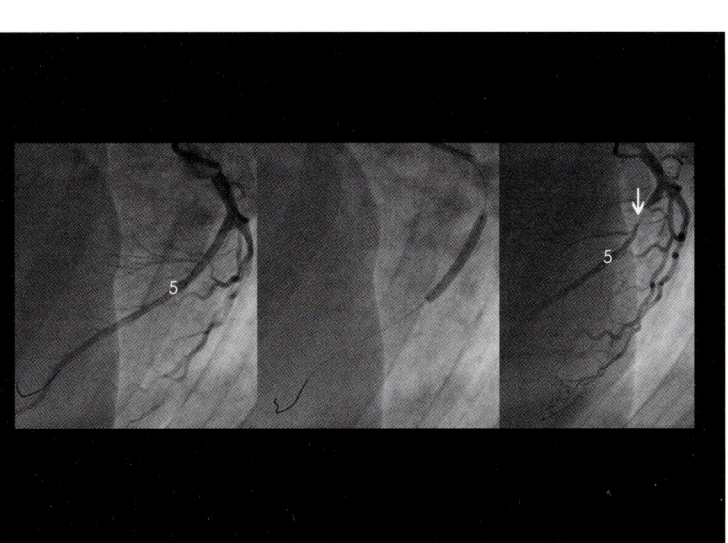

D. 左冠状动脉前室间支重度狭窄置入的支架

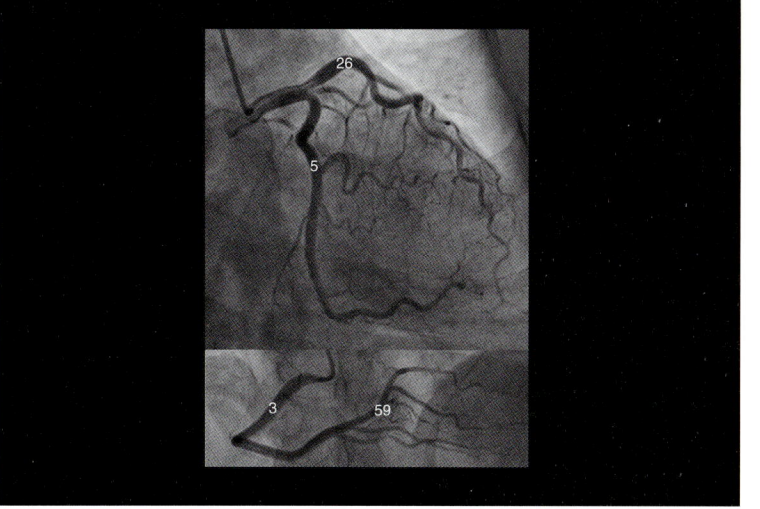

E. 正常左、右冠状动脉 DSA 图像

关键结构：胸导管，前室间支。

此断面经 T8-9 椎间盘。

后纵隔内，胸导管位于脊柱左前方，食管、奇静脉和胸主动脉之间。胸导管是全身最大的淋巴导管，在机体淋巴液和乳糜液的转运过程中起着非常重要的作用，全身约 70% 的淋巴液和乳糜液都通过它转运入血。胸导管损伤，轻者可导致水电解质失衡、免疫功能紊乱和营养不良，重者可危及患者的生命[88]。胸导管上段与左纵隔胸膜相邻，下段与右纵隔胸膜相邻，当食管癌手术或胸导管损伤时，上段常合并左侧乳糜胸，下段损伤常引起右侧乳糜胸[89]。胸导管胸部一般在第 5 胸椎高度，在食管与半奇静脉末端之间，由脊柱右前方斜向左前方上行。胸导管转向左侧的位置，4~6 胸椎高度最多，占 64.27%，最高可达第 3 胸椎，最低可在第 11 胸椎水平。该标本在第 9 胸椎平面，半奇静脉汇入奇静脉处，由脊柱右前方转向了左侧。胸导管 MR 水成像显示国人胸导管最大直径平均为 0.42 cm ± 0.09 cm，男性胸导管最大直径略大于女性[90]。前室间支是左冠状动脉的重要分支，自前室间沟内下降，有 50.3% ± 2.9% 的前室间支终止于后室间沟的下 1/3 可与后室间沟内的后室间支吻合。前室间支主要供血范围为左室前壁、前乳头肌、心尖、右室前壁的一部分、室间隔的前 2/3 及心传导系的右束支和左束支的前半。

胸部连续横断层 77（FH.11970）

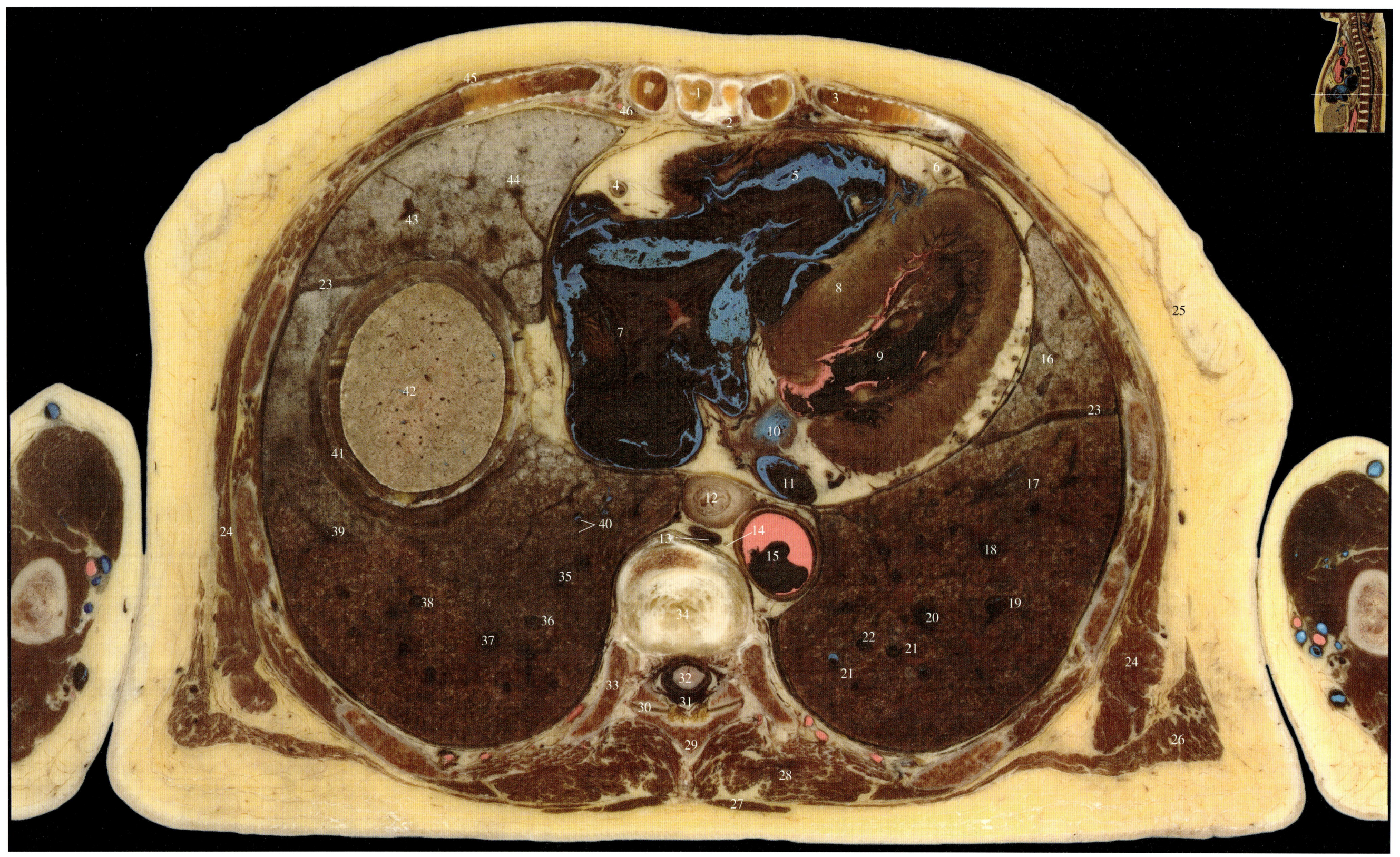

A. 断层标本图像

1. 第 7 肋软骨 7th costal cartilage
2. 剑突 xiphoid process
3. 第 5 肋软骨 5th costal cartilage
4. 右冠状动脉 right coronary artery
5. 右心室 right ventricle
6. 前室间支 anterior interventricular branch
7. 右心房 right atrium
8. 室间隔 interventricular septum
9. 左心室 left ventricle
10. 左心房 left atrium
11. 冠状窦 coronary sinus
12. 食管 esophagus
13. 奇静脉 azygos vein
14. 胸导管 thoracic duct
15. 胸主动脉 thoracic aorta
16. 下舌段（S5）inferior lingular segment
17. 内前底段支气管（B7+8）和动脉（A7+8）medioanterior basal segmental bronchus and artery
18. 内前底段静脉（V7+8）medioanterior basal segmental vein
19. 左肺外侧底段支气管（B9）和动脉（A9）left lateral basal segmental bronchus and artery
20. 左肺外侧底段静脉（V9）left lateral basal segmental vein
21. 左肺后底段支气管（B10）和动脉（A10）left posterior basal segmental bronchus and artery
22. 左肺后底段静脉（V10）left posterior basal segmental vein
23. 斜裂 oblique fissure
24. 前锯肌 serratus anterior
25. 乳腺 mammary gland
26. 背阔肌 latissimus dorsi
27. 斜方肌 trapezius
28. 竖脊肌 erector spinae
29. 棘突 spinous process
30. 关节突关节 zygapophysial joint
31. 硬膜外隙 epidural space
32. 脊髓 spinal cord
33. 第 9 肋骨 9th costal bone
34. T8-9 椎间盘 T8-9 intervertebral disc
35. 右肺内侧底段静脉（V7）right medial basal segmental vein
36. 右肺后底段支气管（B10）和动脉（A10）right posterior basal segmental bronchus and artery
37. 右肺后底段静脉（V10）right posterior basal segmental vein
38. 右肺外侧底段支气管（B9）和动脉（A9）right lateral basal segmental bronchus and artery
39. 前底段静脉（V8）anterior basal segmental vein
40. 内侧段支气管（B7）和动脉（A7）medial basal segmental bronchus and artery
41. 膈 diaphragm
42. 肝 liver
43. 外侧段（S4）lateral segment
44. 内侧段（S5）medial segment
45. 胸大肌 pectoralis major
46. 胸廓内动、静脉 internal thoracic artery and vein
47. 前底段支气管（B8）和动脉（A8）anterior basal segmental bronchus and artery

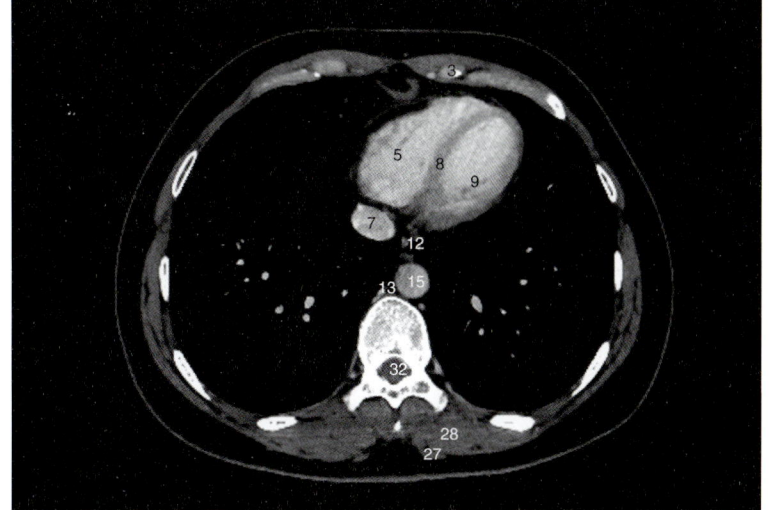

B. CT 纵隔窗增强图像

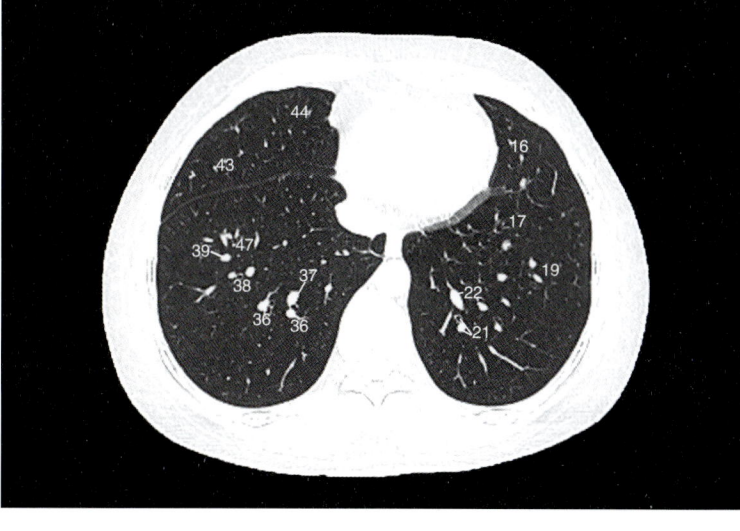

C. CT 肺窗图像

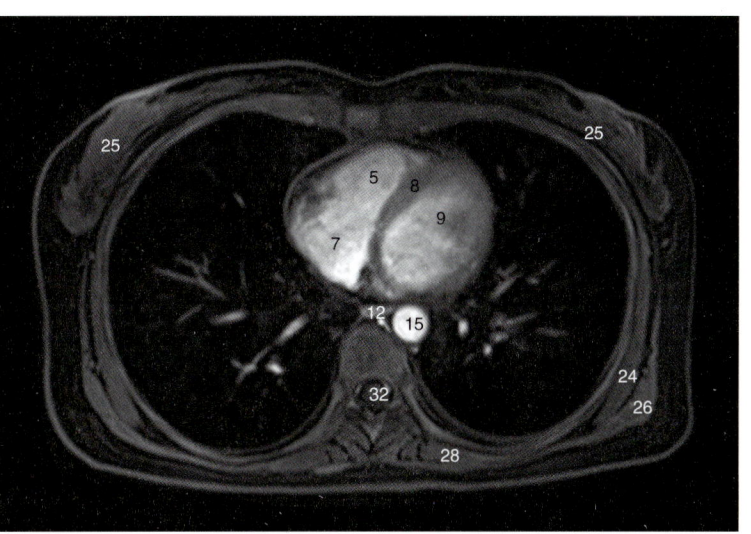

D. MR T1WI 增强图像

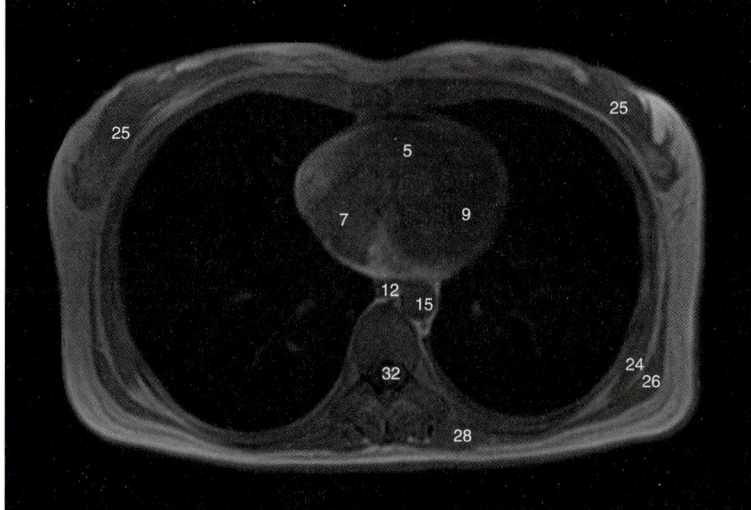

E. MR T1WI 平扫图像

关键结构：右心房，下腔静脉，食管。

断面前方经第 7 胸肋关节，后方经 T8-9 椎间盘。

中纵隔内，左心房即将消失，左房室口、二尖瓣等结构伴随消失，冠状窦向前即将汇入右心房。右心房居于最右侧，腔大而明显。右心房内腔借外侧壁中部的肌性隆起-界嵴分为前部的固有心房和后部的腔静脉窦，前者由原始心房演变而来，后者由原始静脉窦发育而成。界嵴为纵行的肌隆起，其顶部转为横向，连至上腔静脉口的前外面，下部垂直，向下一直延续为下腔静脉瓣。固有心房内壁有高低不平的肌隆起，为梳状肌，腔静脉窦内壁光滑，向下延续为下腔静脉。右心房有 3 个入口，即上腔静脉口、下腔静脉口和冠状窦口，接收由它们输送来的静脉血，右心房的出口即右房室口，有三尖瓣附着，注入右心室[91]。后纵隔内主要有食管、胸主动脉、胸导管及奇静脉等。食管两侧为肺韧带，后方与奇静脉之间有奇静脉食管隐窝，由右胸膜腔深入。脊柱区切及 T8-9 椎间盘下部，椎间盘中间为髓核，周围是纤维环。椎管后方见关节突关节、棘突等。CT 纵隔图像右心房消失，下腔静脉形成，向下穿腔静脉孔进入腹腔，脊柱区见第 9 胸椎椎体、椎弓根、椎弓板及围成的椎管，内有硬脊膜包被的脊髓等结构。

胸部连续横断层 78（FH.11950）

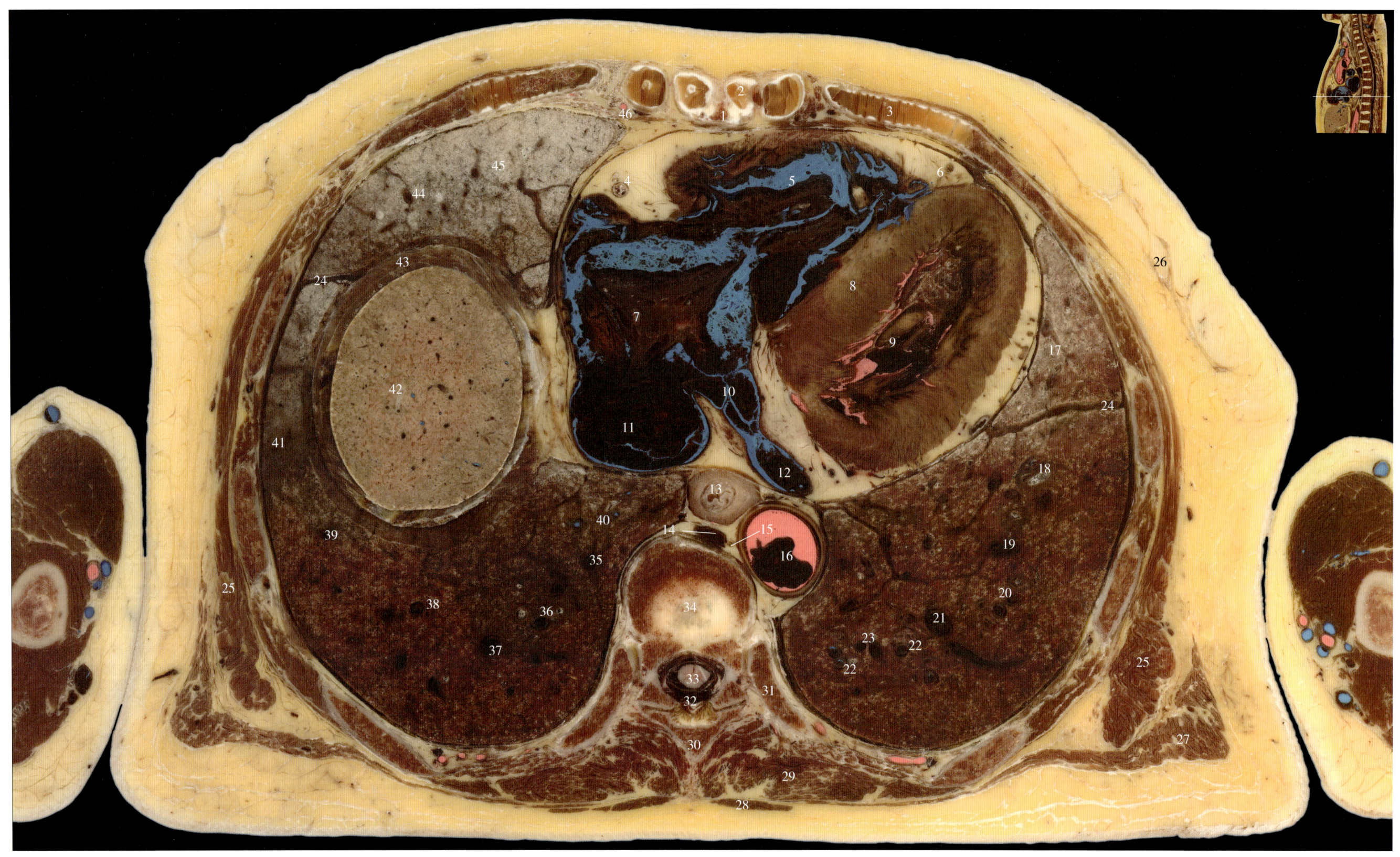

A. 断层标本图像

1. 剑突 xiphoid process
2. 第7肋软骨 7th costal cartilage
3. 第5肋软骨 5th costal cartilage
4. 右冠状动脉 right coronary artery
5. 右心室 right ventricle
6. 前室间支 anterior interventricular branch
7. 右心房 right atrium
8. 室间隔 interventricular septum
9. 左心室 left ventricle
10. 冠状窦口 orifice of coronary sinus
11. 下腔静脉口 orifice of inferior vena cava
12. 冠状窦 coronary sinus
13. 食管 esophagus
14. 奇静脉 azygos vein
15. 胸导管 thoracic duct
16. 胸主动脉 thoracic aorta
17. 下舌段（S5）inferior lingular segment
18. 内前底段支气管（B7+8）和动脉（A7+8）medioanterior basal segmental bronchus and artery
19. 内前底段静脉（V7+8）medioanterior basal segmental vein
20. 左肺外侧底段支气管（B9）和动脉（A9）left lateral basal segmental bronchus and artery
21. 左肺外侧底段静脉（V9）left lateral basal segmental vein
22. 左肺后底段支气管（B10）和动脉（A10）left posterior basal segmental bronchus and artery
23. 左肺后底段静脉（V10）left posterior basal segmental vein
24. 斜裂 oblique fissure
25. 前锯肌 serratus anterior
26. 乳腺 mammary gland
27. 背阔肌 latissimus dorsi
28. 斜方肌 trapezius
29. 竖脊肌 erector spinae
30. 棘突 spinous process
31. 第9肋骨 9th costal bone
32. 硬膜外隙 epidural space
33. 脊髓 spinal cord
34. T8-9椎间盘 T8-9 intervertebral disc
35. 内侧底段静脉（V7）medial basal segmental vein
36. 右肺后底段支气管（B10）和动脉（A10）right posterior basal segmental bronchus and artery
37. 右肺后底段静脉（V10）right posterior basal segmental vein
38. 右肺外侧底段支气管（B9）和动脉（A9）right lateral basal segmental bronchus and artery
39. 前底段静脉（V8）anterior basal segmental vein
40. 内侧底段支气管（B7）和动脉（A7）medial basal segmental bronchus and artery
41. 前底段（S8）anterior basal segment
42. 肝 liver
43. 膈 diaphragm
44. 外侧段（S4）lateral segment
45. 内侧段（S5）medial segment
46. 胸廓内动脉 internal thoracic artery

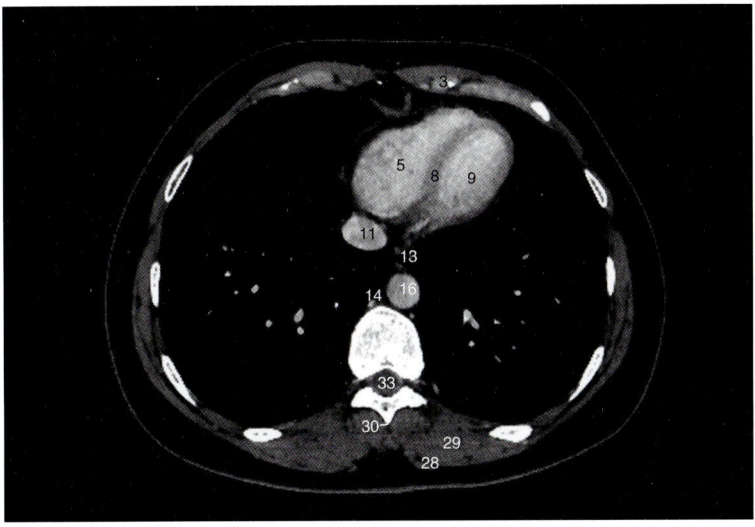

B. CT 纵隔窗增强图像

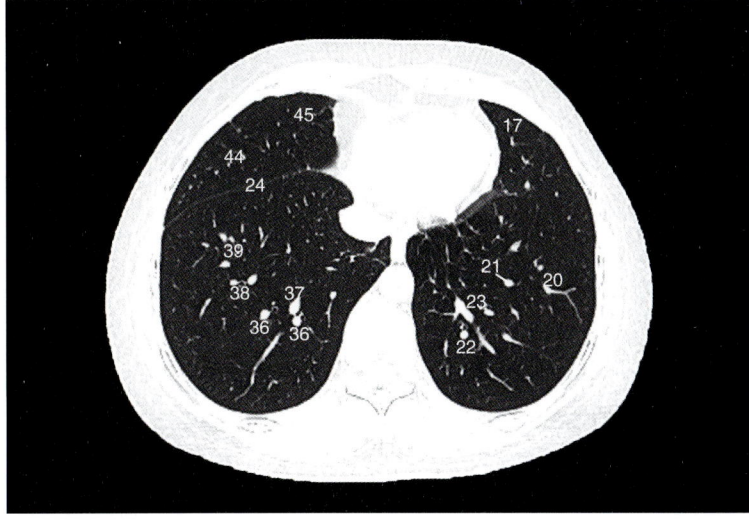

C. CT 肺窗图像

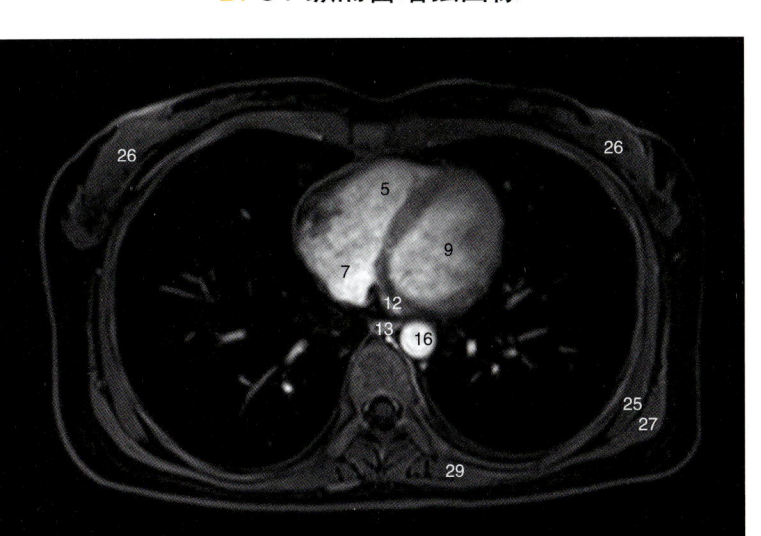

D. MR T1WI 增强图像

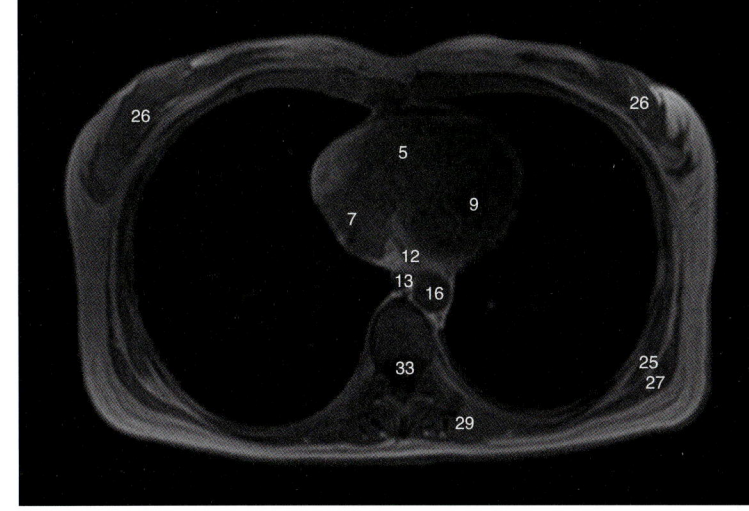

E. MR T1WI 平扫图像

关键结构：房室交点，冠状窦，奇静脉。

此断面后方经T8-9椎间盘和第9胸椎椎体上部。

脊柱区后部仍可见椎管内脊髓及被膜、肋头关节、关节突关节、棘突等结构。在中纵隔内，左心房消失，冠状窦经冠状窦口汇入右心房。在心脏后面，后室间沟、后室间沟与冠状沟相交处称房室交点，是心表面的重要标志，也是左、右心房与左、右心室在心后面相互交汇部位。冠状动脉经此区形成"U"形弯曲，并发出一小支动脉分布至房室结。冠状窦位于此区，回流心脏的大部分静脉血入右心房，窦口常有一个半月形的冠状窦瓣。两肺底结构出现，右肺内仍可见内、外侧段和内、外、后底段的管道。左肺内为下舌段和内、外、后底段支气管和血管分支。后纵隔内食管、奇静脉、胸导管及胸主动脉位置关系不变。右胸膜腔深入食管和奇静脉之间形成奇静脉食管隐窝，奇静脉食管隐窝越深越容易形成肺大泡，并更容易破裂，从而引起自发性气胸[92]。CT纵隔窗图像可见左心室逐渐缩小，食管前移至胸主动脉前方。肺部结构饱满，斜裂前移，后部为肺下叶各底段结构。

胸部连续横断层 79（FH.11930）

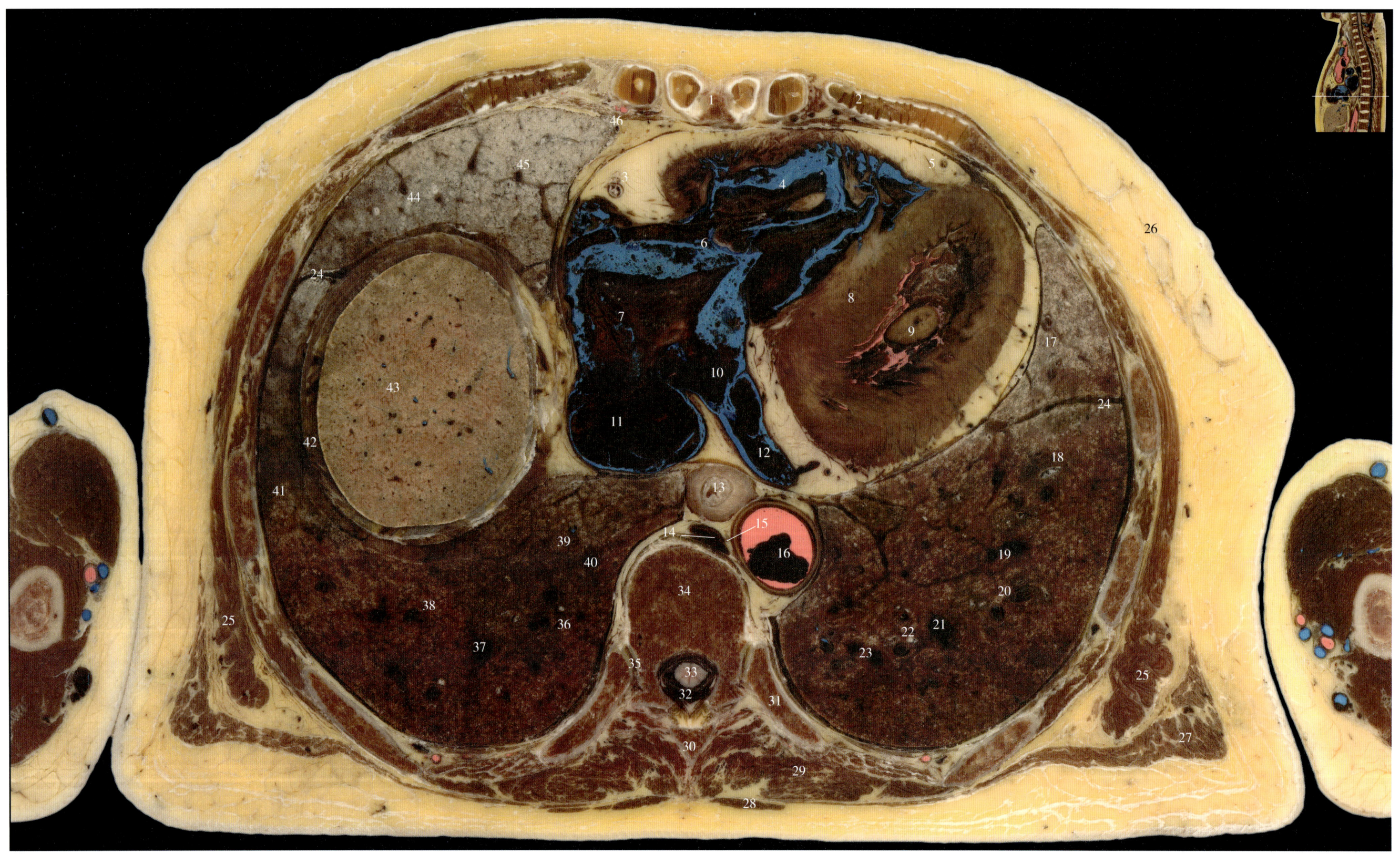

A. 断层标本图像

1. 剑突 xiphoid process
2. 第 5 肋软骨 5th costal cartilage
3. 右冠状动脉 right coronary artery
4. 右心室 right ventricle
5. 前室间支 anterior interventricular branch
6. 三尖瓣 tricuspid valve
7. 右心房 right atrium
8. 室间隔 interventricular septum
9. 左心室 left ventricle
10. 冠状窦口 orifice of coronary sinus
11. 下腔静脉口 orifice of inferior vena cava
12. 冠状窦 coronary sinus
13. 食管 esophagus
14. 奇静脉 azygos vein
15. 胸导管 thoracic duct
16. 胸主动脉 thoracic aorta
17. 下舌段（S5）inferior lingular segment
18. 内前底段支气管（B7+8）和动脉（A7+8）medioanterior basal segmental bronchus and artery
19. 内前底段静脉（V7+8）medioanterior basal segmental vein
20. 左肺外侧底段支气管（B9）和动脉（A9）left lateral basal segmental bronchus and artery
21. 左肺外侧底段静脉（V9）left lateral basal segmental vein
22. 左肺后底段支气管（B10）和动脉（A10）left posterior basal segmental bronchus and artery
23. 左肺后底段静脉（V10）left posterior basal segmental vein
24. 斜裂 oblique fissure
25. 前锯肌 serratus anterior
26. 乳腺 mammary gland
27. 背阔肌 latissimus dorsi
28. 斜方肌 trapezius
29. 竖脊肌 erector spinae
30. 棘突 spinous process
31. 第 9 肋骨 9th costal bone
32. 硬膜外隙 epidural space
33. 脊髓 spinal cord
34. 第 9 胸椎椎体 body of 9th thoracic vertebra
35. 肋头关节 joint of costal head
36. 右肺后底段支气管（B10）和动脉（A10）right posterior basal segmental bronchus and artery
37. 右肺后底段静脉（V10）right posterior basal segmental vein
38. 右肺外侧底段支气管（B9）和动脉（A9）right lateral basal segmental bronchus and artery
39. 内侧底段支气管（B7）和动脉（A7）medial basal segmental bronchus and artery
40. 内侧底段静脉（V7）medial basal segmental vein
41. 前底段（S8）anterior basal segment
42. 膈 diaphragm
43. 肝 liver
44. 外侧段（S4）lateral segment
45. 内侧段（S5）medial segment
46. 胸廓内动脉 internal thoracic artery

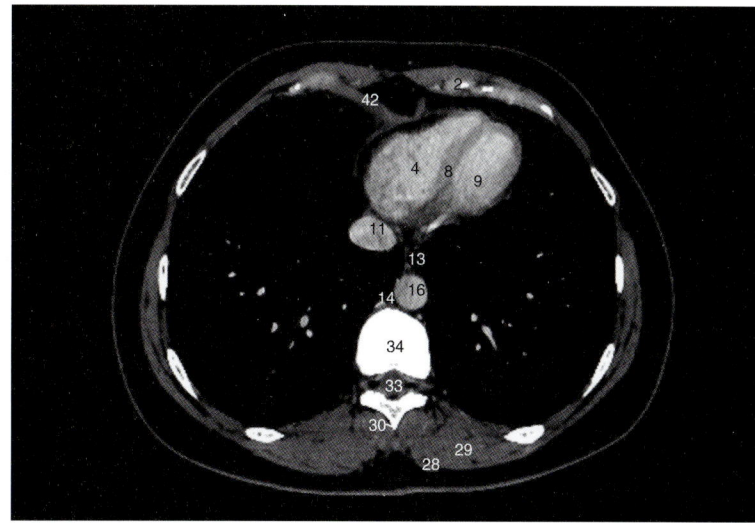

B. CT 纵隔窗增强图像

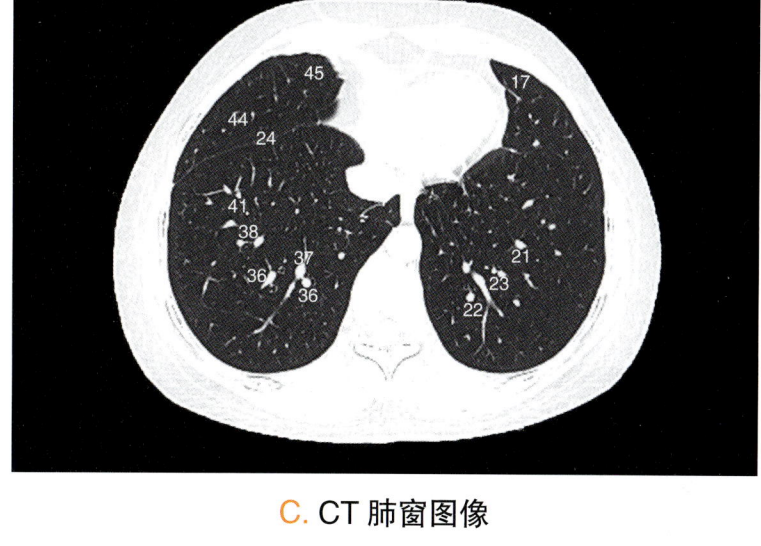

C. CT 肺窗图像

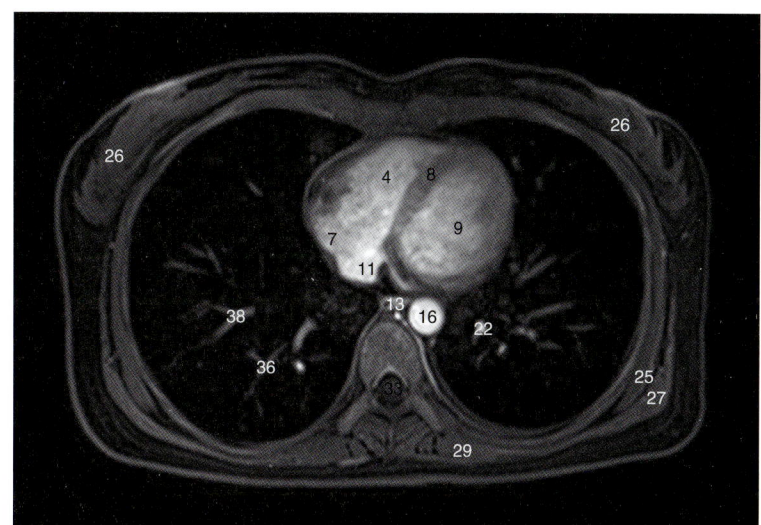

D. MR T1WI 增强图像

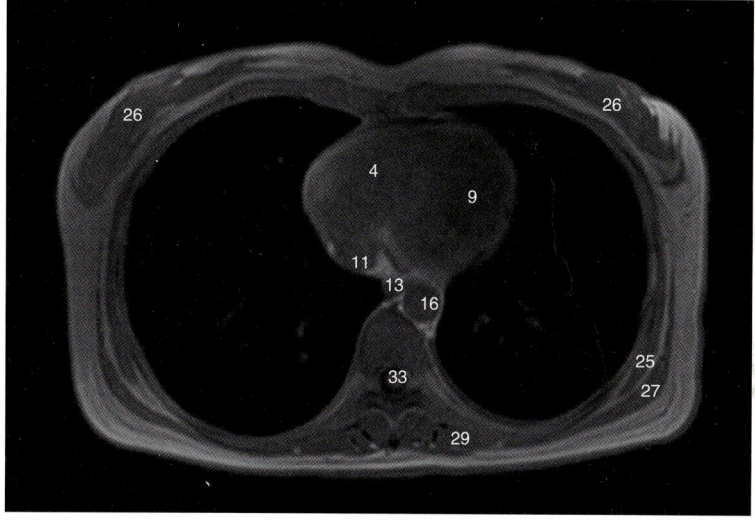

E. MR T1WI 平扫图像

关键结构：膈右穹窿，黄韧带，三尖瓣。

本断面前方经第 7 胸肋关节，后方经第 9 胸椎椎体上份。

中纵隔内仅剩 3 个心腔，左心房已消失。冠状窦汇入右心房，冠状窦口较大，下腔静脉口清晰可见。右心室室腔变小，在右心房与心室之间有三尖瓣复合体，由三尖瓣环、三尖瓣、腱索和乳头肌组成，在功能和结构上成为一个整体，保证血液的单向流动，只能由右心房流入右心室，防止逆流[93]。三尖瓣环是心内最大的瓣膜口，略呈三角形，三尖瓣尖的面积大于三尖瓣环的面积；三尖瓣的前尖、后尖和隔侧尖的面积大小几乎一致。三尖瓣隔侧尖的前上 2/3 不附着于三尖瓣环上，而下移附着在室间隔的膜部和肌部，下移最大的距离在成人为 6.1 mm ± 0.9 mm。左心室前方构成心尖，被第 5 肋遮挡。两肺体积变小，各段内管道细小，几近消失。脊柱区切及第 9 胸椎椎体，其后外侧与第 9 肋的肋头形成肋头关节。椎体前方仍为奇静脉、胸导管、胸主动脉及食管等，食管两侧与肺之间为肺韧带。CT 图像纵隔窗室间隔后方见后室间支，营养左右心室的后壁及室间隔后部。心包前右侧出现膈右穹窿。

胸部连续横断层 80（FH.11910）

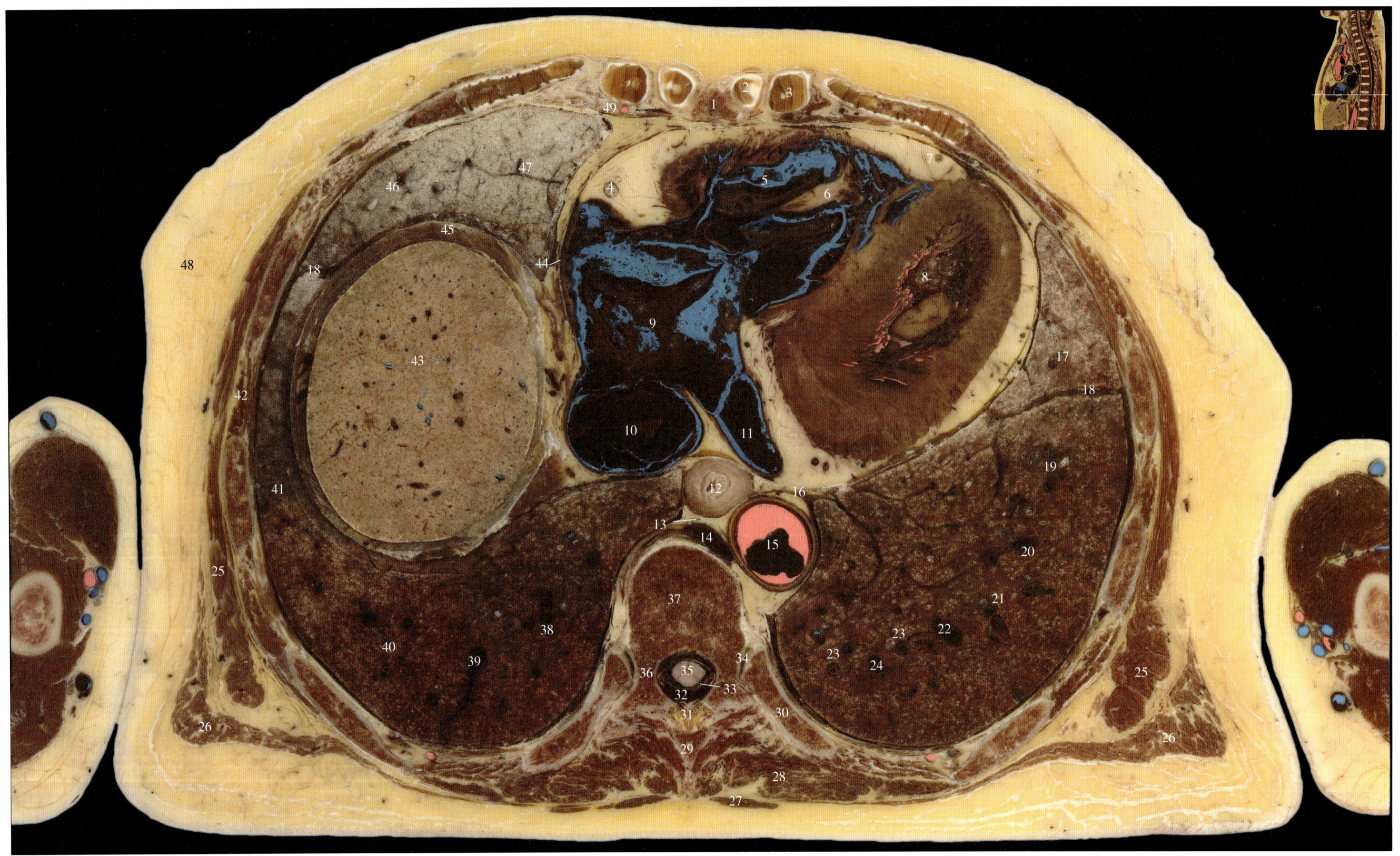

A. 断层标本图像

1. 剑突 xiphoid process
2. 第 7 肋软骨 7th costal cartilage
3. 第 6 肋软骨 6th costal cartilage
4. 右冠状动脉 right coronary artery
5. 右心室 right ventricle
6. 乳头肌 papillary muscle
7. 前室间支 anterior interventricular branch
8. 左心室 left ventricle
9. 右心房 right atrium
10. 下腔静脉 inferior vena cava
11. 冠状窦 coronary sinus
12. 食管 esophagus
13. 胸导管 thoracic duct
14. 奇静脉 azygos vein
15. 胸主动脉 thoracic aorta
16. 肺韧带 pulmonary ligament
17. 下舌段（S5）inferior lingular segment
18. 斜裂 oblique fissure
19. 内前底段支气管（B7+8）和动脉（A7+8）medioanterior basal segmental bronchus and artery
20. 内前底段静脉（V7+8）medioanterior basal segmental vein
21. 左肺外侧底段支气管（B9）和动脉（A9）left lateral basal segmental bronchus and artery
22. 左肺外侧底段静脉（V9）left lateral basal segmental vein
23. 左肺后底段支气管（B10）和动脉（A10）left posterior basal segmental bronchus and artery
24. 左肺后底段静脉（V10）left posterior basal segmental vein
25. 前锯肌 serratus anterior
26. 背阔肌 latissimus dorsi
27. 斜方肌 trapezius
28. 竖脊肌 erector spinae
29. 第 8 胸椎棘突 spinous process of 8th thoracic vertebra
30. 第 9 肋骨 9th costal bone
31. 黄韧带 ligament flava
32. 硬膜外隙 epidural space
33. 硬脊膜 spinal dura mater
34. 肋头关节 joint of costal head
35. 脊髓 spinal cord
36. 椎弓根 pedicle of vertebral arch
37. 第 9 胸椎椎体 body of 9th thoracic vertebra
38. 右肺后底段支气管（B10）和动脉（A10）right posterior basal segmental bronchus and artery
39. 右肺后底段静脉（V10）right posterior basal segmental vein
40. 右肺外侧底段支气管（B9）和动脉（A9）right lateral basal segmental bronchus and artery
41. 前底段（S8）anterior basal segment
42. 肋间肌 intercostal muscle
43. 肝右叶 right lobe of liver
44. 心包腔 pericardial cavity
45. 膈 diaphragm
46. 外侧段（S4）lateral segment
47. 内侧段（S5）medial segment
48. 乳腺 mammary gland
49. 胸廓内动脉 internal thoracic artery
50. 椎间盘 intervertebral disc

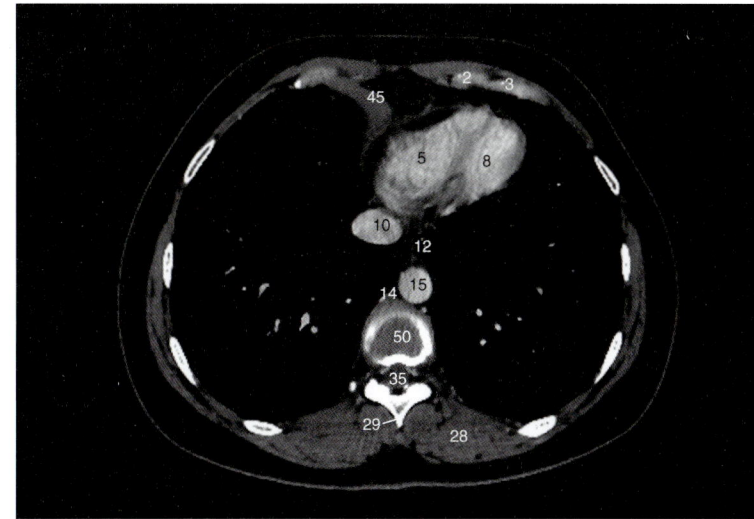

B. CT 纵隔窗增强图像

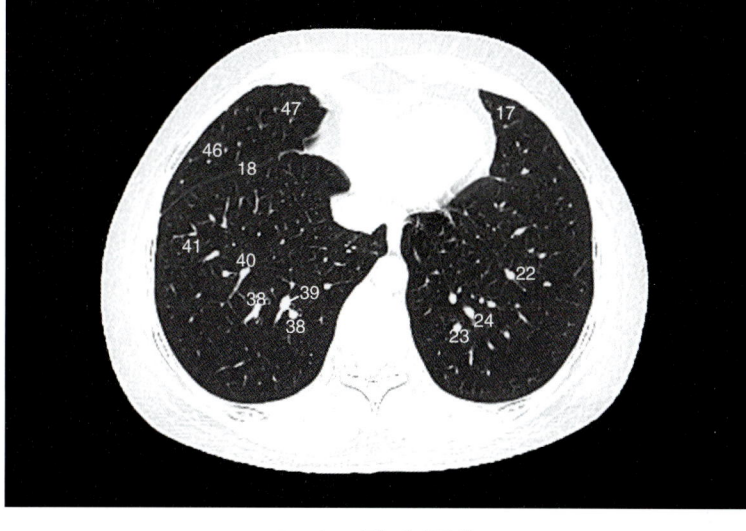

C. CT 肺窗图像

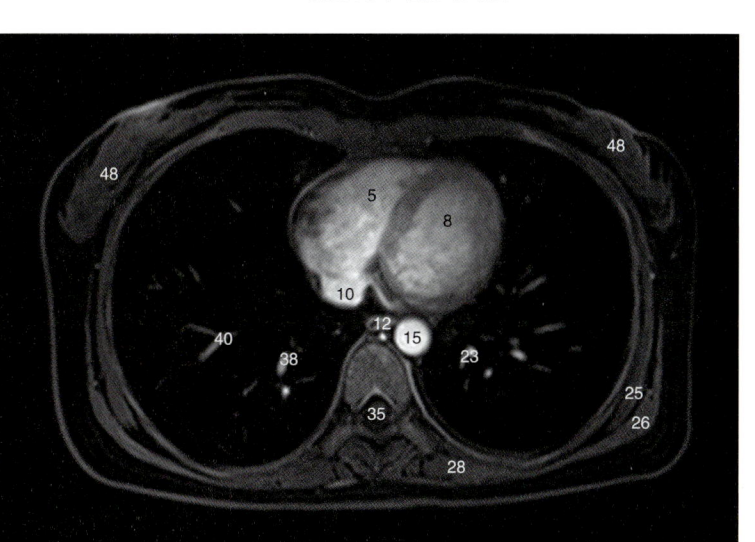

D. MR T1WI 增强图像

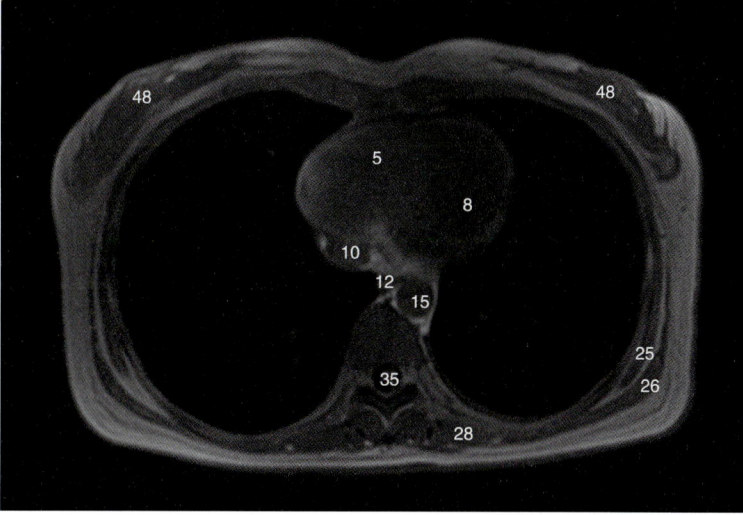

E. MR T1WI 平扫图像

关键结构：冠状窦，膈。

此断面前方经剑突，后方经第 9 胸椎椎体上部。

右心房，左、右心室大致同上一断层，心室内可见乳头肌，右心房前方与右心室之间见右冠状动脉，右心房后方的冠状沟内冠状窦注入右心房，右心房后部的腔静脉窦延续为下腔静脉，向下穿膈的腔静脉孔，向上注入右心房。左、右肺逐渐缩小，两侧肺下叶底段支气管与动脉逐渐消失。膈呈向上隆起的穹隆状，封闭胸腔下口，中央部平坦为中心腱，与心包相贴着，两侧隆凸右高左低，其高低位置因年龄、体位、呼吸状态和腹腔器官充盈程度不同而变化。膈有 3 个裂孔容下腔静脉、食管和主动脉穿过，

其中腔静脉孔位置最高，约平第 8 胸椎平面，有下腔静脉通过。本标本和影像图显示腔静脉孔位置略低，平第 9 胸椎。膈可分为功能不同的肋膈肌和脚膈肌，它们在发育、解剖和功能上均有很大差别，肋膈肌收缩时胸廓下部扩张，起吸气作用，而脚膈肌相反，收缩时胸廓下部缩小，起呼气作用，二者互为拮抗。在临床上可通过膈肌起搏，维持患有膈肌功能障碍患者的自然负压呼吸[94]。CT 图像显示肺部充盈，仍占断面的大部分，两肺下叶底段管道向周边迁移，变细小。右肺前部膈右穹隆出现，中纵隔左、右心室被心包包绕，后纵隔见食管、胸主动脉、奇静脉和半奇静脉等。

胸部连续横断层 81（FH.11890）

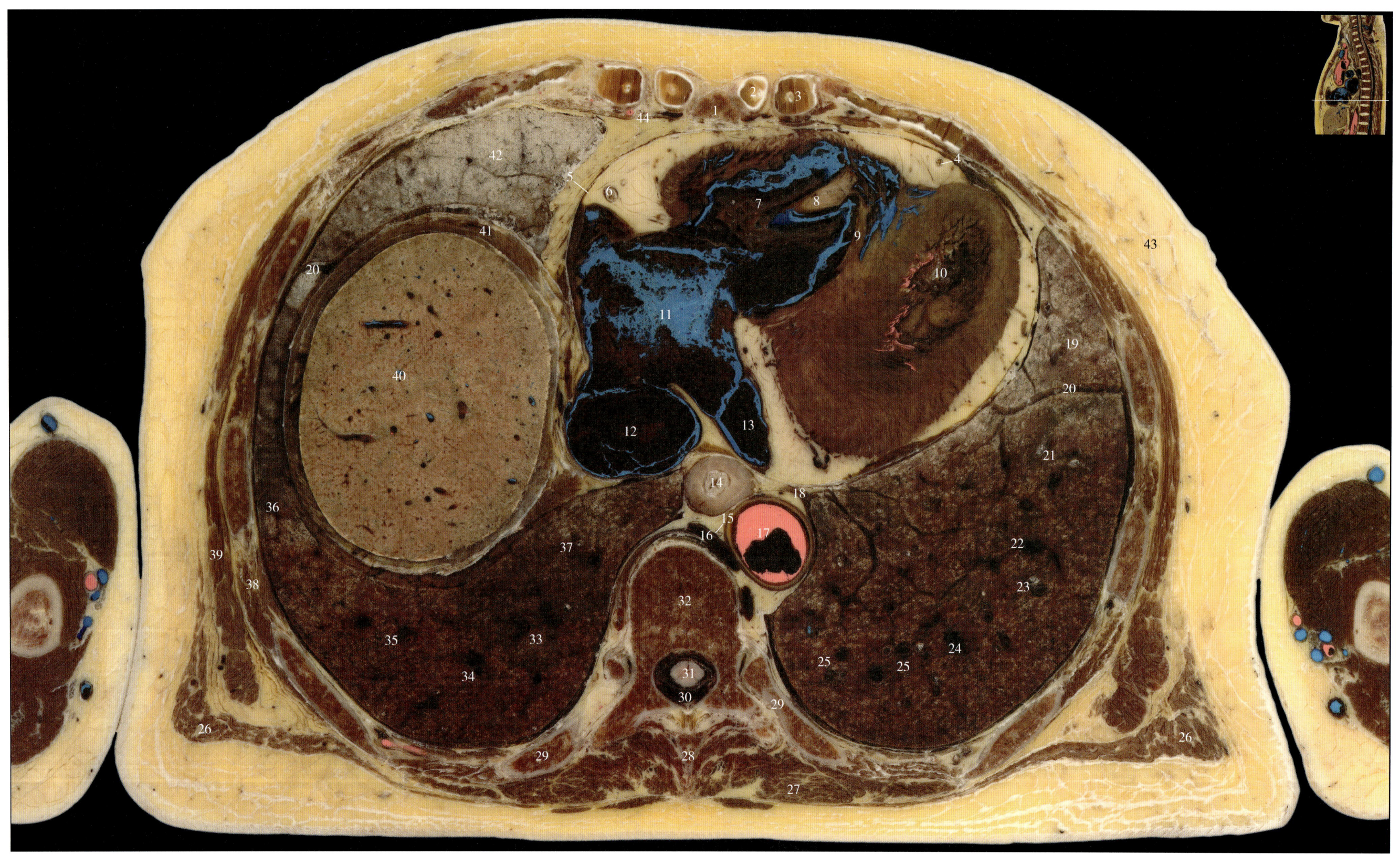

A. 断层标本图像

1. 剑突 xiphoid process
2. 第7肋软骨 7th costal cartilage
3. 第6肋软骨 6th costal cartilage
4. 前室间支 anterior interventricular branch
5. 心包腔 pericardial cavity
6. 右冠状动脉 right coronary artery
7. 右心室 right ventricle
8. 乳头肌 papillary muscle
9. 隔缘肉柱 septomarginal trabecula
10. 左心室 left ventricle
11. 右心房 right atrium
12. 下腔静脉 inferior vena cava
13. 冠状窦 coronary sinus
14. 食管 esophagus
15. 胸导管 thoracic duct
16. 奇静脉 azygos vein
17. 胸主动脉 thoracic aorta
18. 肺韧带 pulmonary ligament
19. 下舌段（S5）inferior lingular segment
20. 斜裂 oblique fissure
21. 内前底段支气管（B7+8）和动脉（A7+8）medioanterior basal segmental bronchus and artery
22. 内前底段静脉（V7+8）medioanterior basal segmental vein
23. 左肺外侧底段支气管（B9）和动脉（A9）left lateral basal segmental bronchus and artery
24. 左肺外侧底段静脉（V9）left lateral basal segmental vein
25. 左肺后底段支气管（B10）和动脉（A10）left posterior basal segmental bronchus and artery
26. 背阔肌 latissimus dorsi
27. 竖脊肌 erector spinae
28. 第8胸椎棘突 spinous process of 8th thoracic vertebra
29. 第9肋骨 9th costal bone
30. 硬膜外隙 epidural space
31. 脊髓 spinal cord
32. 第9胸椎椎体 body of 9th thoracic vertebra
33. 右肺后底段支气管（B10）和动脉（A10）right posterior basal segmental bronchus and artery
34. 右肺后底段静脉（V10）right posterior basal segmental vein
35. 右肺外侧底段支气管（B9）和动脉（A9）right lateral basal segmental bronchus and artery
36. 前底段（S8）anterior basal segment
37. 内侧底段支气管（B7）和动脉（A7）medial basal segmental bronchus and artery
38. 肋间肌 intercostal muscle
39. 前锯肌 serratus anterior
40. 肝右叶 right lobe of liver
41. 膈 diaphragm
42. 右肺中叶 middle lobe of right lung
43. 乳腺 mammary gland
44. 胸廓内动脉 internal thoracic artery
45. 椎间盘 intervertebral disc

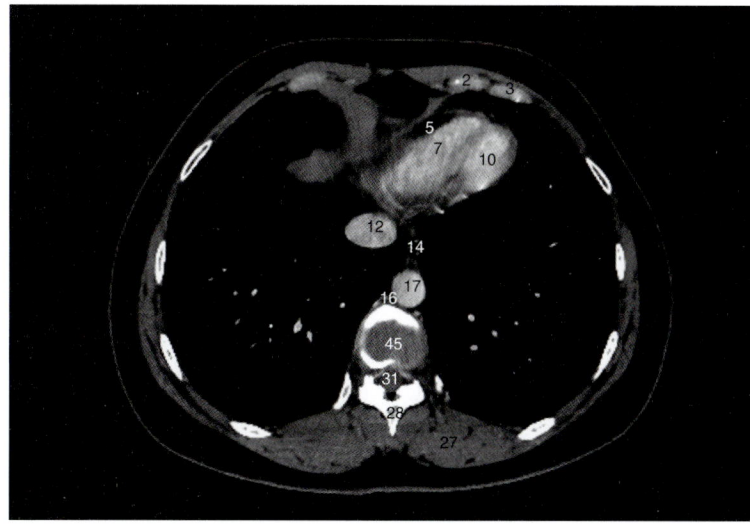

B. CT 纵隔窗增强图像

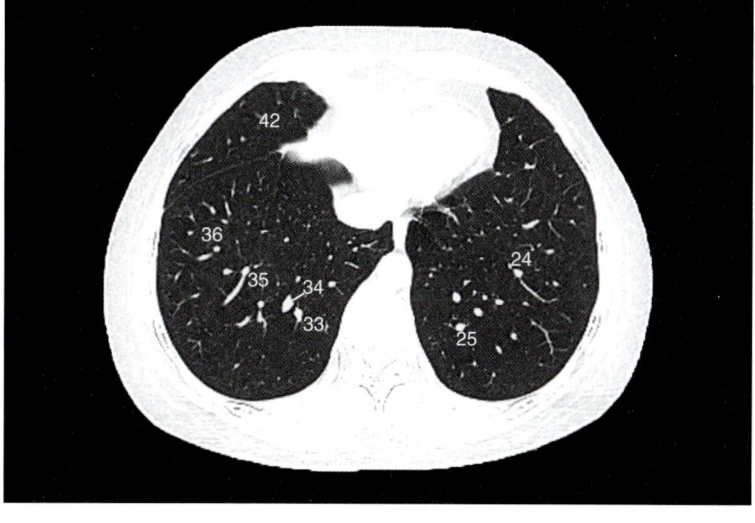

C. CT 肺窗图像

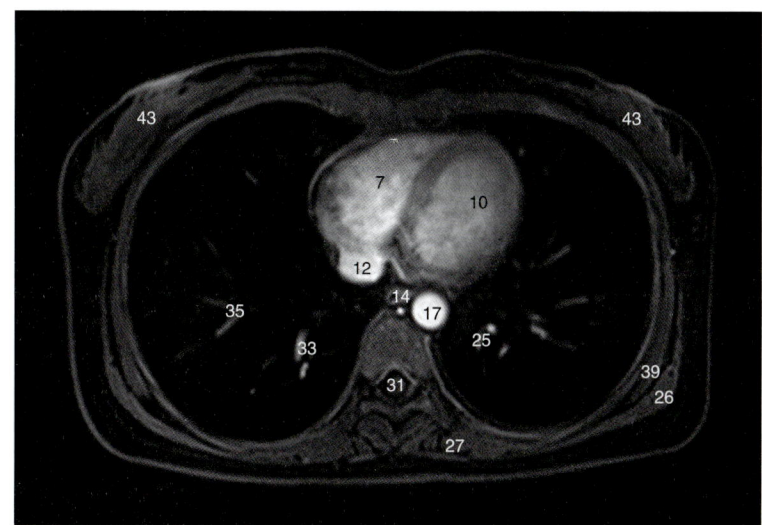

D. MR T1WI 增强图像

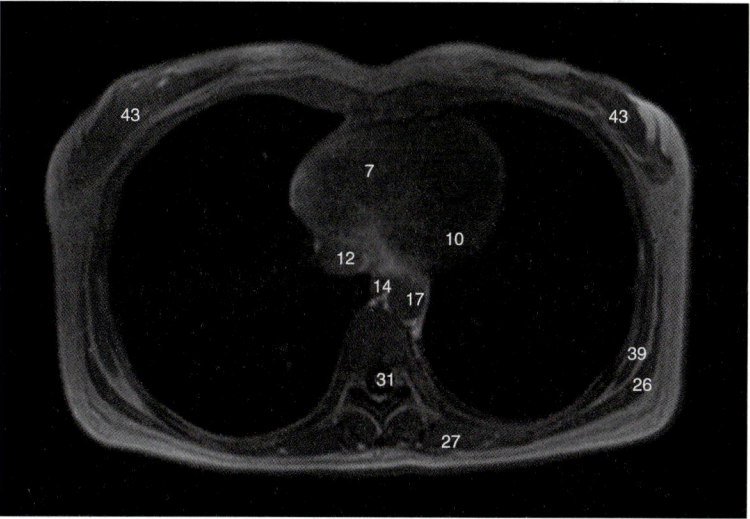

E. MR T1WI 平扫图像

关键结构：心，剑突，隔缘肉柱，奇静脉。

此断面前方经剑突，后方经第9胸椎椎体中份。

中纵隔内仍见3个心腔，右心房及左、右心室腔隙进一步缩小，冠状窦注入右心房。右心室内见前乳头肌和隔缘肉柱，隔缘肉柱又名节制索，自室间隔连至右室前壁的前乳头肌，房室束的右支及供应前乳头肌的血管可通过隔缘肉柱达前乳头肌，在心脏外科手术中，对于有右心室流出道梗阻的患者，对隔缘肉柱的体部及漏斗间隔的隔束和壁束要尽量避免不必要的切除，以免破坏右心室功能及损伤右束支，妨碍心脏复苏[19]。后纵隔内食管向左前方移，走向膈食管裂孔。奇静脉和半奇静脉分别起自右侧和左侧的腰升静脉，沿脊柱两侧上行，约第9胸椎椎体高度经胸主动脉和食管后方，半奇静脉注入奇静脉。CT图像膈穹窿进一步扩大，中纵隔体积缩小，后纵隔和脊柱区仍可见食管、胸主动脉、奇静脉、半奇静脉和椎间盘及椎管内结构。

胸部连续横断层 82（FH.11870）

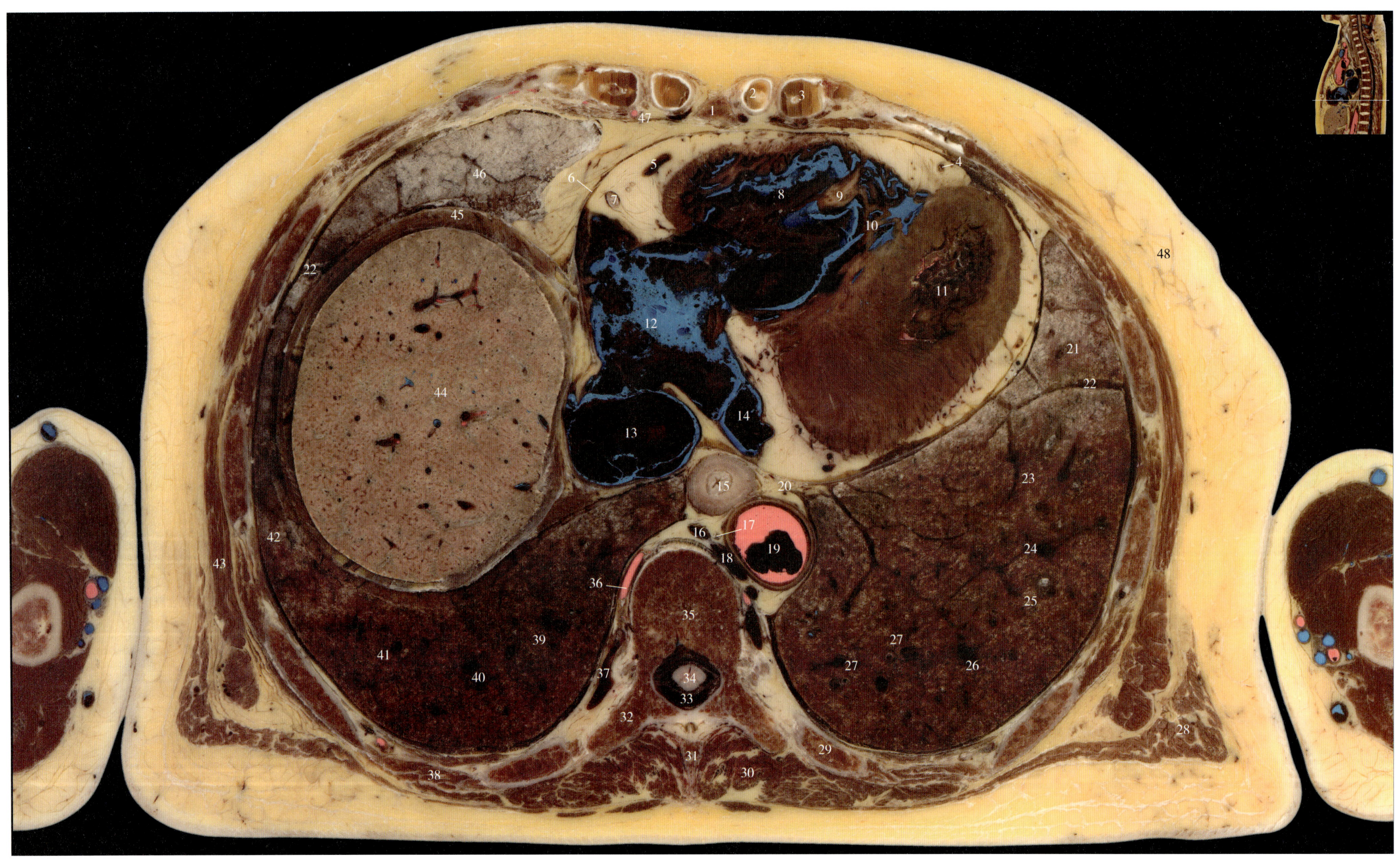

A. 断层标本图像

1. 剑突 xiphoid process
2. 第7肋软骨 7th costal cartilage
3. 第6肋软骨 6th costal cartilage
4. 前室间支 anterior interventricular branch
5. 心小静脉 small cardiac vein
6. 心包腔 pericardial cavity
7. 右冠状动脉 right coronary artery
8. 右心室 right ventricle
9. 前乳头肌 anterior papillary muscles
10. 隔缘肉柱 septomarginal trabecula
11. 左心室 left ventricle
12. 右心房 right atrium
13. 下腔静脉 inferior vena cava
14. 冠状窦 coronary sinus
15. 食管 esophagus
16. 奇静脉 azygos vein
17. 胸导管 thoracic duct
18. 半奇静脉 hemiazygos vein
19. 胸主动脉 thoracic aorta
20. 肺韧带 pulmonary ligament
21. 下舌段（S5）inferior lingular segment
22. 斜裂 oblique fissure
23. 内前底段（S7+8）medioanterior basal segment
24. 内前底段静脉（V7+8）medioanterior basal segmental vein
25. 左肺外侧底段（S9）left lateral basal segment
26. 左肺外侧底段静脉（V9）left lateral basal segmental vein
27. 左肺后底段（S10）left posterior basal segment
28. 背阔肌 latissimus dorsi
29. 第9肋骨 9th costal bone
30. 竖脊肌 erector spinae
31. 棘突 spinous process
32. 横突 transverse process
33. 硬膜外隙 epidural space
34. 脊髓 spinal cord
35. 第9胸椎椎体 body of 9th thoracic vertebra
36. 肋间后动脉 posterior intercostal artery
37. 肋间后静脉 posterior intercostal vein
38. 肋间肌 intercostal muscle
39. 右肺后底段支气管（B10）和动脉（A10）
40. 右肺后底段静脉（V10）right posterior basal segmental vein
41. 右肺外侧底段支气管（B9）和动脉（A9）right lateral basal segmental bronchus and artery
42. 前底段（S8）anterior basal segment
43. 前锯肌 serratus anterior
44. 肝右叶 right lobe of liver
45. 膈 diaphragm
46. 右肺中叶 middle lobe of right lung
47. 胸廓内动脉 internal thoracic artery
48. 乳腺 mammary gland

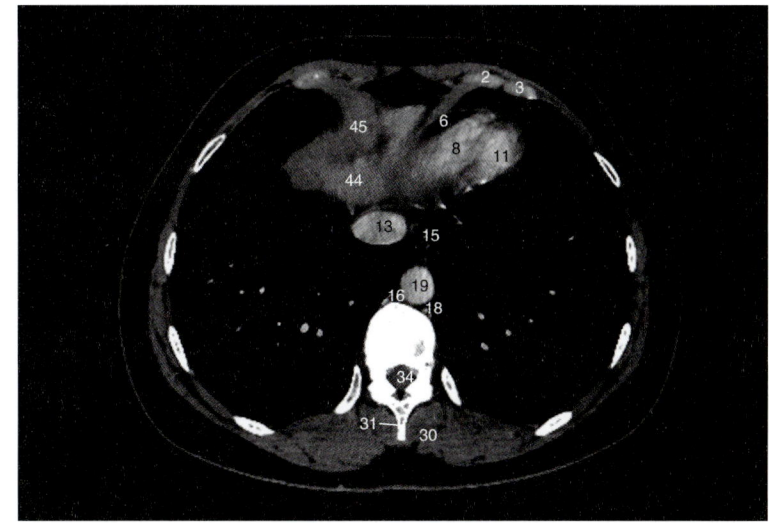

B. CT 纵隔窗增强图像

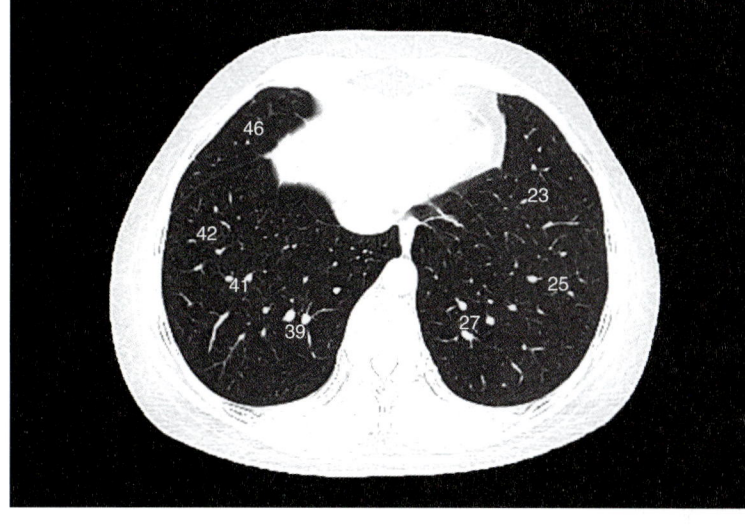

C. CT 肺窗图像

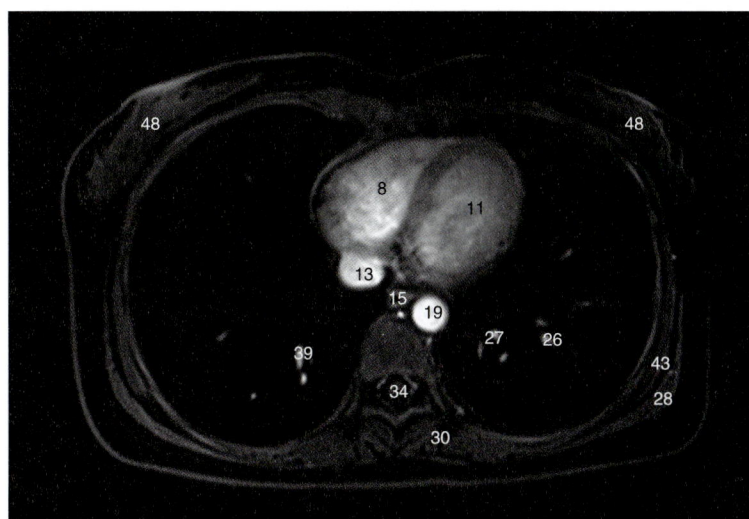

D. MR T1WI 增强图像

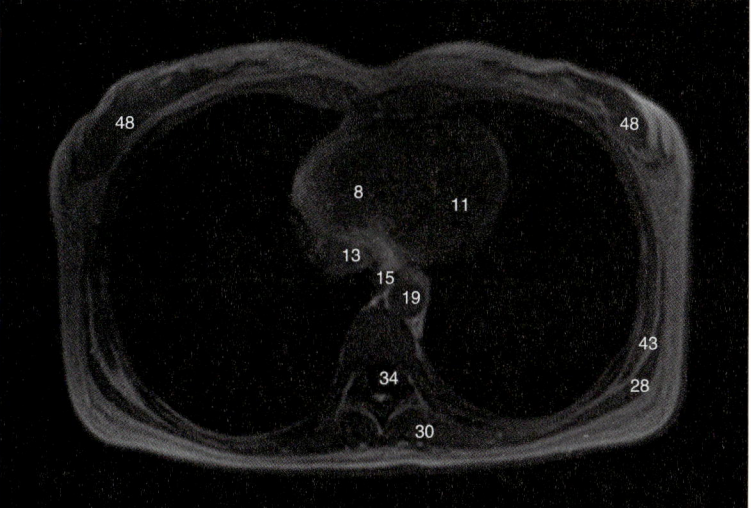

E. MR T1WI 平扫图像

关键结构：剑突，心小静脉，隔缘肉柱。

此断面前方经剑突，后方经第9胸椎椎体中部。

剑突为胸骨最下端的部分，其上端两侧与第7肋骨相接，与胸骨体结合形成剑胸结合，平面后方约平对第9胸椎。中纵隔内左心室室腔进一步缩小，右心房和右心室变化不大，右心室内仍可见前乳头肌和隔缘肉柱，右心室右前方见心小静脉，将进入冠状沟伴行右冠状动脉，注入冠状窦。冠状窦较上一断层变小，下腔静脉逐渐向右侧靠近肝。膈右穹窿和肝右叶较上一断层扩大，左、右肺借肺韧带连于膈和食管的两侧，肺内细小的支气管和血管断面散布其内，肺上叶切除、全肺或肺叶切除、食管手术等均需先切开或切除相应的肺韧带，才能完成手术。后纵隔食管继续左前方移，走向膈食管裂孔，脊柱前方见半奇静脉即将注入奇静脉，胸导管位于胸主动脉和奇静脉之间。CT图像切及肝右叶和膈右穹窿，胸腔中纵隔结构进一步缩小，食管前移。肺内管道细小，主要为肺下叶各底段。

165

胸部连续横断层 83（FH.11850）

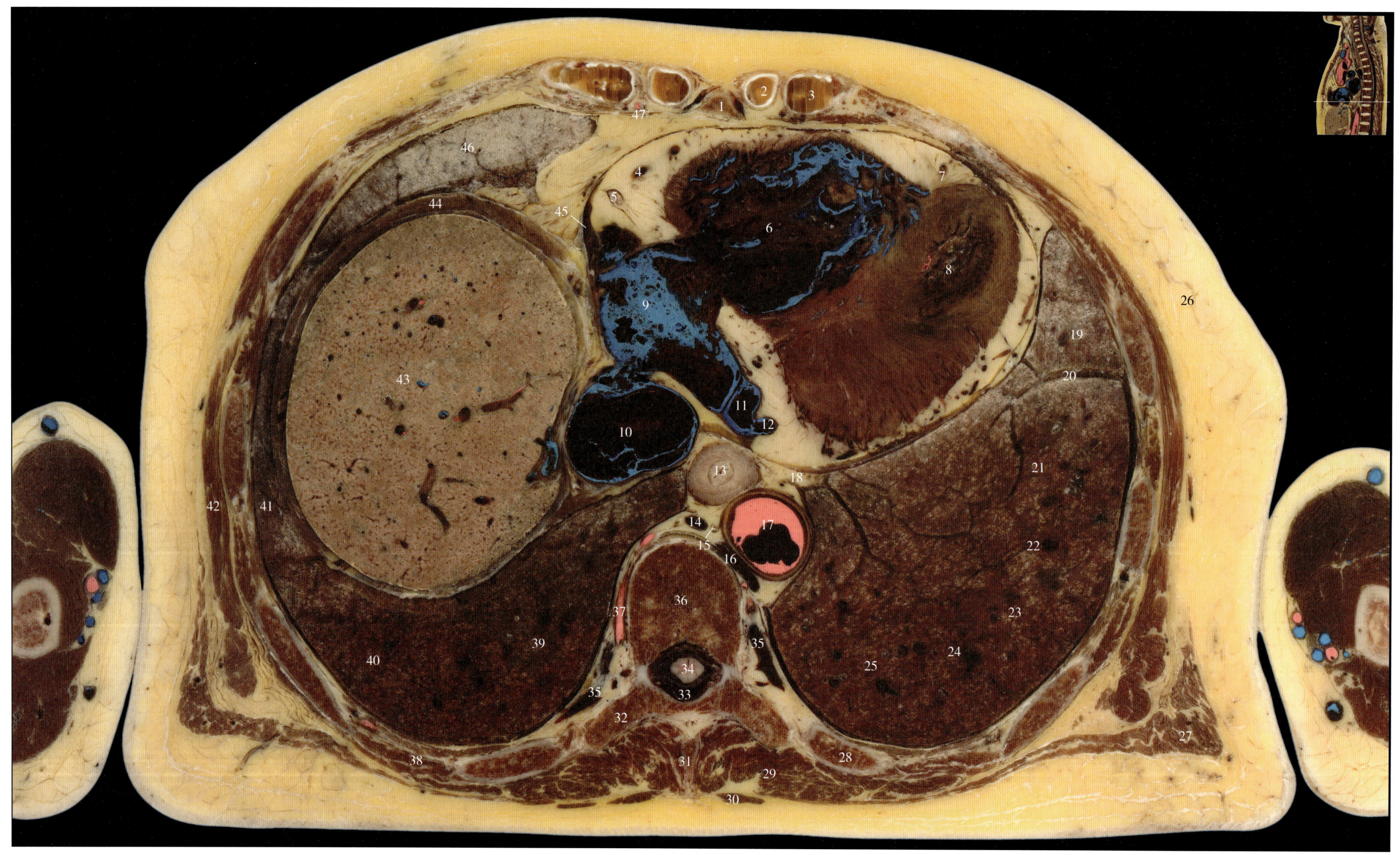

A. 断层标本图像

1. 剑突 xiphoid process
2. 第7肋软骨 7th costal cartilage
3. 第6肋软骨 6th costal cartilage
4. 心小静脉 small cardiac vein
5. 右冠状动脉 right coronary artery
6. 右心室 right ventricle
7. 前室间支 anterior interventricular branch
8. 左心室 left ventricle
9. 右心房 right atrium
10. 下腔静脉 inferior vena cava
11. 冠状窦 coronary sinus
12. 左心室后静脉 posterior vein of left ventricle
13. 食管 esophagus
14. 奇静脉 azygos vein
15. 胸导管 thoracic duct
16. 半奇静脉 hemiazygos vein
17. 胸主动脉 thoracic aorta
18. 肺韧带 pulmonary ligament
19. 下舌段（S5）inferior lingular segment
20. 斜裂 oblique fissure
21. 内前底段（S7+8）medioanterior basal segment
22. 内前底段静脉（V7+8）medioanterior basal segmental vein
23. 左肺外侧底段（S9）left lateral basal segment
24. 左肺外侧底段静脉（V9）left lateral basal segmental vein
25. 左肺后底段（S10）left posterior basal segment
26. 乳腺 mammary gland
27. 背阔肌 latissimus dorsi
28. 第9肋骨 9th costal bone
29. 竖脊肌 erector spinae
30. 斜方肌 trapezius
31. 棘突 spinous process
32. 横突 transverse process
33. 硬膜外隙 epidural space
34. 脊髓 spinal cord
35. 肋间后静脉 posterior intercostal vein
36. 第9胸椎椎体 body of 9th thoracic vertebra
37. 肋间后动脉 posterior intercostal artery
38. 肋间肌 intercostal muscle
39. 右肺后底段支气管（B10）和动脉（A10）right posterior basal segmental bronchus and artery
40. 右肺外侧底段（S9）right lateral basal segment
41. 前底段（S8）anterior basal segment
42. 前锯肌 serratus anterior
43. 肝右叶 right lobe of liver
44. 膈 diaphragm
45. 心包腔 pericardial cavity
46. 右肺中叶 middle lobe of right lung
47. 胸廓内动脉 internal thoracic artery

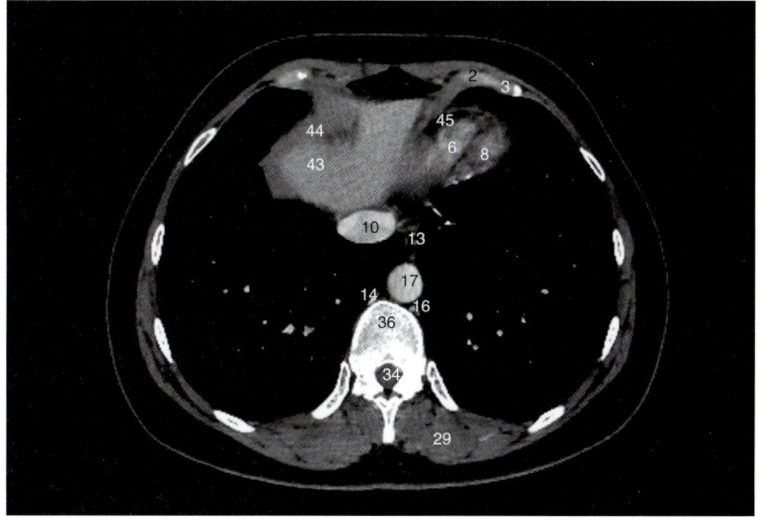

B. CT 纵隔窗增强图像

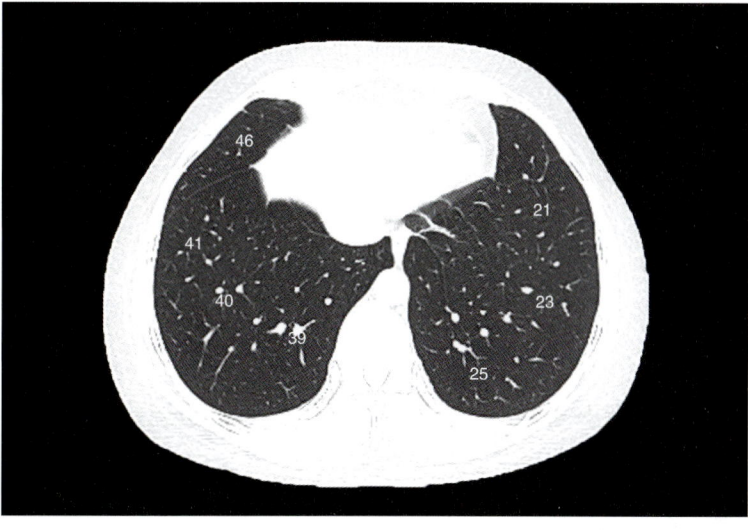

C. CT 肺窗图像

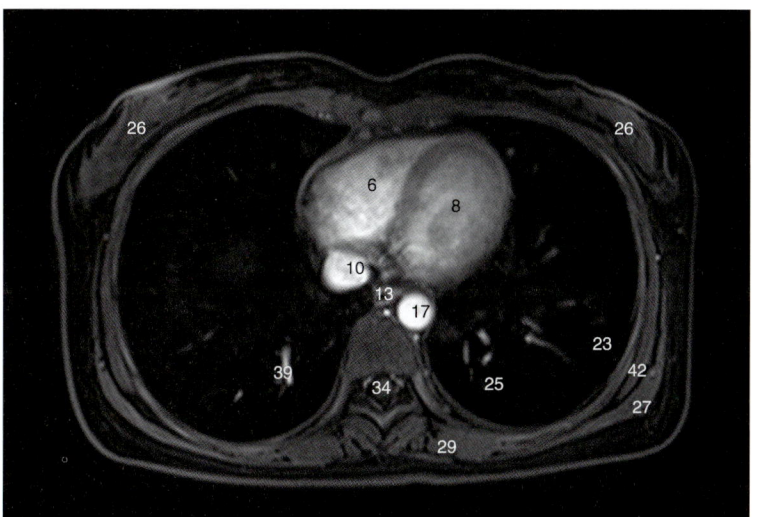

D. MR T1WI 增强图像

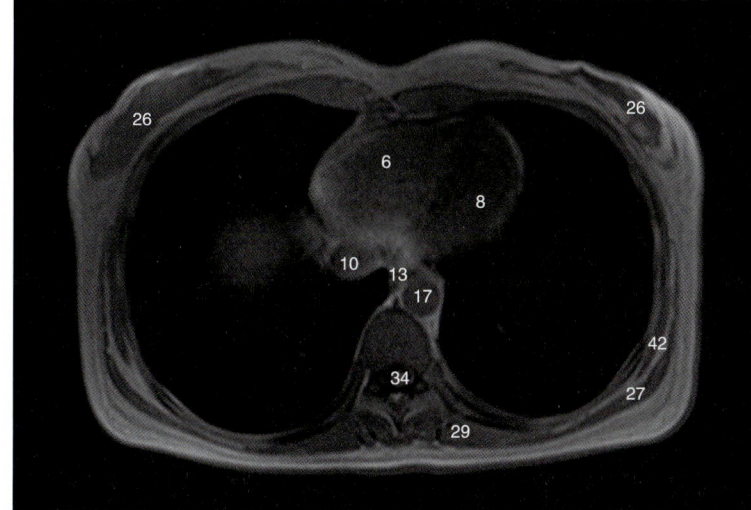

E. MR T1WI 平扫图像

关键结构：前室间支，胸主动脉，肋间后动脉，肋间后静脉。

此断面前方经第剑突上部，后方经第9胸椎椎体中部。

右心房，左、右心室和左、右肺较上一断层变小，左心室内乳头肌消失。右冠状动脉走行在右侧心房和心室之间的冠状沟内，与之伴行的是心小静脉；左右心室的左前方见左冠状动脉的前室间支。冠状窦注入右心房，进一步缩小，可见其属支左心室后静脉注入，收集左心室后壁的静脉血。脊柱两侧和肋间隙见肋间后动、静脉，肋间后动脉发自胸主动脉，肋间后静脉右侧注入奇静脉，左侧注入半奇静脉。膈右穹窿和肝右叶位置大致同上一断层，肝右叶内管道逐渐变得粗大。CT 图像显示膈和肝变大，脊柱区可见胸椎椎体，椎体后外侧与肋头形成的肋头关节，后方的棘突及椎管内的硬膜囊等。椎体前方见奇静脉、半奇静脉和胸主动脉，胸主动脉前方为食管。

胸部连续横断层 84（FH.11830）

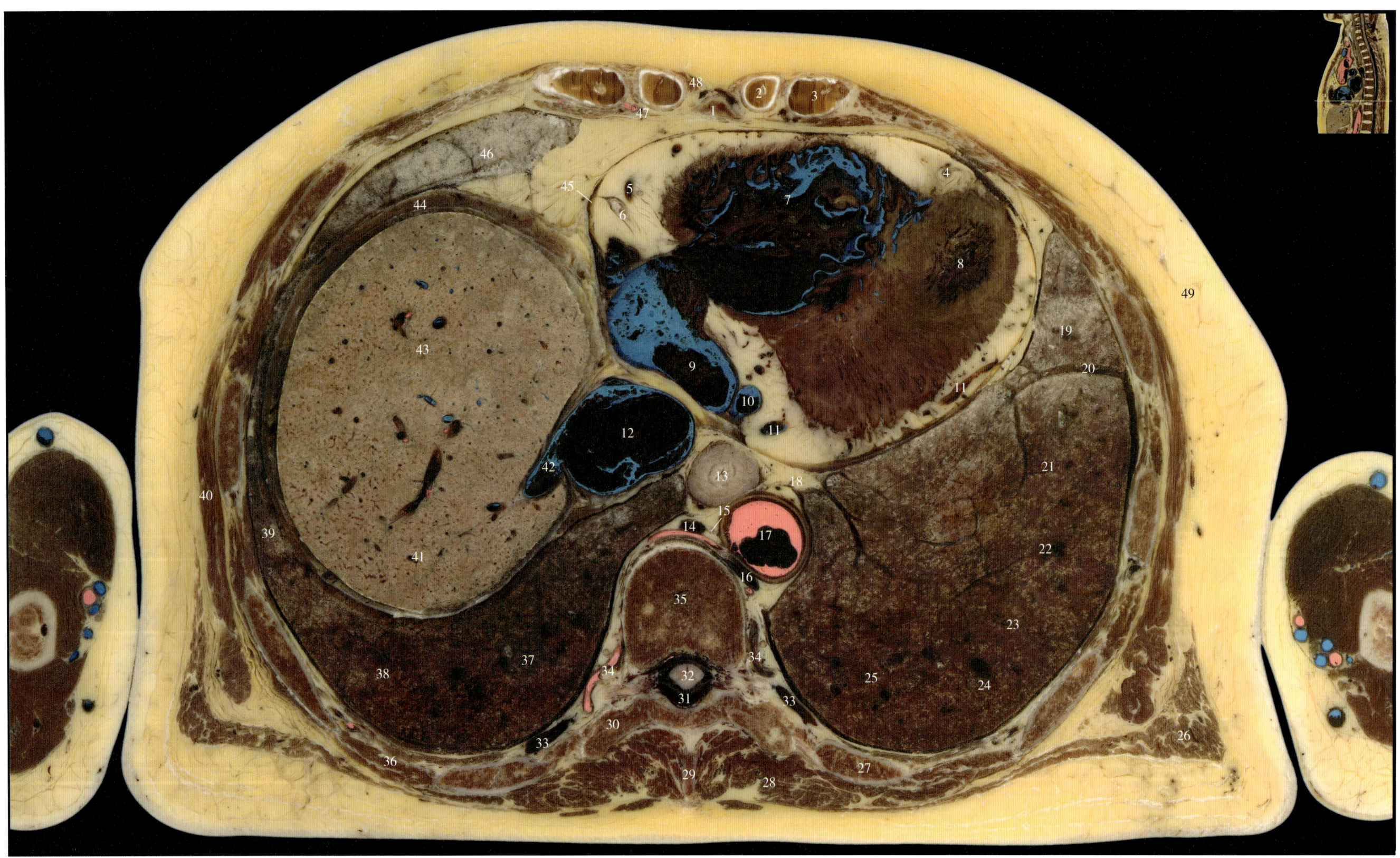

A. 断层标本图像

1. 剑突 xiphoid process
2. 第7肋软骨 7th costal cartilage
3. 第6肋软骨 6th costal cartilage
4. 前室间支 anterior interventricular branch
5. 心小静脉 small cardiac vein
6. 右冠状动脉 right coronary artery
7. 右心室 right ventricle
8. 左心室 left ventricle
9. 右心房 right atrium
10. 冠状窦 coronary sinus
11. 左心室后静脉 posterior vein of left ventricle
12. 下腔静脉 inferior vena cava
13. 食管 esophagus
14. 奇静脉 azygos vein
15. 胸导管 thoracic duct
16. 半奇静脉 hemiazygos vein
17. 胸主动脉 thoracic aorta
18. 肺韧带 pulmonary ligament
19. 下舌段（S5）inferior lingular segment
20. 斜裂 oblique fissure
21. 内前底段（S7+8）medioanterior basal segment
22. 内侧底段静脉（V7）medial basal segmental vein
23. 左肺外侧底段（S9）left lateral basal segment
24. 左肺外侧底段静脉（V9）left lateral basal segmental vein
25. 左肺后底段（S10）left posterior basal segment
26. 背阔肌 latissimus dorsi
27. 第9肋骨 9th costal bone
28. 竖脊肌 erector spinae
29. 棘突 spinous process
30. 横突 transverse process
31. 硬膜外隙 epidural space
32. 脊髓 spinal cord
33. 肋间后静脉 posterior intercostal vein
34. 肋间后动脉 posterior intercostal artery
35. 第9胸椎椎体 body of 9th thoracic vertebra
36. 肋间肌 intercostal muscle
37. 右肺后底段支气管（B10）和动脉（A10）right posterior basal segmental bronchus and artery
38. 右肺外侧底段（S9）right lateral basal segment
39. 前底段（S8）anterior basal segment
40. 前锯肌 serratus anterior
41. 肝右后叶 right posterior lobe of liver
42. 肝右后上缘静脉 right posterior supramarginal vein of liver
43. 肝右前叶 right anterior lobe of liver
44. 膈 diaphragm
45. 心包腔 pericardial cavity
46. 右肺中叶 middle lobe of right lung
47. 胸廓内动脉 internal thoracic artery
48. 腹直肌 rectus abdominis
49. 乳腺 mammary gland
50. 食管旁淋巴结 paraesophageal lymph nodes

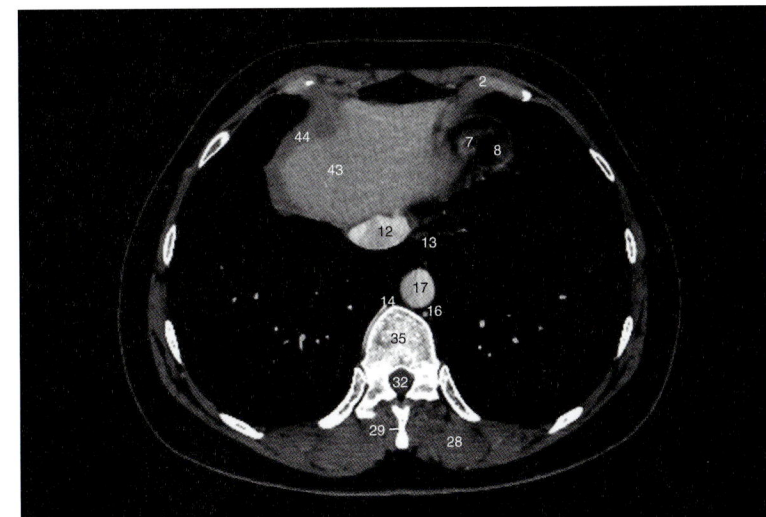

B. CT 纵隔窗增强图像

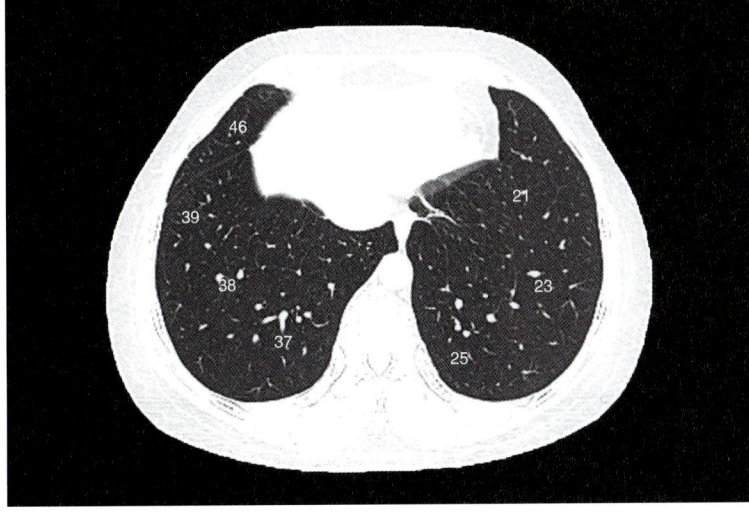

C. CT 肺窗图像

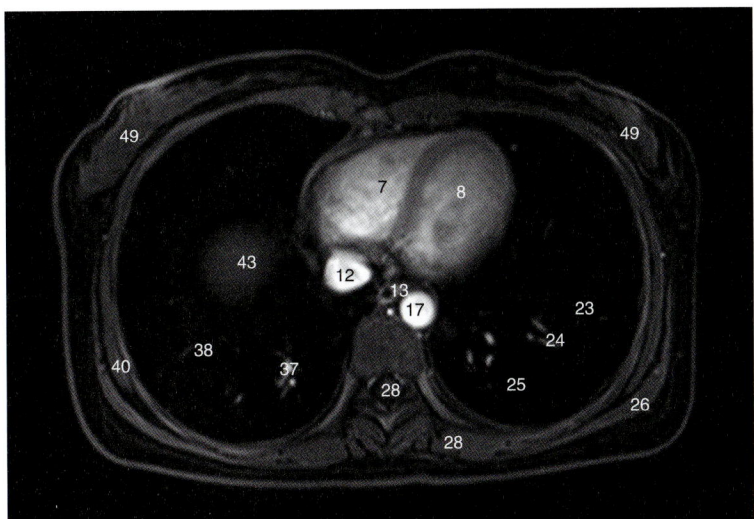

D. MR T1WI 增强图像

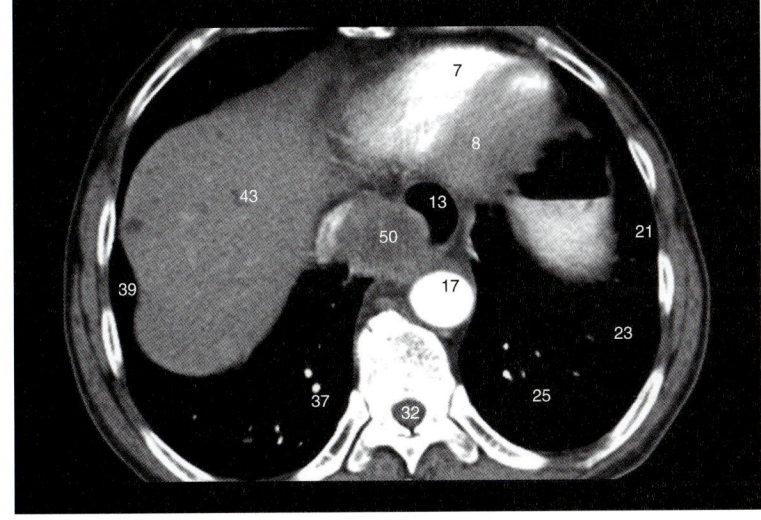

E. 8 区淋巴结转移 CT 图像

关键结构：食管旁淋巴结，冠状窦，食管。

此断面前方经剑突和第7胸肋关节，后方经第9胸椎椎体下部。

右心房变小，左、右心室内部的乳头肌、腱索等结构消失，周围仍可见右冠状动脉、心小静脉、左心室后静脉及前室间支等心脏血管。冠状窦缩小，注入右心房，两肺进一步缩小。食管继续左移，走向膈食管裂孔，在此层面常见食管旁淋巴结（8区），食管旁淋巴结是指邻近食管壁和中线右侧或左侧的淋巴结，不包括气管隆嵴下淋巴结，其上界分别为左肺下叶支气管的上部和右肺中间支气管的下部，其下界为膈，此区域为食管癌好发转移区域[95]。脊柱前方见胸主动脉及其分支肋间后动脉、胸导管及奇静脉和半奇静脉。CT 图像中纵隔心及心包变小，心包与膈中心腱愈着，肝左和肝右静脉注入下腔静脉。因肺部充盈，体积较大，仍可见肺底段细小的管道，右肺中叶即将消失。

胸部连续横断层 85（FH.11810）

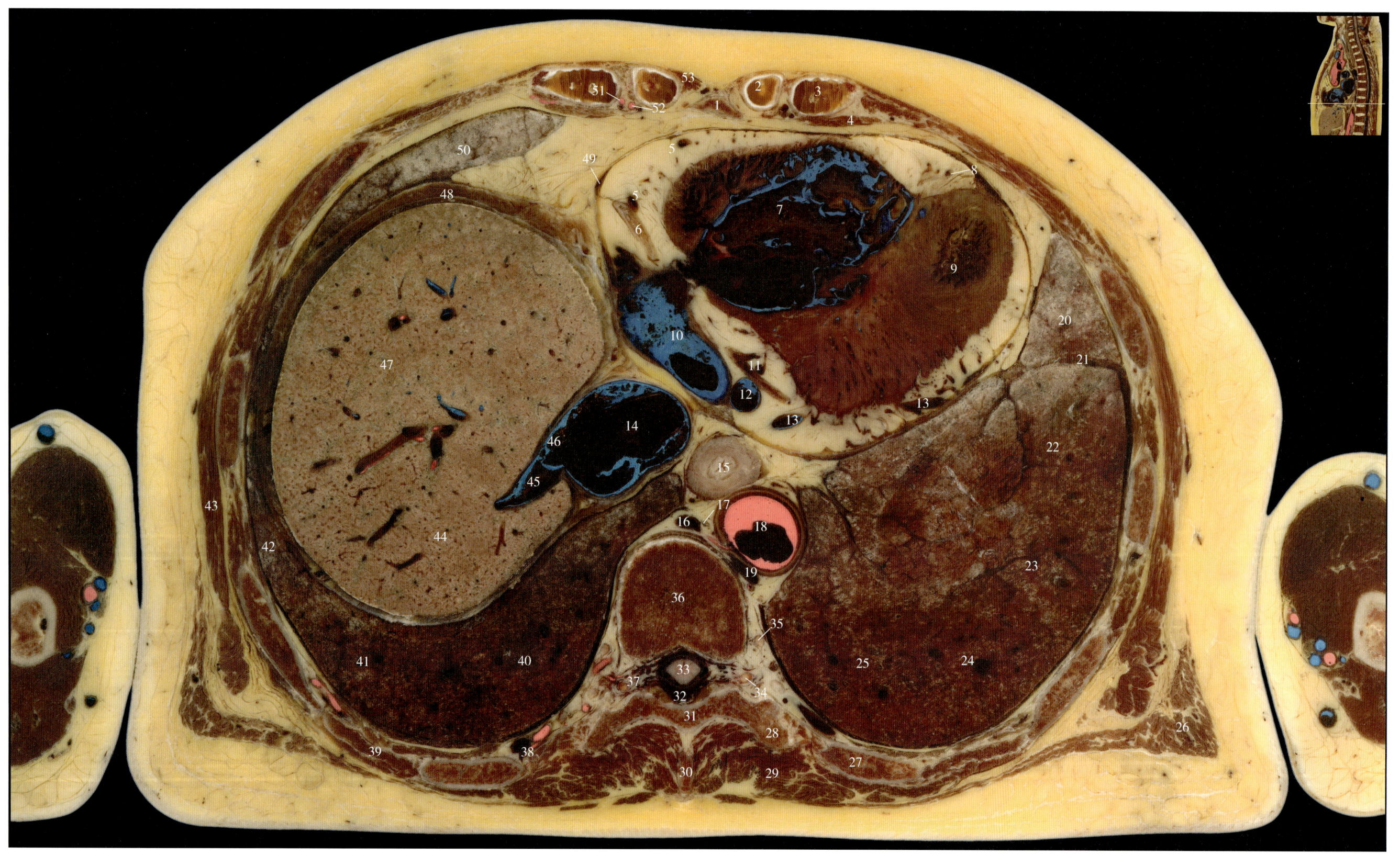

A. 断层标本图像

1. 剑突 xiphoid process
2. 第 7 肋软骨 7th costal cartilage
3. 第 6 肋软骨 6th costal cartilage
4. 胸横肌 transversus thoracis
5. 心小静脉 small cardiac vein
6. 右冠状动脉 right coronary artery
7. 右心室 right ventricle
8. 前室间支 anterior interventricular branch
9. 左心室 left ventricle
10. 右心房 right atrium
11. 右旋支 right circumflex branch
12. 冠状窦 coronary sinus
13. 左室后静脉 posterior vein of left ventricle
14. 下腔静脉 inferior vena cava
15. 食管 esophagus
16. 奇静脉 azygos vein
17. 胸导管 thoracic duct
18. 胸主动脉 thoracic aorta
19. 半奇静脉 hemiazygos vein
20. 下舌段（S5）inferior lingular segment
21. 斜裂 oblique fissure
22. 内前底段（S7+8）medioanterior basal segment
23. 左肺外侧底段（S9）left lateral basal segment
24. 左肺外侧底段静脉（V9）left lateral basal segmental vein
25. 左肺后底段（S10）left posterior basal segment
26. 背阔肌 latissimus dorsi
27. 第 9 肋骨 9th costal bone
28. 横突 transverse process
29. 竖脊肌 erector spinae
30. 棘突 spinous process
31. 椎弓板 lamina of vertebral arch
32. 硬膜外隙 epidural space
33. 脊髓 spinal cord
34. 脊神经节 spinal ganglion
35. 交感干神经节 ganglia of sympathetic trunk
36. 第 9 胸椎椎体 body of 9th thoracic vertebra
37. 椎间孔 intervertebral foramen
38. 肋间后动、静脉 posterior intercostal artery and vein
39. 肋间肌 intercostal muscle
40. 右肺后底段（S10）right posterior basal segment
41. 右肺外侧底段（S9）right lateral basal segment
42. 前底段（S8）anterior basal segment
43. 前锯肌 serratus anterior
44. 肝右后叶 right posterior lobe of liver
45. 肝右后上缘静脉 right posterior supramarginal vein of liver
46. 肝右静脉 right hepatic vein
47. 肝右前叶 right anterior lobe of liver
48. 膈 diaphragm
49. 心包腔 pericardial cavity
50. 右肺中叶 middle lobe of right lung
51. 肌膈动脉 musculophrenic artery
52. 腹壁上动脉 superior epigastric artery
53. 腹直肌 rectus abdominis
54. 肝左内叶 left medial lobe of liver
55. 肝中静脉 middle hepatic vein
56. 肝左静脉 left hepatic vein
57. 乳腺 mammary gland

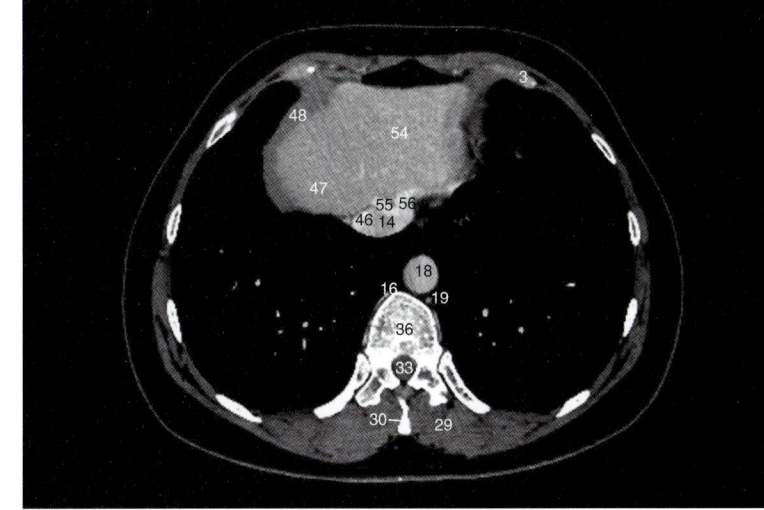

B. CT 纵隔窗增强图像

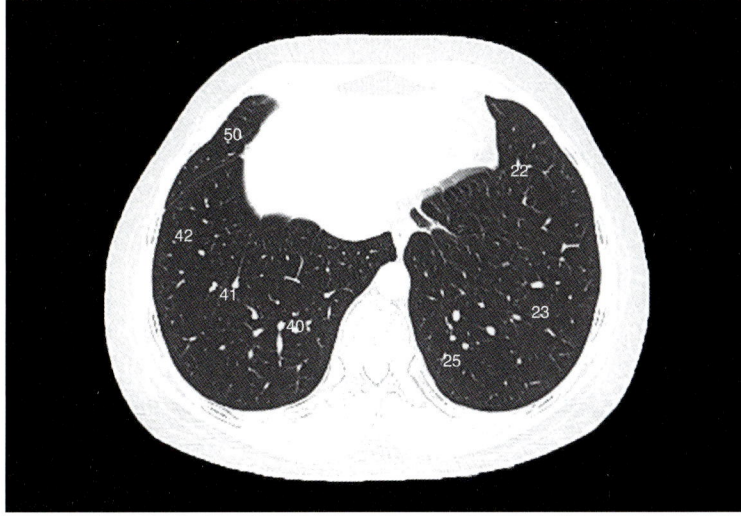

C. CT 肺窗图像

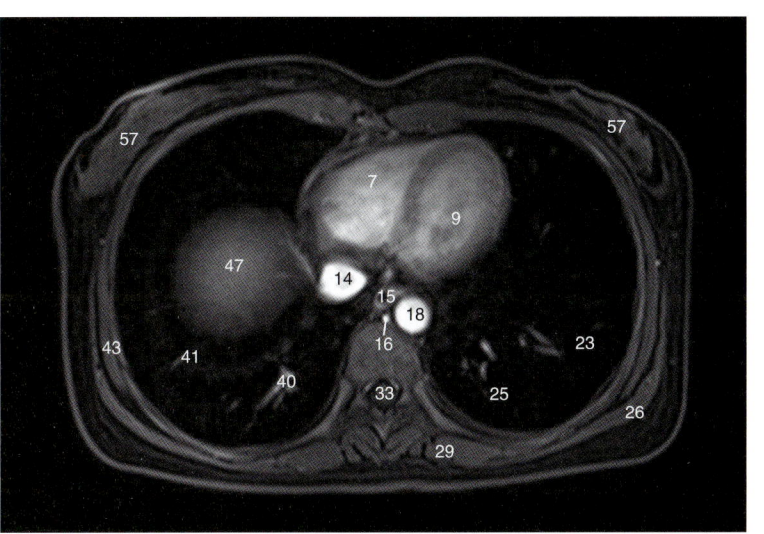

D. MR T1WI 增强图像

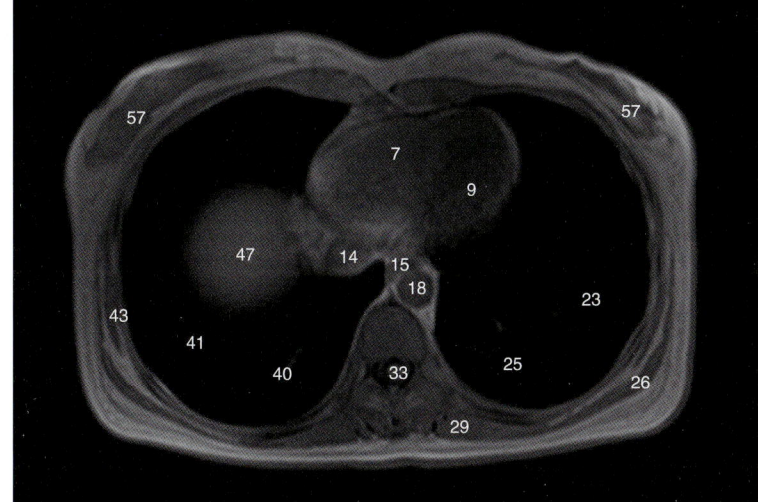

E. MR T1WI 平扫图像

关键结构：右旋支，腹壁上动脉，肌膈动脉。

此断面前方经剑突，后方经第 9 胸椎椎体下部。

右心房缩小明显，即将消失，与心室之间为冠状沟，其内右冠状动脉自右向左行，发出分支右旋支，越过房室交点，营养左心室后壁[96]。其中，右旋支出现率为 94%，大多移行为左室后支，止于房室交点者约为 10%，止于房室交点与左缘之间处者约为 68%，止于左缘者少见。冠状动脉自身特殊的解剖形态可以引起冠状动脉血流动力学改变，进而可导致冠状动脉粥样硬化病变及心肌梗死的发生，临床中冠脉造影检查可有助于心肌梗死患者的病因检查与治疗[97]。食管继续左移，走向膈食管裂孔。膈右穹窿和肝右叶较上一断层变大。下腔静脉位于肝脏面的腔静脉沟内，可见肝右静脉注入。经此层面，胸廓内动脉穿膈进入腹前壁的腹直肌鞘内，移行为腹壁上动脉，并发出分支肌膈动脉，在心外膜消融术的前入路手术中应避免损伤胸廓内动脉和 / 或腹壁上动脉，以免引起纵隔内或上腹部血肿[98]。CT 图像心腔结构消失，心包连于膈中心腱，肺内结构不变。肝脏显示第二肝门结构，肝右静脉、肝左和肝中静脉注入下腔静脉。脊柱区见胸椎、肋头关节等。

胸部连续横断层 86（FH.11790）

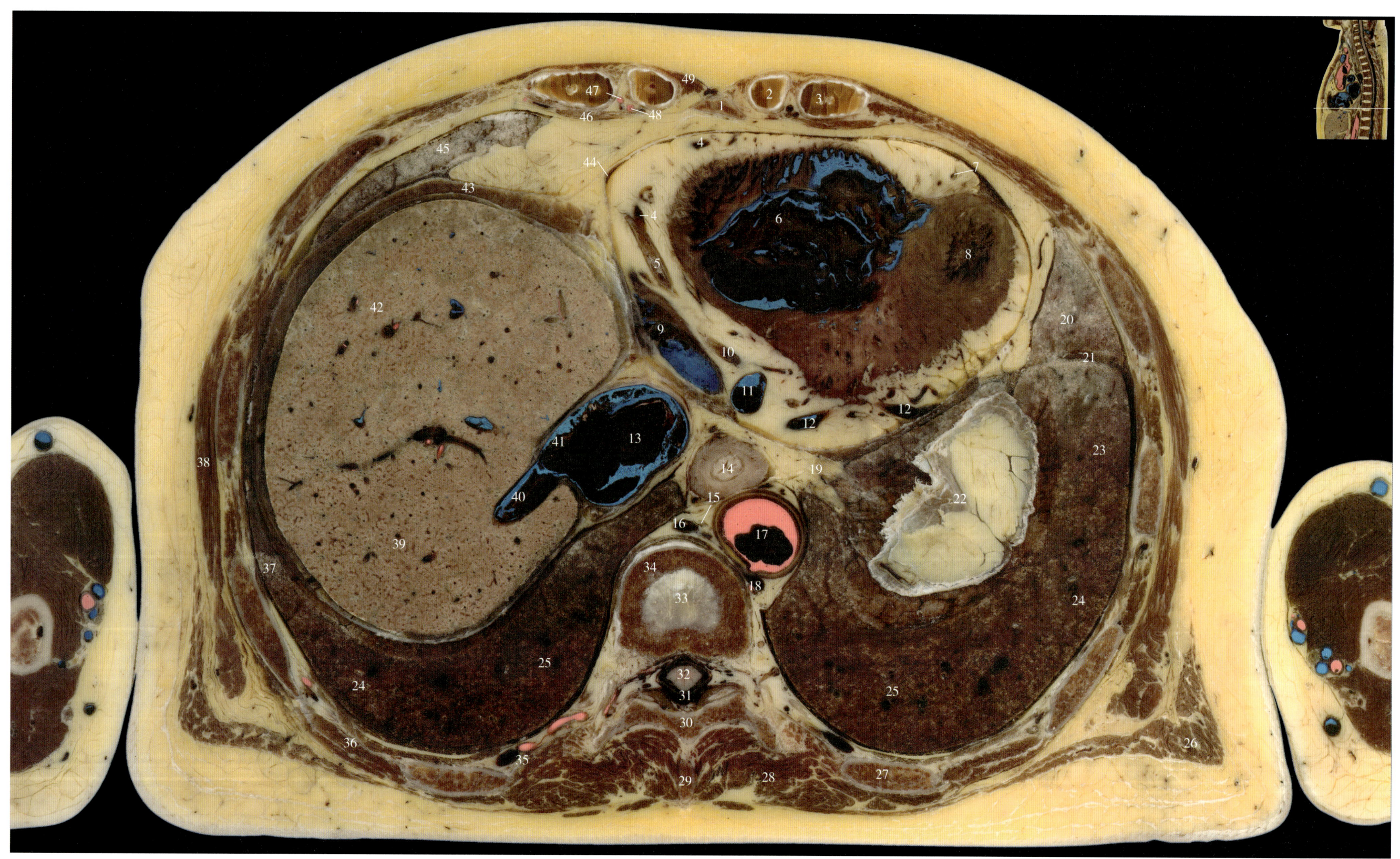

A. 断层标本图像

1. 剑突 xiphoid process
2. 第7肋软骨 7th costal cartilage
3. 第6肋软骨 6th costal cartilage
4. 心小静脉 small cardiac vein
5. 右冠状动脉 right coronary artery
6. 右心室 right ventricle
7. 前室间支 anterior interventricular branch
8. 左心室 left ventricle
9. 右心房 right atrium
10. 右旋支 right circumflex branch
11. 冠状窦 coronary sinus
12. 左室后静脉 posterior vein of left ventricle
13. 下腔静脉 inferior vena cava
14. 食管 esophagus
15. 胸导管 thoracic duct
16. 奇静脉 azygos vein
17. 胸主动脉 thoracic aorta
18. 半奇静脉 hemiazygos vein
19. 肺韧带 pulmonary ligament
20. 下舌段（S5）inferior lingular segment
21. 斜裂 oblique fissure
22. 膈左穹窿 left fornix of diaphragm
23. 内前底段（S7+8）medioanterior basal segment
24. 外侧底段（S9）lateral basal segment
25. 后底段（S10）posterior basal segment
26. 背阔肌 latissimus dorsi
27. 第9肋骨 9th costal bone
28. 竖脊肌 erector spinae
29. 棘突 spinous process
30. 椎弓板 lamina of vertebral arch
31. 硬膜外隙 epidural space
32. 脊髓 spinal cord
33. T9-10椎间盘 T9-10 intervertebral disc
34. 第9胸椎体 body of 9th thoracic vertebra
35. 肋间后动、静脉 posterior intercostal artery and vein
36. 肋间肌 intercostal muscle
37. 前底段（S8）anterior basal segment
38. 前锯肌 serratus anterior
39. 肝右后叶 right posterior lobe of liver
40. 肝右后上缘静脉 right posterior supramarginal vein of liver
41. 肝右静脉 right hepatic vein
42. 肝右前叶 right anterior lobe of liver
43. 膈 diaphragm
44. 心包腔 pericardial cavity
45. 右肺中叶 middle lobe of right lung
46. 胸横肌 transversus thoracis
47. 肌膈动脉 musculophrenic artery
48. 腹壁上动脉 superior epigastric artery
49. 腹直肌 rectus abdominis
50. 肝中静脉 middle hepatic vein
51. 肝左静脉 left hepatic vein
52. 肝左内叶 left medial lobe of liver
53. 乳腺 mammary gland

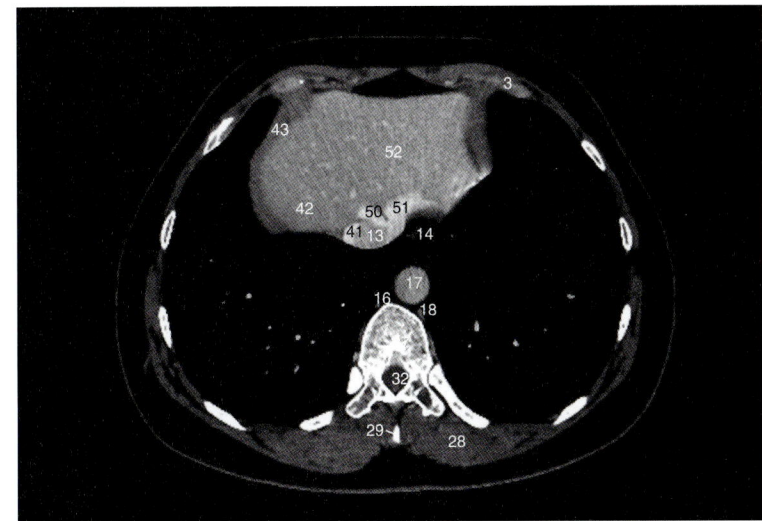

B. CT 纵隔窗增强图像

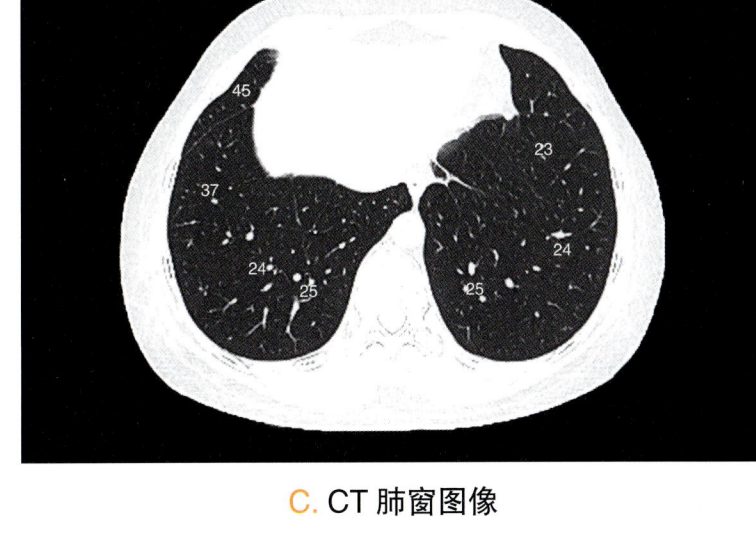

C. CT 肺窗图像

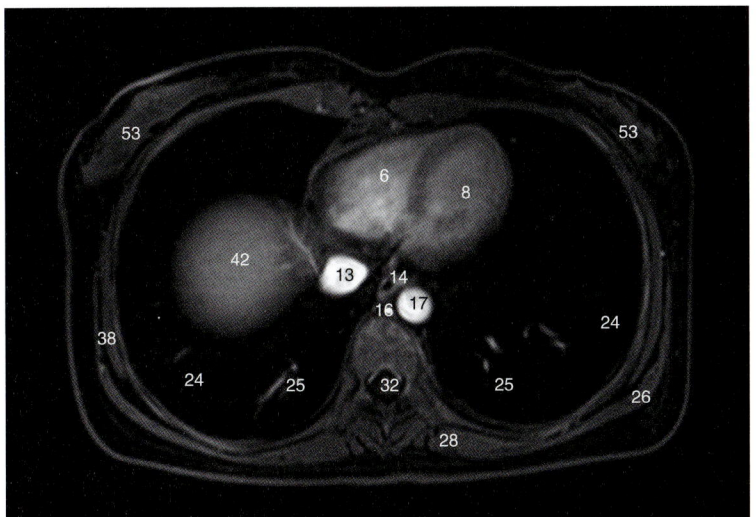

D. MR T1WI 增强图像

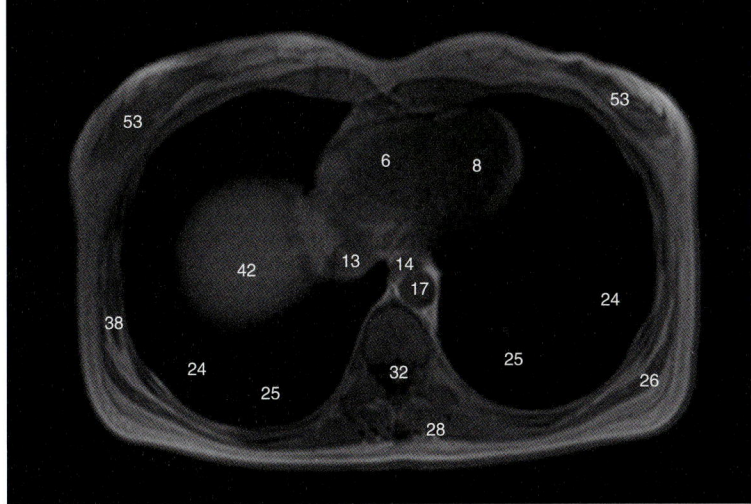

E. MR T1WI 平扫图像

关键结构：右冠状动脉，膈左穹窿，下腔静脉。

此断面经第9胸椎椎体下部和T9-10椎间盘上部。

胸腔内结构进一步缩小，右肺中叶即将消失。左、右心室面积较上一断层变小，右心房即将消失，右冠状动脉主干伴行心小静脉行于右心室后方的冠状沟内，其分支左室后支走向左心室的后方。冠状窦和右心房进一步缩小。膈右穹窿和肝右叶大致同一断层，左侧膈穹窿开始出现，膈左穹窿均低于膈右穹窿，右侧膈穹窿最高点约位于右侧第4肋间隙，左侧膈穹窿最高点约位于左侧第5肋间隙，因受胃、结肠含气量的影响，左侧变化范围较右侧较大。下腔静脉、肝右静脉起始部及右后上缘静脉变化不大。脊柱区切及第9胸椎椎体下缘和T9-10椎间盘，椎体左前方为胸主动脉，前方见奇静脉和半奇静脉，食管继续前移，即将穿食管裂孔。CT图像显示第二肝门层面，有3条肝静脉注入下腔静脉。心包腔结构即将消失，根据肝中静脉分隔左右半肝。两肺主要是下叶底段，随着腹腔结构的增多，进一步缩小。

胸部连续横断层 87（FH.11770）

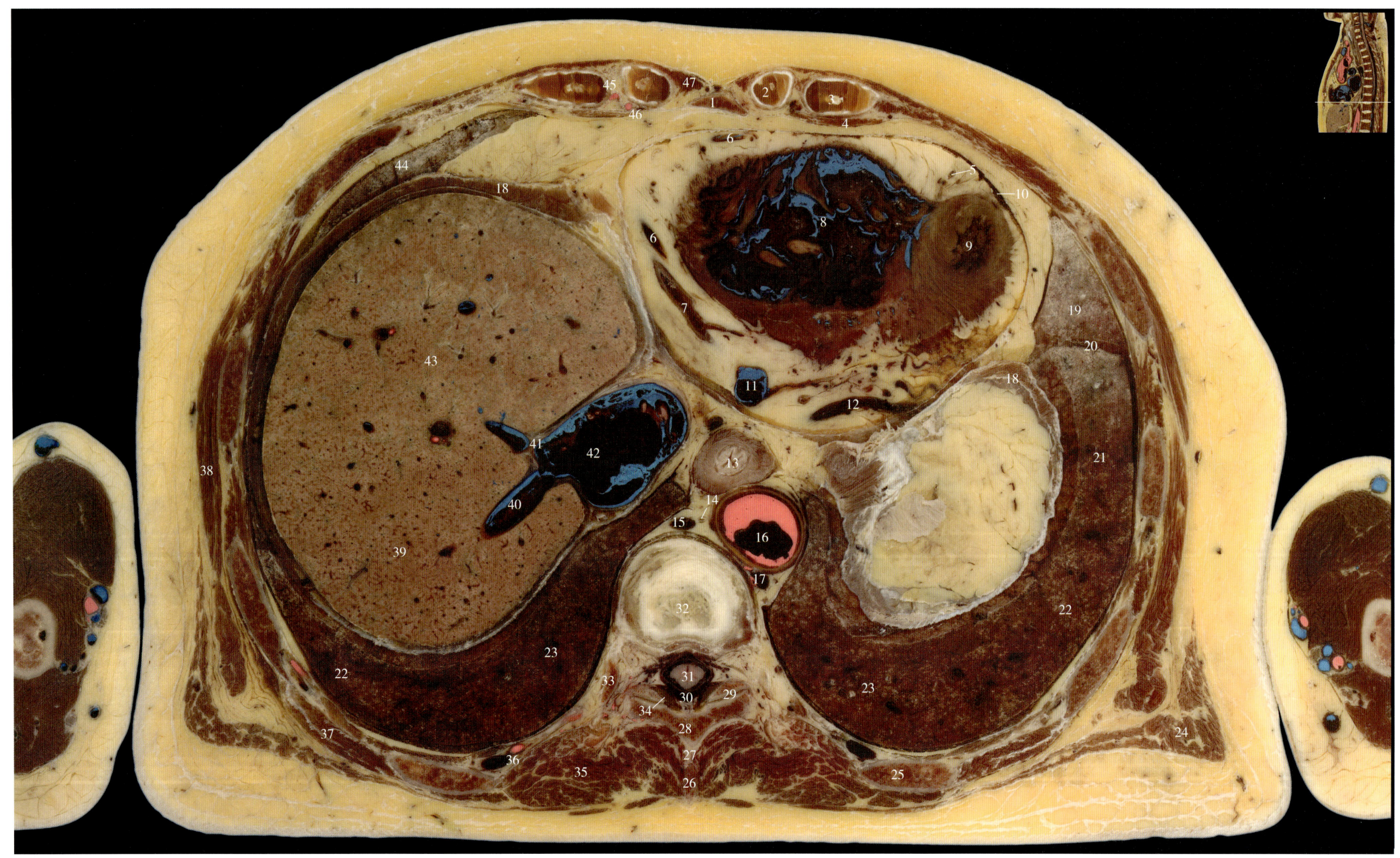

A. 断层标本图像

1. 剑突 xiphoid process
2. 第 7 肋软骨 7th costal cartilage
3. 第 6 肋软骨 6th costal cartilage
4. 胸横肌 transversus thoracis
5. 前室间支 anterior interventricular branch
6. 心小静脉 small cardiac vein
7. 右冠状动脉 right coronary artery
8. 右心室 right ventricle
9. 左心室 left ventricle
10. 心包前下窦 anterior inferior sinus of pericardium
11. 冠状窦 coronary sinus
12. 左室后静脉 posterior vein of left ventricle
13. 食管 esophagus
14. 胸导管 thoracic duct
15. 奇静脉 azygos vein
16. 胸主动脉 thoracic aorta
17. 半奇静脉 hemiazygos vein
18. 膈 diaphragm
19. 下舌段（S5）inferior lingular segment
20. 斜裂 oblique fissure
21. 内前底段（S7+8）medioanterior basal segment
22. 外侧底段（S9）lateral basal segment
23. 后底段（S10）posterior basal segment
24. 背阔肌 latissimus dorsi
25. 第 9 肋骨 9th costal bone
26. 棘突 spinous process
27. 棘间韧带 interspinous ligament
28. 椎弓板 lamina of vertebral arch
29. 关节突关节 zygapophysial joint
30. 硬膜外隙 epidural space
31. 脊髓 spinal cord
32. T9-10 椎间盘 T9-10 intervertebral disc
33. 第 10 肋骨 10th costal bone
34. 黄韧带 ligamenta flava
35. 竖脊肌 erector spinae
36. 肋间后动、静脉 posterior intercostal artery and vein
37. 肋间肌 intercostal muscle
38. 前锯肌 serratus anterior
39. 肝右后叶 right posterior lobe of liver
40. 肝右后上缘静脉 right posterior supramarginal vein of liver
41. 肝右静脉 right hepatic vein
42. 下腔静脉 inferior vena cava
43. 肝右前叶 right anterior lobe of liver
44. 右肺中叶 middle lobe of right lung
45. 肌膈动脉 musculophrenic artery
46. 腹壁上动脉 superior epigastric artery
47. 腹直肌 rectus abdominis
48. 前底段（S8）anterior basal segment
49. 肝中静脉 middle hepatic vein
50. 肝左静脉 left hepatic vein
51. 肝左内叶 left medial lobe of liver
52. 乳腺 mammary gland

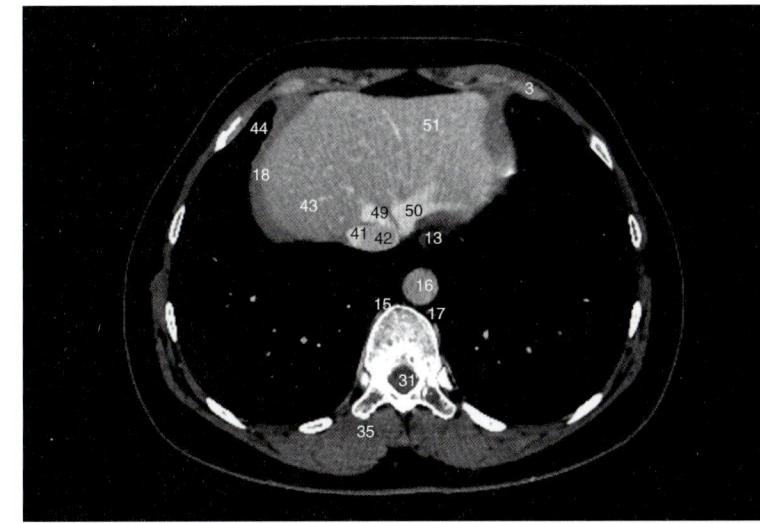

B. CT 纵隔窗增强图像

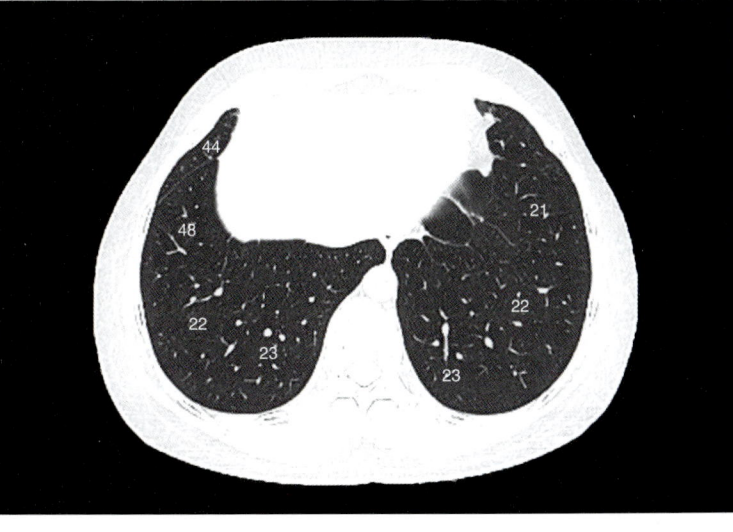

C. CT 肺窗图像

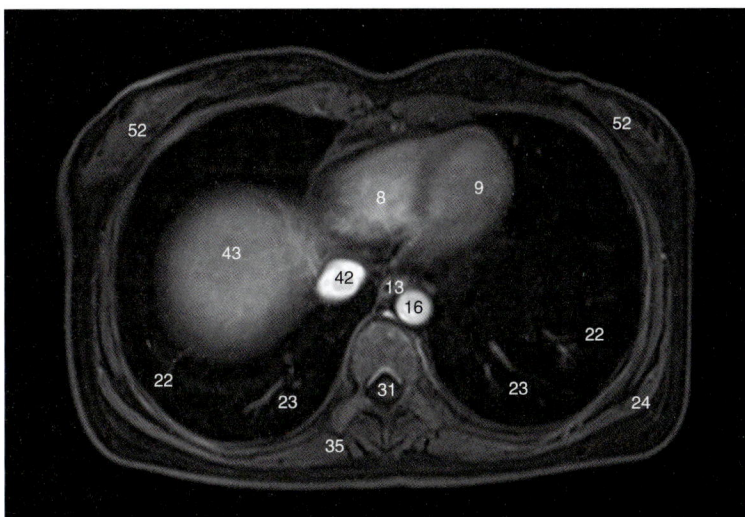

D. MR T1WI 增强图像

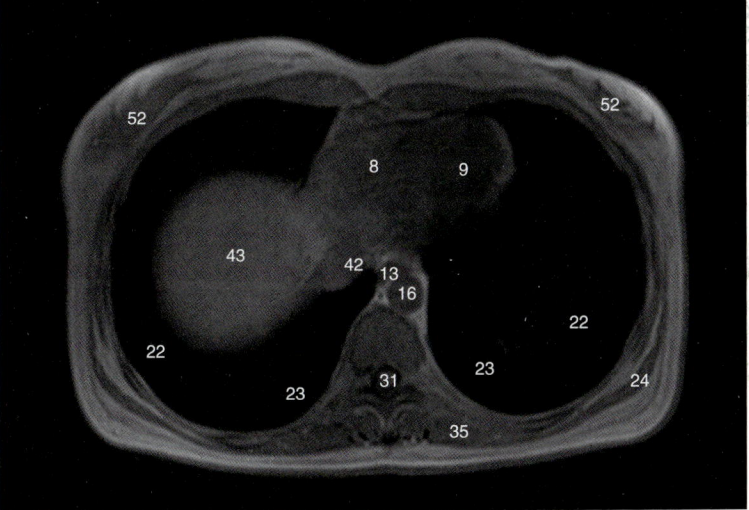

E. MR T1WI 平扫图像

关键结构：左室后静脉，右冠状动脉。

此断面前方经剑突，后方经 T9-10 椎间盘。

右心房消失，左、右心室及两侧肺较上一断层变小，右心室后方的冠状沟内，心小静脉伴随右冠状动脉。冠状窦较上一断层变小，即将消失。膈右穹窿、膈左穹窿及肝右叶较上一断层变大，胃底结构即将出现。较上一断面，左室后静脉走行更加明显，此静脉位于左心室的膈面，在心中静脉的左侧，收集左心室壁的静脉血，上行直接注入心冠状窦或注入心大静脉。许国卿等[99]对左室电极导线植入在不同冠状静脉分支血管与左室起搏部位的关系研究发现，左室电极或双极电极导线植入左室后静脉更容易起搏心尖部。下腔静脉位于肝脏面的腔静脉沟内，肝右静脉主干部分切及。食管、胸主动脉、奇静脉、半奇静脉和胸导管位置变化不大。脊柱区切及 T9-10 椎间盘，后方椎管内见脊髓及其被膜，关节突关节及椎弓板等。CT 图像上心包几近消失，肺仍可见下叶底段，肝断面最大，下腔静脉及 3 条肝静脉清晰可辨。

胸部连续横断层 88（FH.11750）

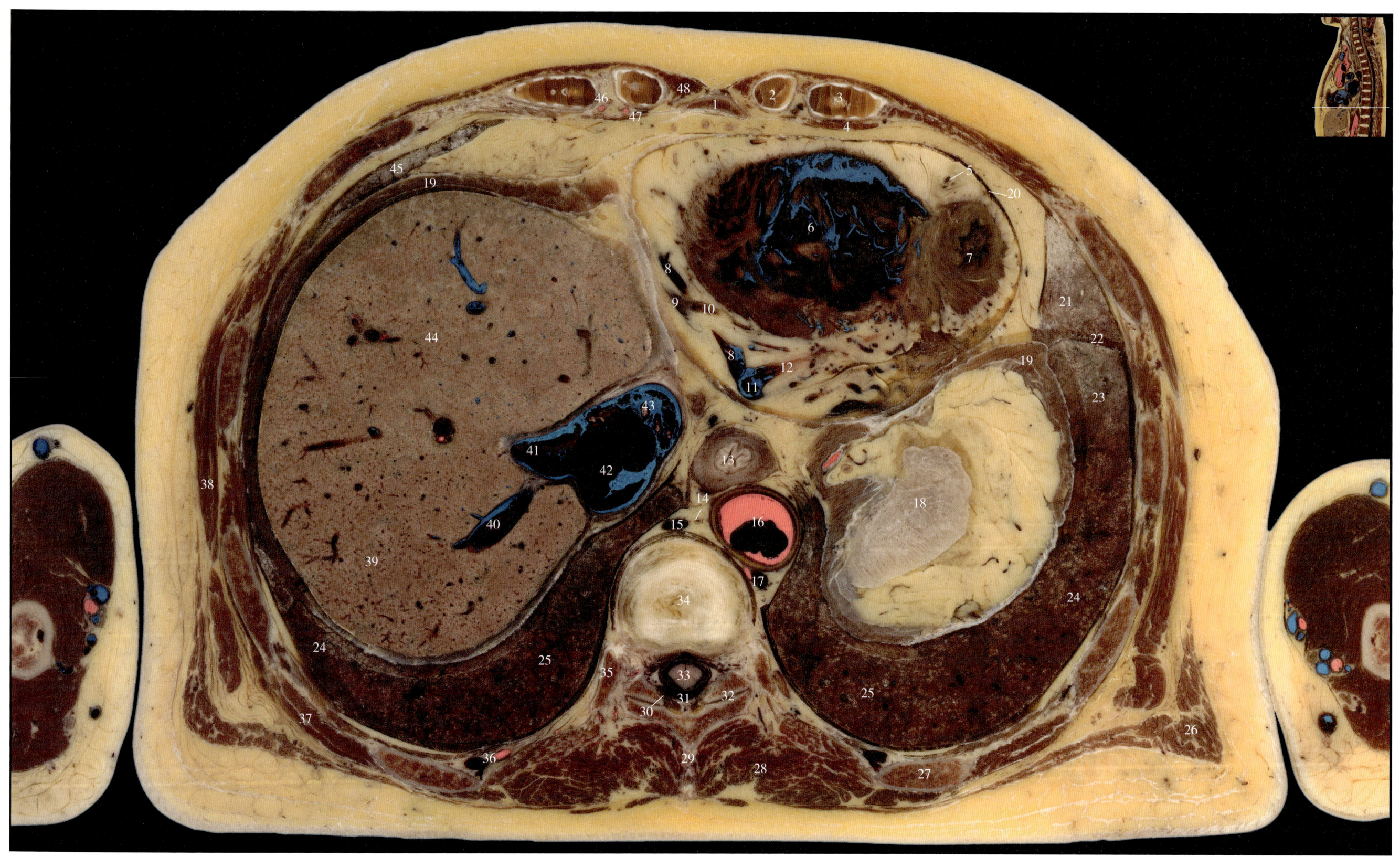

A. 断层标本图像

1. 剑突 xiphoid process
2. 第 7 肋软骨 7th costal cartilage
3. 第 6 肋软骨 6th costal cartilage
4. 胸横肌 transversus thoracis
5. 前室间支 anterior interventricular branch
6. 右心室 right ventricle
7. 左心室 left ventricle
8. 心小静脉 small cardiac vein
9. 右冠状动脉 right coronary artery
10. 后室间支 posterior interventricular branch
11. 冠状窦 coronary sinus
12. 心中静脉 middle cardiac vein
13. 食管 esophagus
14. 胸导管 thoracic duct
15. 奇静脉 azygos vein
16. 胸主动脉 thoracic aorta
17. 半奇静脉 hemiazygos vein
18. 胃底 fundus of stomach
19. 膈 diaphragm
20. 心包前下窦 anterior inferior sinus of pericardium
21. 下舌段（S5）inferior lingular segment
22. 斜裂 oblique fissure
23. 内前底段（S7+8）medioanterior basal segment
24. 外侧底段（S9）lateral basal segment
25. 后底段（S10）posterior basal segment
26. 背阔肌 latissimus dorsi
27. 第 9 肋骨 9th costal bone
28. 竖脊肌 erector spinae
29. 棘间韧带 interspinous ligament
30. 黄韧带 ligamenta flava
31. 硬膜外隙 epidural space
32. 关节突关节 zygapophysial joint
33. 脊髓 spinal cord
34. T9-10 椎间盘 T9-10 intervertebral disc
35. 第 10 肋骨 10th costal bone
36. 肋间后动、静脉 posterior intercostal artery and vein
37. 肋间肌 intercostal muscle
38. 前锯肌 serratus anterior
39. 肝右后叶 right posterior lobe of liver
40. 肝右后上缘静脉 right posterior supramarginal vein of liver
41. 肝右静脉 right hepatic vein
42. 下腔静脉 inferior vena cava
43. 肝左静脉 left hepatic vein
44. 肝右前叶 right anterior lobe of liver
45. 右肺中叶 middle lobe of right lung
46. 肌膈动脉 musculophrenic artery
47. 腹壁上动脉 superior epigastric artery
48. 腹直肌 rectus abdominis
49. 肝中静脉 middle hepatic vein
50. 肝左内叶 left medial lobe of liver
51. 乳腺 mammary gland

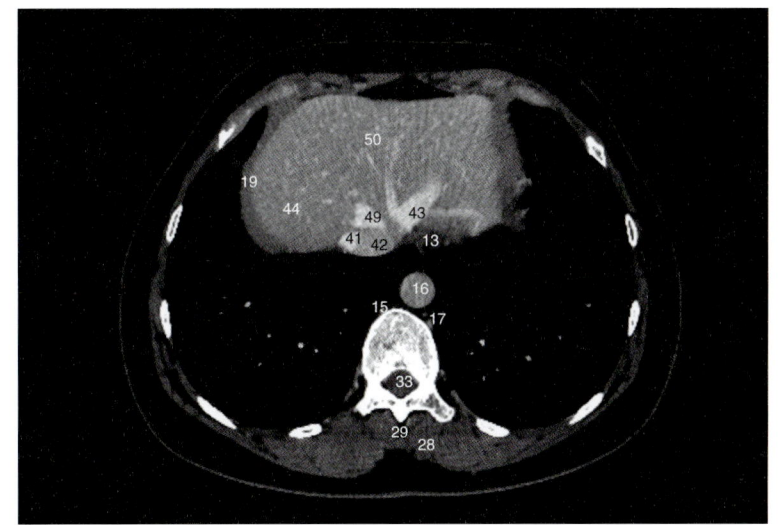

B. CT 纵隔窗增强图像

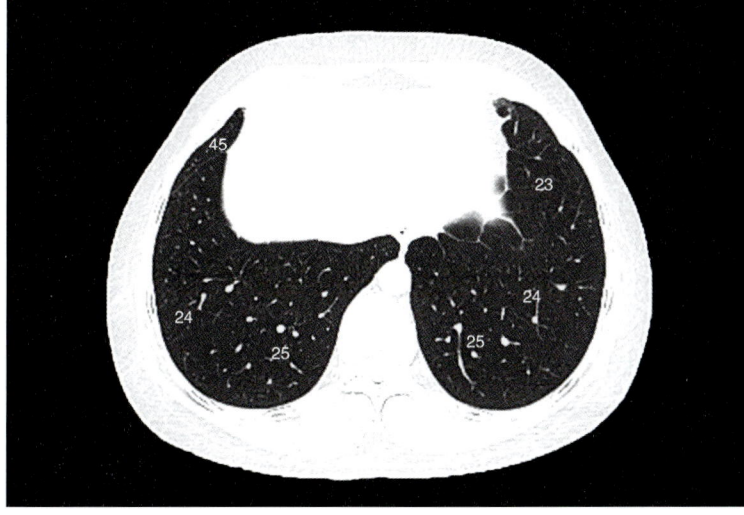

C. CT 肺窗图像

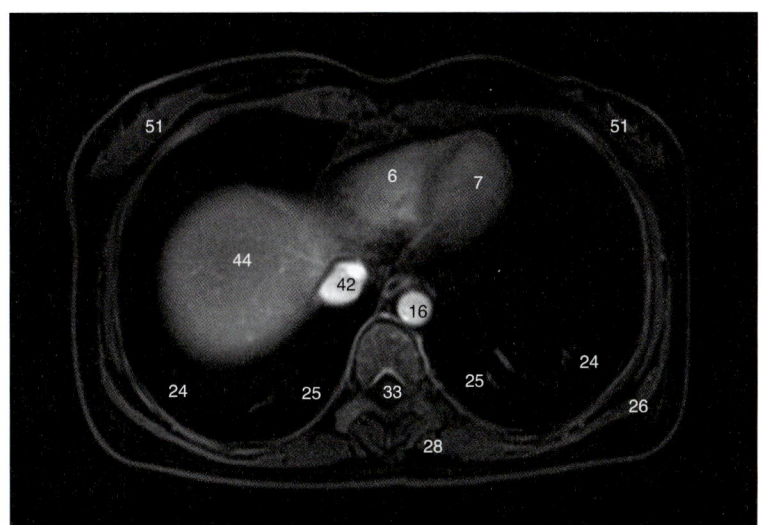

D. MR T1WI 增强图像

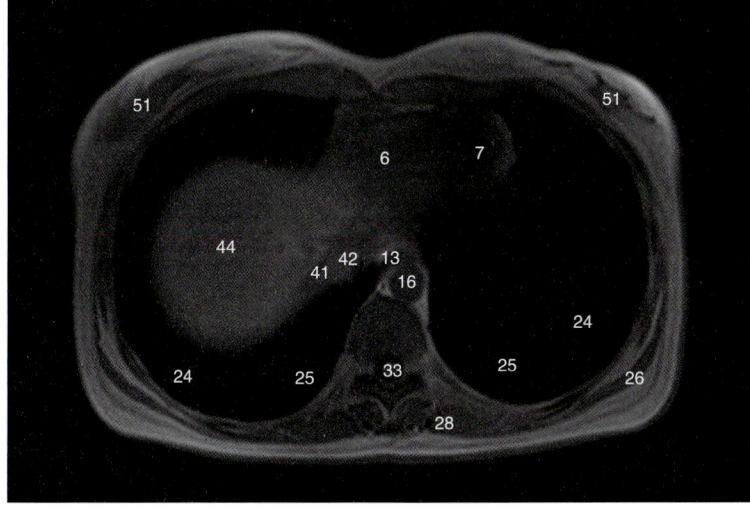

E. MR T1WI 平扫图像

关键结构：冠状窦，心小静脉，心中静脉。

此断面前方经剑突，后方经 T9-10 椎间盘下份。

胸腔内结构进一步缩小，右心室右后方见心小静脉伴行右冠状动脉，右冠状动脉在房室交点处分为后室间支和右旋支，后室间支走行于后室间沟，其出现的概率为 98%，多数止于后室间沟下 1/3[96]。冠状窦到底部，即将消失，有心小静脉和心中静脉汇入。膈右穹窿、膈左穹窿及肝右叶较上一断层变大。由于膈穹窿凸向上，故膈的下方和内侧为腹腔，而胸腔则居其上方和外侧。食管进一步左移至胸主动脉前方，走向膈食管裂孔。在腹腔内，肝占据右侧，胃底首次出现于膈左穹窿的下内侧。下腔静脉位于肝脏面的腔静脉沟内，肝右静脉主干及右后上缘静脉位置不变。CT 图像显示前部心结构消失，3 条肝静脉进入肝内，分隔不同的肝段和肝叶。肺主要为下叶，脊柱区和后纵隔结构变化不大。

胸部连续横断层 89（FH.11730）

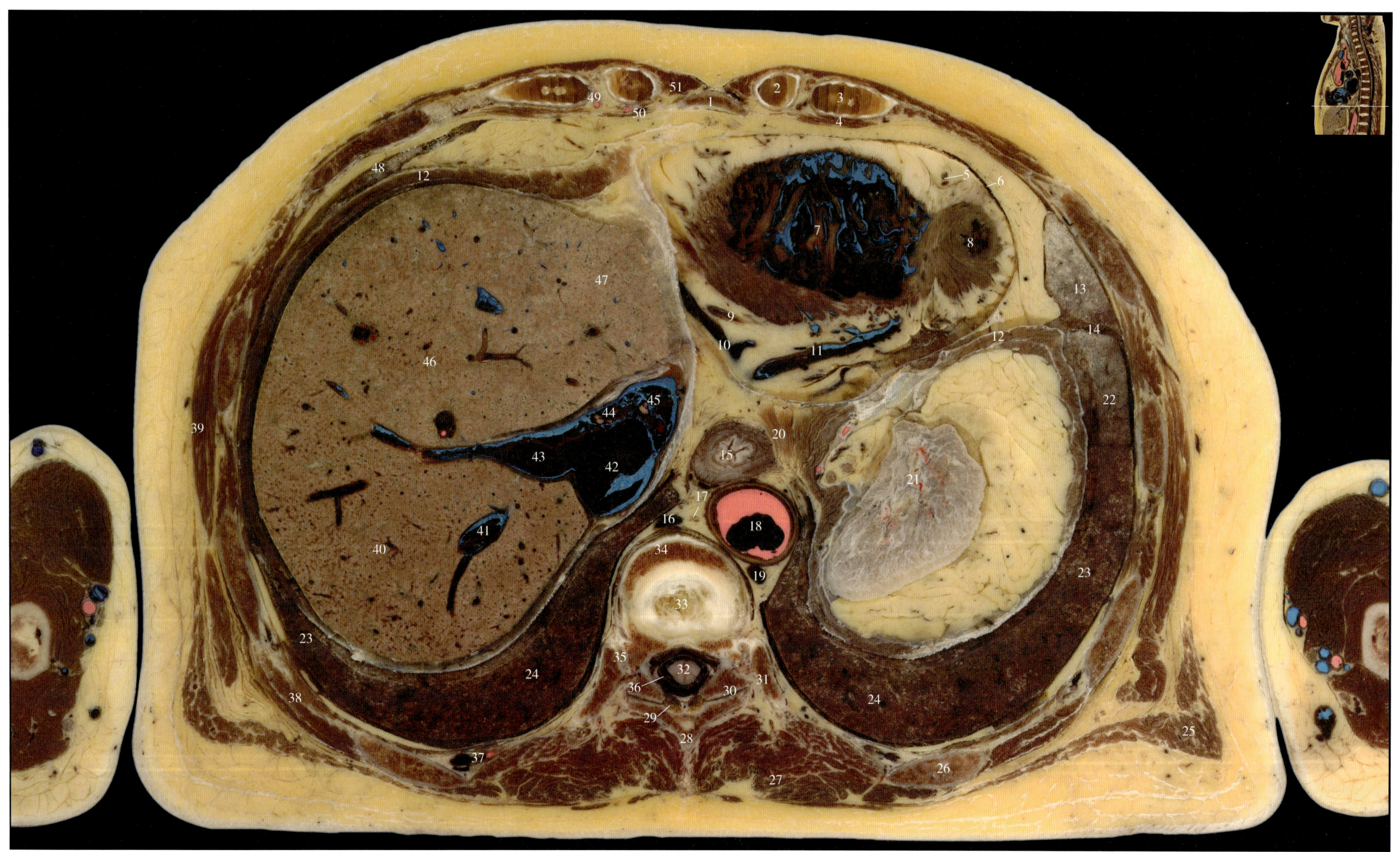

A. 断层标本图像

1. 剑突 xiphoid process
2. 第 7 肋软骨 7th costal cartilage
3. 第 6 肋软骨 6th costal cartilage
4. 胸横肌 transversus thoracis
5. 前室间支 anterior interventricular branch
6. 心包前下窦 anterior inferior sinus of pericardium
7. 右心室 right ventricle
8. 左心室 left ventricle
9. 后室间支 posterior interventricular branch
10. 心小静脉 small cardiac vein
11. 心中静脉 middle cardiac vein
12. 膈 diaphragm
13. 下舌段（S5）inferior lingular segment
14. 斜裂 oblique fissure
15. 食管 esophagus
16. 奇静脉 azygos vein
17. 胸导管 thoracic duct
18. 胸主动脉 thoracic aorta
19. 半奇静脉 hemiazygos vein
20. 右膈脚 right crus of diaphragm
21. 胃底 fundus of stomach
22. 内前底段（S7+8）medioanterior basal segment
23. 外侧底段（S9）lateral basal segment
24. 后底段（S10）posterior basal segment
25. 背阔肌 latissimus dorsi
26. 第 9 肋骨 9th costal bone
27. 竖脊肌 erector spinae
28. 棘突 spinous process
29. 黄韧带 ligamenta flava
30. 关节突关节 zygapophysial joint
31. 第 10 肋骨 10th costal bone
32. 脊髓 spinal cord
33. T9-10 椎间盘 T9-10 intervertebral disc
34. 第 10 胸椎椎体 body of 10th thoracic vertebra
35. 肋头关节 joint of costal head
36. 硬脊膜 spinal dura mater
37. 肋间后动、静脉 posterior intercostal artery and vein
38. 肋间肌 intercostal muscle
39. 前锯肌 serratus anterior
40. 肝右后叶 right posterior lobe of liver
41. 肝右后上缘静脉 right posterior supramarginal vein of liver
42. 下腔静脉 inferior vena cava
43. 肝右静脉 right hepatic vein
44. 肝中静脉 middle hepatic vein
45. 肝左静脉 left hepatic vein
46. 肝右前叶 right anterior lobe of liver
47. 肝左内叶 left medial lobe of liver
48. 右肺中叶 middle lobe of right lung
49. 肌膈动脉 musculophrenic artery
50. 腹壁上动脉 superior epigastric artery
51. 腹直肌 rectus abdominis
52. 乳腺 mammary gland

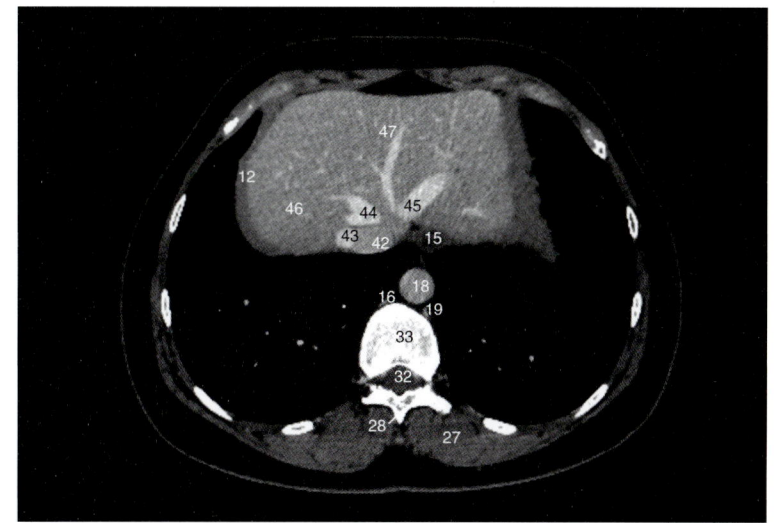

B. CT 纵隔窗增强图像

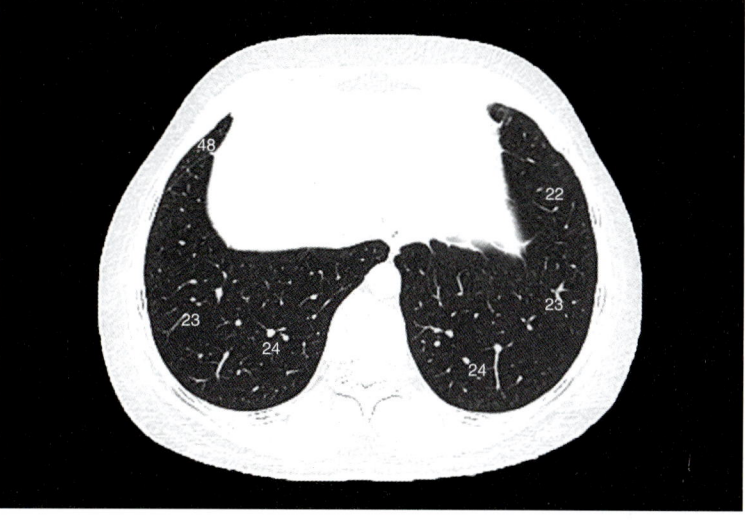

C. CT 肺窗图像

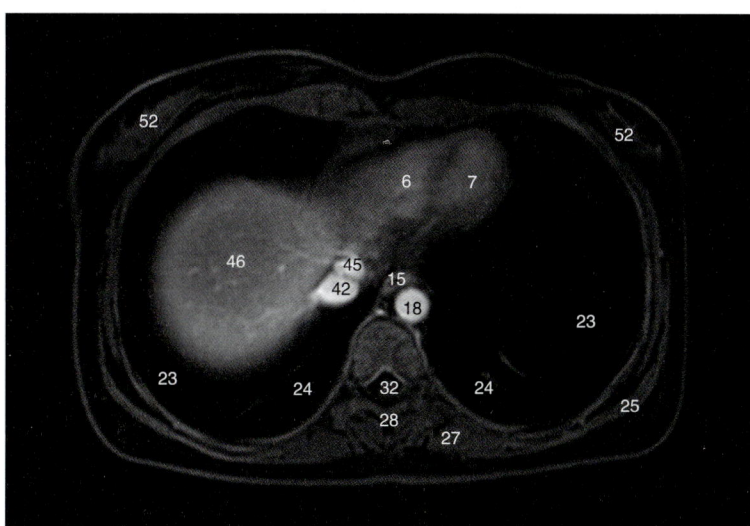

D. MR T1WI 增强图像

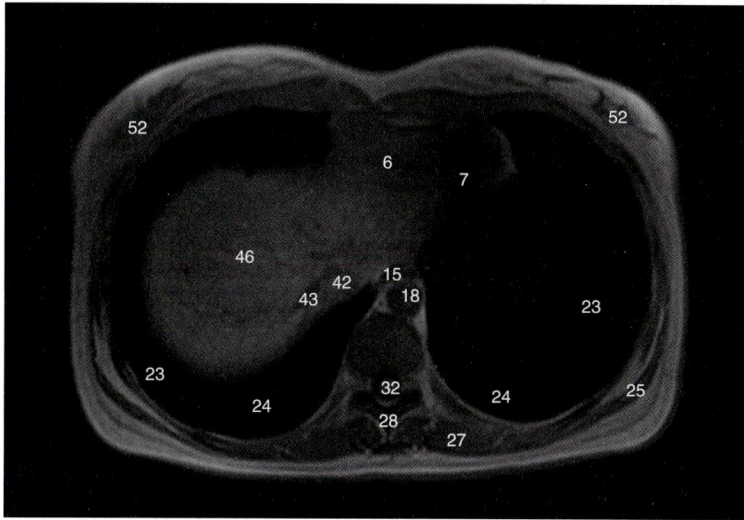

E. MR T1WI 平扫图像

关键结构：后室间支，心小静脉，心中静脉。

此断面前方经剑突，后方经 T9-10 椎间盘下部和第 10 胸椎椎体上部。

胸腔内结构进一步缩小，左心室即将消失，冠状窦消失，见其属支心小静脉和心中静脉。心中静脉起于心尖部，伴行右冠状动脉的后室间支走行于左右心室之间的后室间沟内，注入冠状窦的末端，收集左右心室后壁、室间隔后部、心尖和部分心室前壁的静脉血。心小静脉起于心下缘，在冠状沟内伴右冠状动脉向左注入冠状窦右端或心中静脉。膈及腹腔内结构较上一断层变大。脊柱区切及 T9-10 椎间盘和第 10 胸椎椎体前部，食管位于胸主动脉前方，即将穿膈的食管裂孔。CT 图像胸腔结构仍为肺下叶底段，右肺中叶即将消失。3 条肝静脉走向肝内，肝左叶内有肝左静脉的属支左叶间静脉注入，分隔肝左内叶和左外叶。食管穿膈的食管裂孔，进入腹腔。

胸部连续横断层90（FH.11710）

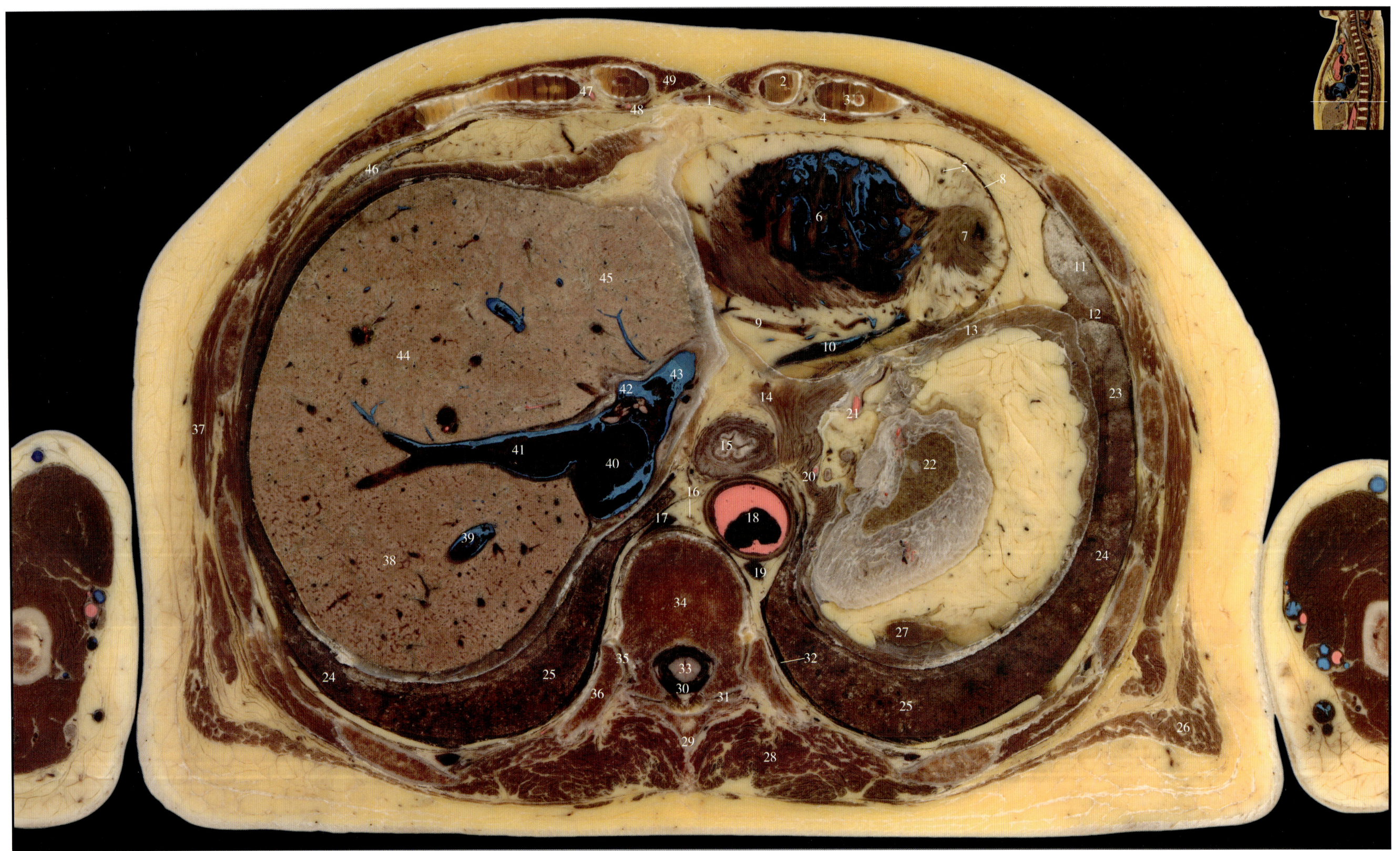

A. 断层标本图像

1. 剑突 xiphoid process
2. 第 7 肋软骨 7th costal cartilage
3. 第 6 肋软骨 6th costal cartilage
4. 胸横肌 transversus thoracis
5. 前室间支 anterior interventricular branch
6. 右心室 right ventricle
7. 心尖 cardiac apex
8. 心包前下窦 anterior inferior sinus of pericardium
9. 后室间支 posterior interventricular branch
10. 心中静脉 middle cardiac vein
11. 下舌段（S5）inferior lingular segment
12. 斜裂 oblique fissure
13. 膈 diaphragm
14. 右膈脚 right crus of diaphragm
15. 食管 esophagus
16. 胸导管 thoracic duct
17. 奇静脉 azygos vein
18. 胸主动脉 thoracic aorta
19. 半奇静脉 hemiazygos vein
20. 左膈脚 left crus of diaphragm
21. 左膈下动脉 left inferior phrenic artery
22. 胃底 fundus of stomach
23. 内前底段（S7+8）medioanterior basal segment
24. 外侧底段（S9）lateral basal segment
25. 后底段（S10）posterior basal segment
23. 肋间肌 intercostal muscle
26. 背阔肌 latissimus dorsi
27. 脾 spleen
28. 竖脊肌 erector spinae
29. 棘突 spinous process
30. 硬膜外隙 epidural space
31. 关节突关节 zygapophysial joint
32. 胸膜腔 pleural cavity
33. 脊髓 spinal cord
34. 第 10 胸椎椎体 body of 10th thoracic vertebra
35. 肋头关节 joint of costal head
36. 第 10 肋骨 10th costal bone
37. 前锯肌 serratus anterior
38. 肝右后叶 right posterior lobe of liver
39. 肝右上缘静脉 right posterior supramarginal vein of liver
40. 下腔静脉 inferior vena cava
41. 肝右静脉 right hepatic vein
42. 肝中静脉 middle hepatic vein
43. 肝左静脉 left hepatic vein
44. 肝右前叶 right anterior lobe of liver
45. 肝左内叶 left medial lobe of liver
46. 右肺中叶 middle lobe of right lung
47. 肌膈动脉 musculophrenic artery
48. 腹壁上动脉 superior epigastric artery
49. 腹直肌 rectus abdominis
50. 乳腺 mammary gland

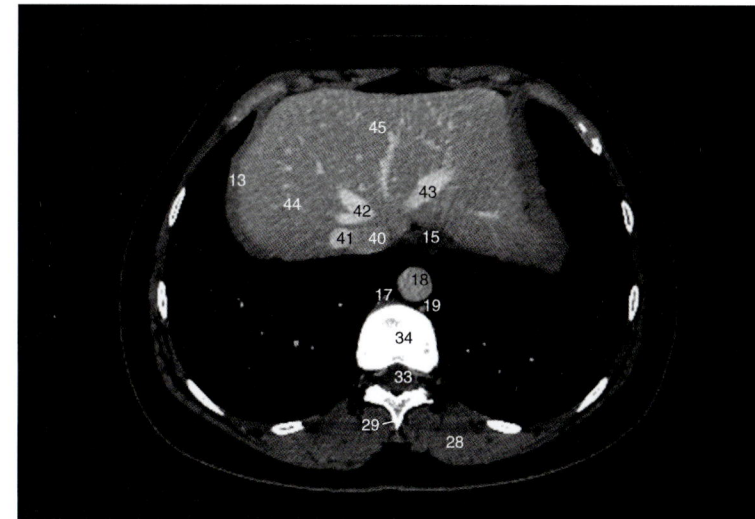

B. CT 纵隔窗增强图像

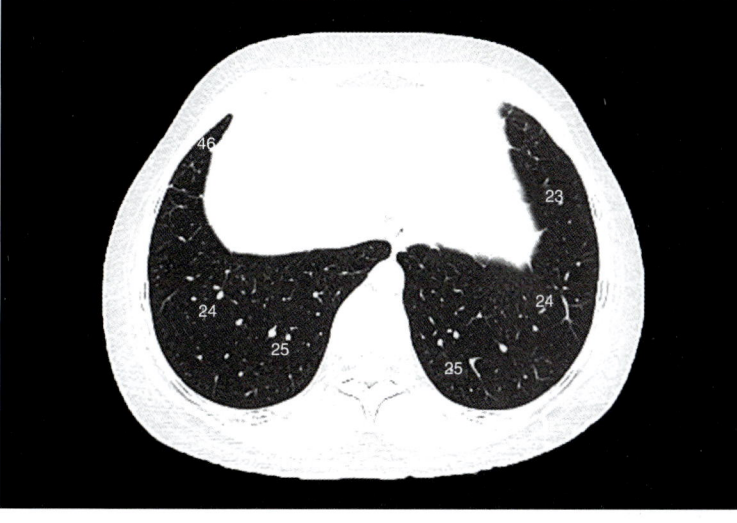

C. CT 肺窗图像

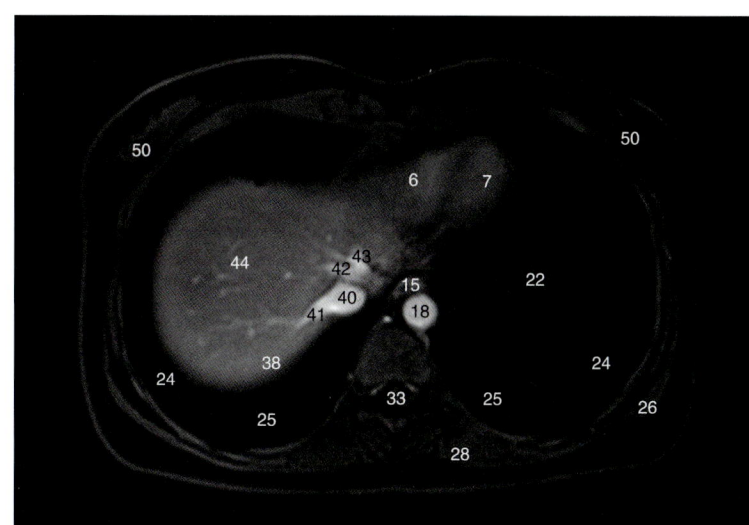

D. MR T1WI 增强图像

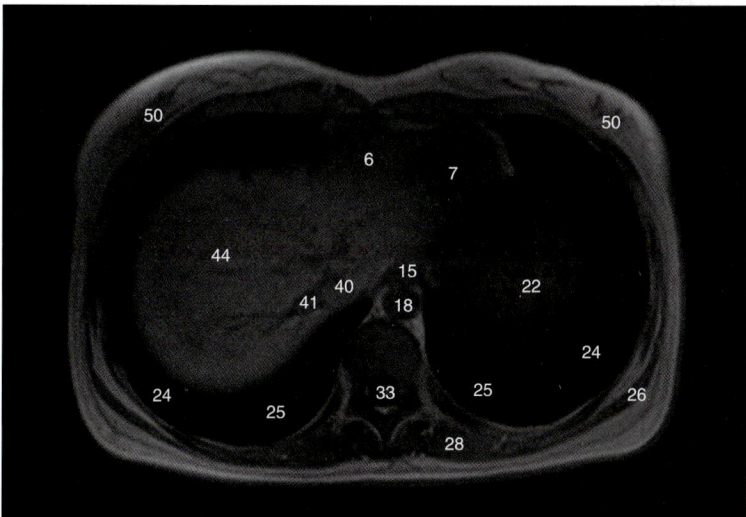

E. MR T1WI 平扫图像

关键结构：膈，右膈脚，食管裂孔。

此断面前方经剑突，后方经第 10 胸椎椎体上部和肋头关节。

膈左、右穹窿进一步扩大，分隔胸腔和腹腔结构。膈的中央为中心腱，肌部前份为胸骨部，周围为肋部，后方的腰部形成左、右膈脚。右膈脚形成的肌纤维环绕食管裂孔，收缩时可起到钳制食管的作用，若肌环发育不良，腹部器官可自此处突入胸腔形成食管裂孔疝[100]。食管裂孔约平第 10 胸椎，有食管和迷走神经前、后干通过。胸腔内心室后方为走向后室间沟的后室间支和伴行的心中静脉。两侧肺下叶呈 "C" 形包绕在后外侧边缘。于此断面上，肝仍为第二肝门，可见肝右静脉主干，分隔右前叶和右后叶。腹腔左侧胃底段增大，在大网膜后方出现脾。CT 图上两肺底缩小，前部为膈和肝，食管腹段左移逐渐移行于胃贲门。脊柱区经过第 10 胸椎椎体，椎管内为脊髓及其被膜。

胸部连续横断层 91（FH.11690）

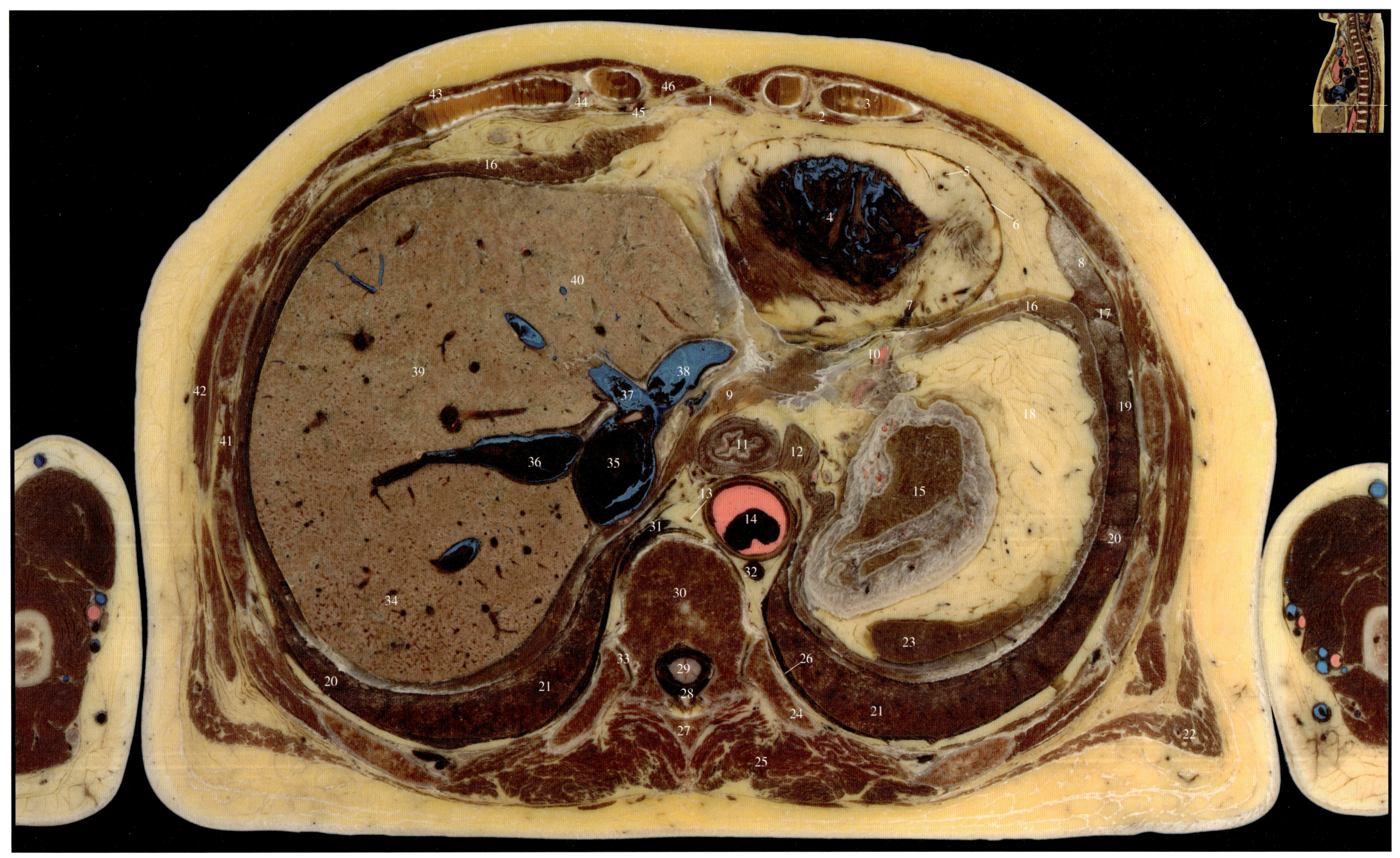

A. 断层标本图像

1. 剑突 xiphoid process
2. 胸横肌 transversus thoracis
3. 第 6 肋软骨 6th costal cartilage
4. 右心室 right ventricle
5. 前室间支 anterior interventricular branch
6. 心包前下窦 anterior inferior sinus of pericardium
7. 心中静脉 middle cardiac vein
8. 下舌段（S5）inferior lingular segment
9. 右膈脚 right crus of diaphragm
10. 左膈下动脉 left inferior phrenic artery
11. 食管 esophagus
12. 左膈脚 left crus of diaphragm
13. 胸导管 thoracic duct
14. 胸主动脉 thoracic aorta
15. 胃底 fundus of stomach
16. 膈 diaphragm
17. 斜裂 oblique fissure
18. 大网膜 greater omentum
19. 内前底段（S7+8）medioanterior basal segment
20. 外侧底段（S9）lateral basal segment
21. 后底段（S10）posterior basal segment
22. 背阔肌 latissimus dorsi
23. 脾 spleen
24. 第 10 肋骨 10th costal bone
25. 竖脊肌 erector spinae
26. 胸膜腔 pleural cavity
27. 第 9 胸椎棘突 spinous process of 9th thoracic vertebra
28. 硬膜外隙 epidural space
29. 脊髓 spinal cord
30. 第 10 胸椎椎体 body of 10th thoracic vertebra
31. 奇静脉 azygos vein
32. 半奇静脉 hemiazygos vein
33. 肋头关节 joint of costal head
34. 肝右后叶 right posterior lobe of liver
35. 下腔静脉 inferior vena cava
36. 肝右静脉 right hepatic vein
37. 肝中静脉 middle hepatic vein
38. 肝左静脉 left hepatic vein
39. 肝右前叶 right anterior lobe of liver
40. 肝左内叶 left medial lobe of liver
41. 肋间肌 intercostal muscle
42. 前锯肌 serratus anterior
43. 腹外斜肌 obliquus externus abdominis
44. 肌膈动脉 musculophrenic artery
45. 腹壁上动脉 superior epigastric artery
46. 腹直肌 rectus abdominis
47. 椎间盘 intervertebral disc
48. 前底段（S8）anterior basal segment

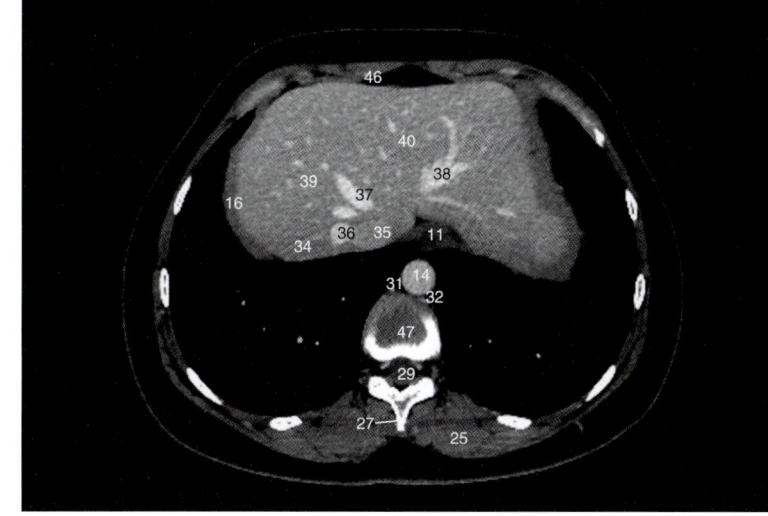

B. CT 纵隔窗增强图像

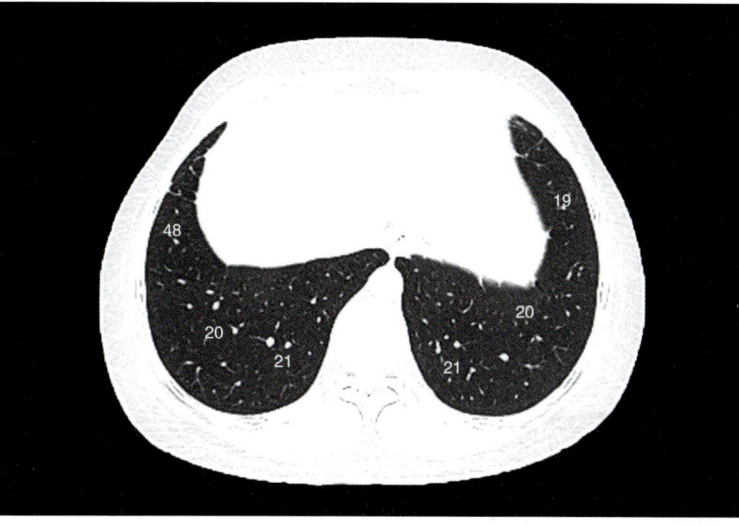

C. CT 肺窗图像

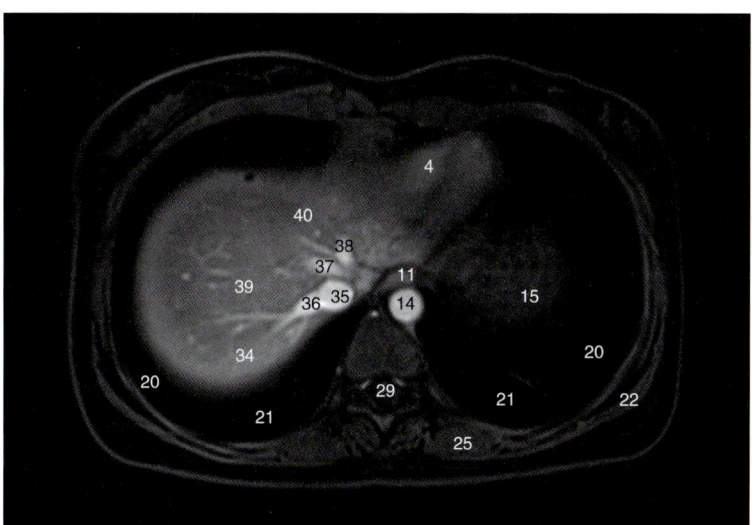

D. MR T1WI 增强图像

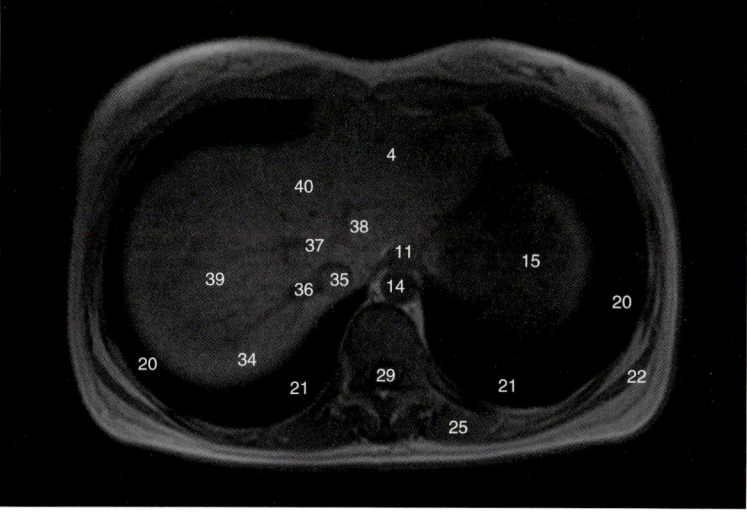

E. MR T1WI 平扫图像

关键结构：膈脚，左膈下动脉，胃膈韧带。

此断面前方经剑突，后方经第 10 胸椎椎体上部。

胸腔内，左心室即将消失，心血管仍可见前方的前室间支和后方的后室间支及心中静脉。双肺下叶较上一断层明显变小，依旧呈 "C" 形围绕于胸腔后外侧。食管下行于胸主动脉前方，正在穿越膈的食管裂孔。食管两侧为左、右膈脚，左膈下动脉自发出后向下至左膈脚贴近腹腔动脉起点的位置穿膈肌进入腹腔，返折后向左上方，经左膈脚的前方，过食管腹段的后方，沿途分别向肾上腺上极、下极和胃的上部发出分支[101]。胃膈韧带右层向右续于食管前方的腹膜，左层连系于膈。胃膈韧带左、右层之间的胃面无腹膜覆盖，称胃裸区。CT 图像显示的肝左叶较大，内有肝左静脉及其分支，食管位于腹主动脉前方，即将连于贲门。脊柱区至 T10-11 椎间盘，后方为椎间孔、椎弓板及椎管及其内容物等。胸腔结构依然是肺下叶位于膈的后外侧。

胸部连续横断层 92 (FH.11670)

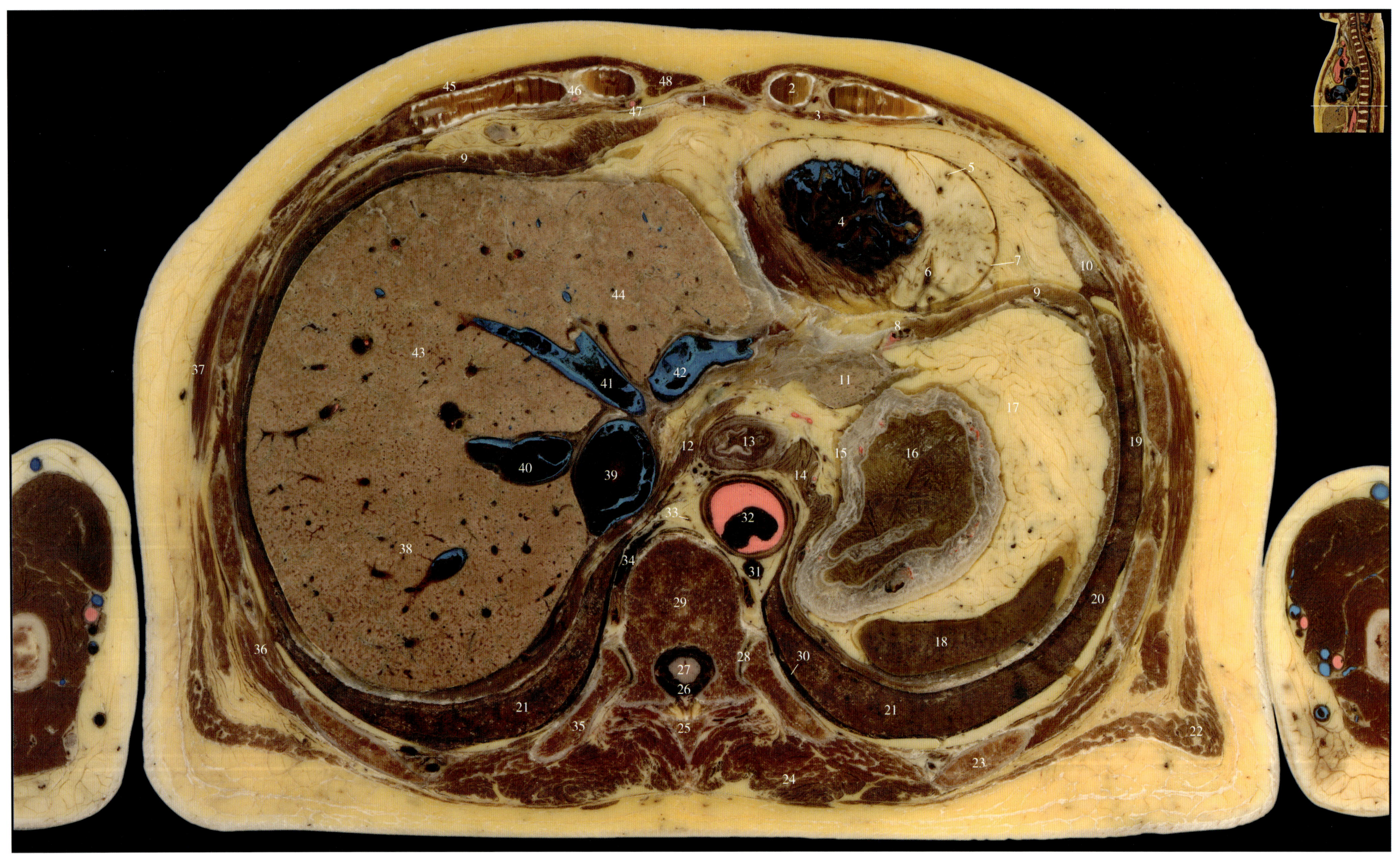

A. 断层标本图像

1. 剑突 xiphoid process
2. 第7肋软骨 7th costal cartilage
3. 胸横肌 transversus thoracis
4. 右心室 right ventricle
5. 前室间支 anterior interventricular branch
6. 心中静脉 middle cardiac vein
7. 心包腔 pericardial cavity
8. 左膈下动脉 left inferior phrenic artery
9. 膈 diaphragm
10. 下舌段（S5）inferior lingular segment
11. 肝左外叶 left lateral lobe of liver
12. 右膈脚 right crus of diaphragm
13. 食管 esophagus
14. 左膈脚 left crus of diaphragm
15. 胃裸区 gastric bare area
16. 胃底 fundus of stomach
17. 大网膜 greater omentum
18. 脾 spleen
19. 内前底段（S7+8）medioanterior basal segment
20. 外侧底段（S9）lateral basal segment
21. 后底段（S10）posterior basal segment
22. 背阔肌 latissimus dorsi
23. 第9肋骨 9th costal bone
24. 竖脊肌 erector spinae
25. 第9胸椎棘突 spinous process of 9th thoracic vertebra
26. 硬膜外隙 epidural space
27. 脊髓 spinal cord
28. 肋头关节 joint of costal head
29. 第10胸椎椎体 body of 10th thoracic vertebra
30. 胸膜腔 pleural cavity
31. 半奇静脉 hemiazygos vein
32. 胸主动脉 thoracic aorta
33. 胸导管 thoracic duct
34. 肋间后静脉 posterior intercostal vein
35. 第10肋骨 10th costal bone
36. 肋间肌 intercostal muscle
37. 前锯肌 serratus anterior
38. 肝右后叶 right posterior lobe of liver
39. 下腔静脉 inferior vena cava
40. 肝右静脉 right hepatic vein
41. 肝中静脉 middle hepatic vein
42. 肝左静脉 left hepatic vein
43. 肝右前叶 right anterior lobe of liver
44. 肝左内叶 left medial lobe of liver
45. 腹外斜肌 obliquus externus abdominis
46. 肌膈动脉 musculophrenic artery
47. 腹壁上动脉 superior epigastric artery
48. 腹直肌 rectus abdominis
49. 椎间盘 intervertebral disc
50. 前底段（S8）anterior basal segment

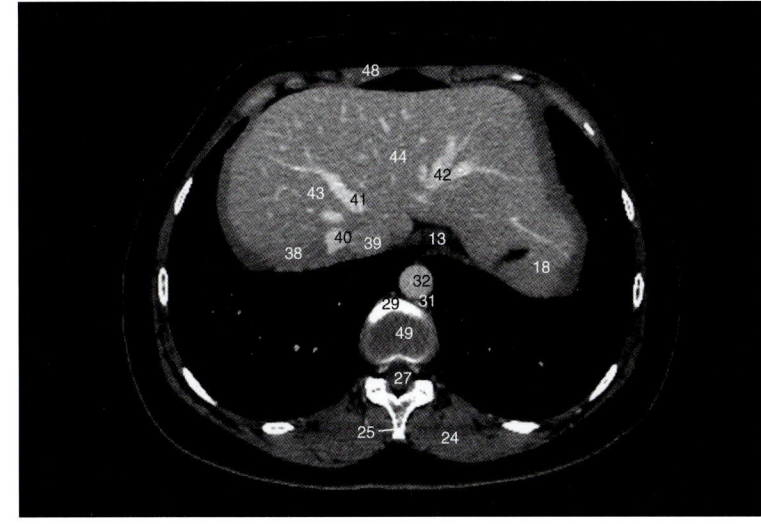

B. CT 纵隔窗增强图像

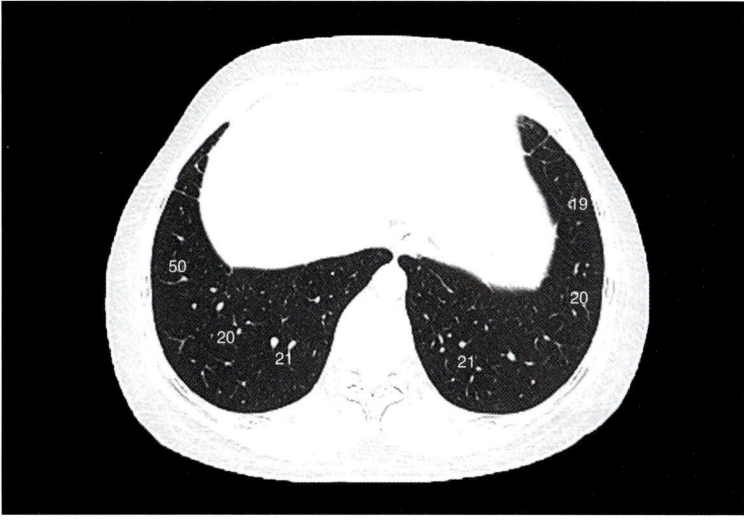

C. CT 肺窗图像

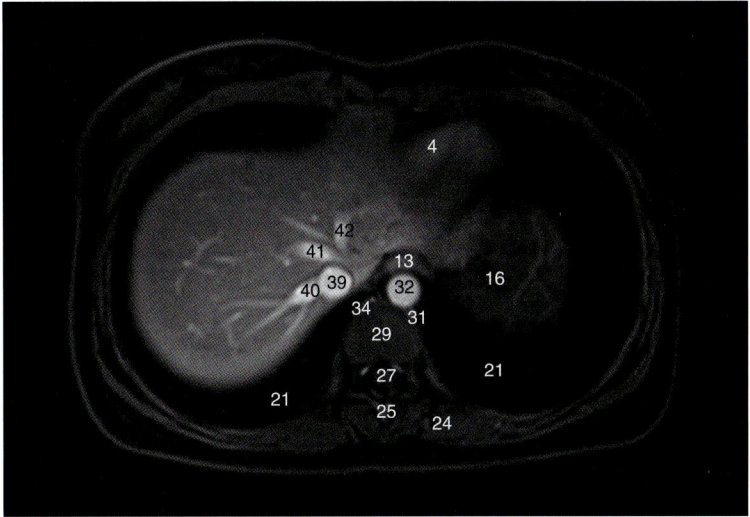

D. MR T1WI 增强图像

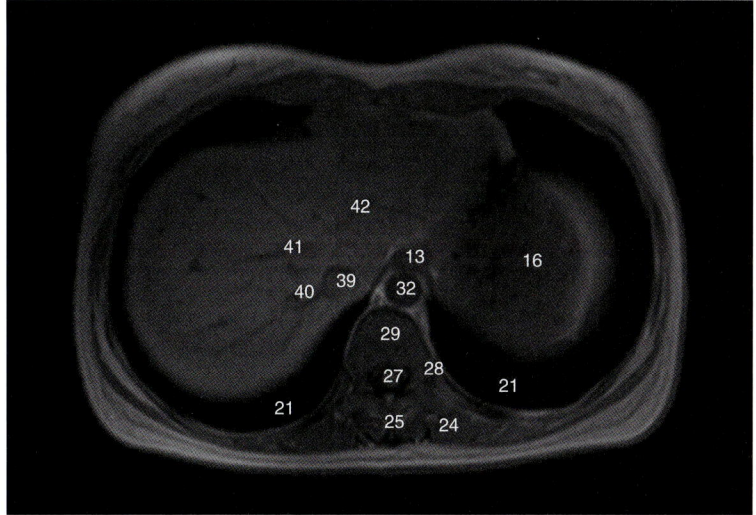

E. MR T1WI 平扫图像

关键结构：剑突，胸骨下角，剑肋角。

此断面前方经剑突，后方经第10胸椎椎体上部。

剑突两侧为第7肋软骨和第6肋软骨，其前方有腹直肌附着。自剑突根部，两侧沿肋软骨向下达第10肋软骨的弓状缘，称为肋弓，与剑突根部之间的形成的角称为胸骨下角，为70°~110°。剑突与肋弓构成剑肋角，心包穿刺时常选择左侧剑肋角呈45°向上进针，可避免损伤胸膜，相对较为安全[102]。胸腔前部见中纵隔心与心包及心包外的脂肪，后部为双肺下叶，呈"C"形位于膈的后外侧，膈胸膜与胸廓内面的肋胸膜之间为肋膈隐窝。膈的腰部为左、右膈脚，位于食管两侧。腹腔内脏器仍为肝、胃底和脾，较上一断层增大，肝左外叶出现在胃底前内侧。脊柱区椎体后外侧见肋头关节。第10胸椎椎体两侧近上缘处，通常各有一全肋凹，与第10肋头关节面形成肋头关节。CT图像显示脊柱区为椎体之间的椎间盘，前方见胸主动脉、奇静脉和半奇静脉，脾出现。

胸部连续横断层 93（FH.11650）

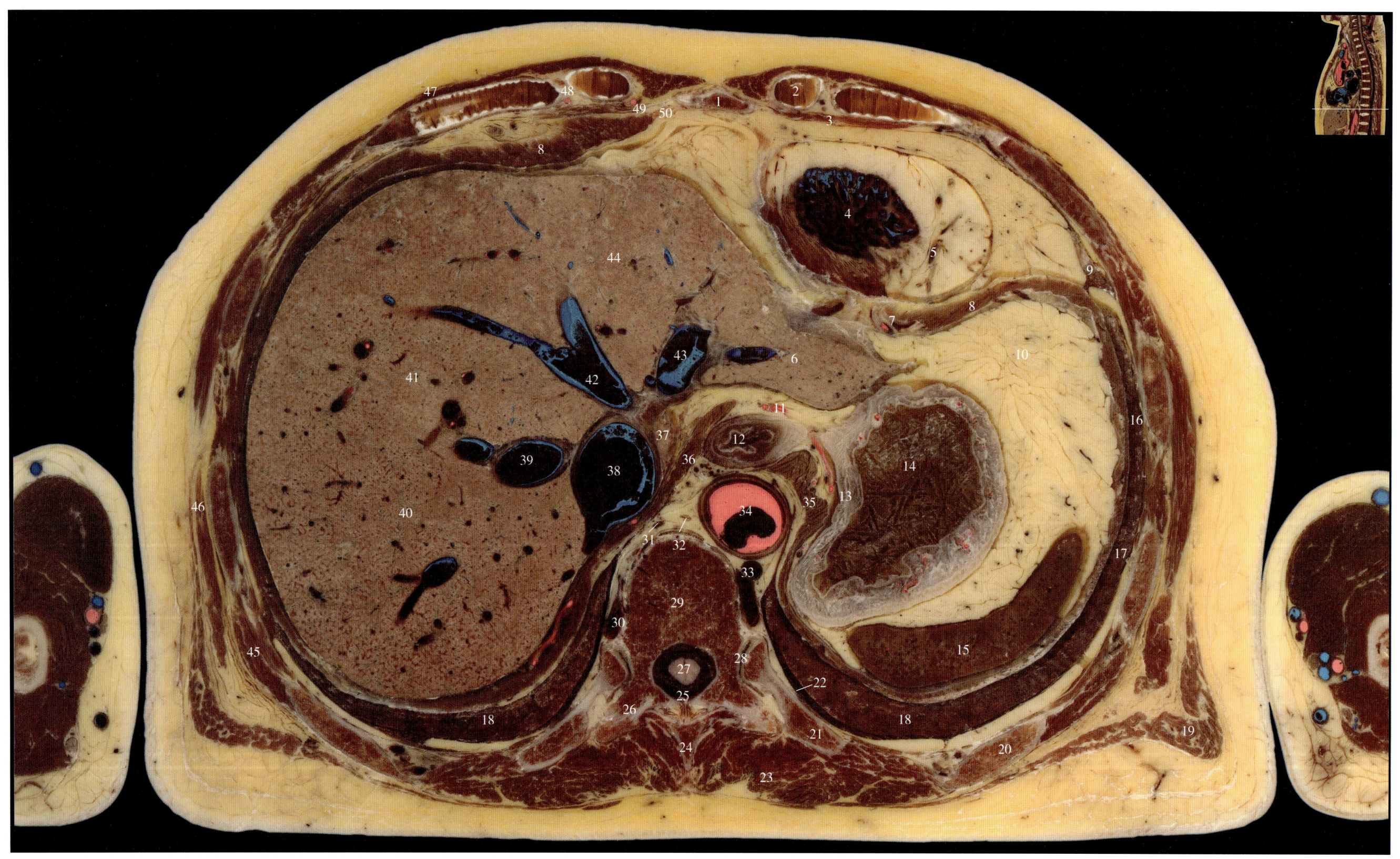

A. 断层标本图像

1. 剑突 xiphoid process
2. 第 7 肋软骨 7th costal cartilage
3. 胸横肌 transversus thoracis
4. 右心室 right ventricle
5. 心中静脉 middle cardiac vein
6. 肝左外叶 left lateral lobe of liver
7. 左膈下动脉 left inferior phrenic artery
8. 膈 diaphragm
9. 下舌段（S5）inferior lingular segment
10. 大网膜 greater omentum
11. 胃左动脉食管支 esophageal branch of left gastric artery
12. 食管 esophagus
13. 胃裸区 gastric bare area
14. 胃底 fundus of stomach
15. 脾 spleen
16. 内前底段（S7+8）medioanterior basal segment
17. 外侧底段（S9）lateral basal segment
18. 后底段（S10）posterior basal segment
19. 背阔肌 latissimus dorsi
20. 第 9 肋骨 9th costal bone
21. 第 10 肋骨 10th costal bone
22. 胸膜腔 pleural cavity
23. 竖脊肌 erector spinae
24. 第 9 胸椎棘突 spinous process of 9th thoracic vertebra
25. 硬膜外隙 epidural space
26. 横突 transverse process
27. 脊髓 spinal cord
28. 肋头关节 joint of costal head
29. 第 10 胸椎椎体 body of 10th thoracic vertebra
30. 肋间后静脉 posterior intercostal vein
31. 奇静脉 azygos vein
32. 胸导管 thoracic duct
33. 半奇静脉 hemiazygos vein
34. 胸主动脉 thoracic aorta
35. 左膈脚 left crus of diaphragm
36. 右膈脚 right crus of diaphragm
37. 肝尾状叶 caudate lobe of liver
38. 下腔静脉 inferior vena cava
39. 肝右静脉 right hepatic vein
40. 肝右后叶 right posterior lobe of liver
41. 肝右前叶 right anterior lobe of liver
42. 肝中静脉 middle hepatic vein
43. 肝左静脉 left hepatic vein
44. 肝左内叶 left medial lobe of liver
45. 肋间肌 intercostal muscle
46. 前锯肌 serratus anterior
47. 腹外斜肌 obliquus externus abdominis
48. 肌膈动脉 musculophrenic artery
49. 腹壁上动脉 superior epigastric artery
50. 胸肋三角 sternocostal triangle
51. 前底段（S8）anterior basal segment

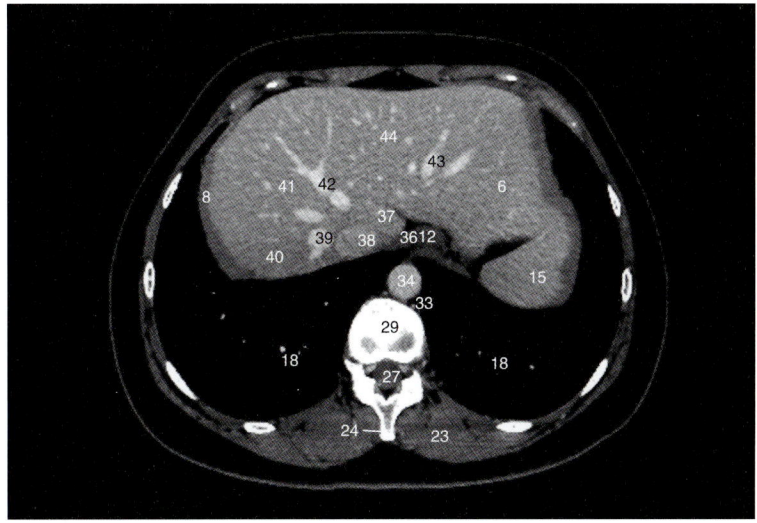

B. CT 纵隔窗增强图像

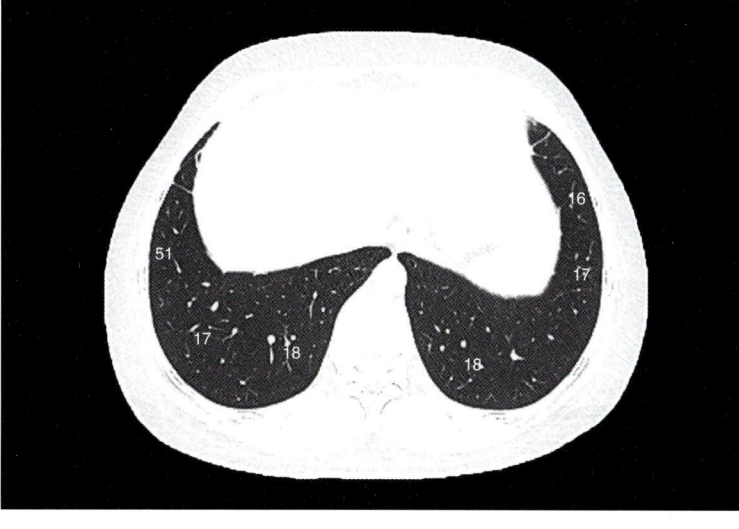

C. CT 肺窗图像

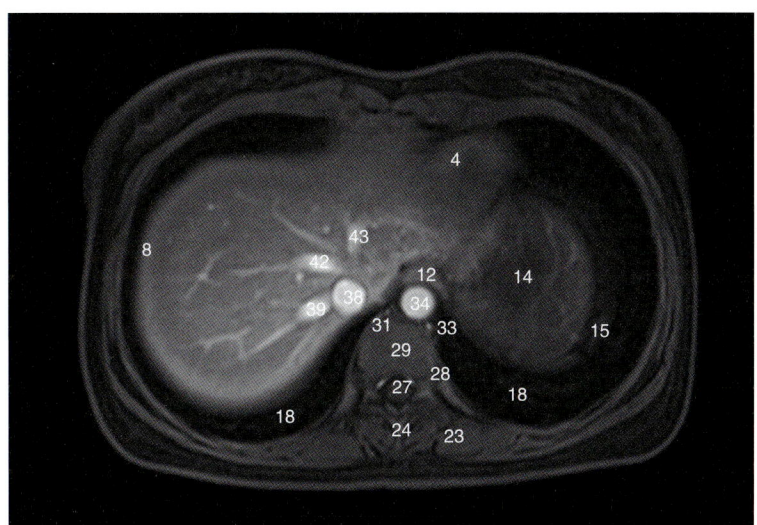

D. MR T1WI 增强图像

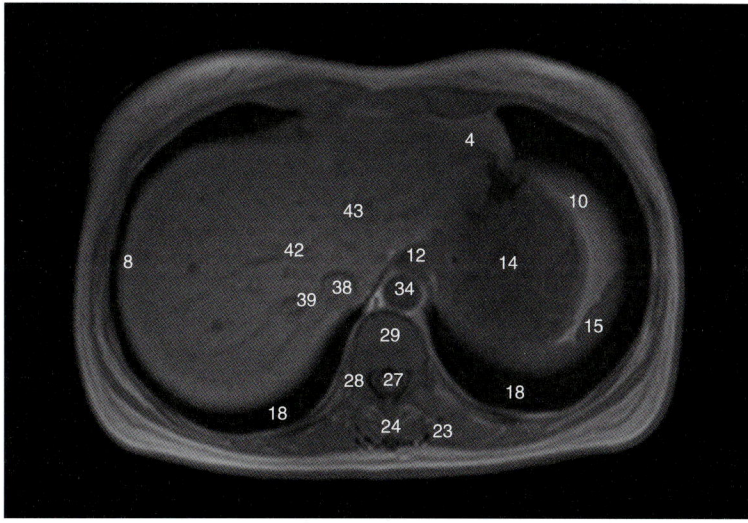

E. MR T1WI 平扫图像

关键结构：肋膈隐窝，胸肋三角。

此断面前方经剑突，后方经第 10 胸椎椎体中部。

膈分隔胸、腹腔的脏器，其前部为膈的胸骨部，附着于剑突后方，由 2 个小束构成，两束之间于正中线上有不明显的裂隙。膈的肋部为膈最广大的起点，以多个肌齿起自下位 6 个肋软骨内面。胸骨部与肋部起点之间为胸肋三角，内有腹壁上动、静脉和淋巴管通过。胸肋三角是膈的薄弱区，胸、腹之间仅隔以两侧浆膜，是膈疝容易发生的部位。胸腔内，心与双肺较上一断层明显变小，右肺下缘前部大部分消失，胸壁与膈之间的胸膜腔形成肋膈隐窝。腹腔内，肝尾状叶首次出现于下腔静脉左前方，并向左突入网膜囊上隐窝。3 条肝静脉进入肝内，分隔肝的左外叶、左内叶、右前叶和右后叶。肝、胃底和脾均较上一断层进一步增大，食管腹部即将连于胃的贲门，胃小弯侧可见胃左动脉食管支。胃裸区较上一断层增宽，位于胃膈韧带左、右层之间，与膈之间形成左膈下腹膜外间隙，内有血管、迷走神经后干和淋巴结分布，左肾上腺也位于此间隙。

胸部连续横断层 94（FH.11630）

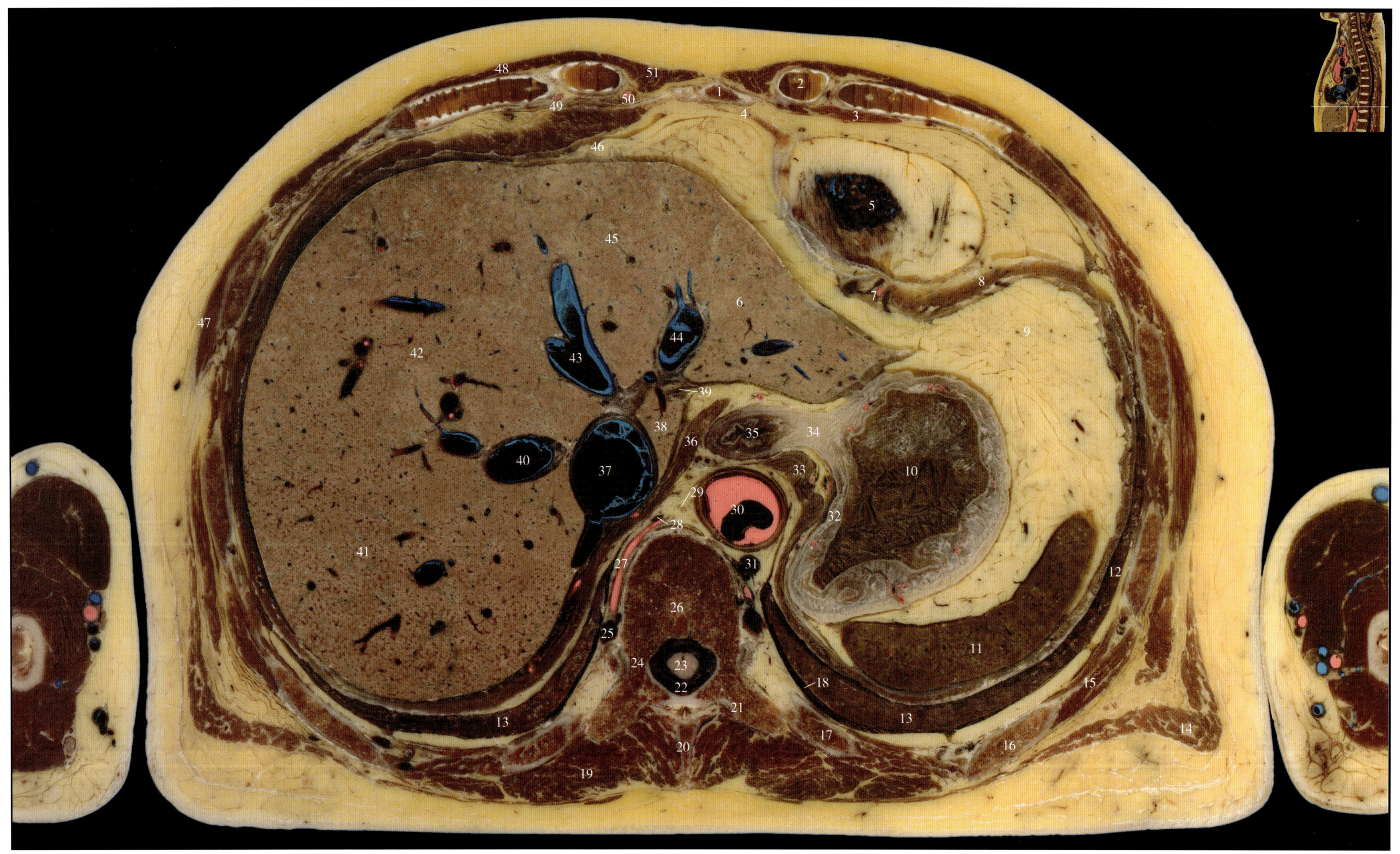

A. 断层标本图像

1. 剑突 xiphoid process
2. 第7肋软骨 7th costal cartilage
3. 胸横肌 transversus thoracis
4. 胸肋三角 sternocostal triangle
5. 右心室 right ventricle
6. 肝左外叶 left lateral lobe of liver
7. 左膈下动脉 left inferior phrenic artery
8. 膈 diaphragm
9. 大网膜 greater omentum
10. 胃底 fundus of stomach
11. 脾 spleen
12. 外侧底段（S9）lateral basal segment
13. 后底段（S10）posterior basal segment
14. 背阔肌 latissimus dorsi
15. 肋间肌 intercostal muscle
16. 第9肋骨 9th costal bone
17. 第10肋骨 10th costal bone
18. 胸膜腔 pleural cavity
19. 竖脊肌 erector spinae
20. 棘突 spinous process
21. 横突 transverse process
22. 硬膜外隙 epidural space
23. 脊髓 spinal cord
24. 椎弓根 pedicle of vertebral arch
25. 肋间后静脉 posterior intercostal vein
26. 第10胸椎椎体 body of 10th thoracic vertebra
27. 肋间后动脉 posterior intercostal artery
28. 奇静脉 azygos vein
29. 胸导管 thoracic duct
30. 胸主动脉 thoracic aorta
31. 半奇静脉 hemiazygos vein
32. 胃裸区 gastric bare area
33. 左膈脚 left crus of diaphragm
34. 贲门部 cardiac part of stomach
35. 食管腹部 abdominal part of esophagus
36. 右膈脚 right crus of diaphragm
37. 下腔静脉 inferior vena cava
38. 肝尾状叶 caudate lobe of liver
39. 静脉韧带裂 fissure for ligamentum venosum
40. 肝右静脉 right hepatic vein
41. 肝右后叶 right posterior lobe of liver
42. 肝右前叶 right anterior lobe of liver
43. 肝中静脉 middle hepatic vein

44. 肝左静脉 left hepatic vein
45. 肝左内叶 left medial lobe of liver
46. 肝镰状韧带 falciform ligament of liver
47. 前锯肌 serratus anterior
48. 腹外斜肌 obliquus externus abdominis
49. 肌膈动脉 musculophrenic artery
50. 腹壁上动脉 superior epigastric artery
51. 腹直肌 rectus abdominis

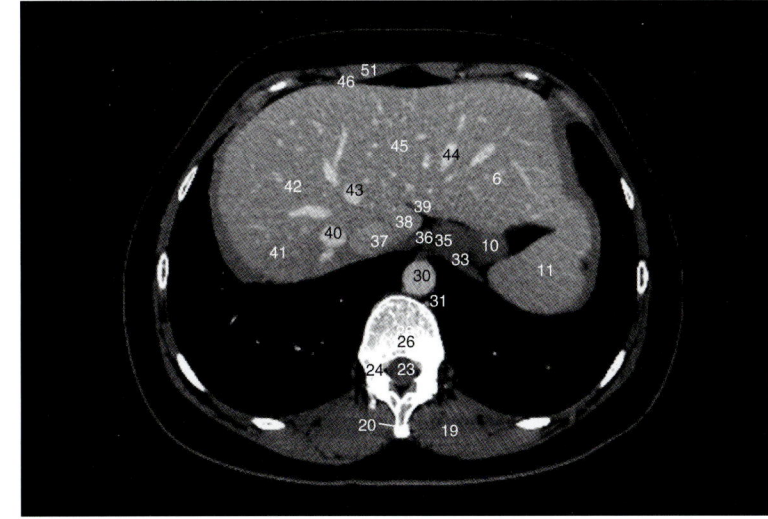

B. CT 纵隔窗增强图像

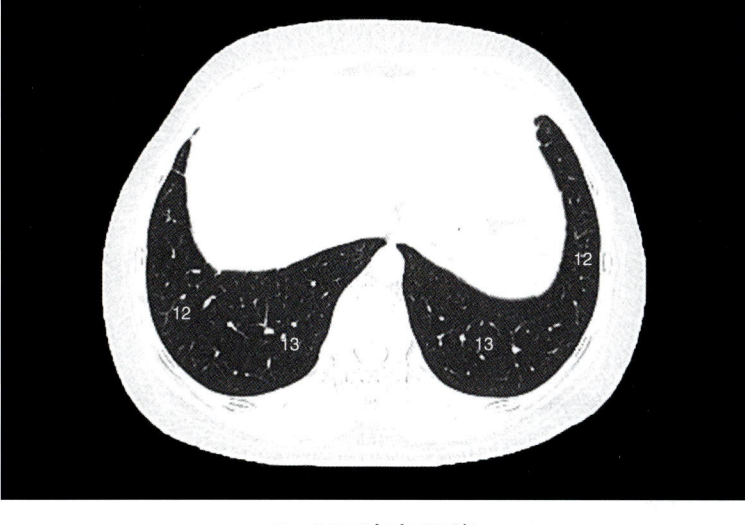

C. CT 肺窗图像

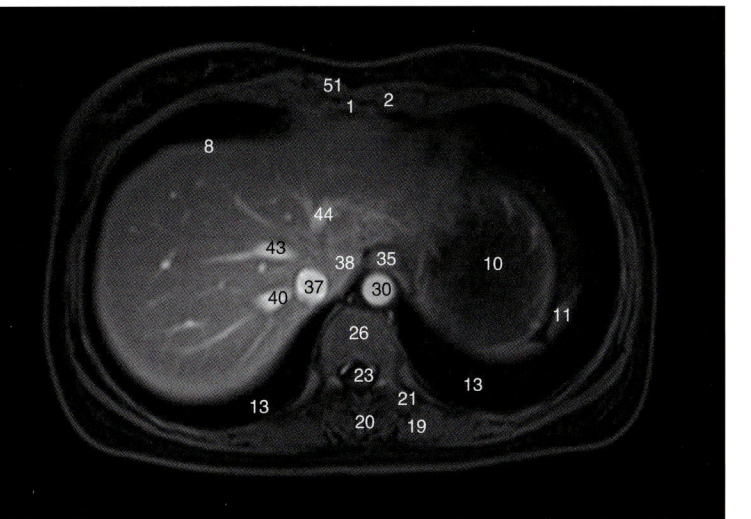

D. MR T1WI 增强图像

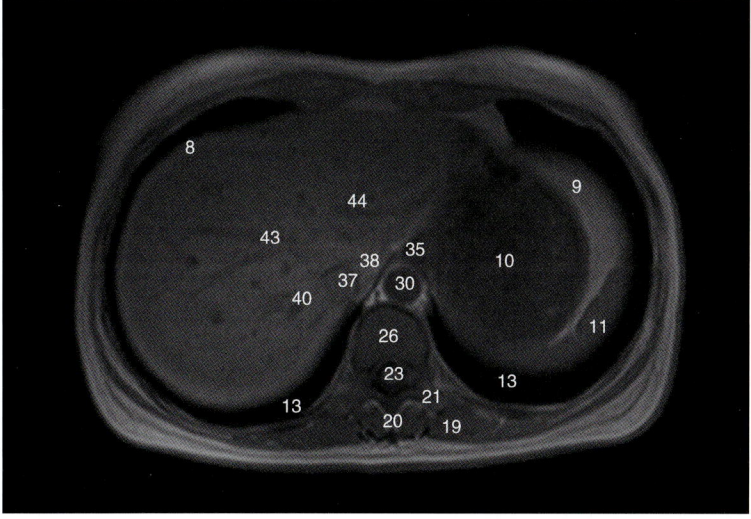

E. MR T1WI 平扫图像

关键结构：肋间后动、静脉，胸椎。

此断面前方经剑突下部，后方经第10胸椎椎体中部。

胸椎椎体横断面呈心形，前面凸后面凹，椎体静脉在椎体中部向后汇入椎体后静脉。椎体前方有前纵韧带，后方有后纵韧带，可限制脊柱的过度后伸和前屈。胸椎椎弓根短而窄，椎弓板后外侧的突起为横突，向后的突起为棘突。胸椎棘突呈叠瓦状突向后下，同一断面可见到2个棘突断层，上位胸椎棘突较小，居后；下位胸椎棘突较大，在前，两棘突之间有棘间韧带相连[20]。椎体两侧见肋间后动、静脉，肋间后动脉发自胸主动脉，肋间后静脉注入奇静脉和半奇静脉。胸腔内，心和肺进一步变小，心仅有右心室，左、右肺仅剩下下叶的一小部分。腹腔内，肝较上一断层进一步增大，并越过中线到左季肋区。胃底及脾的断面较上一断层增大。此断面可见到食管腹部连于胃的贲门，胃裸区较上一断层增宽。肝右静脉继续向外侧移行，肝中静脉及其属支向前外侧走行，肝左静脉则继续移位到左前侧。CT图像显示腹腔内脏器主要为肝、胃和脾，胸腔内为肺下叶，胸、腹腔由膈分开。

胸部连续横断层 95（FH.11610）

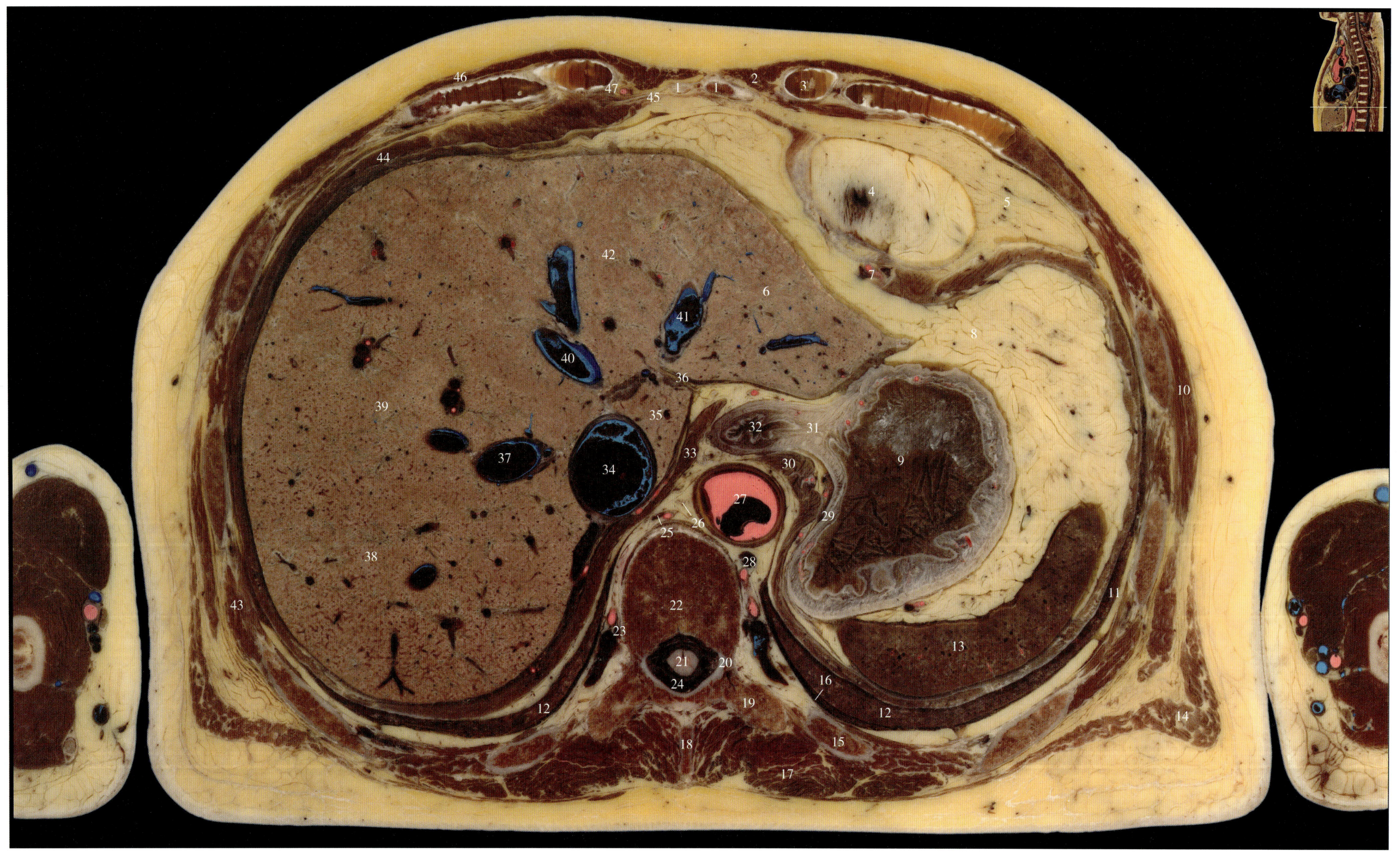

A. 断层标本图像

1. 剑突 xiphoid process
2. 腹直肌 rectus abdominis
3. 第 7 肋软骨 7th costal cartilage
4. 心 heart
5. 心包外脂肪 extrapericardial fat
6. 肝左外叶 left lateral lobe of liver
7. 左膈下动脉 left inferior phrenic artery
8. 大网膜 greater omentum
9. 胃底 fundus of stomach
10. 前锯肌 serratus anterior
11. 外侧底段（S9）lateral basal segment
12. 后底段（S10）posterior basal segment
13. 脾 spleen
14. 背阔肌 latissimus dorsi
15. 第 10 肋骨 10th costal bone
16. 胸膜腔 pleural cavity
17. 竖脊肌 erector spinae
18. 棘突 spinous process
19. 横突 transverse process
20. 椎弓根 pedicle of vertebral arch
21. 脊髓 spinal cord
22. 第 10 胸椎椎体 body of 10th thoracic vertebra
23. 肋间后动、静脉 posterior intercostal artery and vein
24. 硬膜外隙 epidural space
25. 奇静脉 azygos vein
26. 胸导管 thoracic duct
27. 胸主动脉 thoracic aorta
28. 半奇静脉 hemiazygos vein
29. 胃裸区 gastric bare area
30. 左膈脚 left crus of diaphragm
31. 胃贲门 cardia of stomach
32. 食管腹部 abdominal part of esophagus
33. 右膈脚 right crus of diaphragm
34. 下腔静脉 inferior vena cava
35. 肝尾状叶 caudate lobe of liver
36. 静脉韧带裂 fissure for ligamentum venosum
37. 肝右静脉 right hepatic vein
38. 肝右后叶 right posterior lobe of liver
39. 肝右前叶 right anterior lobe of liver
40. 肝中静脉 middle hepatic vein
41. 肝左静脉 left hepatic vein
42. 肝左内叶 left medial lobe of liver
43. 肋间肌 intercostal muscle
44. 膈 diaphragm
45. 胸肋三角 sternocostal triangle
46. 腹外斜肌 obliquus externus abdominis
47. 腹壁上动脉 superior epigastric artery

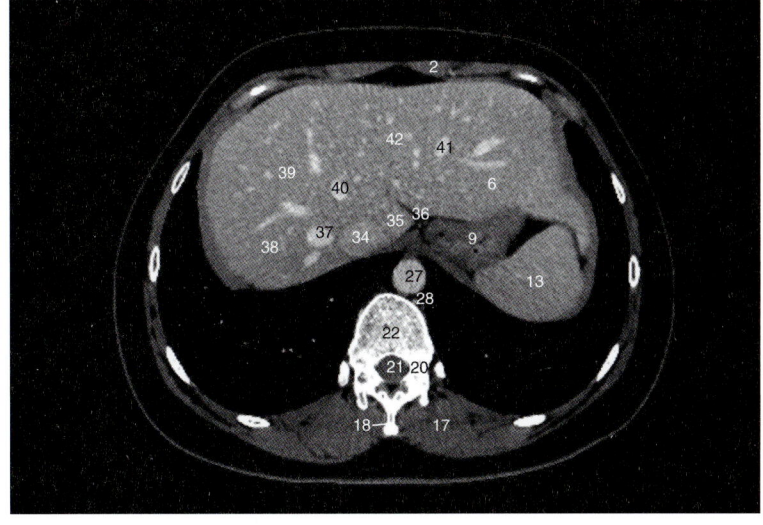

B. CT 纵隔窗增强图像

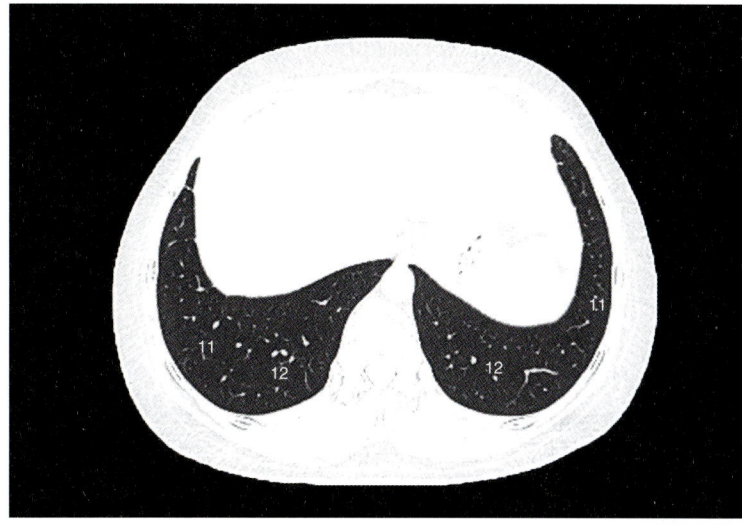

C. CT 肺窗图像

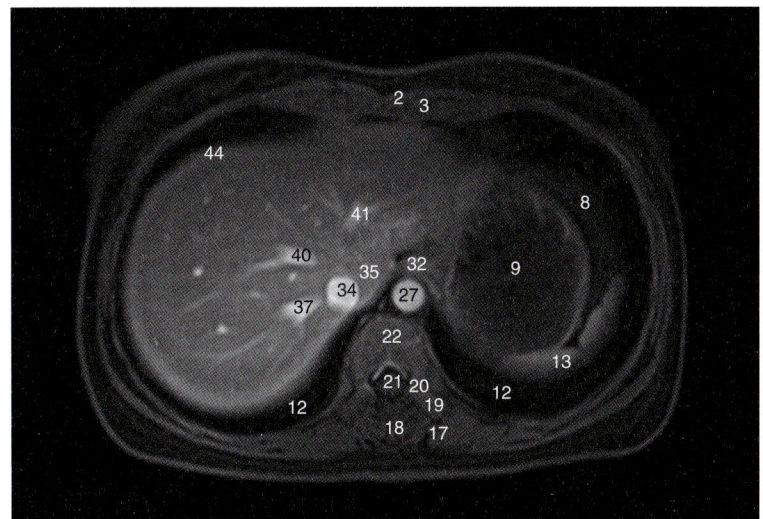

D. MR T1WI 增强图像

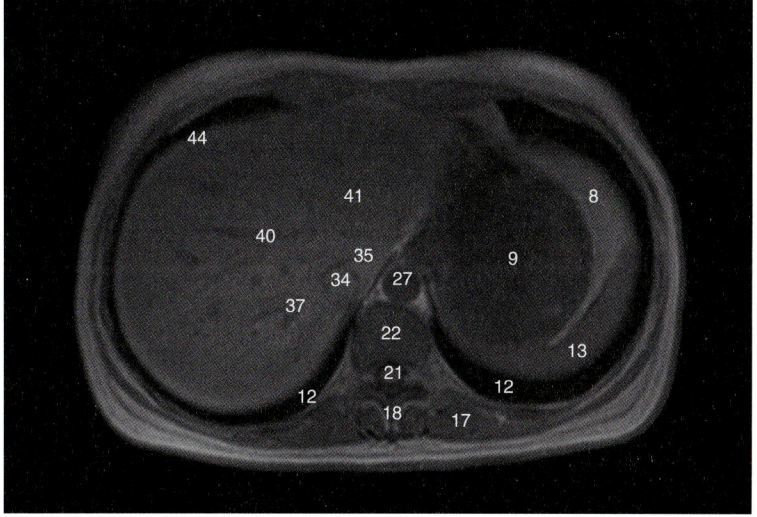

E. MR T1WI 平扫图像

关键结构：胸肋三角，心包脂肪垫。

此断面前方经剑突下部，后方经第 10 胸椎椎体中部。

胸腔前部为右心室下部及心包腔，纤维心包形成心包的外层，由致密结缔组织构成，与膈的中心腱相愈着。纤维心包外面与胸膜之间有心包外脂肪形成的心包脂肪垫，为肥胖老年人正常的生理表现，CT 表现为心膈角部位堆积的团块状、三角形脂肪密度影，外缘边界清楚，内缘与心包关系密切，临床上常易误认为心包积液或胸膜腔积液。心包脂肪垫的体积与冠状动脉的钙化有密切关系，可作为冠状动脉钙化评分及冠心病的评价指标[103]。胸腔后部左、右肺仅剩下叶的下缘后部，肺下缘较锐利。腹腔内，在肝前方与膈之间出现镰状韧带，肝镰状韧带右侧、肝右叶前外侧面、膈与肝冠状韧带上层之间为右肝上间隙；肝镰状韧带左侧、肝左外叶前面与膈之间为左肝上前间隙。肝为第二肝门下方层面，下腔静脉位于肝脏面的腔静脉沟内，3 条肝静脉进入肝内，肝右静脉继续向外侧移行，分隔肝右前叶和右后叶，肝中静脉及其属支向前外侧走行，肝左静脉则继续移向左前方。

胸部连续横断层 96（FH.11590）

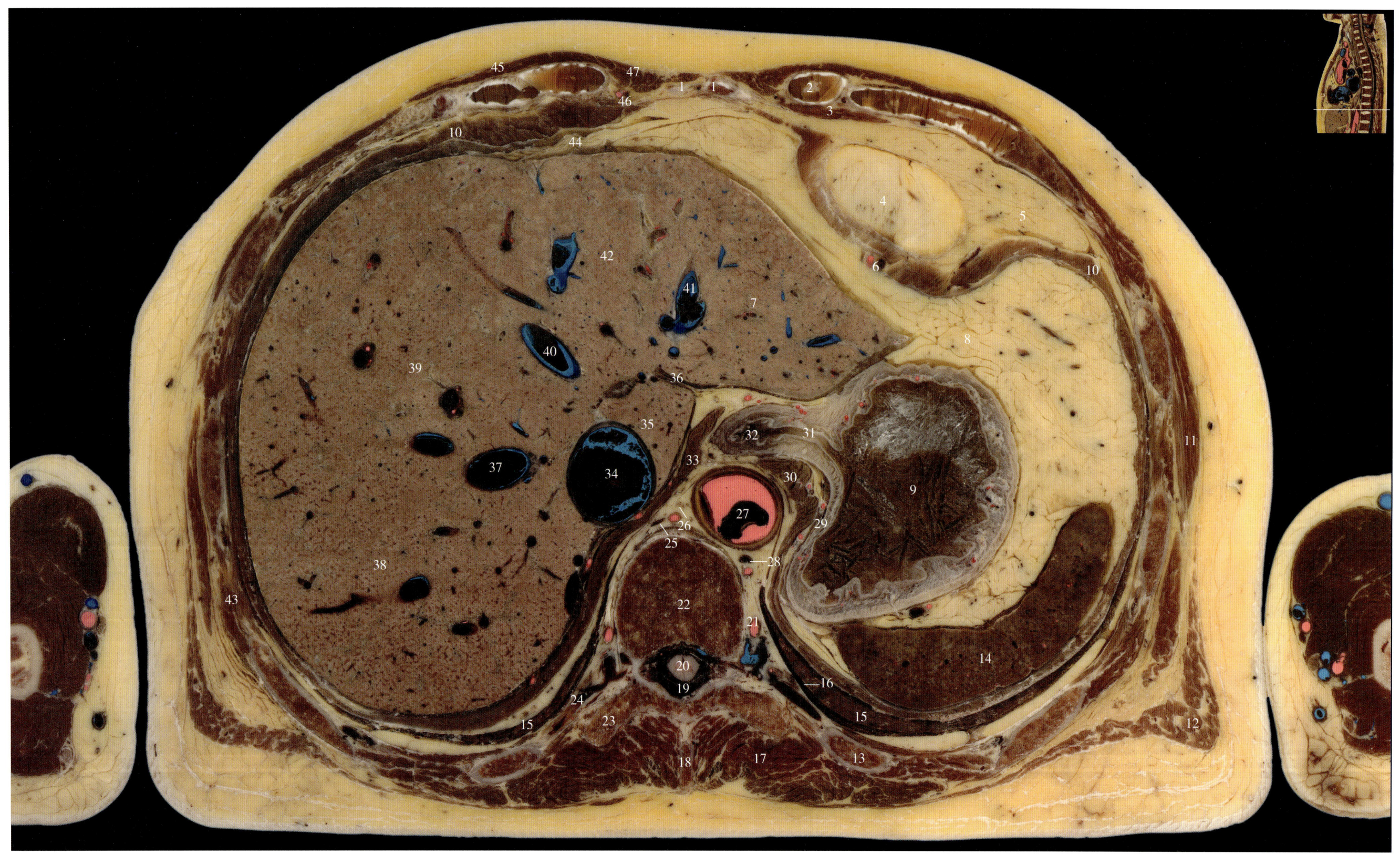

A. 断层标本图像

1. 剑突 xiphoid process
2. 第 7 肋软骨 7th costal cartilage
3. 胸横肌 transversus thoracis
4. 心包内脂肪 pericardial fat
5. 心包外脂肪 extrapericardial fat
6. 左膈下动、静脉 left inferior phrenic artery and vein
7. 肝左外叶 left lateral lobe of liver
8. 大网膜 greater omentum
9. 胃底 fundus of stomach
10. 膈 diaphragm
11. 前锯肌 serratus anterior
12. 背阔肌 latissimus dorsi
13. 第 10 肋骨 10th costal bone
14. 脾 spleen
15. 后底段（S10）posterior basal segment
16. 胸膜腔 pleural cavity
17. 竖脊肌 erector spinae
18. 第 9 胸椎棘突 spinous process of 9th thoracic vertebra
19. 硬膜外隙 epidural space
20. 脊髓 spinal cord
21. 肋间后动脉 posterior intercostal artery
22. 第 10 胸椎椎体 body of 10th thoracic vertebra
23. 横突 transverse process
24. 肋间后静脉 posterior intercostal vein
25. 奇静脉 azygos vein
26. 胸导管 thoracic duct
27. 胸主动脉 thoracic aorta
28. 半奇静脉 hemiazygos vein
29. 胃裸区 gastric bare area
30. 左膈脚 left crus of diaphragm
31. 胃贲门 cardia of stomach
32. 食管腹部 abdominal part of esophagus
33. 右膈脚 right crus of diaphragm
34. 下腔静脉 inferior vena cava
35. 肝尾状叶 caudate lobe of liver
36. 静脉韧带裂 fissure for ligamentum venosum
37. 肝右静脉 right hepatic vein
38. 肝右后叶 right posterior lobe of liver
39. 肝右前叶 right anterior lobe of liver
40. 肝中静脉 middle hepatic vein
41. 肝左静脉 left hepatic vein
42. 肝左内叶 left medial lobe of liver
43. 肋间肌 intercostal muscle
44. 肝镰状韧带 falciform ligament of liver
45. 腹外斜肌 obliquus externus abdominis
46. 腹壁上动脉 superior epigastric artery
47. 腹直肌 rectus abdominis
48. 肝门静脉左支矢状部 sagittal portion of left hepatic portal vein
49. 外侧底段（S9）lateral basal segment

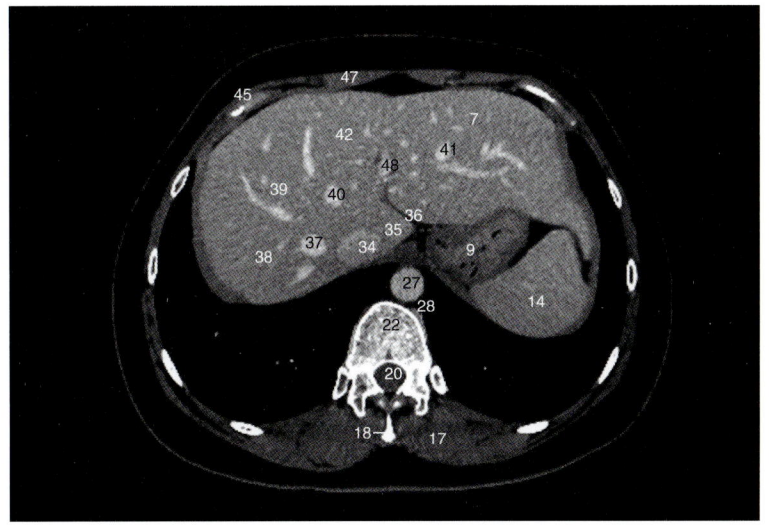

B. CT 纵隔窗增强图像

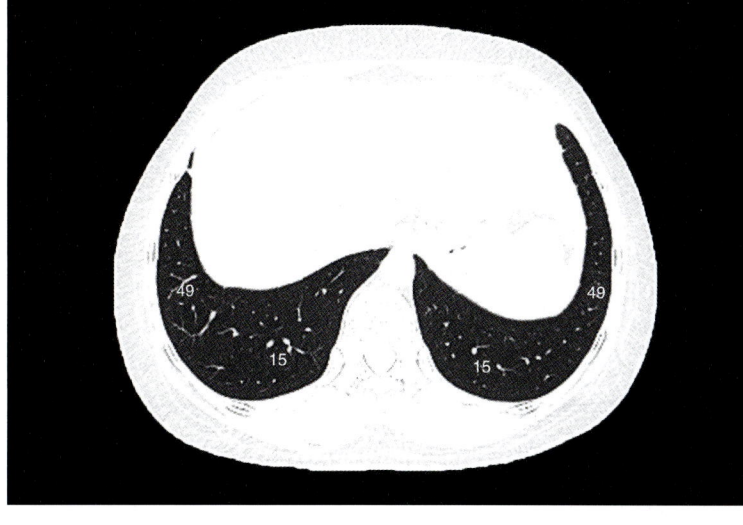

C. CT 肺窗图像

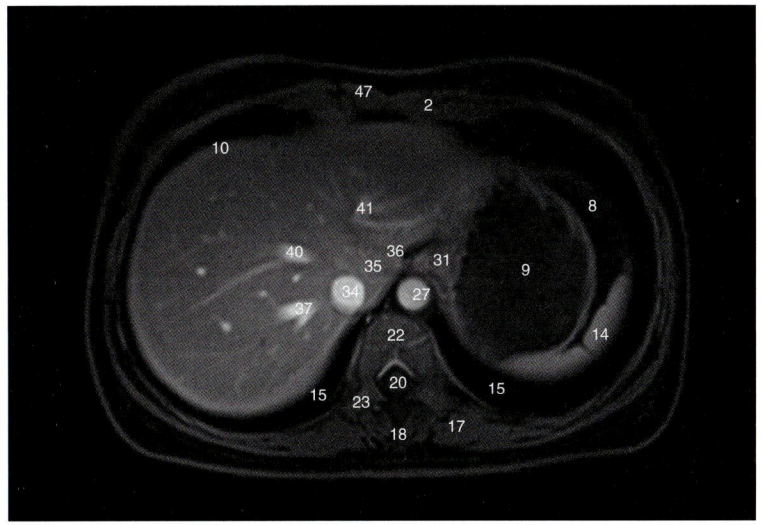

D. MR T1WI 增强图像

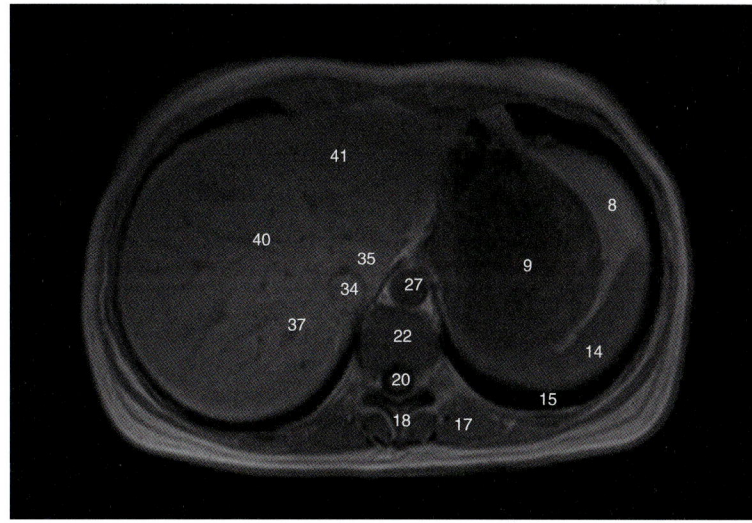

E. MR T1WI 平扫图像

关键结构：膈下动脉，静脉韧带裂。

此断面前方经剑突，后方经第 10 胸椎椎体下部。

胸腔内结构越来越小，心消失，仍可见心包腔，分隔心包内和外的脂肪。膈分隔胸、腹腔脏器，心包后方见左膈下动、静脉伴行。膈下动脉多发自腹腔干或腹主动脉，亦可发自肾动脉或肝左动脉。左、右膈下动脉分别经膈左右脚的前方，至膈的中心腱分支分布于膈肌和腹壁，中途还发出肾上腺上动脉营养肾上腺。膈下静脉一般与膈下动脉伴行，汇入下腔静脉。腹腔内，肝左叶及肝尾状叶较上一断层增大，尾状叶前面与左外叶之间为静脉韧带裂，小网膜的肝胃韧带部分起始于其右端，并分其为前后两部。静脉韧带裂前部向左通胃肝隐窝，二者合称左肝下前间隙。静脉韧带裂后部为网膜囊上隐窝的一部分，包绕肝尾状叶。肝中静脉分隔左、右半肝，肝右静脉是右半肝的分界标志，分隔肝右前叶与肝右后叶。肝左叶依据左叶间静脉分为肝左内叶与肝左外叶。影像学图像显示腹腔内结构肝、胃和脾体积进一步增大，脊柱区见胸椎椎体、椎弓根、椎管及其内容物、横突、棘突及肋头关节等。

胸部连续横断层 97 (FH.11570)

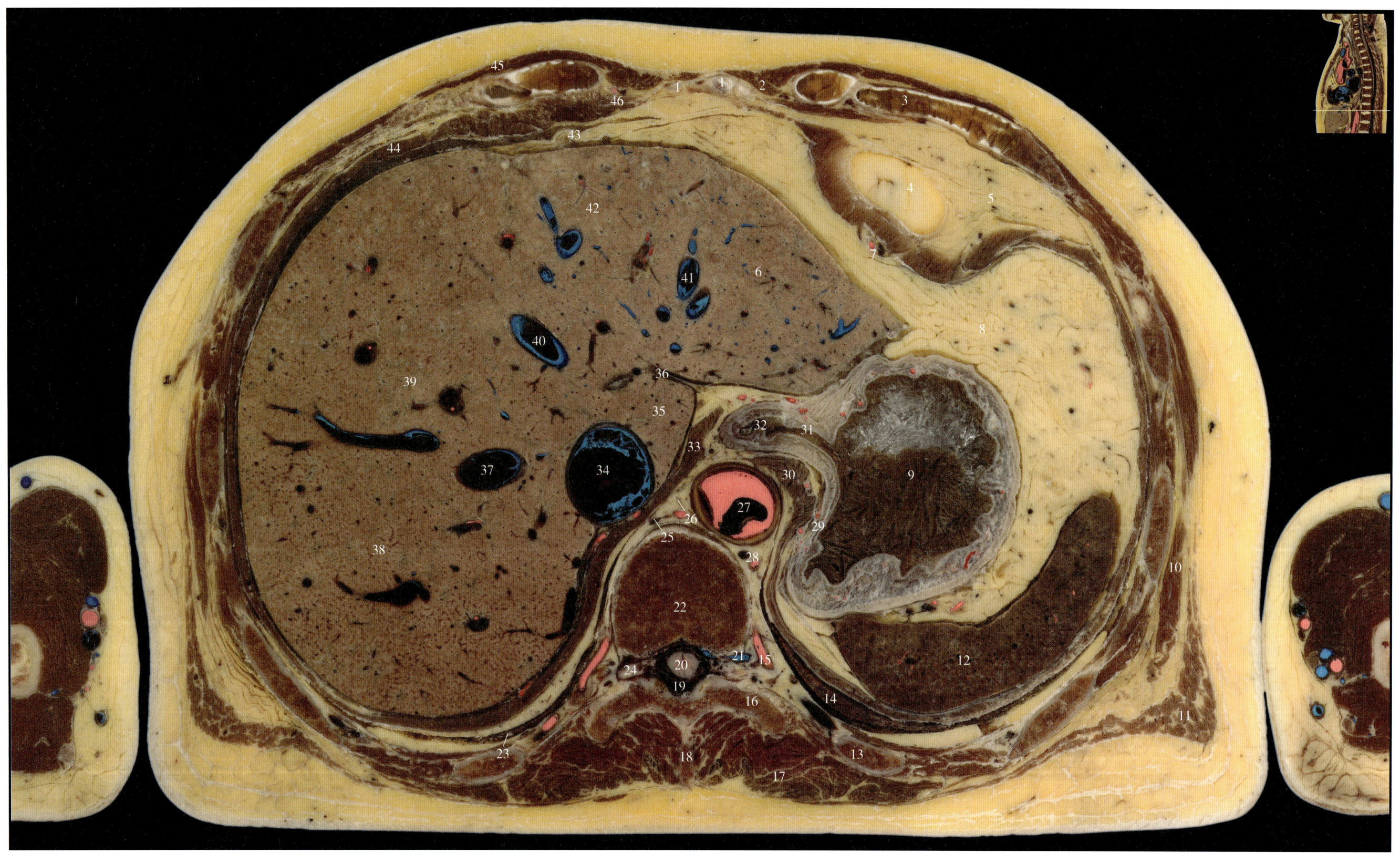

A. 断层标本图像

1. 剑突 xiphoid process
2. 腹直肌 rectus abdominis
3. 第 6 肋软骨 6th costal cartilage
4. 心包内脂肪 pericardial fat
5. 心包外脂肪 extrapericardial fat
6. 肝左外叶 left lateral lobe of liver
7. 左膈下动脉 left inferior phrenic artery
8. 大网膜 greater omentum
9. 胃底 fundus of stomach
10. 前锯肌 serratus anterior
11. 背阔肌 latissimus dorsi
12. 脾 spleen
13. 第 10 肋骨 10th costal bone
14. 后底段（S10）posterior basal segment
15. 肋间后动脉 posterior intercostal artery
16. 横突 transverse process
17. 竖脊肌 erector spinae
18. 第 9 胸椎棘突 spinous process of 9th thoracic vertebra
19. 硬膜外隙 epidural space
20. 脊髓 spinal cord
21. 椎间静脉 intervertebral vein
22. 第 10 胸椎椎体 body of 10th thoracic vertebra
23. 肋膈隐窝 costodiaphragmatic recess
24. 脊神经 spinal nerve
25. 奇静脉 azygos vein
26. 胸导管 thoracic duct
27. 胸主动脉 thoracic aorta
28. 半奇静脉 hemiazygos vein
29. 胃裸区 gastric bare area
30. 左膈脚 left crus of diaphragm
31. 胃贲门 cardia of stomach
32. 食管腹部 abdominal part of esophagus
33. 右膈脚 right crus of diaphragm
34. 下腔静脉 inferior vena cava
35. 肝尾状叶 caudate lobe of liver
36. 静脉韧带裂 fissure for ligamentum venosum
37. 肝右静脉 right hepatic vein
38. 肝右后叶 right posterior lobe of liver
39. 肝右前叶 right anterior lobe of liver
40. 肝中静脉 middle hepatic vein
41. 肝左静脉 left hepatic vein
42. 肝左内叶 left medial lobe of liver
43. 肝镰状韧带 falciform ligament of liver
44. 膈 diaphragm
45. 腹外斜肌 obliquus externus abdominis
46. 腹壁上动脉 superior epigastric artery
47. 肝门静脉左支矢状部 sagittal portion of left hepatic portal vein
48. 外侧底段（S9）lateral basal segment
49. 蛛网膜下隙 subarachnoid space

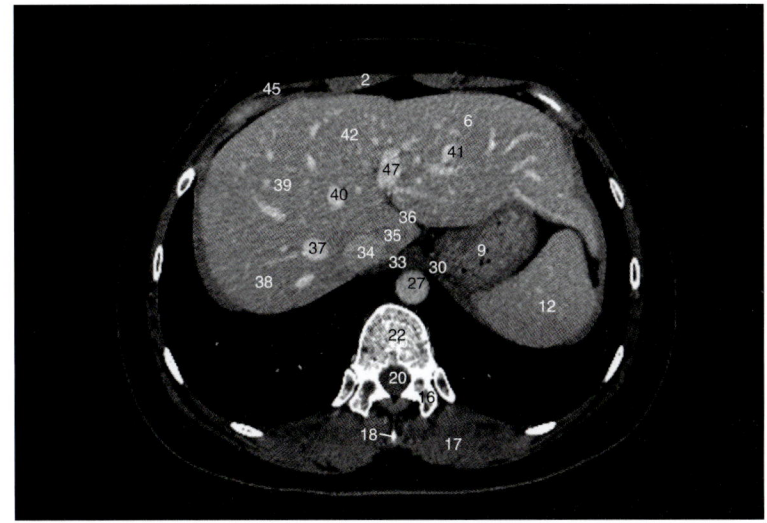

B. CT 纵隔窗增强图像

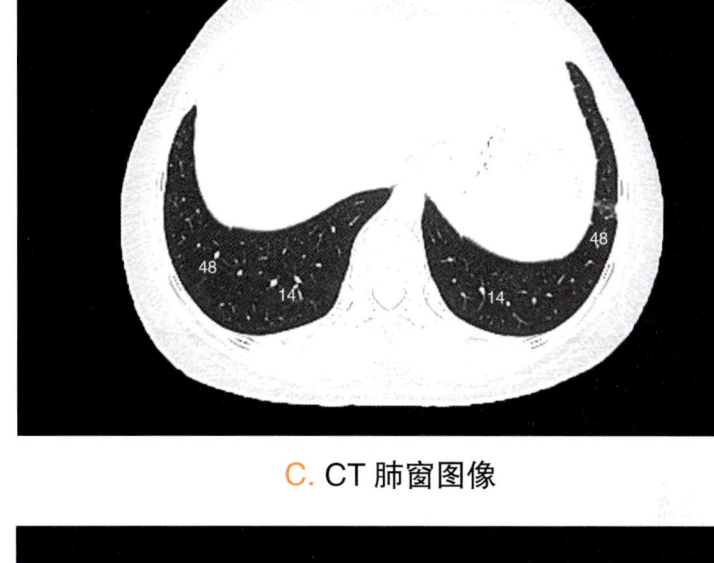

C. CT 肺窗图像

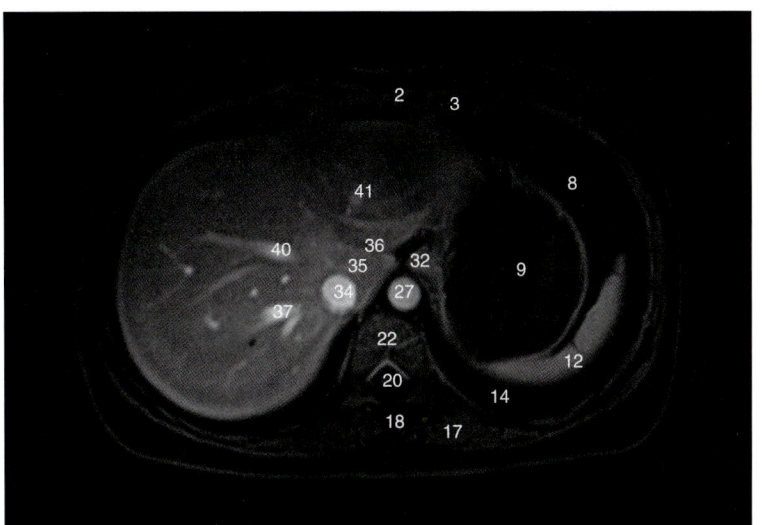

D. MR T1WI 增强图像

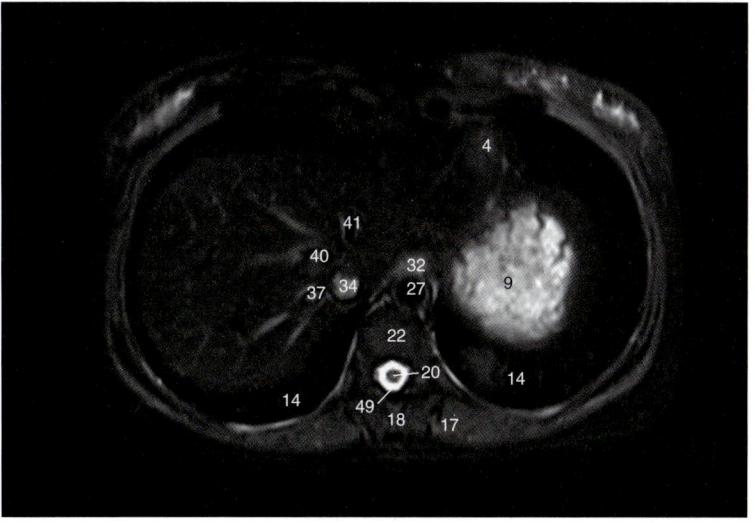

E. MR T2WI 抑脂图像

关键结构：椎间孔，椎间静脉，椎静脉丛。

此断面后方经第 10 胸椎椎体下部。

胸椎椎体后方为椎管和椎间孔（管），椎间孔位于相邻椎弓根之间，有一定的长度，因此又称椎间管，内有椎间静脉和脊神经根穿出。脊柱区周围的椎静脉系由椎内、外静脉丛及其连接其间的椎体静脉和椎间静脉组成，该静脉系缺乏静脉瓣，是沟通颅内、外和上、下腔静脉系的重要途径，在静脉回流中其调节作用。当盆、腹、胸腔等部位发生感染、肿瘤或有寄生虫时，可经椎静脉丛侵入颅内或其他远位器官。椎内静脉丛位于椎管内硬膜外隙，主要接受由椎骨和脊髓回流的静脉血，分为前、后两部分。椎外静脉丛攀附于脊柱周围，与椎内静脉丛通过椎体静脉和椎间静脉等吻合，汇入肋间后静脉等。椎间静脉引流脊髓和椎内、外静脉丛的静脉血，汇入肋间后静脉。临床上可用椎间孔镜进行椎间盘突出、椎管狭窄等微创手术治疗，手术时注意椎间静脉、脊神经根等，避免损伤[104]。膈的左前方，胸腔内心包到其下部，仍可见心包内、外脂肪充填，其前方为第 6 肋。右肺下缘已消失，左肺仍可见下缘小部分，即将消失。腹腔内，肝的静脉走向外周，肝左静脉分出左叶间支，作为左外叶和左内叶的分界。尾状叶前方为静脉韧带裂，其右侧与胃之间为肝胃韧带，内有胃左动脉的分支。CT 图像胸腔内结构为位于后部的两侧肺下叶，脊柱区见椎体及两侧的肋头关节。

胸部连续横断层 98（FH.11550）

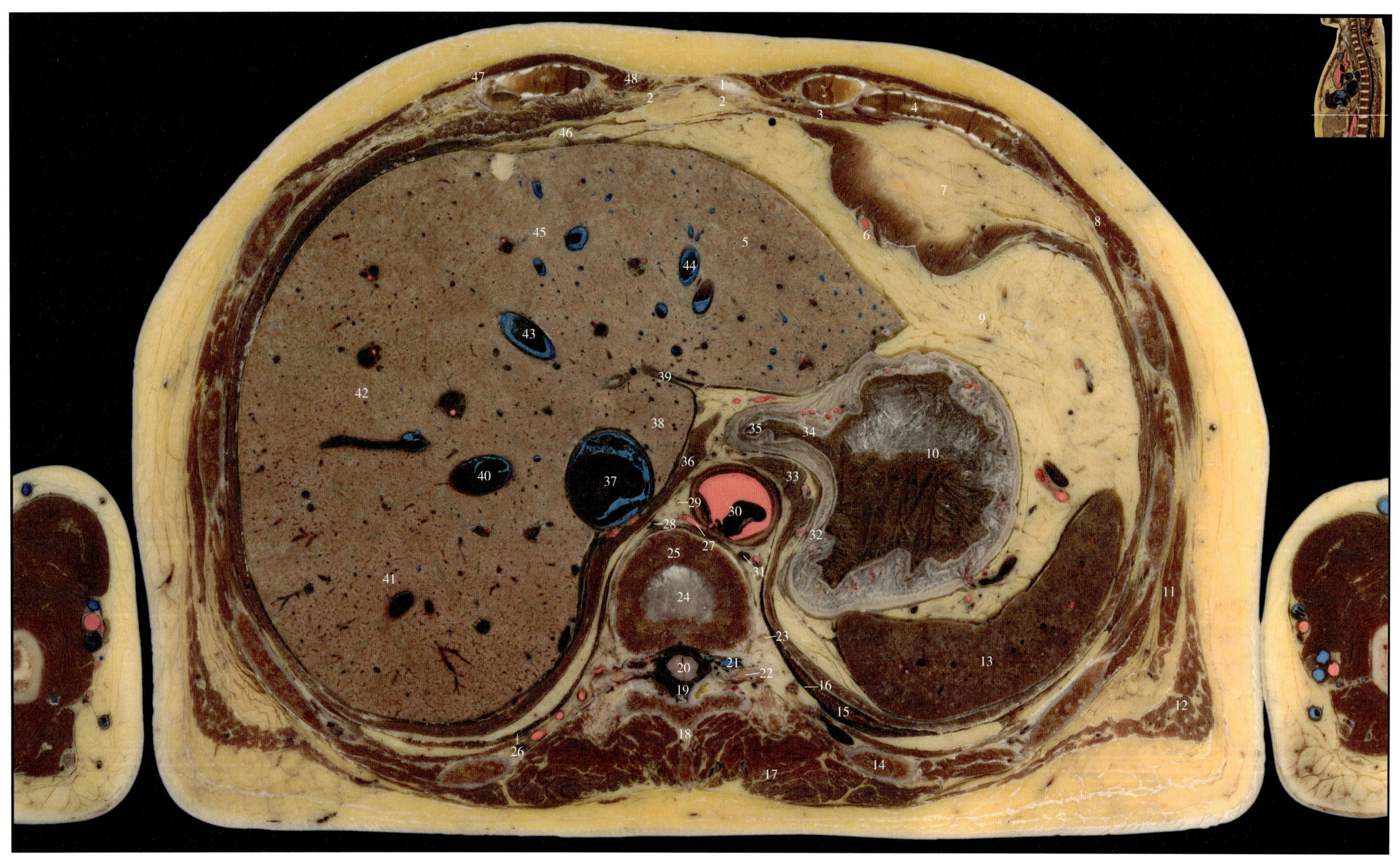

A. 断层标本图像

1. 剑突 xiphoid process
2. 膈的胸骨部 sternal part of diaphragm
3. 胸横肌 transversus thoracis
4. 第6肋软骨 6th costal cartilage
5. 肝左外叶 left lateral lobe of liver
6. 左膈下动脉 left inferior phrenic artery
7. 心包外脂肪 extrapericardial fat
8. 肋间肌 intercostal muscle
9. 大网膜 greater omentum
10. 胃底 fundus of stomach
11. 前锯肌 serratus anterior
12. 背阔肌 latissimus dorsi
13. 脾 spleen
14. 第10肋骨 10th costal bone
15. 后底段（S10） posterior basal segment
16. 胸膜腔 pleural cavity
17. 竖脊肌 erector spinae
18. 棘突 spinous process
19. 硬膜外隙 epidural space
20. 脊髓 spinal cord
21. 椎间静脉 intervertebral vein
22. 脊神经节 spinal ganglion
23. 交感干神经节 ganglia of sympathetic trunk
24. T10-11椎间盘 T10-11 intervertebral disc
25. 第10胸椎椎体 body of 10th thoracic vertebra
26. 肋膈隐窝 costodiaphragmatic recess
27. 肋间后动脉 posterior intercostal artery
28. 奇静脉 azygos vein
29. 胸导管 thoracic duct
30. 胸主动脉 thoracic aorta
31. 半奇静脉 hemiazygos vein
32. 胃裸区 gastric bare area
33. 左膈脚 left crus of diaphragm
34. 胃贲门 cardia of stomach
35. 食管腹部 abdominal part of esophagus
36. 右膈脚 right crus of diaphragm
37. 下腔静脉 inferior vena cava
38. 肝尾状叶 caudate lobe of liver
39. 静脉韧带裂 fissure for ligamentum venosum
40. 肝右静脉 right hepatic vein
41. 肝右后叶 right posterior lobe of liver
42. 肝右前叶 right anterior lobe of liver
43. 肝中静脉 middle hepatic vein
44. 肝左静脉 left hepatic vein
45. 肝左内叶 left medial lobe of liver
46. 肝镰状韧带 falciform ligament of liver
47. 腹外斜肌 obliquus externus abdominis
48. 腹直肌 rectus abdominis
49. 肝门静脉左矢状部 sagittal portion of left hepatic portal vein
50. 外侧底段（S9） lateral basal segment

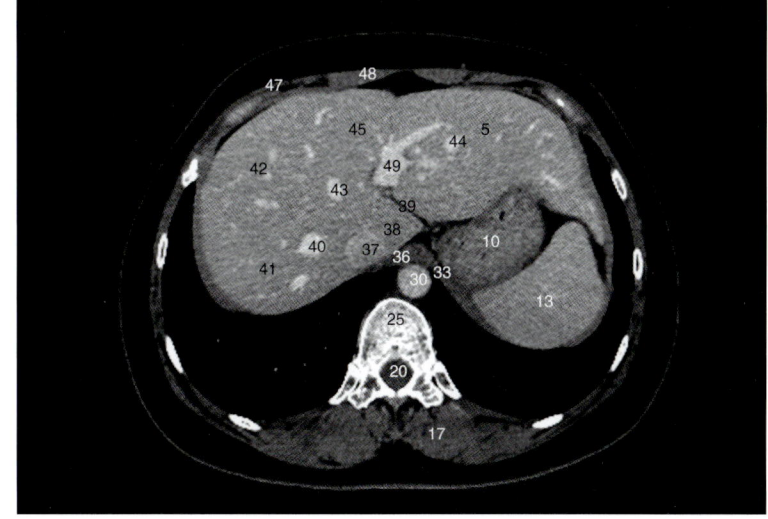

B. CT 纵隔窗增强图像

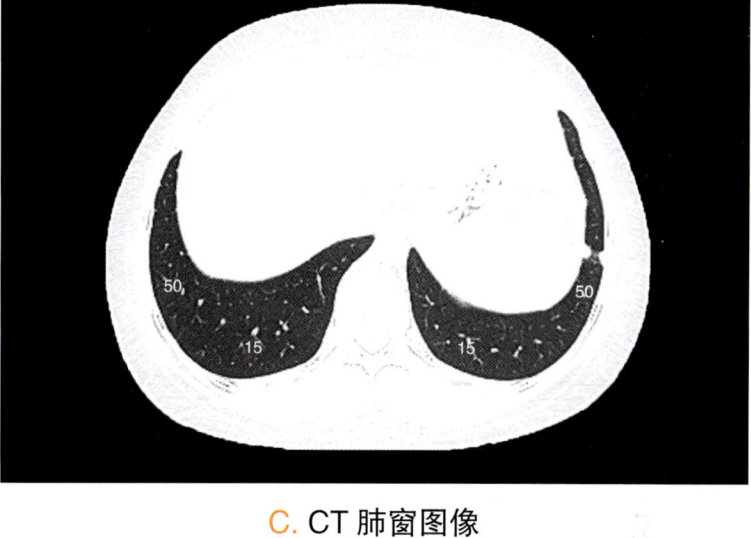

C. CT 肺窗图像

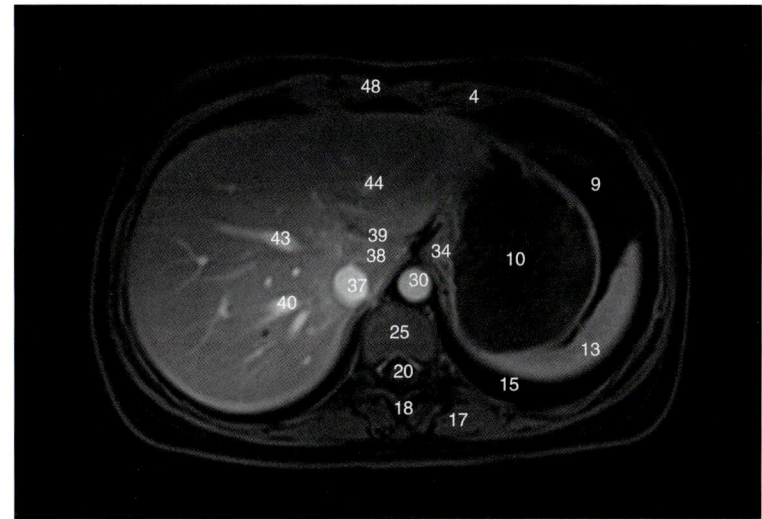

D. MR T1WI 增强图像

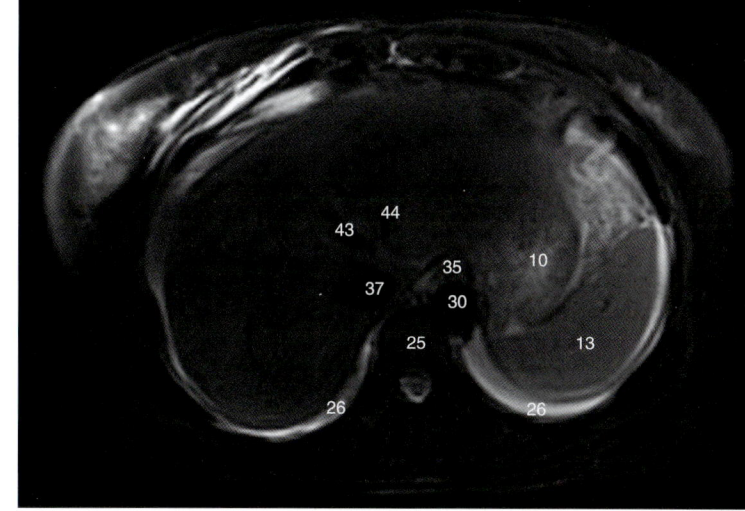

E. 胸膜腔积液 MR 图像

关键结构：肋膈隐窝，交感干神经节。

此断面后方经第10胸椎椎体下部和T10-11椎间盘上部。

椎体后方为椎管、椎间孔及内容物，椎体两侧有交感干神经节，又称椎旁神经节，位于椎体两侧，与节间支连接成交感干。胸部又称为胸神经节，通常有10~12对，多呈扁三角形，位于相应的肋头前方。穿过第5~9胸神经节的节前纤维向前下方走行合成内脏大神经，沿椎体和肋间血管的前方下行，穿过膈脚进入腹腔，终于腹腔神经节，节后纤维随神经丛分布到肝、胆、胰、脾、肾等腹腔脏器。临床上对反复发作的慢性胰腺炎、胰腺癌、上腹部腹膜后肿瘤等导致的反复发作、难以控制的上腹部疼痛可行内脏大神经切断术进行治疗[102]。胸腔后部，膈与胸壁之间的胸膜腔为肋膈隐窝，又称肋膈窦，为胸膜壁层的肋胸膜和膈胸膜返折处，左右各一，自剑突向后下至脊柱两侧，呈半环形，后部较深，是胸膜腔最低处，深度一般可达2个肋和肋间隙，胸膜腔积液首先积聚于此处。因肋膈隐窝后部较深，引流和抽液比较彻底，胸膜腔积液时，临床上常选择肩胛线第8或第9肋间隙进针抽取。但由于抽出液体后受压下降的膈可再度回升，所以穿刺部位不要低于第9肋间隙。胸膜腔积液 MR T2图像可见胸部病变时位于肋膈隐窝内呈高信号的胸膜腔积液。

胸部连续横断层 99（FH.11530）

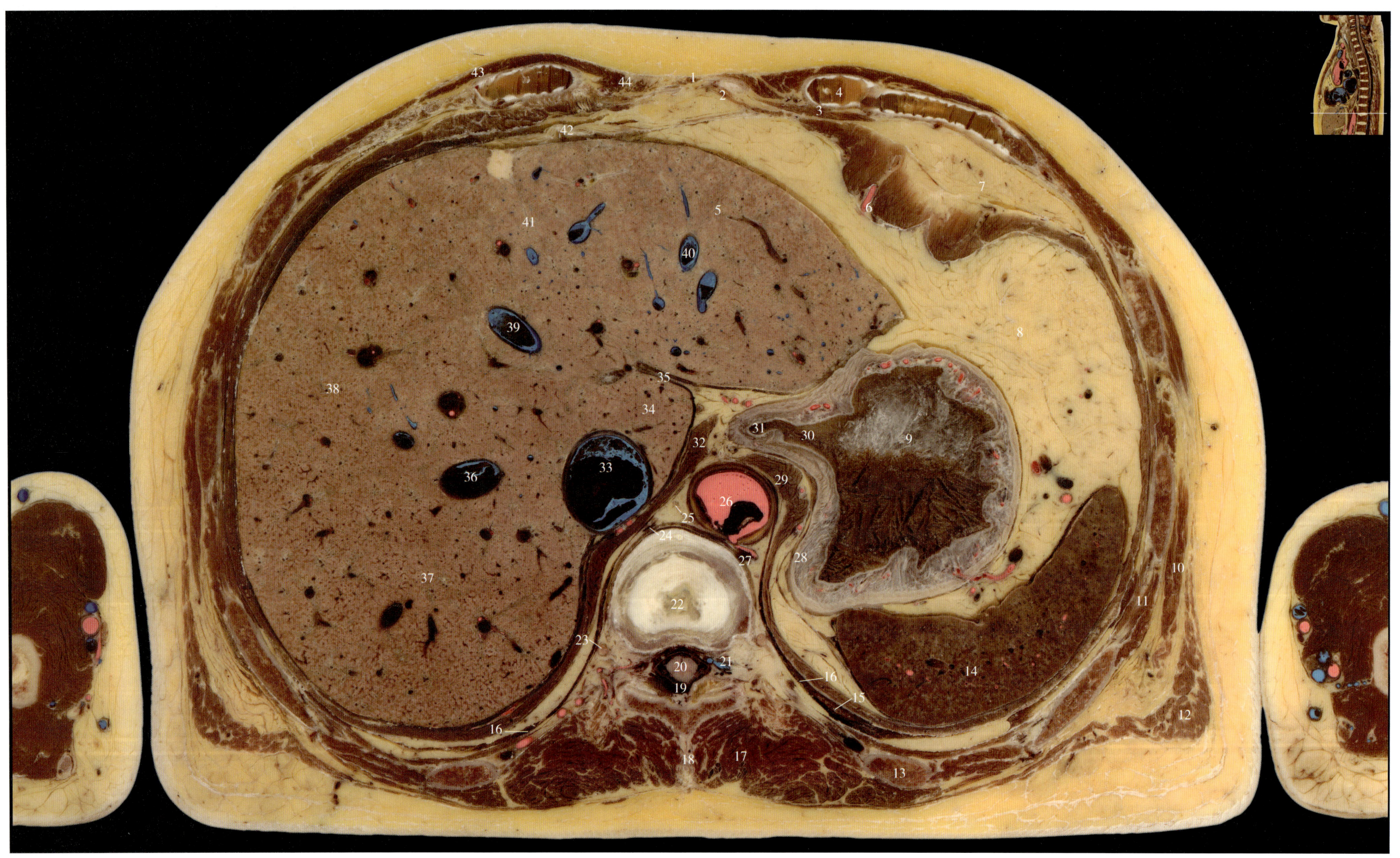

A. 断层标本图像

1. 腹白线 linea alba
2. 膈的胸骨部 sternal part of diaphragm
3. 胸横肌 transversus thoracis
4. 第 7 肋软骨 7th costal cartilage
5. 肝左外叶 left lateral lobe of liver
6. 左膈下动脉 left inferior phrenic artery
7. 心包外脂肪 extrapericardial fat
8. 大网膜 greater omentum
9. 胃底 fundus of stomach
10. 前锯肌 serratus anterior
11. 肋间肌 intercostal muscle
12. 背阔肌 latissimus dorsi
13. 第 9 肋骨 9th costal bone
14. 脾 spleen
15. 后底段（S10） posterior basal segment
16. 肋膈隐窝 costodiaphragmatic recess
17. 竖脊肌 erector spinae
18. 棘间韧带 interspinous ligament
19. 硬膜外隙 epidural space
20. 脊髓 spinal cord
21. 椎间静脉 intervertebral vein
22. T10-11 椎间盘 T10-11 intervertebral disc
23. 交感干神经节 ganglia of sympathetic trunk
24. 奇静脉 azygos vein
25. 胸导管 thoracic duct
26. 胸主动脉 thoracic aorta
27. 半奇静脉 hemiazygos vein
28. 胃裸区 gastric bare area
29. 左膈脚 left crus of diaphragm
30. 胃贲门 cardia of stomach
31. 食管腹部 abdominal part of esophagus
32. 右膈脚 right crus of diaphragm
33. 下腔静脉 inferior vena cava
34. 肝尾状叶 caudate lobe of liver
35. 静脉韧带裂 fissure for ligamentum venosum
36. 肝右静脉 right hepatic vein
37. 肝右后叶 right posterior lobe of liver
38. 肝右前叶 right anterior lobe of liver
39. 肝中静脉 middle hepatic vein
40. 肝左静脉 left hepatic vein
41. 肝左内叶 left medial lobe of liver
42. 肝镰状韧带 falciform ligament of liver
43. 腹外斜肌 obliquus externus abdominis
44. 腹直肌 rectus abdominis
45. 肝门静脉左支矢状部 sagittal portion of left hepatic portal vein
46. 肝圆韧带裂 fissure for ligamentum teres hepatis
47. 外侧底段（S9） lateral basal segment
48. 蛛网膜下隙 subarachnoid space

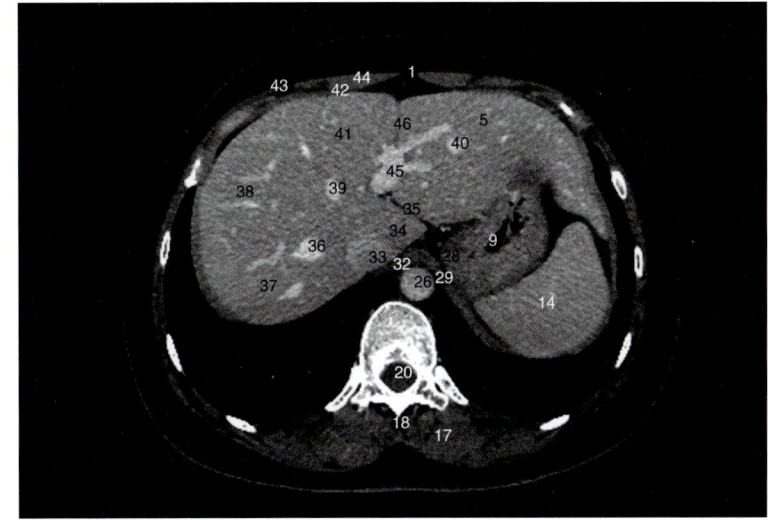

B. CT 纵隔窗增强图像

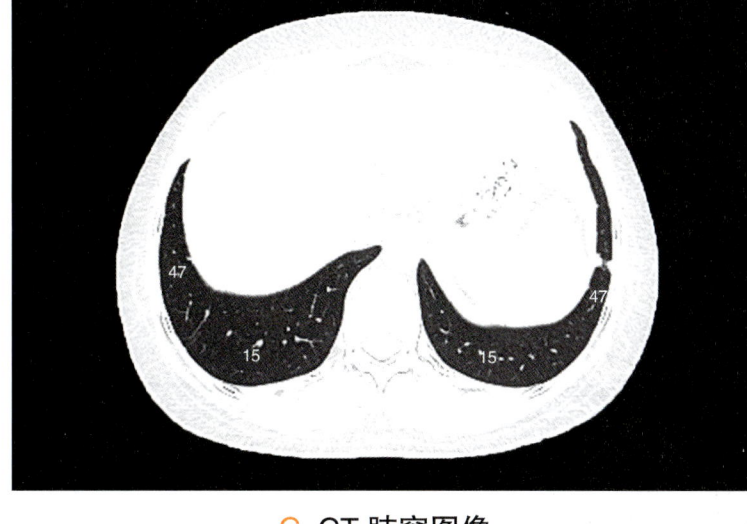

C. CT 肺窗图像

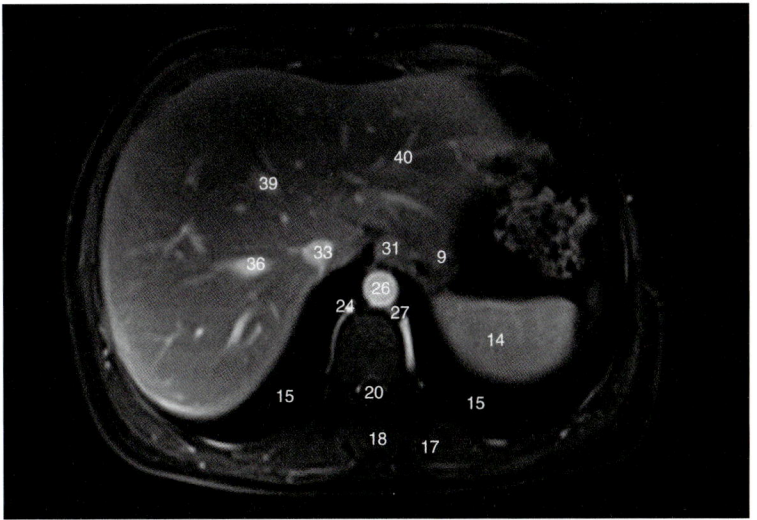

D. MR T1WI 增强图像

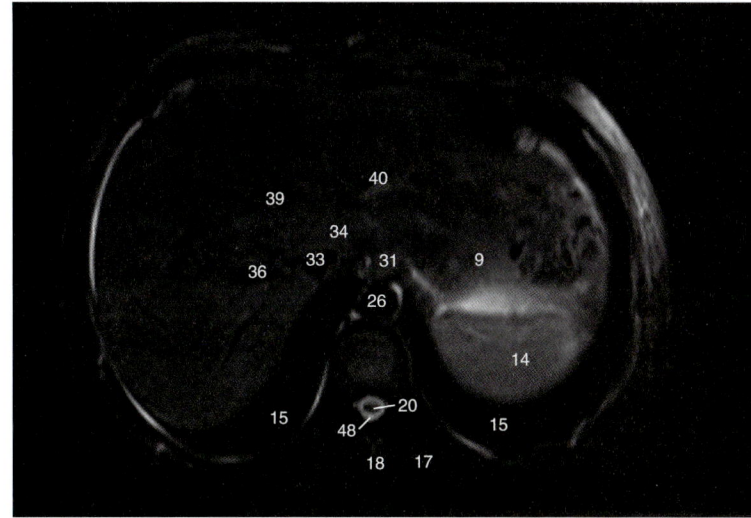

E. MR T2WI 抑脂图像

关键结构：椎间盘，交感干神经节。

此断后方经 T10-11 椎间盘上部。

椎间盘由髓核、纤维环、Sharpey 纤维和透明软骨终板组成。髓核位于中央偏后，呈半透明胶状外观，主要由软骨基质和胶原纤维构成，出生时含水量为 80%~90%，随着年龄增长含水量逐渐下降，并逐渐为纤维软骨样物质代替。纤维环由多层纤维软骨按同心圆排列组成，位于髓核周围，其含水量较髓核低。纤维环后部相对薄弱，髓核易向后外侧和后方突出，压迫脊神经根或脊髓而出现相应症状，称椎间盘突出症。Sharpey 纤维是椎间盘的最外层，主要由胶原纤维组成，无软骨基质。透明软骨终板紧贴于椎体的上、下面，构成髓核的上、下界。CT 图像上，椎间盘密度低于椎体，髓核和纤维环难以区分。在 MR T1WI 图像上外纤维环和 Sharpey 纤维呈低信号，而内纤维环和髓核呈较高信号；MR T2WI 图像上髓核呈高信号，可与外周的纤维环识别。椎间盘的形状、大小与所连结的椎体上下面相似，其厚薄各部不同，胸上部最薄，腰部最厚，颈腰部前厚后薄，而胸部椎间盘则与此相反。另外，椎间盘厚度及大小随年龄而有差异[40]。椎间盘可缓冲外力对脊柱的震动及增加脊柱的运动幅度。影像学图像肺下叶进一步缩小，位于断面后部，胃与膈之间为胃裸区。肝左、肝中、肝右静脉走行于离下腔静脉较远侧的肝实质中，其长轴均指向下腔静脉。

胸部连续横断层 100（FH.11510）

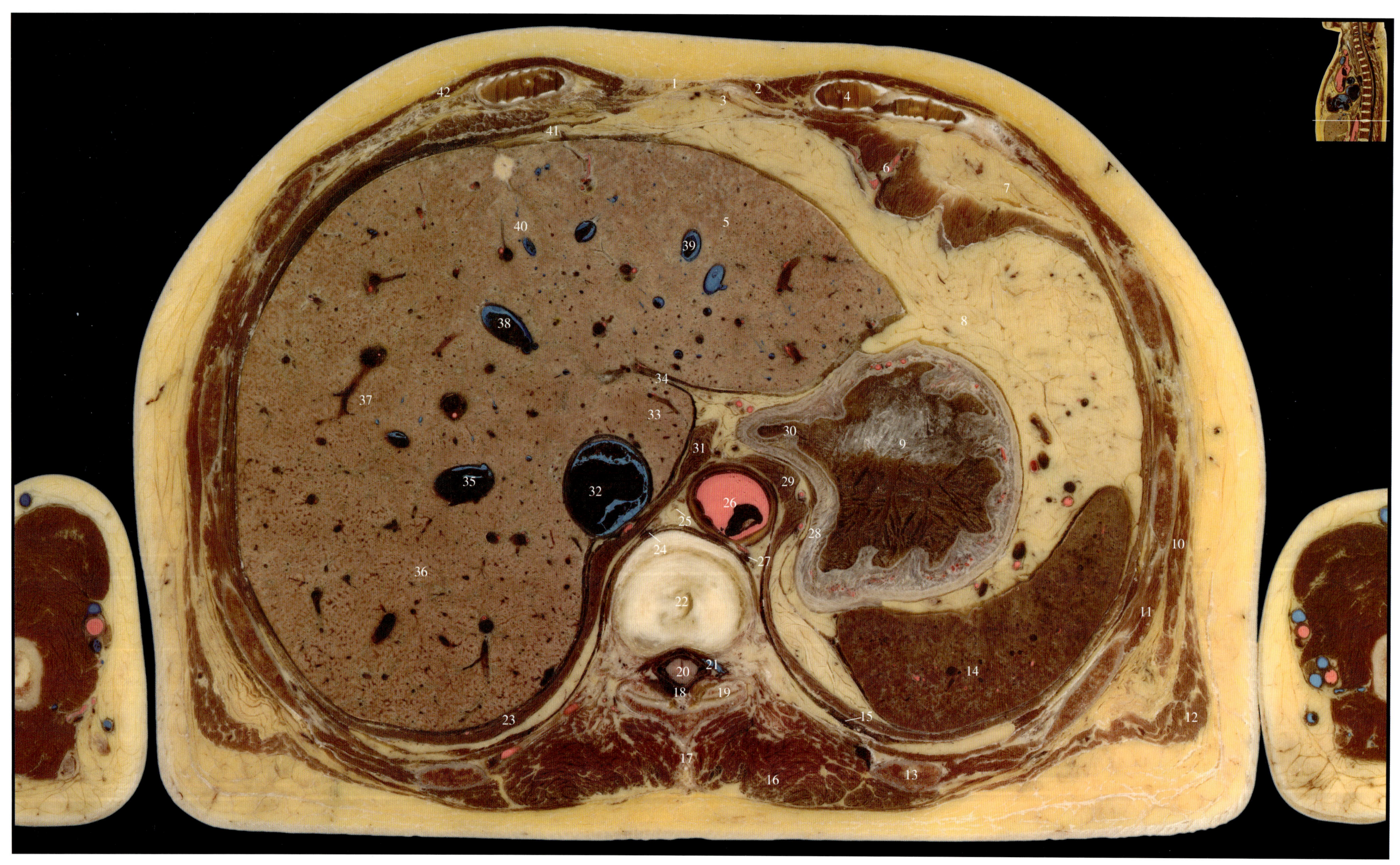

A. 断层标本图像

1. 腹白线 linea alba
2. 腹直肌 rectus abdominis
3. 膈的胸骨部 sternal part of diaphragm
4. 第 7 肋软骨 7th costal cartilage
5. 肝左外叶 left lateral lobe of liver
6. 左膈下动脉 left inferior phrenic artery
7. 心包外脂肪 extrapericardial fat
8. 大网膜 greater omentum
9. 胃底 fundus of stomach
10. 前锯肌 serratus anterior
11. 肋间肌 intercostal muscle
12. 背阔肌 latissimus dorsi
13. 第 10 肋骨 10th costal bone
14. 脾 spleen
15. 肋膈隐窝 costodiaphragmatic recess
16. 竖脊肌 erector spinae
17. 棘间韧带 interspinous ligament
18. 硬膜外隙 epidural space
19. 关节突关节 zygapophysial joint
20. 脊髓 spinal cord
21. 椎间静脉 intervertebral vein
22. T10-11 椎间盘 T10-11 intervertebral disc
23. 膈 diaphragm
24. 奇静脉 azygos vein
25. 胸导管 thoracic duct
26. 胸主动脉 thoracic aorta
27. 半奇静脉 hemiazygos vein
28. 胃裸区 gastric bare area
29. 左膈脚 left crus of diaphragm
30. 胃贲门 cardia of stomach
31. 右膈脚 right crus of diaphragm
32. 下腔静脉 inferior vena cava
33. 肝尾状叶 caudate lobe of liver
34. 静脉韧带裂 fissure for ligamentum venosum
35. 肝右静脉 right hepatic vein
36. 肝右后叶 right posterior lobe of liver
37. 肝右前叶 right anterior lobe of liver
38. 肝中静脉 middle hepatic vein
39. 肝左静脉 left hepatic vein
40. 肝左内叶 left medial lobe of liver
41. 肝镰状韧带 falciform ligament of liver
42. 腹外斜肌 obliquus externus abdominis
43. 肝门静脉左支矢状部 sagittal portion of left hepatic portal vein
44. 肝圆韧带裂 fissure for ligamentum teres hepatis
45. 后底段（S10） posterior basal segment
46. 外侧底段（S9） lateral basal segment
47. 蛛网膜下隙 subarachnoid space

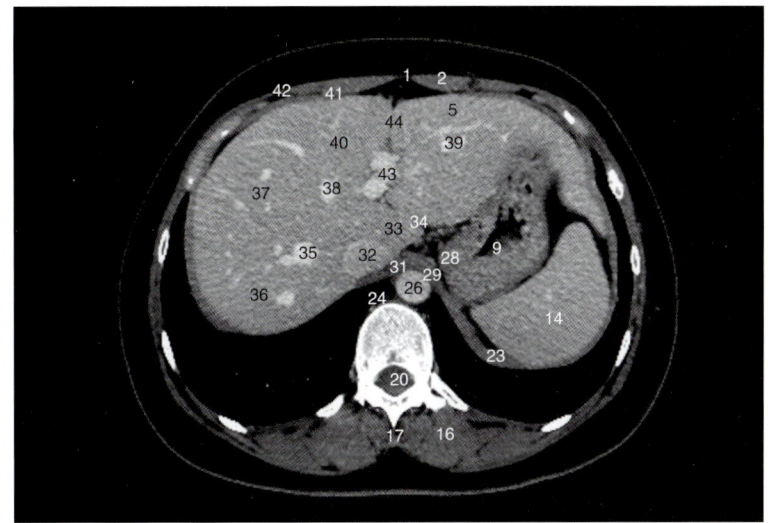

B. CT 纵隔窗增强图像

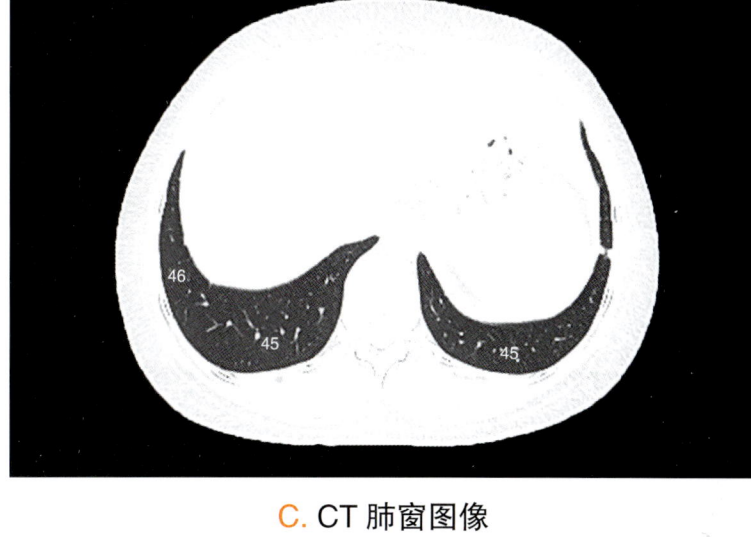

C. CT 肺窗图像

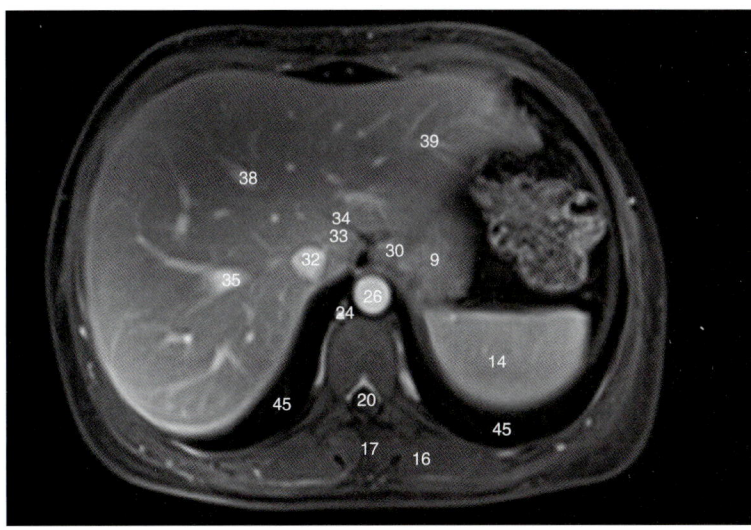

D. MR T1WI 增强图像

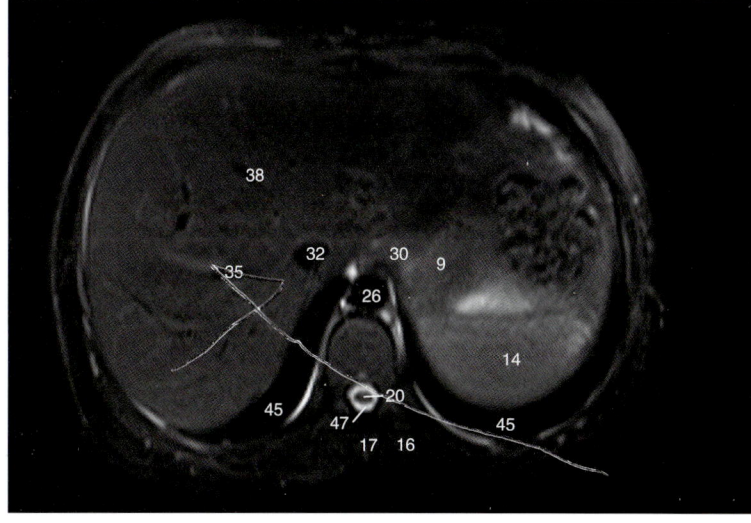

E. MR T2WI 抑脂图像

关键结构：蛛网膜下隙，硬膜囊，硬膜外隙。

此断面后部经 T10-11 椎间盘中部。

前部剑突消失，中线两侧为腹直肌。椎间盘后方为椎管，椎管内有脊髓及其被膜，软脊膜与蛛网膜之间为蛛网膜下隙，充满脑脊液，在 MR T1 图像为低信号，MR T2 图像为高信号。脊髓蛛网膜与硬脊膜之间的硬膜下隙在 CT、MR 图像中不显影，故可将这两层被膜看作一层结构。硬脊膜厚而致密，由结缔组织构成，与其内的蛛网膜一起形成长筒状的囊腔，称为硬膜囊，其内包绕脊髓、脊神经根、终丝和脑脊液等。硬脊膜与椎管内面的骨膜之间为硬膜外隙，内有椎内静脉丛、脂肪及神经根等，略呈负压，临床上进行硬膜外麻醉，就是将药物注入此间隙，以阻滞神经根内的神经传导[20]。椎管两侧为椎间管，有椎间静脉和脊神经根穿出。本断面胸腔内结构仅可见膈左前方的心包外脂肪和膈后外侧的肋膈隐窝。腹腔内，食管腹部消失，贲门连接胃底。胃与静脉韧带裂之间为小网膜，有胃左动脉的支。胸主动脉发出肋间后动脉进入肋间隙。CT 图像中肝内见肝门静脉左支矢状部和肝圆韧带裂，胸腔内结构为两肺下叶，脊柱区见椎体、椎弓根、椎弓板、棘突及肋头关节等。

胸部连续横断层 101（FH.11490）

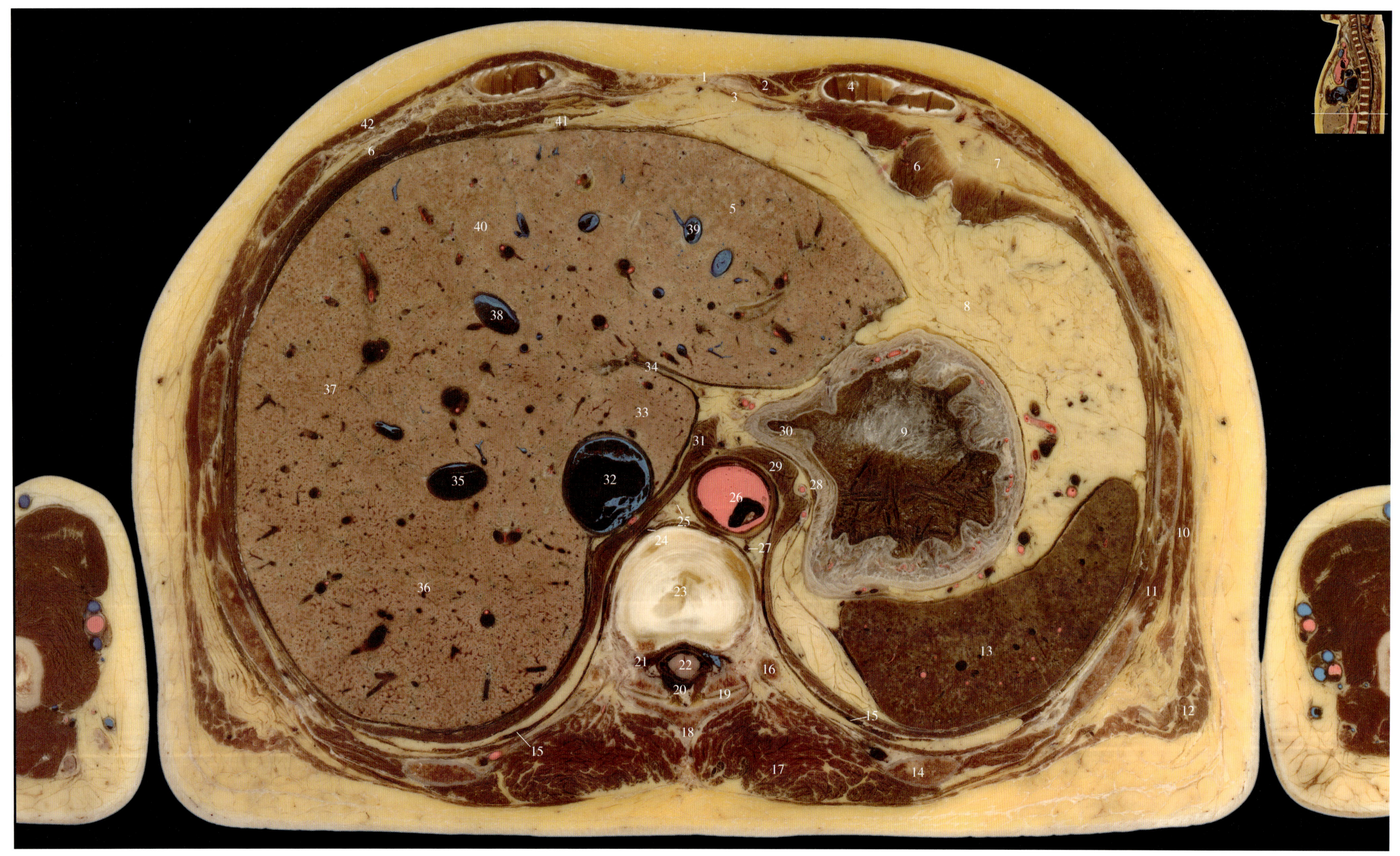

A. 断层标本图像

1. 腹白线 linea alba
2. 腹直肌 rectus abdominis
3. 膈的胸骨部 sternal part of diaphragm
4. 第 7 肋软骨 7th costal cartilage
5. 肝左外叶 left lateral lobe of liver
6. 膈 diaphragm
7. 心包外脂肪 extrapericardial fat
8. 大网膜 greater omentum
9. 胃底 fundus of stomach
10. 前锯肌 serratus anterior
11. 肋间肌 intercostal muscle
12. 背阔肌 latissimus dorsi
13. 脾 spleen
14. 第 10 肋骨 10th costal bone
15. 肋膈隐窝 costodiaphragmatic recess
16. 第 11 肋骨 11th costal bone
17. 竖脊肌 erector spinae
18. 棘突 spinous process
19. 关节突关节 zygapophysial joint
20. 硬膜外隙 epidural space
21. 椎间孔 intervertebral foramen
22. 脊髓 spinal cord
23. T10-11 椎间盘 T10-11 intervertebral disc
24. 奇静脉 azygos vein
25. 胸导管 thoracic duct
26. 胸主动脉 thoracic aorta
27. 半奇静脉 hemiazygos vein
28. 胃裸区 gastric bare area
29. 左膈脚 left crus of diaphragm
30. 胃贲门 cardia of stomach
31. 右膈脚 right crus of diaphragm
32. 下腔静脉 inferior vena cava
33. 肝尾状叶 caudate lobe of liver
34. 静脉韧带裂 fissure for ligamentum venosum
35. 肝右静脉 right hepatic vein
36. 肝右后叶 right posterior lobe of liver
37. 肝右前叶 right anterior lobe of liver
38. 肝中静脉 middle hepatic vein
39. 肝左静脉 left hepatic vein
40. 肝左内叶 left medial lobe of liver
41. 肝镰状韧带 falciform ligament of liver
42. 腹外斜肌 obliquus externus abdominis
43. 肝门静脉左支矢状部 sagittal portion of left hepatic portal vein
44. 肝圆韧带裂 fissure for ligamentum teres hepatis
45. 后底段（S10）posterior basal segment

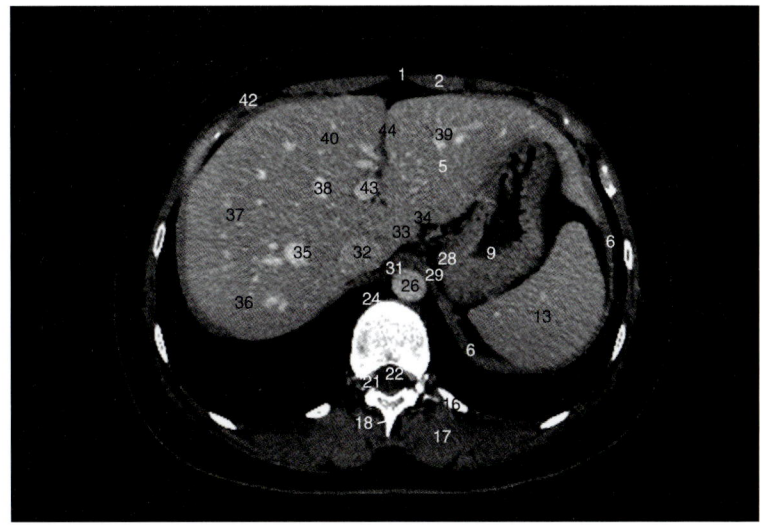

B. CT 纵隔窗增强图像

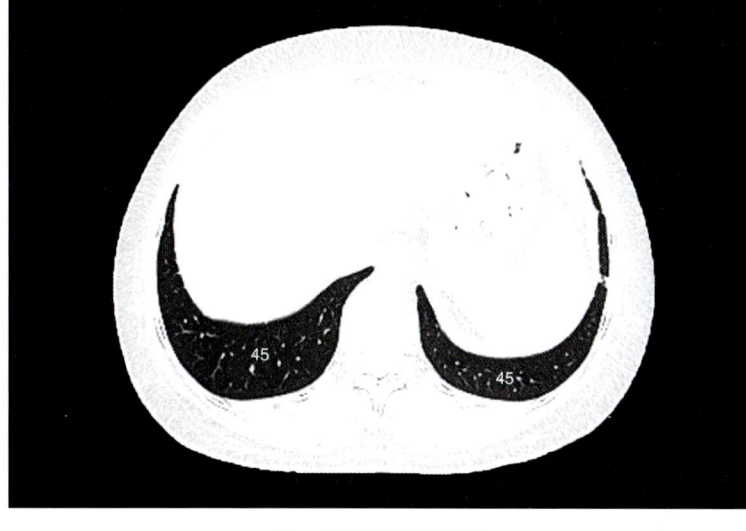

C. CT 肺窗图像

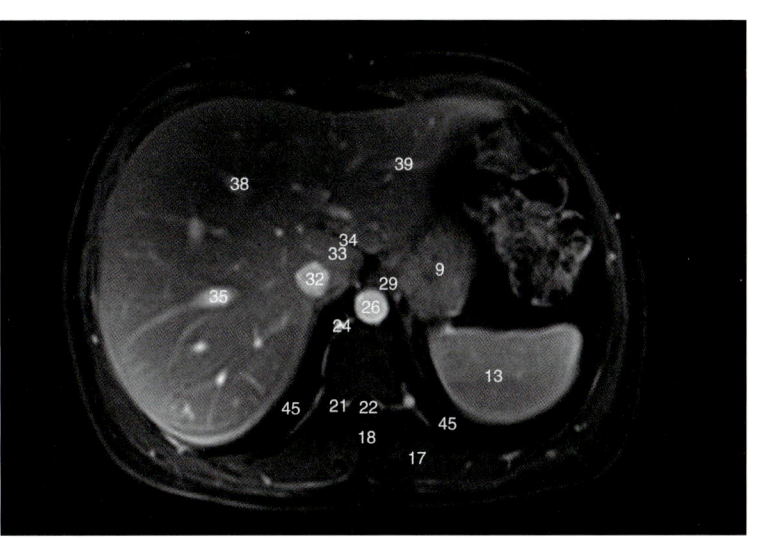

D. MR T1WI 增强图像

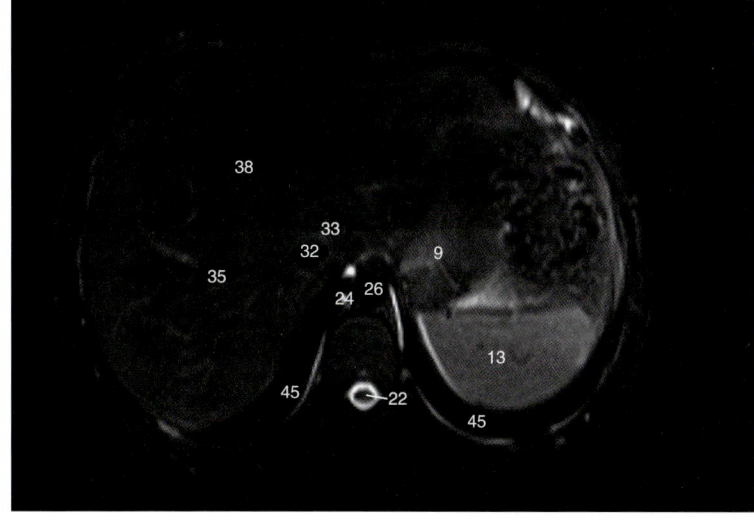

E. MR T2WI 抑脂图像

关键结构：膈脚后间隙，椎间盘，关节突关节。

此断面后部经 T10-11 椎间盘。

胸腔内结构近消失，仅可见膈左前方的心包外脂肪和膈后外侧的肋膈隐窝。腹腔内为上腹部脏器，如肝、胃和脾。下腔静脉位于肝脏面的腔静脉沟内，肝内静脉走向外周，分隔肝的各叶和段，肝门静脉的分支位于各肝叶和肝段内，越来越粗大。肝静脉韧带裂和胃之间为小网膜。左、右膈脚环绕胸主动脉两侧，其后方和椎体前方之间为膈脚后间隙，横断面呈三角形，正常该间隙由脂肪组织充填，内有主动脉、神经、淋巴结、乳糜池、胸导管、奇静脉和半奇静脉等。当膈脚后间隙发生炎症和肿瘤时，可导致其内的淋巴结肿大；主动脉破裂时，可导致该间隙淤血；肝硬化时，可导致间隙内奇静脉和半奇静脉曲张；内分泌病变时，该间隙内大量脂肪沉积，这些病变均可引起膈脚后间隙明显增大[105]。椎间盘后方椎管内见脊髓及其被膜，椎管后方见关节突关节，由第 11 胸椎的上关节突和第 10 胸椎的下关节突构成，胸椎的关节突关节呈冠状位，横断面上，关节腔呈横位，下位椎骨的上关节突位于关节腔前方，上位椎骨的下关节突位于关节腔后方。

参考文献

[1] Pawha P,Jiang N,Shpilberg K,et al. Gross and Radiographic Anatomy. Anesthesiology and Otolaryngology,2012,12:3-33.

[2] Raveendran VL,Kamalamma GK.Inferior cervical ganglion and stellate ganglion-concepts revisited.Journal of Evolution of Medical and Dental Sciences,2018,7 (13):1653-1658.

[3] Inari H,Teruya N,Kishi M,et al. Clinicopathological features of breast cancer patients with internal mammary and/or supraclavicular lymph node recurrence without distant metastasis. BMC Cancer,2020,20 (1):171-180.

[4] Palumbo VD,Fazzotta S,Fatica F,et al. Pancoast tumour :current therapeutic options. Clin Ter,2019,170 (4):e291-e294.

[5] 郑克,陈文斌,朱思琪,等. 高风险甲状腺手术中神经监测对喉返神经保护的研究现状与进展. 中国现代普通外科进展,2019,22(8):623-627.

[6] Liu N,Chen B,Li L,et al. Mechanisms of recurrent laryngeal nerve injury near the nerve entry point during thyroid surgery:a retrospective cohort study. Int J Surg,2020,83:125-130.

[7] 李兵,叶亦致,李泽斌,等. 喉返神经与非返性喉返神经临床应用解剖学研究进展. 解剖学杂志,2020,43 (3):235-238.

[8] Pandey NN,Bhambri K,Kumar S. Rare and anomalous retro-oesophageal course of the left brachiocephalic vein in tetralogy of fallot:evaluation on CT angiography with relevant embryology. Heart Lung Circ,2020,29 (1):e14-e16.

[9] Choi Y,Chung SB,Kim MS. Prevalence and anatomy of aberrant right subclavian artery evaluated by computed tomographic angiography at a single institution in Korea. J Korean Neurosurg Soc,2019,62 (2):175-182.

[10] El-Sherief Ahmed H,Lau Charles T,Carter Brett W,et al. Staging Lung Cancer:Regional Lymph Node Classification. Radiologic clinics of North America,2018,56 (3):399-409.

[11] Story L,Zhang T,Uus A,et al. Antenatal thymus volumes in fetuses that deliver <32 weeks gestation:an MRI pilot study. Acta Obstet Gynecol Scand,2020,Online ahead of print.

[12] Wang Y,Zhu L,Xia W,et al. Anatomy of lymphatic drainage of the esophagus and lymph node metastasis of thoracic esophageal cancer. Cancer Manag Res,2018,10:6295-6303.

[13] Tjan-Heijnen V,Viale G. The lymph node and the metastasis. N Engl J Med,2018,378 (21):2045-2046.

[14] Dey Hazra RO,Reich AR,Hanhoff M,et al. Injuries of the sternoclavicular joint. Unfallchirurg,2020,123 (11):879-889.

[15] Madabushi R,Tewari S,Gautam S K,et al. Serratus anterior plane block:a new analgesic technique for post-thoracotomy pain. Pain Physician,2015,18 (3):E421-E424.

[16] Tavares MR,Cruz JA,Waisberg DR,et al. Lymph node distribution in the central compartment of the neck:an anatomic study. Head Neck,2014,36 (10):1425-1430.

[17] 申虹,魏伯俊,彭振兴. 气管前间隙病变的诊断及手术治疗. 中华耳鼻咽喉头颈外科杂志,2016(06):451-453.

[18] Rizeq YK,Many BT,Vacek JC,et al. Diaphragmatic paralysis after phrenic nerve injury in newborns. J Pediatr Surg,2020,55 (2):240-244.

[19] Susan Standring.格氏解剖学. 41版. 丁自海,刘树伟,译. 济南:山东科学技术出版社,2017.

[20] 陈鑫. 冠状动脉旁路移植术的现状和展望. 中华外科杂志,2020,58 (5):321-325.

[21] Flores-Funes D,Aguilar-Jiménez J,Martínez-Gálvez M,et al. The problem of axillary staging in breast cancer after neoadjuvant chemotherapy. Role of targeted axillary dissection and types of lymph node markers. Cirugia Espanola,2020,27 (11):4488-4499.

[22] 舒畅,李鑫. 主动脉弓部疾病的治疗方法概述及其进展. 中华血管外科杂志,2018,3 (1):8-11.

[23] Azizova A,Onder O,Arslan S,et al. Persistent left superior vena cava:clinical importance and differential diagnoses. Insights Imaging,2020,11 (1):110.

[24] Abdelrahman H,Al-Thani H,Al-Sulaiti M,et al. Clinical presentation and surgical treatment of retrosternal goiter:a case series study. Qatar Med J,2020,2020 (1):13.

[25] 杨开清,李光明,羊惠君. 主动脉弓及其邻近结构的横断层解剖. 华西医科大学学报,1999,30 (1):47-49.

[26] Colin PE,Deprez L,Cousin F. Oily Ascites revealing a spontaneous rupture of a mature ovarian cystic teratoma. Journal of the Belgian Society of Radiology,2020,104 (1):50-51.

[27] Winter R,Steinböck M,Leinich W,et al. The reverse latissimus dorsi flap:An anatomical study and retrospective analysis of its clinical application. Journal of plastic,reconstructive & aesthetic surgery:JPRAS,2019,72 (7):1084-1090.

[28] 唐东方,高文,谭德炎. 肺叶、肺段淋巴结引流的解剖学特征. 中华胸部外科电子杂志,2018,5 (1):10-15.

[29] Hansen T,Nilsson M,Lindholm D,et al. Normal radiological lymph node appearance in the thorax. Dis Esophagus,2019,32 (10):1-6.

[30] Kuperberg SJ,Shostak E. High-riding superior pericardial recess:a key pitfall in misinterpretation during CT evaluation of the mediastinum. J Bronchology Interv Pulmonol,2019,26 (1):71-73.

[31] Basile A,Bisceglie P,Giulietti G,et al. Prevalence of "high-riding" superior pericardial recesses on thin-section 16-MDCT scans. European Journal of Radiology,2006,59 (2):265-269.

[32] Al-Mnayyis A,Al-Alami Z,Altamimi N,et al. Azygos lobe:prevalence of an anatomical variant and its recognition among postgraduate physicians. Diagnostics (Basel),2020,10(7):470.

[33] Meng S,Liu G,Wang S,et al. Nodal involvement pattern in clinical stage IA non-small cell lung cancer according to tumor location. Cancer Manag Res,2020,12 :7875-7880.

[34] Lu D,Li CL,Lv WF,et al. Diagnostic value of multislice computerized tomography angiography for aortic dissection:A comparison with DSA. Exp Ther Med,2017,13(2):405-412.

[35] 管政,李琼,刘士远. 国人主支气管长度及内径与体质量指数

相关性的 CT 研究. 实用放射学杂志, 2015, 31 (10):1613-1616.

[36] 中国解剖学会体质调查委员会. 中国人解剖学数值. 北京：人民卫生出版社, 2002:5.

[37] 张苗, 王涛, 赵新亚, 等. 多层螺旋 CT 血管造影在右肺上叶动脉解剖中的应用. 医学影像学杂志, 2016, 26 (3):435-438.

[38] Klimek-Piotrowska W, Hołda MK, Piątek K, et al. Normal distal pulmonary vein anatomy. Peer J, 2016, 4:e1579.

[39] 刘树伟, 王怀经, 柳澄, 等. 右肺门支气管和血管在横断面上的配布特点. 中国临床解剖学杂志, 2004, 22 (5):457-462.

[40] 刘树伟. 断层解剖学. 3 版. 北京：高等教育出版社, 2017.

[41] 雷晓燕, 郭佑民, 许贵平, 等. 中心肺动脉血流速度的 MRI 测量研究. 中国医学影像技术, 2006, 22 (3):409-412.

[42] 张兆明, 王守安, 刘树伟. 左肺上叶尖后段静脉的多层螺旋 CT. 解剖学杂志, 2009, 32 (6):736-739.

[43] 王丽华, 李润明, 郭佑民. 正常成人肺动脉分支心动周期不同时相影像对比研究. 实用放射学杂志, 2006, 22 (10):1182-1185.

[44] Beigel R, Wunderlich NC, Ho SY, et al. The left atrial appendage: anatomy, function, and noninvasive evaluation. JACC Cardiovasc Imaging, 2014, 7 (12):1251-65.

[45] 杨志宏, 丁仲如, 吴弘, 等. 经皮穿刺封堵左心耳的应用解剖. 中国临床解剖学杂志, 2005, 23 (02):167-169.

[46] 杨延坤, 郑宏, 孙鑫, 等. 64 排螺旋 CT 心脏增强扫描在左心耳解剖形态评价中的应用. 实用放射学杂志, 2014, 30 (4):584-587.

[47] 刘树伟, 王怀经. 左肺门支气管和血管在横断面上的配布特点. 中国临床解剖学杂志, 2006, 24 (4):351-354.

[48] Heřmanová Z, Ctvrtlík F, Heřman M. Incomplete and accessory fissures of the lung evaluated by high-resolution computed tomography. Eur J Radiol, 2014, 83(3):595-599.

[49] 徐冰, 迟永堃, 李晓婷, 等. 64 排螺旋 CT 观察肺裂变异. 中国医学影像技术, 2011, 27 (05):975-978.

[50] Sreenivasulu K, Anilkumar P, Gaiqwad MR. Morphological anatomy of accessory fissures in lungs. Indian J Tuberc, 2012, 59(1):28-31.

[51] 王佑怀, 张在沛, 李兴富, 等. 右肺斜裂水平裂的 CT 应用解剖. 中国临床解剖学杂志, 2001, 19 (1):43-45.

[52] 赵凤敏, 陈文军, 谢晓霞, 等. 心包窦、心包隐窝及心包间隙影像横断解剖. 中国 CT 和 MRI 杂志, 2007, 5 (2):20-21.

[53] Madden ME. Introduction to Sectional Anatomy. 3rd ed. Philadelphia:Lippincott Williams & Wilkins, 2013.

[54] 王守安, 张兆明, 刘树伟, 等. 左肺上、下舌段静脉的多层螺旋 CT 研究. 中华解剖与临床杂志, 2009, 14 (6):400-403.

[55] Rissi R, Marques MJ, Neto HS. Checking the shape and lobation of the right atrial appendage in view of their clinical relevance. Anat Sci Int, 2019, 94(4):324-329.

[56] 王玉, 王宜芹, 丁承宗. 320 排动态容积 CT 在评价冠状动脉解剖结构方面的价值. 中国中西医结合影像学杂志, 2014, 12 (4):369-371.

[57] Khwansang N, Chentanez V. Anatomic variations of coronary arteries:origins, branching patterns, and abnormalities. Asian Biomedicine, 2019, 12 (3):117-123.

[58] 李国照, 高明, 谢明伟, 等. 正常引流肺静脉解剖变异的多层螺旋 CT 血管成像研究. 中华解剖与临床杂志, 2016, 21 (3):200-203.

[59] Ravenel JG, Erasmus JJ. Azygoesophageal recess. J Thorac Imaging, 2002, 17 (3):219-226.

[60] Akahashi T, Murakawa T, Fukami T, et al. Pneumothorax after left pneumonectomy:accentuated negative pressure at azygoesophageal recess by a mediastinal shift and rotation. Eur J Cardiothorac Surg, 2010, 37 (5):1222.

[61] 陈光平, 董海娜, 叶再挺, 等. 多层螺旋 CT 成像对右肺中叶肺段与亚段肺动脉管径的评价. 解剖学报, 2012, 43 (1):72-76.

[62] Klimek-Piotrowska W, Hołda MK, Piątek K, et al. Normal distal pulmonary vein anatomy. Peer J, 2016, 14 (4):e1579.

[63] 宗刚军, 白元, 秦永文, 等. 经导管主动脉瓣及肺动脉瓣置换的应用解剖. 中国临床解剖学杂志, 2008, 26 (3):252-254.

[64] Alkadhi H, Wildermuth S, Plass A, et al. Aortic stenosis:comparative evaluation of 16-detector row CT and echocardiography. Radiology, 2006, 240 (1):47-55.

[65] 张祖志, 吴鹏, 申国明. 主动脉窦与心包横窦的应用解剖研究. 解剖与临床, 2007, 12 (01):21-22.

[66] Verschakelen JA, De Wever W. Computed tomography of the lung. 2nd ed. Berlin:Springer, 2018.

[67] 陈光祥, 漆军, 黄新文, 等. 64 层螺旋 CT 在肺静脉解剖学研究中的应用. 中国临床医学影像杂志, 2009, 20 (08):599-602.

[68] Mori S, Tretter JT, Spicer DE, et al. What is the real cardiac anatomy? Clin Anat, 2019, 32 (3):288-309.

[69] Kauczor HU, Wielpütz MO. MRI of the Lung. 2nd ed. Switzerland:Springer, 2018.

[70] Godwin JD, Vock P, Osborne DR. CT of the pulmonary ligament. Am J Roentgenol, 1983, 141 (2):231-236.

[71] 余建群, 杨志刚, 杨开清. 肺韧带对下胸部疾病螺旋 CT 表现的影响及其解剖学基础. 中华放射学杂志, 2003, 37 (1):67-69.

[72] Olivetti L. Atlas of Imaging Anatomy. New York:Springer, 2015.

[73] Fletcher SW, Black W, Harris R, et al. Report of the international workshop on screening for breast cancer. Natl Cancer Inst, 1993, 85(20):1644-1656.

[74] Zonderland HM, Coerkamp EG, Hermans J, et al. Diagnosis of breast cancer:contribution of US as an adjunct to mammography. Radiology, 1999, 213(2):413-422.

[75] 孙占国, 唐光才, 范新文. 64 层螺旋 CT 显示冠状静脉系统形态学的研究. 中华老年心脑血管杂志, 2008, 10 (10):744-747.

[76] 丁自海, 张希. 临床解剖学·胸部分册. 2 版. 北京：人民卫生出版社, 2014.

[77] Kim AM, Hunter TA, McQuillan BF, et al. Imaging in congenital and hereditary abnormalities of the interventricular septum:clinical anatomy and diagnostic clues. J Thorac Imaging, 2018, 33 (3):147-155.

[78] 马小静, 何亚峰, 陈鑫. 心血管影像解剖图谱. 北京：人民卫生出版社, 2018.

[79] 何伟红, 谭理连, 李志铭. 320 排螺旋 CT 观察正常心脏二尖瓣. 中国医学影像技术, 2010, 26 (11):2099-2102.

[80] Carrascosa PM, Capunay CM, Deviggiano A, et al. Clinical Atlas of cardiac and aortic CT and MRI. Switzerland:Springer, 2019.

[81] 刘树伟. 人体断层解剖学. 北京：高等教育出版社, 2006.

[82] Hoit BD. Anatomy and physiology of the pericardium. Cardiol Clin, 2017, 35 (4):481-490.

[83] Rodriguez ER, Tan CD. Structure and anatomy of the human pericardium. Prog Cardiovasc Dis, 2017, 59 (4):327-340.

[84] 陶然, 钟震亚, 田国忠. 食管胸部下段器官外供血动脉的解剖学观测. 解剖学研究, 2007, 29 (6):457-458.

[85] Medrano-Gracia P, Ormiston J, Webster M, et al. A computational atlas of normal coronary artery anatomy. Euro Intervention, 2016, 12 (7):845-854.

[86] Altin C, Kanyilmaz S, Koc S, et al. Coronary anatomy, anatomic variations and anomalies:a retrospective coronary angiography study. Singapore Med J, 2015, 56 (6):339-345.

[87] Kwong RY, Jerosch-Herold M, Heydari B. Cardiovascular Magnetic Resonance Imaging. 2nd ed. New York:Springer. 2019.

[88] 张金周, 郑鑫林, 张建华. 胸导管手术的研究现状. 中国胸心血管外科临床杂志, 2016, 23(4):399-402.

[89] Bourgeois P, Munck D, Sales F, et al. Anomalies of thoracic lymph duct drainage demonstrated by lymphoscintigraphy and review of the literature about these anomalies. Eur J Surg Oncol, 2008, 34 (5):553-555.

[90] 陈朔, 许乙凯. 胸导管的磁共振水成像研究. 国际医学放射学杂志, 2012, 35 (6):533-535.

[91] Dahou A, Levin D, Reisman M, et al. Anatomy and Physiology of the Tricuspid Valve. JACC Cardiovasc Imaging, 2019, 12 (3):458-

468.

[92] Tsuyoshi T,Mitsuaki K,Hideki K,et al. A deep azygoesophageal recess may increase the risk of secondary spontaneous pneumothorax. Surg Today,2017,47 (9):1147-1152.

[93] Sakon Y,Murakami T,Fujii H,et al. New insight into tricuspid valve anatomy from 100 hearts to reappraise annuloplasty methodology. Gen Thorac Cardiovasc Surg,2019,67:758–764.

[94] Kocjan J,Adamek M,Gzik-Zroska B,et al. Network of breathing. Multifunctional role of the diaphragm:a review. Adv Respir Med,2017,85 (4):224-232.

[95] Niwa Y,Koike M,Hattori M,et al. Short-term outcomes after conventional transthoracic esophagectomy. Nagoya J Med Sci,2016,78 (1):69-78.

[96] Collet C,Grundeken MJ,Asano T,et al. State of the art:coronary angiography. Euro Intervention,2017,25,13 (6):634-643.

[97] Max B Sayers. Diagnostic coronary angiography:past,present and future. Br J Hosp Med,2018,79 (2):66-67.

[98] Nagamatsu Y,Mori S,Fukuzawa K,et al. Anatomical characteristics of the superior epigastric artery for epicardial ablation using the anterior approach. J Cardiovasc Electrophysiol,2019,30 (8):1339-1340.

[99] 许国卿,于海波,梁延春,等. 左室电极导线植入不同冠状静脉分支血管与左室起搏部位关系. 临床军医杂志,2019,47 (10):1063-1066.

[100] Roman S,Kahrilas PJ. The diagnosis and management of hiatus hernia. BMJ,2014,349 (23):g6154.

[101] 向展华,孙善全,梅勇,等. 左膈下动脉及其分支的应用解剖学观察. 重庆医学,2012,41 (35):3695-3696.

[102] 刘正津. 胸心外科临床解剖学. 济南：山东科学技术出版社,2000.

[103] Torkian P,Langroudi TF,Negarestani AM,et al. A new approach to cardiac fat volume assessment and the correlation with coronary artery calcification. Rom J Intern Med,2020,58 (2):81-91.

[104] Gkasdaris G,Tripsianis G,Kotopoulos K,et al. Clinical anatomy and significance of the thoracic intervertebral foramen:A cadaveric study and review of the literature. J Craniovertebr Junction Spine,2016,7(4):228-235.

[105] Federle MP,Rosado-de-Christenson ML,Woodward PJ,et al. Diagnostic and surgical imaging anatomy:chest,abdomen,pelvis. Manitoba:Amirsys,2007.

索 引

B

半奇静脉 hemiazygos vein　165~203
背阔肌 latissimus dorsi　105~203
贲门部 cardiac part of stomach　189
臂丛 brachial plexus　3~39
臂丛后束 posterior cord of brachial plexus　41~57
臂丛内侧束 medial cord of brachial plexus　41~57
臂丛外侧束 lateral cord of brachial plexus　41~57

D

大网膜 greater omentum　183~203
大圆肌 teres major　49~129
第 10 肋骨 10th costal bone　175~203
第 10 胸椎椎体 body of 10th thoracic vertebra　179~197
第 11 肋骨 11th costal bone　203
第 1 肋骨 1st costal bone　3~9,31~45
第 1 胸椎椎体 body of 1st thoracic vertebra　3~13
第 2 肋骨 2nd costal bone　5~59
第 2 肋软骨 2nd costal cartilage　51~69
第 2 胸神经 2nd thoracic nerve　21
第 2 胸椎椎体 body of 2nd thoracic vertebra　15~31
第 3 肋骨 3rd costal bone　21~85
第 3 肋软骨 3rd costal cartilage　87~95,99~107
第 3 肋肋关节 3rd sternocostal joint　91~97
第 3 胸神经 3rd thoracic nerve　39
第 3 胸椎椎体 body of 3rd thoracic vertebra　33~49
第 4 肋骨 4th costal bone　41~91,133~137
第 4 肋软骨 4th costal cartilage　115~121,125~131
第 4 胸神经 4th thoracic nerve　57,59

第 4 胸椎椎体 body of 4th thoracic vertebra　51~67
第 5 肋骨 5th costal bone　61~77,85~89,93~103,109
第 5 肋软骨 5th costal cartilage　139~149,155~159
第 5 胸椎椎体 body of 5th thoracic vertebra　71~85
第 6 肋骨 6th costal bone　81~93,103,121,123
第 6 肋软骨 6th costal cartilage　151,153,161~183,195,197
第 6 胸神经 6th thoracic nerve　99
第 6 胸椎椎体 body of 6th thoracic vertebra　91~105
第 7 肋骨 7th costal bone　101,107~117,143~147
第 7 肋软骨 7th costal cartilage　155~193,199~203
第 7 胸椎椎体 body of 7th thoracic vertebra　113~127
第 8 颈神经 8th spinal nerve　5
第 8 肋骨 8th costal bone　131~129,143~147
第 8 胸椎棘突 spinous process of 8th thoracic vertebra　161,163
第 8 胸椎椎体 body of 8th thoracic vertebra　135~149
第 9 肋骨 9th costal bone　149~179,185~189,199
第 9 胸椎棘突 spinous process of 9th thoracic vertebra　183~187,193,195
第 9 胸椎椎体 body of 9th thoracic vertebra　159~173
第 3 肋骨 3rd costal bone　77

E

二尖瓣 mitral valve　131~153

F

房间隔 interatrial septum　133~153
肺动脉干 pulmonary trunk　75~103
肺韧带 pulmonary ligament　125,135~153,161~169,173
肺韧带淋巴结（9区） pulmonary ligament lymph nodes　127~133
腹白线 linea alba　199~203
腹壁上动脉 superior epigastric artery　171~195

腹外斜肌 obliquus externus abdominis　183~203
腹直肌 rectus abdominis　169~203

G

肝 liver　151~159
肝镰状韧带 falciform ligament of liver　189,193~203
肝门静脉左支矢状部 sagittal portion of left hepatic portal vein　193~203
肝尾状叶 caudate lobe of liver　187~203
肝右后上缘静脉 right posterior supramarginal vein of liver　169~181
肝右后叶 right posterior lobe of liver　169~203
肝右静脉 right hepatic vein　171~203
肝右前叶 right anterior lobe of liver　169~203
肝右叶 right lobe of liver　161~167
肝圆韧带裂 fissure for ligamentum teres hepatis　199~203
肝中静脉 middle hepatic vein　171~203
肝左静脉 left hepatic vein　171~203
肝左内叶 left medial lobe of liver　171~203
肝左外叶 left lateral lobe of liver　185~203
冈上肌 supraspinatus　3~21
冈下肌 infraspinatus　3~117
隔缘肉柱 septomarginal trabecula　163,165
膈 diaphragm　151~195,201,203
膈的胸骨部 sternal part of diaphragm　197~203
膈神经 phrenic nerve　3~33
膈神经和心包膈血管 phrenic nerve and pericardiacophrenic vessels　35~97
膈右穹窿 right fornix of diaphragm　149,173
肱二头肌 biceps brachii　87~93
肱二头肌长、短头 long and short heads of biceps brachii　69~85
肱二头肌长头 long head of biceps brachii　41,47,51,57~67
肱二头肌短头 short head of biceps brachii　27~67
肱骨 humerus　21~93

肱骨头 head of humerus　　3~19
肱三头肌 triceps brachii　　47~53
关节盘 articular disc　　21~25
关节突关节 zygapophysial joint　　5,7,21~25,41~45,61~65,83~87,127,153,155,175~181,201,203
冠状窦 coronary sinus　　133~177
冠状窦口 orifice of coronary sinus　　157,159

H

横突 transverse process　　3~13,23~57,67~77,89~97,143~149,165~171,187~195
横突棘肌 transversospinales　　5~141
后底段（S10）posterior basal segment　　173~203
后段动脉（A2）posterior segmental artery　　77,75
后段静脉（V2）posterior segmental vein　　41~77
后段支气管（B2）posterior segmental bronchus　　77
后段支气管（B2）和动脉（A2）posterior segmental bronchus and artery　　59~65,69~75
后室间支 posterior interventricular branch　　151,153,177~181
黄韧带 ligament flava　　47,49,125,147~151,161,175~179
喙肱肌 coracobrachialis　　27~93
喙突 coracoid process　　7~25

J

肌膈动脉 musculophrenic artery　　171~189
棘肌 spinales　　5~141
棘间韧带 interspinous ligament　　11,79,101,153,175,177,199,201
棘突 spinous process　　3~9,21~29,43~53,65~69,73~79,87~101,143~159,165~181,189,191,197,203
脊神经 spinal nerve　　143~147,171,195,197
脊髓 spinal cord　　3~21,25~35,39~203
甲状腺下静脉 inferior thyroid vein　　5~17
尖段动脉（A1）apical segmental artery　　57~75
尖段静脉（V1）apical segmental vein　　49~77,85
尖段静脉尖支（V1）apical branch of apical segmental vein　　29~71
尖段支气管（B1）apical segmental bronchus　　57~75
尖段支气管（B1）和动脉（A1）apical segmental bronchus and artery　　41~55
尖后段动脉（A1+2）apicoposterior segmental artery　　41,55,67~75,83,85,89,93
尖后段静脉（V1+2）apicoposterior segmental vein　　43~81,87,91
尖后段静脉段内支（V1+2）intrasegmental ramus of apicoposterior segmental vein　　67~79
尖后段支气管（B1+2）apicoposterior segmental bronchus　　67~87
尖后段支气管（B1+2）和动脉（A1+2）apicoposterior segmental bronchus and artery　　41~65
肩关节腔 cavity of shoulder joint　　3~7,11~19,23
肩胛冈 spine of scapula　　3~21
肩胛骨 scapula　　5,9,21~133
肩胛骨下角 inferior angle of scapula　　135
肩胛上静脉 suprascapular vein　　7~13
肩胛提肌 levator scapulae　　3~39
肩胛下动脉 subscapular artery　　27~53
肩胛下肌 subscapularis　　5,9~121
剑突 xiphoid process　　155~197
腱索 tendinous cord　　143,145,149~153
降主动脉 descending aorta　　67~71
交感干神经节 ganglia of sympathetic trunk　　149,197,199
交感干神经节 ganglia of sympathetic trunk　　171
界嵴 crista terminalis　　133
颈长肌 longus colli　　3~9
颈夹肌 splenius cervicis　　3~25,29
颈静脉弓 jugular venous arch　　17
颈前静脉 anterior jugular vein　　3~15
颈外静脉 external jugular vein　　3,5
静脉韧带裂 fissure for ligamentum venosum　　189~203

L

肋膈隐窝 costodiaphragmatic recess　　195~203
肋横突关节 costotransverse joint　　27,29,49~53,73,75,115,143~147
肋间后动、静脉 posterior intercostal artery and vein　　63,65,81,83,175,179,143~147,151,171,173,177,191
肋间后动脉 posterior intercostal artery　　37~45,49~61,91,95,97,103,165~169,189,193~197
肋间后静脉 posterior intercostal vein　　77,165~169,185~189,193
肋间肌 intercostal muscle　　153,161~193,197~203
肋间内、外肌 intercostales interni and externi　　7~41,47~75,79~103
肋间内肌 intercostales interni　　43,45,145,149,151
肋间外肌 intercostales externi　　43,45,145,147
肋间最内肌 intercostales intimi　　7~41,47~59
肋头关节 joint of costal head　　13~17,27~31,47~53,71,73,91~95,159,161,179~187
肋头关节 joints of costal head　　115,151
菱形肌 rhomboideus　　3~89,127,129
隆嵴下淋巴结（7区）subcarinal lymph nodes　　77~107

N

内侧底段动脉（A7）medial basal segmental artery　　111,123,125
内侧底段静脉（V7）medial basal segmental vein　　131~159,169
内侧底段支气管（B7）和动脉（A7）medial basal segmental bronchus and artery　　127,135~159,163
内侧底段支气管（B7）medial basal segmental bronchus　　113,123,125,131,133
内侧段（S5）medial segment　　151~161
内侧段动脉（A5）lateral segmental artery　　109~123
内侧段静脉（V5）medial segmental vein　　135
内侧段静脉（V5）medial segmental vein　　137,147~149
内侧段支气管（B5）和动脉（A5）medial segmental bronchus and artery　　125~149
内侧段支气管（B5）medial segmental bronchus　　111~123
内前底段（S7+8）medioanterior basal segment　　165~187
内前底段动脉（A7+8）medioanterior basal segmental artery　　111
内前底段动脉（A7+8）medioanterior basal segmental artery　　105~109,113~167
内前底段动脉（A7+8）medioanterior basal segmental artery　　99~103
内前底段支气管（B7+8）medioanterior basal segmental bronchus　　121~129,133~137
内前底段支气管（B7+8）medioanterior basal segmental bronchus　　115~119,131
内前底段支气管（B7+8）和动脉（A7+8）medioanterior basal segmental bronchus and artery　　139~163

P

脾 spleen　　181~203

Q

奇静脉 azygos vein　　67~183,187~203
奇静脉弓 arch of azygos vein　　61~69
奇静脉食管隐窝 azygoesophageal recess　　79~127
气管 trachea　　3~69
气管膜壁 membranous wall　　23
髂肋肌 iliocostalis　　23~141
前底段（S8）anterior basal segment　　153,157~187
前底段动脉（A8）anterior basal segmental artery　　131,133
前底段静脉（V8）anterior basal segmental vein　　135~157
前底段支气管（B8）和动脉（A8）anterior basal segmental bronchus and artery　　135~155
前底段支气管（B8）anterior basal segmental bronchus　　131,133,137
前段静脉（V3）anterior segmental artery　　73

208

前段支气管（B3）和动脉（A3）anterior segmental bronchus and artery　43,47~59
前锯肌 serratus anterior　5~203
前乳头肌 anterior papillary muscles　165
前室间支 anterior interventricular branch　103~185
前斜角肌 scalenus anterior　3~17
前纵隔淋巴结（3a）anterior mediastinal lymph nodes　43
前纵隔淋巴结（3a）anterior mediastinal lymph nodes　45
前纵隔淋巴结（3a）anterior mediastinal lymph nodes　47~55

R

乳头肌 papillary muscle　137~153,161,163
乳腺 mammary gland　105~181

S

三尖瓣 tricuspid valve　139~153,159
三角肌 deltoid　3~25
上段静脉（V6）superior segmental vein　101
上段支气管（B6）superior segmental bronchus　101,103
上后锯肌 serratus posterior superior　3~49
上气管旁淋巴结（2区）upper paratracheal lymph nodes　17,19,33
上腔静脉 superior vena cava　41~113
上腔静脉口 orifice of superior vena cava　115,117
上舌段动脉（A4）superior lingular segmental artery　91,97~107
上舌段支气管（B4）superior lingular segmental bronchus　95,97,101~107
上舌段支气管（B4）和动脉（A4）superior lingular segmental bronchus and artery　93,109~125
上叶支气管 superior lobar bronchus of left lung　89
上叶支气管下干 inferior trunk of superior lobar bronchus　97
舌动脉干（A4+5）lingular arterial trunk　97~101
舌静脉干（V4+5）lingular venous trunk　103~145
升主动脉 ascending aorta　67~127
食管 esophagus　3~187
食管腹部 abdominal part of esophagus　189~199
食管旁淋巴结 paraesophageal lymph nodes　169
室间隔 interventricular septum　131,133,147~159
室间隔肌部 muscular part of interventricular septum　143,145
室间隔膜部 membranous part of interventricular septum　135~145
竖脊肌 erector spinae　3,143~203
水平裂 horizontal fissure　95~105
锁骨 clavicle　3~19

锁骨下肌 subclavius　3~13
锁骨胸骨端 sternal end of clavicle　21~29

T

T10-11 椎间盘 T10-11 intervertebral disc　199,197,201,203
T1-2 椎间盘 T1-2 intervertebral disc　11~17
T2-3 椎间盘 T2-3 intervertebral disc　29~35,47~53
T4-5 椎间盘 T4-5 intervertebral disc　67~71
T5-6 椎间盘 T5-6 intervertebral disc　87~91,107
T6-7 椎间盘 T6-7 intervertebral disc　109,111
T7-8 椎间盘 T7-8 intervertebral disc　129~133
T8-9 椎间盘 T8-9 intervertebral disc　151~157
T9-10 椎间盘 T9-10 intervertebral disc　173~179
头臂干 brachiocephalic trunk　9~45
头静脉 cephalic vein　9~61

W

外侧底段（S9）lateral basal segment　173~201
外侧段（S4）lateral segment　151~161
外侧段动脉（A4）lateral segmental artery　107~119
外侧段静脉（V4）lateral segmental vein　117~149
外侧段支气管（B4）和动脉（A4）lateral segmental bronchus and artery　121~149
外侧段支气管（B4）lateral segmental bronchus　111~119
外后底段静脉（V9+10）posterolateral basal segmental vein　131
胃贲门 cardia of stomach　191~203
胃底 fundus of stomach　177~203
胃裸区 gastric bare area　185~203
胃左动脉食管支 esophageal branch of left gastric artery　187

X

下腔静脉 inferior vena cava　161~203
下腔静脉口 orifice of inferior vena cava　157,159
下舌段（S5）inferior lingular segment　155~187
下舌段动脉（A5）inferior lingular segmental artery　103~107,119~125,147~149,153
下舌段静脉（V5）inferior lingular segmental vein　121,123,151
下舌段支气管（B5）和动脉（A5）inferior lingular segmental bronchus and artery　35,37,47~61,127~131,143~153
下舌段支气管（B5）inferior lingular segmental bronchus　101,105~125,

133~141
斜方肌 trapezius　3~167
斜角支 diagonal branch　109
斜裂 oblique fissure　65~183
心 heart　191
心包内脂肪 pericardial fat　193,195
心包前下窦 anterior inferior sinus of pericardium　175~183
心包腔 pericardial cavity　161~173,185
心包上隐窝 superior recess of pericardium　55,59,63,67~93
心包外脂肪 extrapericardial fat　191~203
心大静脉 great cardiac vein　109~131
心尖 cardiac apex　181
心小静脉 small cardiac vein　165~179
心中静脉 middle cardiac vein　177~187
星状神经节 stellate ganglion　3,5
胸背动脉 thoracodorsal artery　55~61
胸大肌 pectoralis major　3~141,145~155
胸导管 thoracic duct　3~69,75~79,83~203
胸骨柄 manubrium sterni　21~61
胸骨甲状肌 sternothyroid　3~27
胸骨角 sternal angle　67
胸骨颈静脉切迹 jugular notch of sternum　17
胸骨舌骨肌 sternohyoid　3~41
胸骨体 body of sternum　61~65,69~153
胸横肌 transversus thoracis　171~189,193,197,199
胸肩峰动脉 thoracoacromial artery　21~29
胸交感神经节 thoracic sympathetic ganglion　7~11,21,23,41,101
胸廓内动、静脉 internal thoracic artery and vein　33~35,43~45,53,57,61,65~107,115,127~129,145,149,151~155
胸廓内动脉 internal thoracic artery　5~9,17~31,37~41
胸肋三角 sternocostal triangle　187~191
胸膜顶 cupula of pleura　3,5
胸膜腔 pleural cavity　17,19,33,37,71,181~197
胸锁关节 sternoclavicular joint　27,31
胸锁关节腔 cavity of sternoclavicular joint　29
胸锁乳突肌 sternocleidomastoid　3~15,19
胸外侧静脉 lateral thoracic vein　63~153
胸腺 thymus　17~101
胸小肌 pectoralis minor　13~107
胸主动脉 thoracic aorta　73~203
胸主动脉食管支 esophageal branch of thoracic aorta　143,145
旋肱后动脉 posterior circumflex humeral artery　43,47,49
旋肩胛动、静脉 circumflex scapular artery and vein　55,57,65,67

209

旋肩胛静脉 circumflex scapular vein　69
旋支 circumflex branch　109~153
旋支 left circumflex coronary artery　129

Y

腋动、静脉 axillary artery and vein　79~91
腋动脉 axillary artery　17~77
腋静脉 axillary vein　17~77
腋淋巴结 axillary lymph nodes　35~39,43~47,51,57~69
硬脊膜 spinal dura mater　41,45,161,179
硬膜外隙 epidural space　9~21,25,33,39,43,47~119,123,125,129~177,181~203
右肺底段上静脉 right superior basal vein　129~137
右肺底段下静脉 right inferior basal vein　129~137
右肺底段总静脉 right common basal vein　131
右肺动脉 right pulmonary artery　79~101
右肺段淋巴结（13R）right segmental lymph nodes　115
右肺后底段（S10）right posterior basal segment　171
右肺后底段动脉（A10）right posterior basal segmental artery　105~137
右肺后底段动脉（A10）right posterior basal segmental bronchus　139
右肺后底段静脉（V10）right posterior basal segmental vein　139~165
右肺后底段支气管（B10）right posterior basal segmental bronchus　131~139
右肺后底段支气管（B10）right posterior basal segmental bronchus　119~129,137
右肺后底段支气管（B10）和动脉（A10）right posterior basal segmental bronchus and artery　141~169
右肺后段动脉（A2）right posterior segmental artery　79~87
右肺后段静脉（V2）right posterior segmental vein　79~97
右肺后段支气管（B2）right posterior segmental bronchus　79,81
右肺后段支气管（B2）和动脉（A2）right posterior segmental bronchus and artery　67
右肺基底干支气管 right common basal bronchus　105~117
右肺尖 apex of right lung　5~13,21
右肺尖段静脉（V1）right apical segmental vein　79~83,87~91
右肺尖前段静脉（V1+3）right apicoanterior segmental vein　93~97
右肺门淋巴结（10R）right hilar lymph nodes　81
右肺内侧底段动脉（A7）right medial basal segmental artery　113~121,129
右肺内侧底段静脉（V7）right medial basal segmental vein　155
右肺内侧底段支气管（B7）right medial basal segmental bronchus　115~121,129
右肺内前外侧底段动脉（A7+8+9）right common trunk of medial, anterior and lateral basal segmental arteries　105~113
右肺前底段动脉（A8）right anterior basal segmental artery　117~129

右肺前底段支气管（B8）right anterior basal segmental bronchus　121~129
右肺前段动脉（A3）right anterior segmental artery　77~89
右肺前段动脉（A3）和支气管（B3）right anterior segmental artery and bronchus　93
右肺前段静脉（V3）right anterior segmental vein　87~111
右肺前段支气管（B3）right anterior segmental bronchus　77~89
右肺前段支气管（B3）和动脉（A3）right anterior segmental bronchus and artery　61~75,91,95~99
右肺前外侧底段动脉（A8+9）right anterolateral basal segmental artery　115,119~129,137
右肺前外侧底段支气管（B8+9）right anterolateral basal segmental bronchus　119,125~129
右肺前外侧底段支气管（B8+9）和动脉（A8+9）right anterolateral basal segmental bronchus and artery　131~135
右肺前外后底段支气管（B8+9+10）right common trunk of anterior, lateral and posterior basal segmental bronchi　119~123
右肺前外后底段支气管（B8+9+10）right common trunk of anterior, lateral, posterior basal segmental bronchi　113~117
右肺上段动脉（A6）right superior segmental artery　91~99,105,113
右肺上段静脉（V6）right superior segmental vein　105~121
右肺上段支气管（B6）right superior segmental bronchus　97,107~113
右肺上叶 superior lobe of right lung　15~19,23~39
右肺上叶动脉 right superior lobar artery　77~87
右肺上叶静脉 right superior lobar vein　99~115
右肺上叶支气管 superior lobar bronchus of right lung　73~83
右肺外侧底段（S9）right lateral basal segment　167~171
右肺外侧底段动脉（A9）right lateral basal segmental artery　117~137
右肺外侧底段静脉（V9）right lateral basal segmental vein　139~147
右肺外侧底段支气管（B9）right lateral basal segmental bronchus　131,137
右肺外侧底段支气管（B9）和动脉（A9）right lateral basal segmental bronchus and artery　133~141
右肺外侧底段支气管（B9）right lateral basal segmental bronchus　125
右肺外侧底段支气管（B9）right lateral basal segmental bronchus　121,123,127,129
右肺外侧底段支气管（B9）和动脉（A9）right lateral basal segmental bronchus and artery　143~165
右肺外后底段静脉（V9+10）right posterolateral basal segmental vein　135~139
右肺下叶动脉 right inferior lobar artery　99~117
右肺下叶支气管 right inferior lobar bronchus　103~109
右肺叶间动脉 right interlobar artery　87~103
右肺叶间淋巴结（11R）right interlobar lymph nodes　85,87,91~99
右肺中叶 middle lobe of right lung　163~181

右肺中叶动脉 right middle lobar artery　99~111
右肺中叶静脉 right middle lobar vein　115~119
右肺中叶支气管 right middle lobar bronchus　105~111
右膈脚 right crus of diaphragm　179~203
右冠状动脉 right coronary artery　109,123~177
右喉返神经 right recurrent laryngeal nerve　3~13
右颈总动脉 right common carotid artery　3,5
右迷走神经 right vagus nerve　3~75
右上肺静脉 right superior pulmonary vein　103,107~113
右上气管旁淋巴结（2R）right upper paratracheal lymph nodes　21~29,35
右食管旁淋巴结（8R）right paraesophageal lymph nodes　109~113
右锁骨下动脉 right subclavian artery　3~15
右锁骨下静脉 right subclavian vein　13,15
右头臂静脉 right brachiocephalic vein　3~39
右下肺静脉 right inferior pulmonary vein　113,115,119~129
右下气管旁淋巴结（4R）right lower paratracheal lymph nodes　39~75
右心耳 right auricle　95~117
右心房 right atrium　119~131,135~173
右心室 right ventricle　105~189
右胸廓内动脉 right internal thoracic artery　3
右旋支 right circumflex branch　171,173
右叶间淋巴结（11R）right interlobar lymph nodes　83,89,101
右缘支 right marginal branch　151
右主支气管 right principal bronchus　71~79

Z

中间支气管 intermediate bronchus　81~101
中斜角肌 scalenus medius　3~11
蛛网膜下隙 subarachnoid space　147,195,199,201
主动脉窦 aortic sinus　129~135
主动脉弓 aortic arch　47~65
主动脉弓旁淋巴结（6区）paraaortic lymph nodes　63~67
主动脉弓下淋巴结（5区）subaortic lymph nodes　69~79
椎弓板 lamina of vertebral arch　15~19,35~41,55~63,77~85,99~103,125,127,143~153,161,171~175,189,191
椎间静脉 intervertebral vein　195~201
椎间孔 intervertebral foramen　3,19,23,81,121,171,203
椎间盘 intervertebral disc　161,163,183,185
最长肌 longissimus　5~141
左侧外侧底段支气管（B9）和动脉（A9）left lateral basal segmental bronchus and artery　145
左肺底段上静脉 left superior basal vein　127,129

左肺底段下静脉 left inferior basal vein　127,129
左肺底段总静脉 left common basal vein　125
左肺动脉 left pulmonary artery　69~87
左肺后底段（S10）left posterior basal segment　165~171
左肺后底段动脉（A10）left posterior basal segmental artery　111~135
左肺后底段静脉（V10）left posterior basal segmental vein　131~161
左肺后底段支气管（B10）left posterior basal segmental bronchus　131~135
左肺后底段支气管（B10）和动脉（A10）left posterior basal segmental bronchus and artery　137~163
左肺后底段支气管（B10）left posterior basal segmental bronchus　119~129
左肺基底干支气管 left common basal bronchus　105~113
左肺尖 apex of left lung　11~21
左肺门淋巴结（10L）left hilar lymph nodes　81~85
左肺内前外侧底段动脉（A7+8+9）left common trunk of medial, anterior and lateral basal segmental arteries　111~123
左肺前底段静脉（V8）left anterior basal segmental vein　129
左肺前段动脉（A3）left anterior segmental artery　69~81
左肺前段静脉（V3）left anterior segmental vein　75~99
左肺前段支气管（B3）left anterior segmental bronchus　61~89
左肺上段动脉（A6）left superior segmental artery　85~103
左肺上段静脉（V6）left superior segmental vein　97,105~119
左肺上段支气管（B6）left superior segmental bronchus　95~99
左肺上段支气管（B6）和动脉（A6）left superior segmental bronchus and artery　105~111
左肺上叶 superior lobe of left lung　23~39
左肺上叶支气管 superior lobar bronchus of left lung　91~95
左肺上叶支气管上干 superior trunk of left superior lobar bronchus　85~93
左肺上叶支气管下干 inferior trunk of left superior lobar bronchus　99~103
左肺外侧底段（S9）left lateral basal segment　165~171
左肺外侧底段动脉（A9）left lateral basal segmental artery　119~133
左肺外侧底段静脉（V9）left lateral basal segmental vein　131~171
左肺外侧底段支气管（B9）和动脉（A9）left lateral basal segmental bronchus and artery　135
左肺外侧底段支气管（B9）left lateral basal segmental bronchus　131,133
左肺外侧底段支气管（B9）和动脉（A9）left lateral basal segmental bronchus and artery　137~163
左肺外侧底段支气管（B9）left lateral basal segmental bronchus　119~129
左肺外后底段动脉（A9+10）left posterolateral basal segmental artery　97~117
左肺外后底段静脉（V9+10）left posterolateral basal segmental vein　133
左肺外后底段支气管（B9+10）left posterolateral basal segmental bronchus　115,117
左肺下叶动脉 left inferior lobar artery　85~109
左肺下叶支气管 left inferior lobar bronchus　95~103

左肺斜裂 oblique fissure of left lung　61,63
左肺叶间淋巴结（11L）left interlobar lymph nodes　87,91~95
左肺叶淋巴结（12L）left lobar lymph nodes　75~93,99~109
左膈脚 left crus of diaphragm　181~203
左膈下静脉 left inferior phrenic vein　193
左膈下动脉 left inferior phrenic artery　181~201
左冠状动脉 left coronary artery　109,111,125
左喉返神经 left recurrent laryngeal nerve　3~69
左颈内静脉 left internal jugular vein　3,5
左颈总动脉 left common carotid artery　5~45
左迷走神经 left vagus nerve　3~73
左上肺静脉 left superior pulmonary vein　93~107
左上气管旁淋巴结（2L）left upper paratracheal lymph nodes　27~31,35~41
左食管旁淋巴结（8L）left paraesophageal lymph nodes　97~107
左室后静脉 posterior vein of left ventricle　171~175
左室后支 posterior branch of left ventricle　151
左锁骨下动脉 left subclavian artery　3~45
左锁骨下静脉 left subclavian vein　3,5,15~19
左头臂静脉 left brachiocephalic vein　7~49
左下肺静脉 left inferior pulmonary vein　107~123
左下气管旁淋巴结（4L）left lower paratracheal lymph nodes　59,61~67
左心耳 left auricle　85~111
左心房 left atrium　101~155
左心室 left ventricle　131~179
左心室顶壁 roof of left ventricle　117~129
左心室后静脉 posterior vein of left ventricle　167,169
左胸膜顶 left cupula of pleura　9
左叶间淋巴结（11L）left interlobar lymph nodes　89
左主支气管 left principal bronchus　71~93
左椎动脉 left vertebral artery　3~7
左椎静脉 left vertebral vein　3,5